TREATMENT OF

INJURIES

TO ATHLETES

Don H. O'Donoghue, M.D.

Professor of Orthopedic Surgery,
University of Oklahoma Medical School,
Oklahoma City

Illustrated

W. B. SAUNDERS COMPANY
Philadelphia   London

THIS BOOK IS DEDICATED TO

MY WIFE, CHRIS,

who has been my constant stimulation and inspiration

Preface

I have given a great deal of thought to the advisability of including a bibliography in this volume. The material in this book is in large part basic. No claim is made for originality of concept or of procedures. Indeed, it is so fundamental that proper acknowledgment is well nigh impossible. I give full credit to my confreres, both present and past, for all I know about the subject. I had at first considered that I might credit those procedures which are generally understood to have been advanced by a specific man. Further consideration made it seem unjustifiable to credit some things but to leave the greater number unacknowledged. So a very grateful bow is offered to those members of the medical profession who take the pains to reduce their thinking to print and so make it available for all who want to, and can, read. By the same token, the thoughts in this book are freely available to anyone and no credit need be given me. My reward will be in your perusal of this book.

I also owe a debt of gratitude to the American athlete. That which in the beginning was an interesting sideline in a life devoted largely to pediatric orthopedics, has burgeoned to become perhaps my major interest. The young athlete with his tremendous enthusiasm and his desire to recover is a stimulation to anyone who has the privilege of caring for him. He makes a splendid antidote to the rapidly increasing group of "free loaders" who would rather be supported by their brothers than return to work.

Finally, I must express my sincere appreciation to the Athletic Department of the University of Oklahoma, which has to my personal knowledge never permitted selfish considerations to interfere in any way with the proper medical management of its athletes. It has presented a shining example which has spread throughout our state and has been particularly valuable in our successful efforts to improve the overall care of the young athlete in our public schools. The combined efforts of school administrators, teachers, coaches, trainers and physicians are resulting in a steady improvement in this vital area which will be rewarded manyfold by notable improvement in the physical condition of our people.

DON H. O'DONOGHUE, M.D.

Oklahoma City, Oklahoma

Contents

PART III.   THE TREATMENT OF INJURIES IN SPECIFIC AREAS

Introduction

A BOOK devoted entirely to injuries to a special group must have justification. Why injuries to athletes alone? Why not just injuries in general? Certainly the athlete is a human being, subject to the same frailties as the rest of the race, and one might reasonably expect him to be treated in the same manner. Could not the physician refer for guidance to one or more of the multitude of books that have been written on the subject of injury?

The very fact that you are reading this book to some extent justifies it. Obviously you recognize the athletic injury as a special situation—an area in which we as physicians can render a unique service. I believe that a few paragraphs explaining our approach to this stimulating subject will give added meaning to the later sections on specific injuries.

There is, indeed, real significance in the fact that a separate volume on the subject of injuries to athletes is considered to be warranted. Ten years ago this would not have been likely. Lately, however, there has been a tremendous upsurge of interest in this subject, not only among orthopedists, but among physicians in general, and indeed among the laity. An increasing number of postgraduate seminars and medical sessions have been concerned with it. At a postgraduate course on athletic injuries sponsored by the University of Colorado at Denver less than four years ago at which from 30 to 40 registrants were expected, an amazing total of almost 300 very interested and enthusiastic physicians, orthopedists, coaches and trainers appeared. In the following years the attendance was markedly increased. The injuries discussed at this and other meetings have been largely those of college athletes, but there is presently a groundswell in various parts of the country to develop these educational sessions to include secondary school and even grade school athletics.

Organized athletics have been extended to involve a major segment of our youth. In many areas not only the junior high schools but the grade schools partici- pate in competitive sports. Whether or not this is good, it must be recognized as a fait accompli which cannot be ignored. There is no present trend toward less ath- letics. On the contrary, the trend is toward a more inclusive program. Indeed, one of the major criticisms leveled at athletic programs has been their tendency to include the few to the neglect of the many. It should be recalled that in this country the various types of organized athletics, many of them competitive, must serve almost the whole function of physical conditioning whereas in other countries there are various health clubs, hiking clubs, ski societies, etc. Organizations of the latter type have not been popular in the United States. Our citizens are a keenly competitive group, and exercise for exercise's sake, the calisthenic drill, the regimentation into marching clubs, has not appealed to them, one reason being the fact that in other countries these various groups have been used as springboards for political activity. Our youth have an almost paranoid dislike of anything smacking of regimentation. The effort, therefore, must be not to decry athletics and demand less participation but, on the contrary, to demand greater participation and then see to it that the whole background of organized athletics is improved.

There can be no denying that competitive athletics have a great appeal to the mass of our people. However, the public is more inclined to look at the score, to observe the outstanding player, and to foster the competitive contest than to direct its attention toward those facets of the program which are best calculated to return the major good to the greatest number. Comparatively little attention outside the confines of sport itself has been paid to conditioning or to prevention of injury. An occasional blare of publicity follows a major injury to a stellar athlete or the un- timely death of a budding prep school player. Occasionally this triggers a lay maga- zine article on the importance of equipment or the value of physical conditioning as important factors in the prevention of injury. The greater emphasis, however, is placed on the injury itself. The sport pages eagerly play up injury to the star. Wryly enough, the reporter moans that the star has been disabled by his operation rather than by his injury.

In the final analysis, however, the lay public and, I fear, the majority of our medical profession have little knowledge of the actual processes of training and of the actual mechanics of injury.

COMPETITIVE ATHLETICS: BENEFITS AND RISKS

Why is it important for young men to participate in athletics? Certainly, they do carry an element of risk. Perhaps the solution to the problem of athletic injuries lies in the prayer of the timorous mother that her boy not compete. Abandonment of sports would certainly be the quickest way to prevent injury to the contestant.

In common with many others, I believe there are tangible benefits to be de- rived from athletic competition that greatly outweigh the element of risk. Certainly some of them are obvious. No one seriously doubts that the athlete does develop a stronger, healthier body. Most of the myths of catastrophic sequelae from strenuous athletic activity have been dispelled. "The athlete's heart" is a bogyman which has finally been exorcized. The ex-athlete who "turns fat" has at least postponed his impending adiposity throughout his years of training. The trained athlete is superior to his more sedentary fellow in drive and stamina, better fitted for both work and play.

I think most of us would agree that competitive athletics do have a salutary effect upon the character of the participant. This is particularly true if the programs are so managed that too much emphasis is not placed on winning and sufficient attention is given to the development of the vital ability of the athlete to value his own and respect his opponent's capabilities. The player learns the importance of team participation, that he must sacrifice immediate gain to the final end, that desire is one of the key factors in success. The fact that the word "sportsmanship" seems trite has in no way changed its reality as a trait of character. Team effort as opposed to individual glory, ability to take a job and follow it through, the necessity to take it as well as to dish it out, are all basic measures learned by the successful athlete.

There are certainly material benefits for the athlete in our present educational system that have much importance. Many a young man goes to school on his athletic ability. Much has been said about scholarships, especially by those who know the least about them. Suffice it to say that the athletic scholarship does permit many a lad to finish his education who otherwise would have dropped out of school long before. Who are we to say that the athletic scholarship is not as worthwhile as the scholarship for merit in other fields? In most of the better schools of the country the scholarship athlete maintains a scholastic average higher than the average of his school. A good estimate of the quality of the scholarship program in a given institution can be made from the proportion of the scholarship boys who go ahead to graduation.

So much for the benefit of athletics to the student in school. But after graduation, what? It has been said that the athlete out of school is as a fish out of water. Not so! Many athletes make some form of physical education or a related field their career. The conditioning of our youth depends upon the organized type of athletic training which he gets in the elementary and secondary schools and such organizations as the Y.M.C.A. and Boy Scouts. Without the trained athlete to provide capable leadership these programs would be in sorry straits, indeed. We need these people. Indeed, we will find that much of the physical education of our youth is in the hands of the former athlete. On a more personal plane, many an athlete makes contacts during his school years with men who are seeking his very type of qualifications to man the leading jobs in industry. In 30 odd years of knowing athletes I have seen most of them display the same fine enthusiasm and attain the same success in life that they did in school. Certainly there are real advantages to an athletic program from many standpoints.

Why then is there such bitter opposition to organized competitive athletics as such? Not because of any interference with scholastic pursuits, not because of any moral implications, not because the after-effects of training impair the physique in later life but because of one principal thing, namely, physical injuries. Do athletes get physical injuries? The answer is "Yes, they do." Here is a very real objection to the athletic program—in fact, almost the only real objection. Our youngsters do get injured—on occasion, even seriously or fatally injured. It must be the duty of the medical profession to accept this challenge and do everything in its power to minimize those things which interfere with the goals of the athletic program.

THE ROLE OF THE PHYSICIAN

What can we as physicians do to prevent injury, to minimize temporary disability and to prevent permanent disability? Much indeed has been accomplished in the past few years toward these ends. A few years ago the trainer in the average scholastic institution was a fugitive from the supply room, having graduated into the "wrapping and taping" club largely by osmosis. He had no real knowledge of injuries and his main concern actually was to "keep 'em rollin'." We all remember the famous men who attained a great deal of notoriety by reason of their ability to keep the athlete in the game. Too many times this goal of immediate playing was a more vital one than the final goal of complete recovery of the patient. During this era the doctor was a necessary evil. The player felt that once he reached the doctor his days as an athlete were over. In too many instances this feeling was justified for two very pertinent reasons. First, since the doctor was the last resort, he did not see the player until long after treatment should ideally have been instituted. Second, and I think of almost equal importance, was the sad reality that it was not of any immediate concern to the doctor whether or not the player was an athlete or was able to remain one after treatment was completed. All too often the first recommendation the doctor made was "Well, give up football," or "You must not play any more baseball." This simply tended to confirm the conviction of the player, the coach and the public that athletes and physicians were incompatible. Also, in the past there has been a tendency on the part of the coaching staff to demand that the player continue in spite of injury or be labeled "yellow." The trainer was urged to "tape her up" and "run him back in"—often to the detriment of the player, the team and the game. In our major institutions this is no longer true.

A more enlightened approach has demonstrated that everyone is better served by having the injured player promptly and ably treated, thereby obtaining recovery before he does himself irreparable damage. The successful coach seeks to protect the player and seeks to prevent damage to either body or mind. In the well-run athletic program of today, the coach, trainer, team physician and specialist *all* combine in one effective unit, designed to keep the player well equipped and in ideal condition. In fact, more emphasis is placed and actually more time is spent on preparing a player to participate and on preventing his injury than is spent on treatment. The player, coach, trainer and physician are no longer working at cross purposes in most institutions. Athletic injuries are much less frequent and they are less severe than in the past. The period of disability is shorter. The degree of recovery is more complete. Many factors have combined to cause this vast improvement in the one area where it must be conceded that athletics may have a bad effect.

So we find that once again the physician must become not only the doer but the teacher. The physician with an especial interest in athletes must prepare himself to handle their injuries and he must in turn pass this information on to other physicians. It must be recognized that there is one overriding difference in the management of injuries to athletes. That is, that the patient must get complete recovery from his injury or he is no longer an athlete. True enough, this axiom *should* apply to any injury the doctor sees but nowhere else is it dramatized quite so constantly as in the care of the athlete.

DIAGNOSTIC JUDGMENT

The outstanding consideration in the treatment of athletic injury is early detection, not only of the nature of the injury but of its degree. The optimum time to examine an athlete for injury is as soon as possible after he is hurt. There must be no compromise with this statement. It may be impossible to examine the patient, or to make a complete diagnosis, at once, but if it can be done precious time has been saved. Frequently the initial examination is by the coach, the trainer or the physician on the field. Whoever this is, he must make as careful an evaluation of the injured player's condition as he is capable of doing and must pass this information on to each succeeding link in the chain of therapy. The doctor must conscientiously and objectively examine the player. Does the injury seem serious enough that the boy should not return to the game or should he be strapped up and allowed to play? To err is human but the margin of error can be drastically reduced by comprehensive consideration of the patient's injury. There is no place here for wishful thinking. The player is eager to continue and should not be deprived unnecessarily of this privilege. On the other hand, if continued competition adds to the hazard of injury, he should not be permitted to compete. It is, of course, always better to err on the side of conservatism.

After the injury sidelines the player, what then? The prevalent habit of packing the injured part in ice and delaying examination until a convenient time the next day, or even later, is to be deplored. Your examination as a physician should be done at the earliest possible moment even at considerable inconvenience to yourself, the coach or the player. It should be obvious that the part should be undressed, all taping or strapping removed and a meticulous examination carried out. Frequently, the diagnosis, which will be easy in the early stage, becomes exceedingly difficult as pain increases apprehension and swelling, edema and hemorrhage interfere with an accurate evaluation of the injury. If consultation with a specialist is needed, seek it promptly so that the specialist, too, may be able to take advantage of the optimum time for treatment. The specialist should have enough integrity to be able to cooperate with the referring physician and "take the monkey off his back," as it were, in regard to the severity of the injury. This is particularly true of the decision on whether or not the player should be allowed to compete, either at once or later.

CONCEPTS OF TREATMENT

Once treatment is decided upon, the physician should proceed to carry it out with confidence. If the treatment is within the capabilities of the team physician, he should be permitted to conduct it. If the specialist's attention is required, the specialist himself should not hesitate to say so. The physician should be encouraged to seek the specialist's advice early and this will be done only when there is good rapport between the player, the referring physician and the specialist.

The following concepts of treatment have proved to be of great value:

1. Make *complete* recovery your goal. While this may not be possible in any given case, it must always be the goal. The athlete is basically in good condition and can well tolerate any reasonable measure if it serves to increase his chances for a complete recovery.

2. Adopt the best method of treatment. Medical evaluation of the nature and extent of injury must be the controlling factor in the choice of treatment. A temporizing attitude will not accomplish the best results. If you really believe that one method is distinctly better than another you should recommend it and then carry it out. This must be an entirely objective decision. How often do we hear the statement, "Well, perhaps this knee would be better operated but I'll put it in a cast," or "We really should have put the boy on crutches but . . . ."

3. Avoid expediency. Outside influence must not be permitted to outweigh sound medical judgment. Many pressing factors will tend to influence the doctor's decision. All concerned are extremely unwilling to believe that the player is really hurt but the boy's desire to compete, his fear of failing his teammates, the parents' desire to see their son excel, the coach's hope that the player is not really hurt—all must be ignored if the proper conclusion is to be reached. Procrastination, vacillation, so-called "conservative" attitudes, must not prevail. Temporary convenience must be sacrificed for the ultimate goal.

4. Be prompt with your treatment. A definitive decision as to the proper method of treatment must be made at the earliest possible moment and then carried out. We have been able to show conclusively that delay very often spells the difference between success and failure of treatment.

5. Last and not least, the physician—not the player, not the coach, not the parents, but the physician—must recognize the value of competitive athletics. He must believe that to this particular patient it is vital that he be restored to competitive athletics. If he fails in this, the patient-doctor relationship suffers and rapport is lost. The doctor who deprecates the player's ambition should not be treating him.

Will such a program be accepted? Yes, but not without some educational effort on the part of the doctor. He must be able to show conclusively that the program is better not only for the doctor, but for the school, the coach and especially for the player. This will require time. He must be interested and capable. As his program develops, those most concerned will recognize the benefits. They will observe that the sprained ankle responds to treatment, that a short, complete lay-off is followed by normal ability as opposed to an ineffectual season. The coach will note that prompt treatment restores the player more rapidly and permits more actual playing in the long run and so is better for the team. The player will not fear the doctor who has a sympathetic and understanding attitude. He notes that his buddy gets well. He also expects to get well and will accept the physician's recommendation for treatment. He may fear some specific part of the treatment such as the insertion of a needle into a joint but never to the extent of failing to return or refusing the treatment provided he believes that the doctor is sincerely trying to restore him to his normal ability.

These are not idle dreams of Utopia. The type of program described is practical, and has been established in a number of institutions. It must be our aim to make it the rule, not the exception. Nor is a full scale, university type training program necessary. The program does require an able, conscientious coach and a physician who will interest himself in the peculiar problems of the athlete.

PART I

Prevention of Injuries

2

Prevention of Injuries

THE PREVENTION of injuries should be the major goal of any-
one responsible for the physical and mental conditioning of athletes. If we grant
that the athletic program is important from the standpoint of the improvement of
the physical and mental condition of our young people, we must adopt every possible means to see that there is no detrimental effect from the athletic program.
There may be differences of opinion on the benefits of athletics but we cannot deny
that almost the only deleterious effect is physical injury. We spend much time de-
vising ways and means to relieve the effects of injury. If we spent even a small percentage of this time in striving to prevent the injury from occurring, a major portion of our problem would be solved.

Prevention of injuries has many facets. In a university type training program,
more attention will be given to prevention of injuries by one means or another
than to their treatment. In the secondary school programs, someone must be made
responsible for the physical welfare of the players. There has been a steady improvement in this facet of the problem for many years. The trainer has become a skilled
professional person. Unfortunately, most secondary schools cannot afford full-time
trainers. The role of the physician here must be that of advisor to whatever amateur trainer is available. It is neither fair nor advisable to put the whole responsibility of physical conditioning upon the busy coach, however capable he may be.
The coach must of necessity concentrate his attention on the practice session or
on the game. His training duties must be incidental to this. The team physician
should be the one who is especially interested in this problem. He must be willing
to accept the responsibility for it even at some inconvenience to himself. It may
seem very tedious to supervise the details of strapping, wrapping and equipment,
weight control and all of the other facets, but the team physician is not worthy of

the name if he is not willing to do it. This is particularly important in the preseason training period. Prevention of injury is as much the sphere of the doctor as is prevention of disease. The overall aim of the athletic program is to improve the participant. If the program leaves the participant in poorer condition than when he started, it has failed regardless of how many games have been won.

THE INDIVIDUAL PLAYER

Physical Condition (General Health)

Before the prospective player is permitted to enter an athletic program, he should have an intelligent and complete physical examination. It is not necessary to take a multitude of laboratory tests. The general physical examination should, however, provide leads to needed supplemental measures. For example, if there seems to be a defect in vision, a detailed examination of the eye should be recommended. If a cardiac murmur is discovered, it should be investigated. It is not enough simply to examine a player and record the findings. The physician should be willing to give an opinion as to the boy's physical ability to participate in the sports concerned. If he does not feel himself capable of doing this, he should recommend special examinations. It is not proper to request a boy to drop the program simply because the physician does not know whether or not he has a physical defect which would contraindicate his participation. It is almost as bad to err by over-conservatism as it is to overlook serious hazards. Does this functional heart murmur really constitute a hazard? Can this boy's adiposity be controlled? Are this young man's bones to be judged overbrittle because he has had several fractures? To each individual the answers are extremely vital. They must be vital to the examining physician as well.

Once it has been decided that the candidate may compete in athletics, every effort must be made to *improve* his physical condition. He should be given advice as to his diet and told to avoid faddish eating, to avoid overeating and to eat regularly. He should be advised not to snack between meals at the expense of his regular meal. Many young people are subject to constipation. This can usually be completely controlled by regulation of the diet, which is far better than the habitual use of laxatives. An effort should be made to determine the proper weight for the individual player and his diet then is regulated to reach this weight by high caloric regimens for the undernourished and low caloric, high protein diets for the adipose. On every squad there will be several players who are in dire need of regulation in this regard.

The player should be instructed in good living habits. He should get plenty of rest and sleep. The two are not necessarily synonymous. If he has irregular study and sleeping hours, an effort should be made to find a schedule more in keeping with his general surroundings. There is no point in forcing him to go to bed early and get up early if the habit of his family is to go to bed late and get up late. There is nothing magical in certain specific hours of sleep. The benefit is in the number of hours and the degree of relaxation. The well regulated program should permit the player to have 30 to 40 minutes of relative relaxation between practice or competition and eating. It goes without saying that he should be instructed not to eat just before strenuous practice periods. Great emphasis is put on eating before an actual game but too often the practice session is not so well regulated. The play-er's blood may be concentrated in his muscles by extreme physical exercise when it should be busy aiding in the digestion of his food.

The player should be instructed to avoid all drugs except on the specific pre-scription of a physician. This includes intoxicants and nicotine.

Conditioning

The physical conditioning of a player should be a continuous thing. If the player can be kept in good condition throughout the year, one of the major goals of the athletic program will have been accomplished; namely, the improvement of the general condition of the youth of America. Nonetheless, there are certain sports that require concentration of conditioning far beyond the others. Ideally, the conditioning should be fitted to the sport. In our University of Oklahoma pro-gram, for example, the football player is urged to keep in condition the year round. It is fully understood that he probably will not keep in game condition for the full 12 months, but it is fatuous to believe that he can be put in game condition in two or three weeks. Hence, each individual player is instructed when he leaves school exactly what he should do that summer. The following summer conditioning pro-gram for high school athletes is recommended by Ken Rawlinson, Head Trainer, University of Oklahoma, and is quoted directly from his book:*

SUMMER CONDITIONING PROGRAM FOR HIGH SCHOOL ATHLETES

It is my belief that a high school athlete needs even more incentive to carry on a summer conditioning program than a college athlete. There follows a summer or off-season conditioning plan that could be inaugurated in any high school.
 A. Personal letters to the boys.
 B. Physical examination.
 C. Start gradually, reach peak in August.
 D. Give the boys a plan or chart to follow.
  1. Conditioning exercises.
  2. Run (6:30 mile or its equivalent).
  3. Wind sprints.
  4. Step climb, forward and backward.
  5. Specific rehabilitation exercises.
  6. Temperate living.
   a. Sleep—"the great restorer"—a minimum of nine hours. Two hours before mid-night is better than four after.
   b. Good diet.
   c. No intoxicants. The A.M.A. has stated that "alcohol is a detriment to the human organism. Its use in therapeutics, as a tonic, food, or stimulant has no scientific value. It attacks the central nervous system. It is not a food; it is a poison."
   d. No smoking. Nowhere is there any medical evidence that states that it improves an athlete's ability. It actually slows him up. Nicotine is a poison. If one smokes a pack of cigarettes a day for a week, he inhales 400 mg. of nicotine, which in a single injection would kill him instantly.
   e. No drugs. The United States Olympic Committee has recently ruled that any competitor who uses drugs, stimulants, or other substances known as "dope" for any purpose will be disqualified.

The major portion of this conditioning must be carried out by the athlete himself. He cannot be expected to do it without proper direction and instruction. Each boy is given a set of exercises which he is to use three or four times a week

* Rawlinson, Ken: Modern Athletic Training. Englewood Cliffs, New Jersey, Prentice-Hall, Inc., page 25.

until the first part of August and then daily until the beginning of the fall practice. He is encouraged to supplement these exercises by jogging, running for endurance, wind sprints and other types of exercise. He is encouraged to maintain, at least to some degree, his training program by getting rest, sleep, proper food and by avoiding dissipation throughout the summer. Furthermore, each boy is assigned the weight at which he is expected to be when he reports for the first day of practice in the fall. The player is told that he should report in such condition that he could play a game on the first day of practice.

Obviously, such a program cannot be fitted entirely to the secondary school. However, the essence of the program is there. If the boy is to participate in football, he should start conditioning himself early in the summer. It will not suffice simply to tell him to keep himself in shape. He must be given a specific program to follow. Most of the eager young athletes will be glad to carry out such a program if they know what is really expected of them. There is probably less trouble with physical conditioning for football than for any other sport since this is recognized as a rugged sport. It is equally important for the player to be conditioned for such games as basketball, baseball and particularly for track. Many a track career has been nipped in the bud because the participant has not been "brought along" by gradually increasing effort. A single major effort by the broad jumper or the sprinter may be responsible for losing the whole season of competition since he may develop a tenosynovitis of the tendo achillis or a strain of the hamstring muscle or a "march" fracture of the foot or fibula (Fig. 30, page 66). A runner should not be permitted to run the mile under competition until he has many times paced himself through this same distance at a gradually accelerating rate. The baseball player who needs to get his arm as well as his legs in top shape may require a wholly different set of exercises although the goal remains the same. He must not be permitted to exert the maximum strength of any muscle until it has been suitably conditioned for this effort. This is well known as it applies to the pitcher but it may be equally disastrous for the outfielder or third baseman to start his practice with maximum throws to the plate or across to first. These factors are particularly pertinent in secondary school players. These boys have a maximum of desire and a minimum of regulatory common sense. They require supervision and this is one of the major advantages of organized athletics. In a regulated program the player can have supervision and so be gradually developed until his full potential is reached.

It should be noted that the doctor has a real responsibility to try to eliminate any exercise that he feels to be bad, no matter how traditional or popular it may be. Any orthopedist handling injuries knows all too well the danger of the popular "deep knee bends" and "duck waddle." In these exercises as the heel is forcibly jammed against the buttock, there is a real danger of a posterior tear of the medial or lateral meniscus. They have no advantage over three-quarter knee bends. Obviously, all doctors will not agree on what exercises are particularly bad and what are good. The doctor must first inform himself and then have the strength of his conviction in offering his advice to the athletic administration.

There follow examples of exercises for conditioning for certain sports as developed by Mr. Ken Rawlinson, Head Trainer of the University of Oklahoma, and published in his book.*

* Rawlinson, Ken: Modern Athletic Training. Englewood Cliffs, New Jersey, Prentice-Hall, Inc., Chapter III.

CONDITIONING ATHLETES' BODIES

For top performance, body conditioning is absolutely necessary. A conditioned boy is less susceptible to injuries. Conditioning affects:
1. Ability to play.
2. Mental attitude.
3. Determination.
4. Teamwork.
5. Spirit.

Many fail to make the team because they do not have the desire. They will not pay the price to get themselves into shape both physically and mentally. Mental conditioning is a phase often overlooked, but it is very vital. Many athletes do not think it is important, but it goes hand-in-hand with physical conditioning. If an athlete is going to be great, he must have both.

Conditioning at Oklahoma

The conditioning program for the fall season at the University of Oklahoma begins at the close of spring football practice (approximately the middle of April). This portion of the conditioning program must be carried on by the athlete himself. He cannot be expected to do this without proper direction and instruction. It is our firm conviction that if athletes have the desire to be great, they must be and are willing to pay the price to help accomplish their goal.

Basic Principles of Running

An important phase of conditioning is running. Every athlete should learn how to run correctly. Anyone can be taught to run a little faster, if he has the desire. Following are a few suggestions:
1. Relax. The body must be supple to attain best performance.
2. Run on balls of the feet.
3. Point the toes straight ahead. You lose at least one-half inch on each step if toes are not straight ahead.
4. Run in a straight line. It is the shortest distance between two points.
5. Develop your proper stride. The average stride is the height of your body. Lengthen your stride as much as possible but do not overstride. It is worse than an understride.
6. Running angle is important; body leaning, head up, ankles, hips, shoulders and head in a straight line. Do not bend too far backward. You should be in the proper running angle and with the proper stride 12-15 yards from the starting point.
7. Arm action is very important; opposite arm and leg move in unison. Keep arm relaxed and shoot uppercuts to height of shoulder and not beyond center of body. Bring arm back so hand does not go beyond crest of hip, a relaxed piston-like movement.

* * *

Short sprints develop speed.
Distance-running develops endurance.
Running in circles and figure eights strengthens ankles, knees, hips and backs.

* * *

The yearly conditioning program at the University of Oklahoma follows. (Take into consideration that we work on rehabilitation the year round.)

APRIL-MAY:
Workout three times a week. Run, tennis, golf, handball, track, weights and exercises. Assign weights for September weigh-in.

JUNE:
Run two or three times a week, distance-running plus daily exercises. (See below.)

JULY:
Run three to four days a week, distance-running plus a few sprints and daily exercises. (See below.)

AUGUST:
Increase the tempo in everything. Workout five to seven days a week, with emphasis on sprinting (properly warmed up), conditioning drills and football drills.

Daily Exercise Guide

Do five exercises per day for six days a week during the months of June and July. Increase the tempo in August. These exercises are set up specifically to reach every area of the body, and can be done daily in the athlete's room or back yard. He should start exercises by jumping rope.

MONDAY:

Side Bender. Position: Stand with feet apart, hands clasped overhead, arms straight. Bend sideward to the right, bending right knee and slowly going as far as possible. Repeat to left. Repeat ten times each side.

Knee Stretcher. Position: Stand with feet apart, knees slightly flexed and hands on outside of knees. Press knees together with hands. Knees offering resistance. Repeat outward twenty times.

Shoulder Hang. Position: Grasp an overhead crossbar, ladder, tree limb, etc., and hang elbows straight. Hang one minute, relax and repeat ten times. Especially good for boys with acromioclavicular, muscular or nerve shoulder trouble. (If shoulder will permit, walk hand-over-hand across overhead ladder.

Hurdle Spread. Position: Sit in hurdle position with right leg forward. Bend trunk forward and touch right foot with both hands. Repeat forty times, then extend left leg and repeat forty times.

TUESDAY:

Groin Stretch. Position: Stand with feet apart, hands on groin. Bend body obliquely to right and left (forward and backward). Stretch it out.

Bicycle Ride. Position: Support body on shoulders with elbows on ground and hands on hips supporting the body. Move feet and legs in motion necessary for riding a bicycle as rapidly as possible for count of forty. Repeat four to five times.

Stomach Drill. Position: Flat on back with hands under hips, with legs straight together and toes pointed. Raise feet slowly with a slow count of ten until the legs are perpendicular to the ground, lower them slowly halfway and stop; here spread the legs and bring them together eight times, then lower legs to within six inches from the ground and repeat the spread eight times. Raise legs slowly to the perpendicular position and lower them to the ground very slowly. Repeat eight times.

Leg Flexing. Position: Sitting position. With both hands grasp left leg and pull knee up to ear. Relax and repeat with right leg. Repeat rapidly for count of 100.

WEDNESDAY:

Wood Chopper. Position: Stand with feet apart, trunk turned right, hands together and over right shoulder. In a chopping movement bring arms down vigorously between the legs. Uncoil over left shoulder and repeat. Repeat twenty times each side.

Push Up or Push Up and Clap. Position: Flat on stomach with toes dug in and hands flat on ground, clap hands and catch on hands without allowing body to contact ground. Repeat ten to fifteen times.

Quarter Eagles. Position: Feet width of shoulders, parallel, and heels on ground. Bend at knees so thighs are parallel to ground. Maintaining the above base, jump ¼ turns to right and left.

Belly Rock. Position: Face down, hands back of neck. Raise head, chest and feet and rock back and forth seventy-five times.

THURSDAY:

Trunk Twister. Position: Stand with feet apart, hands clasped behind head and elbows back. Bend and bounce downward and simultaneously rotate trunk far to left. Recover and repeat to right. Repeat fifteen times to each side.

All Fours. Position: Face down. Weight on hands and feet, and walk forward, backward, sideward, etc. (crab walk—same exercise with back down).

Burpee. Position: Standing. Assume squat-position with hands on ground, elbows inside knees. Thrust feet and legs backward, weight supported on hands and toes. Return to squat-position, then to starting position. Repeat twenty times.

Sit Up and Paw Dirt. Position: Flat on back with arms extended overhead. Sit up, thrust arms forward and touch toes, knees straight. Return to starting position. Swing legs overhead until feet touch ground behind neck. Dig the dirt with running motion of legs, for fifteen counts. Return to original position and repeat twelve times.

FRIDAY:

Mountain Climber. Position: Squatting with hands on ground, right leg drawn up to chest and left leg extended to rear with knee straight. With a fast cadence extend right foot backward and bring left leg to chest. Repeat twenty-five times.

Wrestler's Bridge. Position: Weight supported on toes and head. Rotate in circles to right and left.

Leg-Back Stretch. Position: Flat on back with arms bracing shoulders against the turn. With knee stiff, raise one leg to perpendicular position and swing it across body until foot touches hand on opposite side, shoulders flat throughout. Repeat twenty times with right, left and both legs (good for low back injuries).

Toe and Heel Dance. Position: One-half squat-position with trunk erect. Remaining in this position, jump with the right heel extended in front and the left toe extended behind. Jump again, reversing the order of the feet. Repeat rapidly forty times. From same position jump with the right heel to the side and left foot in place. Repeat to left.

SATURDAY:

Sacro-Iliac Stretch. Position: Sitting with knees drawn to chest. Lock arms around knees and roll back onto shoulders. Continue to roll and tighten the grip of the arms.

Leg Stretch. Position: Stand erect with hands at sides. Bend forward without bending knees, and touch toes. Repeat 20-30 times. Repeat same with legs crossed.

Groin Stretcher. Position: On knees, hands on hips, stretch backward as far as possible and return. Repeat.

High Step-Dive. Position: Stationary high step run-dive forward, weight on hands and let chest strike ground lightly, then abdomen, thighs and feet. Jump to feet and repeat fifteen times.

SUNDAY—*Optional.*

By September first, the athlete should be in condition to play a regulation game if it were necessary. If he watches his weight, works hard and faithfully, he will have no trouble reporting back in tip-top condition. The athlete should post the daily exercises in his bedroom.

If Post Season Game:
    December—Practice.
    January—Nothing.
    February—Three times a week: Run, exercises, handball, weights, weight assignments for
            spring football.

If No Post Season Game:
    December—Nothing.
    January—Same as February above.
    February—Step up the January program.

MARCH-APRIL:

Spring Practice—Tuesday, Wednesday, Thursday and Saturday for five weeks.

Weight Lifting as Part of the Program

Weight lifting, like any other activity, is an ideal form of exercising if not carried to an extreme. Weight lifting alone is not recommended. It should be a part of an over-all program.

In regard to agility, muscle mass and endurance, Dr. Robert Brashear, orthopedic surgeon of Knoxville, Tennessee, made the following comments in his booklet on "Athletic Injuries": "Whether one is trying to rebuild a weakened muscle postoperatively or whether one is trying to develop a boy's muscles, he must strain his muscles to the ultimate if he is to build muscle mass. We develop grace and agility by handball and boxing, by fancy diving, by the trampoline and even by doing the jitterbug. We develop endurance by running up and down the stadium steps, but we never develop muscle mass except by strain."

A suggested weight-lifting program for football players is as follows:

BUILDING STRENGTH, POWER, BODY BULK

Breathe in deeply when lifting, exhale when lowering. In the first six exercises below, start with 40 to 50 pounds and increase the weight five to ten pounds per session. Athletes should build up to maximum weight, with 15 repetitions of each exercise done in three series of five each. These exercises should be done three times a week, with adequate warm-up before each exercise period (running, stretching exercises, and rope-skipping).

1. To develop spring, initial charge, ankles, body balance and strength:
   Calf Raises. Place weight on back of neck, feet eight inches apart, body straight. Raise up on toes as high as possible.
2. To develop leg power and strength, back strength, explosive power, increase size of thoracic cage (good weight-gaining exercise):
   Knee Bends. Place weight on back of neck, feet 12 to 14 inches apart, heels flat on ground, toes pointed slightly outside, head up, shoulders back, buttocks low. Squat down to *three-fourths* knee flexion, return to starting position. If weight is too heavy, do only a half squat. (Do not do a deep knee bend.)
3. To strengthen upper back muscles, pulling power, shoulder snap, fingers and wrist:
   Rowing Motion. Feet 24 to 30 inches apart, head up and forward, knees straight but not stiff. Lift weight from ground to chest and return.
4. To strengthen lower back, shoulders, wrist and fingers:
   Stiff-Legged Dead Lifts. Bar on floor in front of feet, feet 12 to 15 inches apart, legs and arms straight. Bend at waist and grasp bar in middle of hand grip. Straighten back and lift weights up to low abdomen. Lower weights to ground in same manner as they were picked up.
5. To develop upper body, shoulders, chest, forearm, elbows, and shoulders:
   Bench Press. Lie flat on back (on bench), with feet on ground. Grasp bar on outside edge of grip of bar. Elbows are placed wide and along line of bar. Lower weights straight up, extend elbows.
6. Best all-around strength exercises. Neck, arms, back and legs:
   Place feet under bar and about 12 inches apart, toes slightly outward, head high, back and arms straight, heels down. Bend at knees and grasp bar, arms and back straight. Lift bar to low abdomen, keeping arms and back straight. Lower to ground with same body movements.
7. To build up knee and thigh:
   Quadriceps Lift. Use iron boot or table. Sit on table, knee bent. Lift foot, knee straight. Use maximum weight and lift three series of ten (30 lifts total).
   Hamstring Lift. On stomach or standing, use iron boot and raise knee to right angle. Same technique as quadriceps lift.
8. To build up or prevent shoulder injury:
   Bar Hang. Five chins and two minutes of hanging at arms' length.

Heavy resistance with low repetitions builds strength and high repetitions with less resistance builds endurance.

The Ingredients of Greatness

As part of athletes' mental conditioning, the following qualities and applications can be posted in the training room.

C-oncentration
H-eart
A-ttitude
M-odesty
P-ractice
S-acrifice

Coaching

The coach himself has a responsibility in the program of prevention of injury that can be exercised by no one else. A great deal of the time and effort of the coach must be spent on fundamentals. The player must be taught to improve his agility. He must have extensive work on coordination. He must be instructed as to the proper stance. The player who is constantly alert, whose muscles are in balance, who is prepared for motion in any direction will usually not be hurt. The injury most often comes at a moment when the player is off guard and unprepared for the blow. The coach will instruct him in the way to protect his head and neck in tackling; will show him how to block most effectively and to avoid injury to himself; how best to avoid the bruising block or the damaging tackle. The rules of sport are so designed as to minimize injuries and the coach will advise the players to obey the rules, not only because it is proper but because if everyone obeys the regulations, there is less chance that anyone will be hurt. An illegal maneuver by one player invites retaliation by another. Proper coaching will keep this to a minimum.

Attitude

The attitude of the player is all-important from the standpoint of prevention of injuries. Here the combined efforts of the whole organization are important. The coach, the trainer, the physician, the specialist—all have their parts to play. Attitude is, however, the primary responsibility of the coach and the trainer. The player's desire to play, to excel, to do a good job will stimulate him to carry out those things needed to reach this goal. In order to play well he will recognize that he must be in good condition, and recognition is the first step in accomplishment. The player must have confidence in his own ability. This confidence arises from his knowledge that he is in excellent condition and that he can put out maximum effort without exhaustion or injury. The player must be tough. This does not imply that he must be mean or dirty. It simply means that he must be physically tough so that he can take whatever physical punishment is required to accomplish the desired end. He must be physically stronger per pound than his opponent. This can come only from excellent conditioning. Given the desire to play, self-confidence, mental alertness and a tough physical condition, he must then learn to play with "carefree abandon." This does not mean he should be reckless, but that he should not be apprehensive and fearful. If the coach can inculcate this spirit in the minds of his players, he will find a sharp decrease in the number of disabling injuries among them. This is an extremely important product of physical conditioning.

ENVIRONMENT

It is also important that proper environment for athletics be available since this can be a major deterrent to injury.

The Playing Field

The university programs lay great stress on the condition of the field—not only the game field which is often reserved for weekends, but particularly the practice field. The secondary schools do not have the advantage of adequate funds for constant supervision of their play areas. However, a little rudimentary care and common sense will accomplish a large part of the same objectives. Each sport has its individual field requirement.

In *football* the practice field should be level and preferably firmly sodded. At the beginning of the season before the field is used, it should be carefully screened for all foreign material. If necessary, the squad itself can fan out and cover the field to remove rocks, boards, tin cans, paper, all the objects which may have accumulated on the field during the summer when it was out of use. Whoever mows the area should be instructed to remove all such foreign material, not just avoid it. Of perhaps even greater importance is the necessity for leveling off the field. This does not simply mean that it should not be put on a hillside. It means that small imperfections should be filled. A person is more likely to receive an injury stepping into a gopher hole than he is running into a trench. He can avoid the larger imperfections but may fail to see the smaller ones. A few hours spent in so conditioning the field will be well worthwhile. It may be impossible to do much about the firmness of the terrain once the season starts. However, a little effort in the spring may pay dividends in softening up the soil and obtaining cover with grass. Watering the field, if possible, helps immensely. A good playing surface is far more important than fancy stadiums, decorated goal posts, etc., and comparatively little money spent on the field will produce gratifying results.

I do not believe anyone uses lime to mark the fields any more. Certainly its use should be condemned. Ample room should be provided at the sidelines so that the player does not crash into obstructions such as stakes, brick piles, fence rails and the like as he runs out of bounds. Similarly, ample room should be provided at the ends of the field, extending well beyond the end zone so that the pass receiver does not charge into a stone wall or fall over the curb of the running track. Safety equipment around the field is important. The markers should be nontraumatic. There should be no stakes driven into the ground as permanent markers unless they are flush with the surface. The "chain gang" should be instructed how to throw their rods flat on the ground. Wooden benches should be kept well away from the sidelines. All these things seem quite rudimentary but a season never passes that someone does not receive a serious injury from hazards which could have easily been removed. Other sports, too, have their problems.

The *basketball floor* should be smooth and free from splinters and not too slick. There should be ample room along the sidelines even at the penalty of making the court narrower. Charging into a wall accounts for breaking an arm, leg or skull since the basketball player does not wear much protective equipment. The practice of hanging the goal at one end of the court just at the front of the stage is a dangerous one. There should be ample room to run under the basket at the ends. No foreign material should be allowed on the floor.

The *baseball field* presents equally important problems. Much attention is usually paid to the infield and rightly so since irregularity of the infield causes many "bad bounces" and this is of interest to everyone. Too many times the outfield is a weed patch. Grass is allowed to grow tall enough to conceal bricks, cans and stones which are definite hazards. The sprinting fielder stepping into a hole in the ground receives the same type of injury as the football player but is less able to cope with it because he has less protective armor. The interest of the school in the baseball team can be stimulated by having the younger boys police the outfield.

In *track,* attention should be paid to the running surface. The curb should either be high enough that the runner will avoid it or else low enough that he will not flip his ankles if he hits it.

You may say that these things are not the responsibility of the physician. They are the responsibility of the physician if he feels himself responsible for the prevention of injuries. There is little accomplished by conditioning a player well and then have him break an ankle as he steps into a hole where a dog has dug up a bone.

If it is necessary for play to take place on inadequate areas, certain precautions must be taken. There is no excuse for leaving debris around. This can always be removed. It may be necessary, however, to play basketball on concrete or blacktop. It may be that some of the football fields are "hardpan" and cannot be remedied. In these circumstances more contact padding should be provided. Knee and elbow pads are mandatory. The wearing of full-length stockings may prevent painful abrasions on the legs. Long-sleeved shirts serve a similar purpose.

Balanced Competition

There is considerable controversy over the desirability of competitive athletics in the younger age groups. It is my personal belief after many years of an active orthopedic practice that the youngster is in much less danger under controlled competitive conditions than he is in ordinary backyard play. Certainly this is true from a physical standpoint. We see relatively few grade school youngsters with injuries from football. We see many with injuries from incidental things. The energy of the youngster is such that he is going to expend it doing something. He is safer under supervised athletics than he is walking along the top of a fence, climbing trees or playing in the streets. Neither do I go along with that group of my pediatric colleagues who believe that competition is dangerous for the youngster. From a practical standpoint the youngster is competitive soon after he is born. If the competition can be directed into proper channels, it can be a healthy thing and much more educational than being beaten up by the neighborhood bully. To a youngster the frustration of losing a game is no more severe than that of the baby who breaks a rattle, and it is equally short-lived. This is particularly true if his competition has direction and understanding. He is taught to recognize that someone must lose each time someone else wins.

Competitive athletics does have a real responsibility in regard to equalization of the competitors. Most of the organized programs do this very well. The youngster is regulated not only according to age but according to size so that the 200 pound 14 year old does not compete with the 85 pound 12 year old. This is a distinct improvement over the casual sandlot games which are catch as catch can and usually are dominated by some prematurely developed youngster.

Balanced competition is particularly necessary in the grade schools but also is important in the high schools. A small high school that is dependent upon a relatively small squad must of necessity have boys on the team who are of something less than Olympic capacities. Hence, care should be taken in scheduling games that a team of immature boys does not compete with a juggernaut of excellent, well trained athletes. This is not nearly as pertinent now as it has been in the past. Comparatively few teams now schedule a so-called "warm-up" or "breather." They usually start right out in competition with their equals. Much credit is due the secondary school conferences which make a real effort to match teams of equal capacity against each other. The danger of injury is thus minimized.

EQUIPMENT

Athletic equipment has a great deal to do with prevention of injury. This is especially true of football, and most of our attention will be given to this sport. Good equipment is a must for a football program. We immediately run into the obstacle of an inadequate budget in many schools and in these a happy medium must be sought.

The physician must take a decisive part in directing the equipment phase of the preventive program. To do so he must inform himself, since ill-founded advice based on personal bias is a poor substitute for well informed judgment. The first step is to determine what things are necessary and are within the budgetary capacities of the particular program. There are two somewhat competitive facets of this problem. Certain items of equipment will add to the ability of the player and so are very desirable from the standpoints of both coach and player. However, one should not allow too much emphasis to be placed upon this facet to the disadvantage of protective measures.

For convenience the items of equipment for the football player will be discussed beginning with the headgear and working down. I believe that this plan will serve our purposes better than to attempt to grade them according to necessity. Indication will be given as to the relative importance of the various pieces of equipment.

There have been vast improvements in *headgear* in recent years and these continue. The old felt headgear that fit like a skull cap did little more than dull the blow and is a far cry from the modern plastic suspension helmet of today. The most important single element of the helmet is the system of webbed suspension straps. These straps must fit the head and keep it from contact with the plastic shell, else the whole function of the suspension is lost. The player himself should be instructed about this since only he can really tell whether the fit is proper. The helmet should protect the back of the neck, and should fit so that when the neck is extended the helmet does not drive into the back of the neck but rather slides down it. The front of the helmet should protect the forehead. The ear pieces should fit well over the ears. The orifice for hearing should coincide with the external auditory canal. It is obligatory that some sort of a bar be worn to protect the face. There has been much experimentation with these bars. One of the most effective is a single bar so placed as to make it difficult for the knee or elbow to reach the eye or nose, yet it protects the mouth. Double bars are more expensive and probably are not necessary for routine use, although they may be needed in specific circumstances. Attempts to use a wide plastic bar have failed because the player tries to see through the plastic with resultant distortion of vision. The headgear is the most important single piece of equipment.

The player with a fractured nose or malar bone will require a double bar or "bird cage" to more fully protect the area around the front of his face. The player with an injury to the jaw will need a bar placed lower to protect the mandible. Incidentally, the players must be sternly instructed that they must not grab the bar of their opponent. All of this is designed to protect the wearer of the helmet. Currently there is considerable agitation over the hardness of the helmet as related to the opposing player. The plastic shell is extremely hard. Its blow is cushioned somewhat by the fact that it is not at the end of a rigid pole so that there is a certain recoil element when the head of the player hits the opponent. At present, work is being done to design a helmet with an outer covering that is less traumatic and yet is not too heavy (Fig. 1). (See page 351.)

Injuries to the *neck* are relatively common in football. Most of them are minor but may be quite distressing. Obviously the player should not play with a serious

Figure 1. Protective equipment—neck, face and head. Upper two rows illustrates different types of football face protection. (Courtesy of Rawlinson, "Modern Athletic Training," © 1961 by Prentice-Hall, Inc.)

1. Mouthpiece
2. Headgear snubber—protect bridge of nose
3. Oral screw
4. Tongue forceps
5. Face guards for sports other than football
6. Rolled towel

injury to his neck. After a sprain or during the recovery period it may be desirable to protect his neck against excessive motion. This cannot be well done with adhesive as elsewhere in the body but quite effective use can be made of the so-called "cotton collar." This is actually a quilted pad narrower at one end than the other, wrapped around the neck and fastened with suitable straps to support the chin, mandible and occiput. A very simple substitute is an ordinary turkish towel (Fig. 1) folded lengthwise to about the width of the distance from the angle of the jaw to the shoulders and then wrapped firmly around the neck. This is quite effective in the player who occasionally gets a "pinched nerve" in the neck since it serves to prevent the motion that causes the pinching.

Most modern *shoulder* pads are quite effective in preventing injury to the shoulder girdle. Ideally they should be designed to protect the sternum and clavicles and particularly the acromioclavicular areas. The cap that extends over the deltoid serves to prevent painful contusions in this area. The most important attribute of any shoulder pad is that it fit the wearer. Too frequently the player picks his own pads out of a pile and he is unable to judge a proper fit. Someone should see that the pad actually fits to protect the parts it is designed to cover. A common injury to the front of the arm is the so-called "blocker's spur," which may often be caused by the edge of the shoulder pad itself rather than by the opponent. If the shoulder has been injured, more adequate support can be obtained from the so-called "Big Boy" or a double cantilever pad. A properly fitted foam rubber or plastic pad may be placed judiciously to protect bruised areas. Straps and strings should all be intact. (See Fig. 2.)

Elbow pads are usually not worn unless there is a specific indication. The per-

Figure 2.   Protective equipment—shoulder, arm, elbow and hand. (Courtesy of Rawlinson, "Modern Athletic Training," © 1961 by Prentice-Hall, Inc.)

1. Heavy duty linebacker, big boy shoulder pads
2. Double cantilever shoulder pad (two rolls of paper denote the double cantilever)
3. Protection for under a shoulder pad
4. Home-made bruise pad—takes pressure off the shoulder
5. Shoulder harnesses (dislocations, strains and sprains)
6. All-purpose injury pad with hole cut in top

son with an olecranon bursitis, abrasion over the elbow or something else of this nature should wear a suitably fitted pad. This applies to basketball as well as football.

Simple coaptation foam rubber or plastic splints may be used on the *arm* or *forearm* to protect an injured area (Fig. 3). No unyielding fiber board or plastic splint may be used below the elbow.

A suitable protective pad should be applied to the *hand* over injured areas. Again, great care must be exercised but no rigid pad is permissible. The protective wrapping of the normal hand utilized by the professionals is not popular in high school or university programs. A recently developed plastic foam pad serves to protect the back of the hand and leave the front of the hand free.

Properly fitted shoulder pads protect the upper part of the *chest* quite adequately and we would not ordinarily recommend supplemental chest pads. Fractured ribs are best protected by circumferential strapping or rib binder (Fig. 3). Two points should be stressed. In the first place, circumferential strapping is not compatible with the deep breathing necessary for active participation. In fact, it is designed to prevent deep breathing. In the second place, the fractured rib is not well protected by a contact pad at the tender site since pain in the ribs comes as much from compression or expansion of the chest in any diameter as it does from direct blow. Indeed, compression injury is more likely to hurt than a blow over the tender area. Contusions, however, are troublesome since any direct contact with

Figure 3.   Protective equipment—shoulder, arm, elbow and hand (*continued*). (Courtesy of Rawlinson, "Modern Athletic Training," © 1961 by Prentice-Hall, Inc.)

1. Elbow bruise pad
2. Fracture glove
3. Sternum or chest injury pad—lace to shoulder pads
4. Upper arm bruise pad—fiber and sponge rubber
5. Forearm pad
6. Hand pads
7. Rib belt
8. Resusitube Airway
9. Bandage scissors
10. Tape cutter
11. Handle of a spoon made into a finger splint
12. Felt thumb pads

them causes pain. The contusion may involve the skin or underlying bone and both can be well protected by a fiber pad, one of the most effective being the pad with a sponge rubber or plastic doughnut around its margin which holds the pad away from the injured part. A supply of this type of contact pad is inexpensive and will add to the ease and comfort of the competitor.

Since the *abdomen* is essentially soft there is no requirement for contact padding here. The player with deep abdominal tenderness as from liver or spleen injury should not compete. The back of the abdomen or flanks is best protected by pads built into the pants or a belt type pad that incorporates two contact pads running along either side of the spine to protect the so-called "kidney area" (Fig. 4). The football pants themselves contain padding for the iliac crest and trochanters. Here again, well arranged contact pads may protect tender areas, provided always that the underlying pathology is not such that competition should not be permitted. The athletic supporter is a must and no player should be allowed to practice or compete without one. The popular jockey shorts are not an adequate substitute for a well fitted athletic supporter. If there has been injury to the genitalia with a painful testicle some of the more protective type supporters may be utilized although they are not particularly comfortable and seem awkward to wear.

Most of the football pants incorporate a quadriceps pad that covers the front and lateral aspect of the *thigh*. Many of these pads are quite inadequate. If they

Figure 4.   Protective equipment—groin, pelvis, buttocks and back. (Courtesy of Rawlinson, "Modern Athletic Training," © 1961 by Prentice-Hall, Inc.)

1. Tail piece and hip pad
2. Hip injury pad
3. Low back injury pad
4. Rubber slingshot bandage

5. Hip pad
6. Pads for protection of a bruised hip
7. Back brace

are built into the pants leg, the latter should fit very snugly or the pants should be strapped down with adhesive. A loose thigh pad does far more harm than good since its edge may cause the very injury it is designed to prevent. In case of painful injury the pad may be strapped to the thigh with adhesive, preferably elastic in type. Anything constrictive around the thigh has the potential of reducing its blood supply and causing muscle cramps. This is not nearly so frequent in the thigh as in the calf but it may occur. The strapping should be snug but not tight. The protective pad only prevents contact injury. If the muscle itself is damaged, active movement of the muscle is the danger and this is not prevented by any pad. Similarly, contact pads are useless in protecting the hamstrings against strain either at their attachment to the pelvis or at the musculotendinous junction back of the thigh.

The normal *knee* is usually not strapped to prevent injury. Occasionally the boy who has grown rapidly to 6 feet or so but still has immature joints may feel that his knees are insecure and want to wear some type of protection. It is extremely difficult to protect the knee against the most common type of injury, namely, injury to the medial collateral ligament mechanism due to external rotation of the leg with the knee slightly flexed, with or without forcible contact against the lateral aspect of the knee. The ordinary pull-on elastic bandage is worthless protection here. It may add to the player's feeling of security but if tight enough to do much good it may also constrict his circulation.

If the knee has been injured the protective wrapping becomes important. It then has some design, namely, to prevent recurrence of a particular type of stress injury. Here again, the pull-on or wrap-on elastic bandage is of little value since it does not in any way protect against lateral or rotary stress. One must also question the value of an elastic pull-on bandage that incorporates a short metal bar or hinge either on one or both sides. The bar is not long enough to prevent leverage action of the leg and thigh. It is cumbersome and at best is inconvenient to wear. There are almost as many modifications of knee braces as there are people treating injured knees, a sure indication that none of them is particularly good. Recent developments aim to produce a corset-like brace that is longer and so more effective than those currently available. My own preference is for the octopus type which to some extent simulates the support given by adhesive strapping.

Many players with greater or lesser knee disabilities are attached to one or another type of support. If this support gives them confidence and they feel it helps, I think it is permissible to use it. It will not prevent re-injury. If there is swelling in the knee, particularly effusion, and this is mild enough that it is proper to permit the player to participate, it is proper for him to wear a pull-on or wrap-on elastic bandage in order to prevent further stretching of the suprapatellar pouch. All of these bandages have the doubtful virtue that they restrict flexion of the knee and so may to some extent prevent overstrain by the deep knee bend or duck waddle position.

If the knee actually needs protection for a weak ligament, for example the medial collateral, this can be best obtained by adhesive strapping. Cross strapping of the knee either on one or both sides as illustrated (Fig. 5) gives considerable protection against the knee "springing open" on the injured side. Owing to the bipod nature of the femoral condyles, it is necessary that the condyle of the femur and the tibial plateau actually separate to put stress on the medial collateral ligament and this can be minimized by adequate strapping. The cross-hatch strapping also to some extent restricts rotation of the leg on the thigh and so the familiar position of external rotation-abduction is prevented.

Figure 5.   A method for strapping the knee to support the lateral collateral ligaments. The criss-cross straps should cross in the midline. Maximum support for this dressing is medially and laterally.

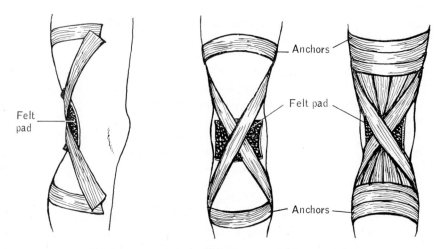

Figure 6.   Strapping of knee to prevent hyperextension.

If the injury to the knee was caused by hyperextension, strapping to prevent hyperextension (Fig. 6) will be much more effective than any permissible brace. Each trainer has his own methods of strapping and one who intends to do this sort of preventive strapping should familiarize himself with the various methods and practice them. Some prefer regular adhesive, others elastic adhesive. Actually, I believe a combination of the two is probably best. The newer type of elastic tape that stretches laterally rather than lengthwise gives much firmer support than the regular elastic type and conforms well to the rounded surfaces. By the very virtue of its firm support, it allows somewhat less mobility.

The knee also needs to be protected against direct contact. Most football pants have a knee pad although in most cases it is woefully inadequate. However, it is far better than nothing and I think every school should have a rigid requirement that these pads be worn. This is even more important in a secondary school. I insist on this requirement in the secondary schools because in these young people the cartilage of the patella and of the femoral condyle is more susceptible to injury and irreparable damage may be done to these areas by direct impact. This is particularly pertinent because many of the fields of play are very hard and the youth is likely to pay for his indiscretion not only by a ruined football season but by permanent damage to the knee. It is the responsibility of the physician, trainer or coach to insist on the wearing of proper protection of the knee against direct contact.

In most sports *leg* protection is not necessary. The exceptions are such games as soccer and hockey. Certain special categories as the baseball catcher are self-evident. Painful areas in the legs may be protected by contact pads.

There has been constant debate as to the virtue of support of the *ankle* during competition. It is my considered opinion that in football every player should have his normal ankles wrapped for every practice or game session. Many players will resist this since they feel it may diminish their agility. When the situation is explained to them, they will almost always accept the wraps gratefully. It is very easy to learn to put on an ankle wrap. The Louisiana wrap (Fig. 7) or some modification

Figure 7. Louisiana ankle wrap. This requires a 100-inch web ankle bandage. The start of the wrap is shown in the upper left drawing and is continued at the upper right, then lower left. At 7 the starting point is reached. The wrap is continued in this same fashion, with overlapping of turns, until the bandage is exhausted. Directly to the right, one complete turn of the bandage is shown. This is not the whole wrap. The bandage may be applied over a heavy sock, as shown, but wrinkles must be avoided.

is perfectly adequate. The wraps are inexpensive. They can be laundered easily and there is no excuse for not insisting on them if the athletic administration concerned agrees they are valuable. The ankle wrap does not restrict ankle motion per se at all since ankle motion is simply dorsal and plantar flexion. It does restrict lateral motion somewhat but even tarsal motion is not greatly restricted. It is protective against excessive tarsal motion, however, and so will effectively reduce the danger of sprain. It is difficult to sprain an ankle that is protected by a well placed ankle wrap unless the force is a major one sufficient to tear the wrapping.

If the ankle has been previously injured, the ankle wrap probably will be inadequate and one should resort to adhesive tape. One should familiarize himself with a good standard method for taping and learn to do it well (Figs. 7 and 8). The tape has the advantage that it may be extended up as high on the leg as is desirable. The greater the protection needed the higher the strapping should go. Since the tape is placed on the skin there is a certain amount of "give" in the bandage but the further the strip extends up the leg the less the resultant play and the firmer the fixation. If the strapping is applied because of an old injury it should vary according to the part to be protected since different types of strapping will be required for the lateral and the medial ligaments (Fig. 9), the arch (Fig. 10), the metatarsal area (Fig. 11), the tendo achillis (Fig. 12) and the dorsiflexors (Fig. 13).

The type of *shoes* is a debatable question. There is no doubt that the high shoe protects the ankle and foot better than the lower one, but many players feel that they are much more active in a low cut shoe. Presumably a low cut shoe plus the ankle wrap should be adequate. However, the high shoes do not replace the ankle

VIEW-1

VIEW-2

VIEW-3

VIEW-4

VIEW-5

VIEW-6

Figure 8.   Taping procedure. (Courtesy of Rawlinson, "Modern Athletic Training,"
© 1961 by Prentice-Hall, Inc.)

wrap. The player cannot be relied upon to lace his shoes tight enough to give support and yet not so tight as to be uncomfortable. I believe the ankle or foot that has been injured should be fitted with a high shoe.

So, too, there is considerable argument about the type of cleat. The value of certain types of cleat will depend a good deal upon the terrain. Many factors argue against long, pointed cleats. They have a real disadvantage upon frozen surfaces or hard ground, as well as upon matted bermuda which may catch the cleat. Some players feel that the hold secured by the pointed cleat on the sod will prevent injury whereas the proponents of the opposite view believe that its very fixation to the ground may encourage injury. In any event the cleat, whatever type is used, should be properly placed on the shoe and should be intact. A broken cleat is a danger not

Figure 13.   Strapping for the dorsiflexors.

the season is under way, however, the routine will be so established that only an occasional inspection will suffice and this can be done in the course of other instruction with the expenditure of little extra time. For example, a method to determine whether or not the athletes actually have their ankles wrapped properly during the practice session is to have them remove their shoes on the field while the coach is talking to them at the end of practice. The players who have their ankles properly wrapped are permitted to go on in and shower at the conclusion of the talk. Those who have not must remain for another work-out. Such measures are not unduly punitive but serve to call attention to the fact that observance of the regulations is important to the staff.

There is nothing more rewarding than to conclude a football season with the players in better condition than when they started. As in all fields of medicine, prevention is far better than cure.

PART II

General
Principles of
Treatment

3

Precepts and Examination

SOME OF THE PRINCIPLES of treatment mentioned in the Introduction merit repetition here. The basic treatment of the athlete is that of any young, healthy human. The most important consideration is that recovery be prompt and, above all, complete. Later in the book the specific treatment for certain conditions will be detailed, but the same basic principles apply to each, modified according to the location and the degree of the injury.

PRECEPTS

Prompt Examination Is Mandatory

Prevention is better than cure; but if injury occurs, the first step must be early recognition of the nature and the severity of the damage. There is usually no better time to determine the extent of an injury than when it happens; the practice of waiting to see is not compatible with the first principle of treatment of athletes, namely, prompt and specific care. As time passes, edema and inflammation supervene to cloud the picture. A careful, complete examination, done early, will often permit definitive treatment days, or even weeks, earlier than the "wait and see" method. Saturday's injuries should not be examined on Monday morning just to suit the convenience of the doctor or others. Once a decision concerning treatment is reached, it should be carried out confidently and completely. If a specialist is needed, he should be consulted early. It is disheartening to examine a patient weeks after his injury and find that the time for proper treatment is long past.

The Goal Must Be 100 Per Cent Recovery

A perfect result may not be possible of attainment in a given case, but if we do not try for it, we will never reach it. The young, well-conditioned athlete will tolerate whatever reasonable measures are necessary to give him complete recovery, and the doctor must resist compromise or unjustified complacency that tends to negate this goal.

Avoid Expediency

Too often, outside influences may overbalance sound judgment. The player's desire to compete, overoptimism, failure to admit the extent of the damage, or hesitation to interfere with school attendance may lead one to adopt a "middle of the road" course. Strict medical evaluation, not temporary convenience, must be the deciding factor.

Adopt the Best Method of Treatment

Here too, a temporizing attitude is fatal to good results. If you really believe the patient needs a cast, use it! If you think he should be on crutches, insist on it! If his ligament needs surgical repair, see to it! The best treatment is early treatment. Time is of the essence in obtaining a complete recovery in most ligament injuries.

Believe in the Value of Competitive Athletics

The physician must recognize that to this patient it is vital that he be restored to athletic competition. If the patient believes that the doctor disparages the importance of athletics, a sympathetic link between patient and doctor is lost. A master violinist would not trust the treatment of his hands to one who believed fiddle playing to be unimportant.

Above All, Treatment Must Be Prompt

Unnecessary delay is not compatible with good results in ligament injuries. "Don't hurry but don't fiddle" is as applicable here as it is in the operating room.

The foregoing precepts will simplify the care of the athlete so that the physician, instead of dreading this responsibility, will learn to look forward to the patient who gives such prompt and gratifying results. It is an interesting fact that most of the principles set forth here are readily applicable to other aspects of medical practice.

EXAMINATION

Time

The optimum time for the first examination of the injured athlete is as soon as possible after the injury. The prevalent custom of making a superficial and hasty examination (often on the field) and then sending the player to the ice bag for several hours is certainly to be deplored. It may not be possible to examine the player at once but the goal should be to examine him as soon as it can be done properly.

Place

Obviously, the first superficial examination of a player will be done on the field or on the sidelines. This can be little more than a cursory evaluation of the severity of the injury. If the injury is of any consequence, proper facilities must be available to make a detailed examination away from the crowd, preferably in a suitable examining room. At this time it will be possible to remove all of the clothing from the part and all of the protective strapping. The knee cannot be examined, for example, through a pair of football pants or over adhesive or elastic strapping. It follows that arrangements must be made to transport the player to suitable surroundings. It is highly desirable that this examination be carried out without the usual cluster of players, parents and fans gathering around and offering gratuitous advice.

Manner

In order to treat injuries to athletes successfully one must cultivate the practice of detailed, meticulous examination. In the case of an extremity injury, an examination should first be carried out on the uninjured extremity for the purpose of comparison. This procedure also can allay to some extent the apprehensions of the injured player and prepare him for the type of examination that is to be carried out on the injured part.

HISTORY

The first step in the examination is the history. Try to obtain as accurate a story as possible from the player or other people concerned as to the mechanism of injury. Did the injury appear to be severe or did it seem mild? Was disability immediate or delayed? Was deformity originally present and later reduced either spontaneously or with help? Did the player feel something slip or tear? Obtaining a careful history may give a vital clue as to the nature of the pathology.

PHYSICAL EXAMINATION

By *observation* note the general appearance at the site of the injury. Observe the location of the swelling, any possible deformity, any damage to the skin or evidence of a direct blow.

By *palpation* determine the degree of underlying tension in the tissues, possible fluctuation caused by hematoma formation, and the presence of local heat, tenderness or crepitation.

By *manipulation* determine the range of pain-free motion, the location of pain on motion, significant instability or abnormal motion. For any given area it is well to develop a routine for examination designed to check all the stabilizing elements of that particular joint. For example, a knee should be checked not only for lateral stability in extension but also for lateral stability in partial flexion and for anteroposterior or rotatory stability. By overlooking any one of these, vital information may be missed in the course of the examination.

X-ray examination should be carried out where fracture is manifest or only suspected. In this day and age there is little excuse for failure to obtain x-ray visualization since this is so readily available. X-ray examination is an art in itself, but it should be noted here that it is of little value to take excellent x-ray pictures if they are not carefully studied and properly evaluated (Fig. 14).

With a complete examination of this character it is the unusual case that will not present a definite clue as to the proper diagnosis. If, for one reason or another, diagnosis cannot be made at the time of the first examination, repeated examinations must be made until the diagnosis is clear. Every effort should be made to make a definitive diagnosis at the first examination since this will permit the institution of specific treatment at once. In any event, re-examination should be made from time to time in order to obtain an exact picture of the progress of the condition. Details of examination of individual parts will be given under appropriate sections. It cannot be overemphasized that successful treatment depends upon accurate diagnosis which in turn depends upon a careful, all-inclusive, atraumatic examination of the injured part.

X-RAY EXAMINATION

X-ray visualization is taken so much for granted now that one cannot justify the omission of this examination if there is any possibility of positive findings. It follows, therefore, that there will be many negative and, to some extent, useless x-ray examinations carried out. However, even if one ignores the medicolegal complications (which he would indeed be bold to do), there is a good argument for generous use of x-ray visualization. The current agitation against overuse of x-ray need not apply to films made for diagnostic purposes, provided they are made under

Figure 14.   An x-ray of the shoulder showing posterior dislocation. To a casual glance, no lesion is apparent. Careful inspection will reveal the head of the humerus medial to the glenoid convexity.

Figure 15.   Patient with left forequarter injury, particularly notable being a fracture of the clavicle in the middle third. An early film (A) shows no evidence of fractured ribs in spite of clinical soreness through this area. A later film (B) (two weeks later) shows fracture of the second and third ribs anteriorly.

proper control with suitable equipment. The extremely rapid x-ray film in common use today entails minimal radiation exposure. To the timorous a few confident words of explanation will allay his fears of over-radiation. One is justified in refusing management of a case in which x-ray visualization is not permitted.

However, it is not sufficient simply to order that the part be x-rayed. Routine x-rays, while they may be of some beauty and value, may not serve at all to rule out the presence of a lesion. The prevalent habit of sending a patient to x-ray, having the film made by the technician or even the radiologist, who has no actual knowledge of the injury suspected, results in many faulty interpretations. The physician should know what he is looking for in the film and so advise the radiolo-

Figure 16.   Exostosis of tibia. Note that the lateral view (A) is negative. The anteroposterior view (B) is inconclusive as to the nature of the mass, whereas the oblique (C) reveals the tumor very distinctly.

gist. He should himself be prepared to position the part to demonstrate the lesion he suspects. If anteroposterior and lateral views are not sufficient, other views should be made. If abnormal motion is suspected, stress x-rays may be desirable. If the original films are negative, repeat films after seven to ten days may be diagnostic. Once the x-ray is made it should be carefully studied, not only immediately but after the film is thoroughly dried and prepared for visualization. If doubt remains, views of the opposite extremity may be valuable or further views of the injured part may be desirable. If the original film is inadequate technically because of overexposure, underexposure, poor positioning, or blurring due to motion, one should not hesitate to request repeat films. With such careful planning and adequate follow-up by the doctor, the x-ray may indeed be a valuable adjunct to the management of a given case. Definite suggestions as to positioning and the use of multiple views will be made when considering specific injuries. (See Figs. 15 and 16.)

LABORATORY EXAMINATION

In the treatment of injuries to athletes, laboratory examination has a relatively small role and will be adequately correlated in the discussion of specific injuries to follow. Ordinarily the athlete is in good general physical condition so that routine blood and urine examinations may be expected to be normal. Special laboratory examinations may be of value in certain specific conditions, but as a rule the physician will obtain little help from laboratory procedures in the diagnosis or treatment of injurias to athletes.

4

Principles in the Management of Specific Injuries

CONTUSION

A CONTUSION MAY BE defined as a direct blow against the integument, causing bruising of the skin and underlying tissues. This results in capillary rupture and an infiltrative type of bleeding followed by edema and inflammatory reaction. The result is local swelling which may be superficial or deep depending upon the nature of the object striking the blow and the location involved. Thus the blow of the patella against the hard ground catches the skin between two hard objects and the resulting damage is to the skin and subcutaneous areas and possibly to the patella. On the other hand, the blow of a hard headgear against the unprotected thigh will catch the muscle between the headgear and the femur. The resulting damage is to the muscle, since the underlying soft tissue effectively protects the skin. The basic pathology is the same regardless of the area involved or the type of the blow.

Proper *treatment* consists of limitation of bleeding by application of cold and a pressure bandage in the early stages, together with immobilization and protection to prevent further injury. This is followed by measures to encourage healing. Local heat, rest and protection are vital at this stage. The area involved and severity of the involvement will determine the specific method utilized in a given case. Basically, the part must be protected from further damage by another direct blow or from overfunction and/or from injudicious methods of treatment. Faradic stimulation, for example, should not be used early in a severely bruised muscle. Unless the bleeding is considerable and of major proportions, the local infiltration of hyaluronidase or local anesthetic is not justified. In extensive contusion, however, particularly of the thigh or back, systemic medication with the various enzyme preparations may be of value. *Rehabilitation* should begin slowly within the limitations of pain and should progress parallel with the healing. Obviously a simple contusion may require but little treatment or rehabilitation, while an extensive contusion in a vital area may tax one's ingenuity to restore function while continuing protection.

HEMATOMA

The athlete is particularly prone to hematoma formation since he regularly exposes himself to the type of trauma likely to cause hematoma. For this discussion a hematoma will be defined as a collection of pooled blood within a relatively restricted area (Fig. 17, *A*). By pooled blood I mean blood not infiltrated through soft tissues but collected in a localized area and maintaining its identity as blood. It can readily be appreciated that this pooling will occur in many situations in many locations and from varying types of trauma since the basic condition from the pathological standpoint is bleeding within the tissues. We do not ordinarily refer to bleeding within an anatomically closed space as a hematoma, as for example in a joint or bursa or within a hollow viscus. In hematoma formation bleeding takes place into the tissues and by virtue of pressure from the hemorrhage the blood makes a space for itself which it wholly fills by pushing other tissue away. This may be extremely extensive as in hematoma formation up and down the fascial planes of the back following a serious vessel rupture in the vicinity of the spine, or it may be extremely localized as in the collection that forms between the skin and the periosteum over the shin.

Diagnosis.   A superficial hematoma is easily recognized but the diagnosis of a deep-seated hematoma may be difficult. Fluctuation is pathognomonic but its presence may indeed be difficult to determine deep in a muscle mass. In doubtful cases diagnostic aspiration is justified.

Treatment.   The treatment of hematoma must of necessity vary widely according to its location and extent. Treatment may be directed toward elimination of the hematoma itself, or toward relieving it because it is causing pressure on an adjacent structure. The general principles of treatment consist of (1) protection against further bleeding; (2) evacuation of the blood; (3) encouragement of absorption of the blood and (4) protection of the part until healing takes place.

During the diagnostic phase, before definitive treatment is begun, pressure dressings should be applied to prevent further bleeding. An ice pack is applied for the same purpose. Once it is determined that there is an aspiratable quantity of blood present, one may appreciably shorten the convalescent time by removing the blood (Fig. 17, *B*). Aspiration demands surgical aseptic technique. A large 15 or 16 gauge needle should be employed since one could hardly expect to evacuate old blood through a 22 gauge needle. Following aspiration the area should be infiltrated with hyaluronidase (Fig. 17, C), which tends to break down the confining wall and hasten the absorption of blood. Any attempt to aspirate a hematoma under any but the most aseptic conditions must be condemned. The dressing room or indeed the average training room is not the place for aspiration since the possibility of infection is particularly great in extravasated blood.

The center of a hematoma is to some extent like the center of an abscess. It may be quite avascular so that the circulating blood does not reach it, and many months may be required for absorption of the blood even in the absence of infection or other complication. The speed of absorption of the hematoma may be increased by diffusion of the hematoma, which is aided by the administration of hyaluronidase and the application of a pressure bandage (Fig. 17, D). These measures lead to more rapid absorption by bringing about greater exposure of the hematoma to the circulating fluids of the body. It has been said that it is unwise to aspirate a hematoma until one is sure the bleeding has stopped since increasing pressure of the hematoma itself will tend to discourage further bleeding. This is fallacious

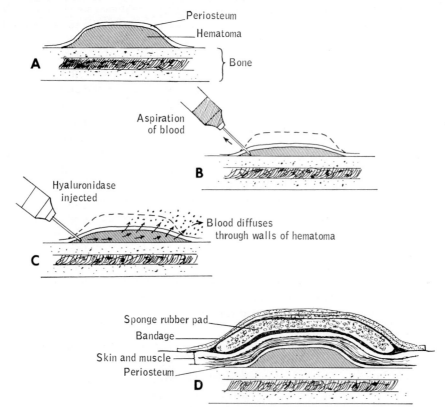

Figure 17. A, Cross section of a hematoma. In this instance the skin and subcutaneous tissue overlie bone and there is a collection of blood underneath the periosteum, well walled off.

B, Needle extending into the hematoma with the blood aspirated and the walls collapsed relatively.

C, Showing hyaluronidase inserted into the hematoma with little arrows indicating the blood was then diffused through the walls.

D, Same hematoma with overlying pressure dressing, indicated by sponge rubber pad and bandage in cross section.

reasoning since the same amount of pressure can readily be applied by external means. The hematoma should be evacuated as completely as possible even at a very early stage and then a pressure bandage will actually keep more pressure on the area than intrinsic pressure from the blood alone could be expected to do.

When the area involved is an actively moving part of the body this part should be protected not only against a direct blow but also against motion, since motion tends to break down the clot within the vessels and to perpetuate the bleeding. Motion also tends to cause irritation throughout the lesion and encourage over-reactive scar formation or calcification. Many a potential case of myositis ossificans has been aborted by careful protection of the part after proper local treatment. It is particularly important in muscle bleeding not to employ the "work it out" technique since this simply encourages further bleeding and promotes calcification. Absorption is also accelerated by the application of heat, which tends to improve the circulation of the area.

Protection against contusion should be continued as long as the area is symptomatic. However, protection against motion may be terminated much sooner. If the hematoma involves muscle or joint or a movable part, mobility can be resumed *within the limits of pain* almost at once. Voluntary pain-free contraction will tend to aid absorption, but forcible exercise of a muscle containing a hematoma will only aggravate the pain. The dividing line between what is a good level of activity and what is deleterious may be very fine, indeed. In many instances the athlete will be prone to minimize his symptoms in order to step up his activity so that real acumen is required in judging how soon full activity may be permitted. Hematomata of more static areas, as under the skin, require protection during periods of bodily contact. The compression bandage should be removed whenever it is obvious that the liquid hematoma is no longer present unless further support is needed because of circulatory embarrassment. It should be noted that following a relatively superficial hematoma there will be gross discoloration of the skin and that this may migrate a considerable distance if a pressure bandage is used. It is not at all unusual in the case of a hematoma over the shin or calf for ecchymoses of the skin to appear about the ankle or even in the foot. Their occurrence is ofttimes alarming to the patient and he should be reassured that it only represents a late stage in the absorption of his hematoma and does not indicate that his condition has grown worse or has extended. It is wise to warn the patient early that he may develop severe discoloration in the skin and that this may take weeks to disappear.

To recapitulate:

1. Diagnosis should be prompt, with aspiration if necessary to make a final determination.

2. The volume of contained blood should be reduced by aspiration, hyaluronidase, pressure, cold first, then heat, and controlled activity.

3. Re-injury should be prevented by protection against trauma or against excessive activity.

4. Resorption should be encouraged by exposing the hematoma to a larger surface area of circulation, by improving the local circulation, and by maintaining the general circulation.

Excessive scar formation or calcification can ofttimes be prevented by these measures.

MYOSITIS OSSIFICANS

Myositis ossificans is a frequent complication of the combination of contusion and hematoma involving the muscle near its origin on bone. The term is often used to include several conditions which may differ considerably. The name would imply inflammation of a muscle followed by ossification. I think this is very infrequently the case. Much more commonly, there is ossification of infiltrated blood along the muscle origin on the bone. The condition may appear as a simple exostosis having a broad base with a sharp extension into the muscle and may seem to be an involvement of the periosteum rather than the muscle (Fig. 18). The muscle is merely displaced by the ossifying mass. In this type of case the etiology is probably partial avulsion of the muscle fibers from the periosteum or even more likely a simple contusion of bone causing subperiosteal hematoma. The mass is pure bone and is firmly attached to the parent bone. In another type of so-called myositis ossificans there is actually a plaque of bone lying within the muscle and separated from the bone by a layer of muscle. It is difficult to determine here just what causes the ossification. The most likely assumption is that some periosteal cells invade the hematoma at the time of injury with formation of true bone and that the condition is not a metaplasia of muscle into bone. A third condition which is also called myositis ossificans is the calcification about a traumatized joint or a fracture site. A hematoma in these locations will calcify as a result of the repeated insult to healing tissue (Fig. 19). In these instances there is no involvement of muscle whatever.

Figure 18. Myositis ossificans. *A,* Well developed, but immature calcification. *B,* Completely mature calcified mass with wide base attached to the bone and spurlike projection into the muscle. *C,* One year after removal. No evidence of recurrence.

Figure 19.   Calcification of a hematoma in a dislocated elbow eight weeks postoperative. This patient was not immobilized and had active forceful manipulation in an effort to
improve motion. Motion is sharply limited and painful. There would have been less calcification if the elbow had been protected two or three weeks and then permitted only gradual motion.

Etiology.   Trauma is almost always the initiating cause of myositis ossificans. In the case of the long muscles the cause may be repeated trauma as occurs
in the upper arm as a result of the constant blows of the blocker in football
(Fig. 18). It may be a single forceful blow as on the quadriceps lateralis or intermedius (Fig. 20) in the anterior thigh, followed by active use. It may consist of
unwise or excessive manipulation of a fractured bone (Fig. 19). In all these
conditions one underlying factor is present, namely, repeated chronic irritation of
an area already damaged. If blood infiltrates into the muscle and the muscle is put
at rest, the chances are that this blood will be absorbed without further complication. If the muscle continues to be irritated by active use, by repeated blows, by
unwise manipulation or by massage, these repeated insults superimpose a new
injury over the early repair and the result is ossification.

Pathology.   The process begins as an infiltrating hematoma either subjacent
to bone or directly involving it. As healing progresses, instead of the orderly formation of scar to be replaced to a greater or lesser extent by normal tissue, osteogenesis
occurs in the scar and it is transformed into bone. This may be an extensive process
or a very mild one depending more upon the extent of the repeated insults than
upon the original injury. This process tends to continue as long as the irritation
continues. When the part is put at rest and the blood supply is improved by local
heat, the ossifying process is arrested. In many instances the bone will be absorbed
and the mass will shrink in size and disappear. In other instances as the bone
formation matures it becomes smaller (Fig. 21) and terminates as normal bone in
the form of an exostosis.

Diagnosis is not difficult once the ossification has matured. It is much more
important to recognize the impending pathology. If following a bruise on the thigh
or arm a diagnosis is made of contusion with hematoma formation, and this condi-

Figure 20.   Calcification in the
quadriceps lateralis which spontaneously
regressed and disappeared.

Figure 21.   A, Calcification in midarm which matured and disappeared within a year (B).
This probably represented bleeding into the periosteum.

Figure 22.   A, Immature calcification in anterior femur. B, Note regression and consolidation of the mass six months later.

tion does not promptly resolve, one should be on guard against formation of bone within the area. This explains why, in the discussion of contusion and hematoma, we insisted that rehabilitation should be carried out within the limits of pain and that reactivation of the area should depend not upon any predetermined time but upon the subsidence of symptoms. X-rays made early will be negative and should be repeated after two or three weeks if the symptoms persist. I have seen many cases in which the clinical examination demonstrated to my satisfaction a calcified mass within the muscle but the x-ray showed only a little cloudiness (Fig. 22). The symptoms have disappeared under proper management and the result was a small flake of calcium either on the bone or in the underlying muscle. More often it was complete resolution.

Treatment.   The early treatment of myositis ossificans is preventive and not surgical. *There is no place for operative treatment in the early stage of myositis ossificans.* As the impending condition is recognized the muscle should be put at rest. Physical therapy in the form of heat is permissible but no passive manipulation should be done. Some active motion may be permitted within the restriction of the splint, but only if it is painless. So treated, the condition may well subside and become asymptomatic. Granted, there may be considerable temporary stiffness of the part and considerable time will have elapsed but a crippling condition will have been averted.

Rehabilitation should be carried out well within the limits of pain, at least for the first several months. Should the patient be seen after the ossification has occurred, the same treatment is instituted, namely, rest and inductive heat.

In the early stage, particularly in myositis ossificans about a long bone, the appearance is frequently that of a new growth, with characteristic laminations of ossification or sometimes the stellate sunray effect which may simulate osteogenic sarcoma. One should not ignore the history of trauma in a case of suspected bone tumor (Fig. 23). There have been many cases of myositis ossificans mistakenly treated by operation for bone tumor and major tragedies have resulted. This is particularly prone to occur because the biopsy of an early myositis ossificans will reveal actively growing young bone, very similar to callus. This may be indistinguishable by the pathologist from a neoplasm. Careful attention to the symptoms and above all to the course of the lesion is of value. Since myositis ossificans runs

Figure 23.   Fatigue fracture. *A,* Early film shows periosteal proliferation suggestive of tumor. *B,* There is increased periosteal proliferation but the fracture line now appears. *C,* Healing stage. The fracture line disappearing.

a relatively short course, at least in the expanding stage, a period of watchful waiting is justified in case of any doubt. In the meantime the part is put at rest and films are made at two-week intervals. Myositis will show diminution of calcification or maturity of the margins, quite different from the development of an osteogenic type tumor. Operation even for the purpose of biopsy may be disastrous (Fig. 24). A few weeks delay probably will be of little importance in the development of an osteogenic tumor.

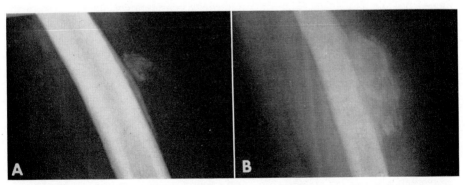

Figure 24.   *A,* Early myositis ossificans. Rather typical case but operated on elsewhere when misdiagnosed as a malignancy. *B,* X-ray a few weeks postoperative showing marked increase in the size of the mass due to the meddlesome surgery. This should be left alone for at least six more months or longer if the mass does not appear to be mature. (Note two types of involvement in the first view: calcification along the periosteum and the oval mass completely separated from the periosteum.)

As the healing progresses and the bone becomes more mature, more activity can be permitted, again restricted by pain. There is no place for passive stretching, certainly within six months, and the physiotherapist or trainer must be carefully instructed so that their urge to hasten rehabilitation will be controlled. One must rigorously resist the use of the knife. Under the exigencies of sport, everyone is anxious to have the player rehabilitated and may feel that the sooner the operation is done the quicker will be the recovery. This is one instance in which the reverse is true. Recovery will be quite prompt following removal of a mature exostosis whereas it will be indefinitely postponed by an attempt at removal of forming bone.

OPEN WOUNDS

This category of injury includes a wide range of conditions of varying severity from a simple scratch on the skin to a compound fracture. A simple classification of breaks in the skin begins with an *abrasion*, which may be defined as a scraping and sliding injury to the skin usually accompanied by a contusion as the integument is caught between an external object and underlying structures. In the ordinary abrasion the full continuity of the skin has not actually been broken through. A *laceration* is a wound of the skin caused by a relatively sharp object so that the skin is actually cut through its full thickness. A *puncture wound* is one made by a penetrating object which pierces all layers of the skin. *Vesiculation* is blistering caused by mechanical, thermal or chemical burning in which the layers of the skin are separated by an exudation of fluid.

Abrasion

An abrasion, which was defined as a scraping injury to the skin, may be of any grade of severity from a simple excoriation of the skin by the opponent's headgear to very extensive damage. The major abrasions will occur over areas of the body where there is firm underlying tissue, particularly bone. Areas commonly injured are the shin, the knee, the iliac crest, the elbow and the back of the hand. Abrasions in themselves are not particularly serious but their complications may indeed become a problem. The most immediate consideration, once injury to the deeper structures has been ruled out, is the prevention of infection. It cannot be overemphasized that the player should be carefully instructed to report any break on the skin that occurs on the playing field. The combination of an open wound and mother earth has very serious connotations from the standpoint of local and generalized infection.

Treatment. The first step in the management of abrasion is prevention by providing adequate playing fields. Contact sports should not be played on concrete, cinder tracks, or rough irregular ground with rocks and glass in the soil. The requirements for player protection will vary directly with the nature of the terrain. Thus, a player on a well groomed, heavily sodded playing field may need but little protection whereas one playing on hard, poorly sodded ground or on abrasive surfaces should have protection such as elbow pads, long sleeved jerseys and long socks.

Once an abrasion occurs it should be reported promptly and as promptly treated. When this is done an abrasion usually is of little importance. The first step in treatment is to clean the skin and there is no better cleansing agent than soap and water. There seems to be no real virtue in a surgical soap (such as the hexachlorophene soaps) for a single wash since the unique value of these preparations is in the build-up of the antiseptic in the skin by repeated washings. Ordinary bland white soap and water is entirely adequate, thorough cleansing being the important factor. The soap acts as a solvent for grease and embedded dirt. If necessary one can brush out ground-in dirt with a soft brush so that when the washing is complete the wound is fresh looking with no embedded foreign material. Some attention to detail at this first washing will save a great deal of later effort.

If a wound has been properly cleaned the application of a topical antiseptic is of doubtful value. In the ordinary abrasion we do not recommend painting with iodine, merthiolate or other chemical. If the surface is not too moist a protective spray such as tincture of benzoin may be applied, in order to reduce pain. Such a spray tends to seal the wound and yet permits exudation of fluids. The application of collodion over such an area is to be condemned since it may simply seal in the infected fluids. The use of a bland ointment preferably with a water-soluble base is recommended if the surface is "weepy." Greasy ointments should be avoided. There is no objection to having an antibiotic in the ointment such as sulfathiazole in Aquaphor, or Furacin. It should be borne in mind that such preparations may cause sensitivity and local reaction and even delay healing.

A suitable dressing and pad are applied to prevent re-injury since disability from an extensive abrasion that has been repeatedly crusted over and peeled off may last for several weeks and materially impair the activity of the athlete, particularly if the abrasion is on an area such as the knee, ankle or hand. The amount of protection necessary will vary a great deal with the severity of the abrasion, its location and its extent. Protection must be (1) against direct trauma and (2) against active overuse of the skin. The latter is particularly pertinent in an abrasion over the extensor surface of a joint such as the knee. Should infection ensue, warm moist packs, rest, elevation and suitable antibiotics are indicated. Great care should be taken in the dressing room in handling the infected wound since one infection may spread to many other players.

Laceration

As defined, a laceration is a separation of the skin with relatively sharp edges. Ordinarily in athletics this is not a cleanly incised wound as with a knife or razor blade; instead, it is a combination of a contusion and a lacerated wound in which the lacerated edge is jagged and irregular. These wounds, too, may be of any degree, from an extensive tearing of the skin with considerable separation of the skin edges to a fissure-like injury with but little external evidence of damage.

Treatment. After it has been determined that there is no underlying injury, the first goal in management is to obtain a clean wound. A laceration caused by a blow of a blunt object against a sharp underlying bone as in the eyebrow represents simply a splitting of the skin without penetration and is probably amply cleaned by the bleeding which accompanies it. On the other hand, a laceration caused by a broken cleat or the sharp equipment of the opposing player is potentially dirty and should not be closed without ample cleansing. A wound that has had direct contact with the ground must be promptly and thoroughly cleansed. The player should be taken to the dressing or treatment room and the wound very carefully explored for foreign material. If necessary, procaine may be injected along the wound edges to facilitate this examination. If the wound appears clean with no penetrating foreign matter it is unwise to scrape out the interior of the wound with an abrasive—and a gauze compress qualifies as such. Simple flushing of the wound with saline or 0.5 per cent procaine solution will usually be adequate.

Next, the wound edges are carefully inspected. Often the wound is not cut cleanly through the skin at a right angle but is a slicing type with a very thin edge on one side and a thick sloping edge on the other. In this instance careful minimal trimming of the skin margins in order to get sharp edge-to-edge contact will speed up healing and prevent excess scar formation. If it is felt essential that the player return promptly to the game, he may have a preliminary suture and then a definitive suture immediately after competition is over. From the medical standpoint this course is much inferior to proper closure of the wound in the first place but it is to be preferred to leaving a jagged wound imperfectly sutured. If there are undermined edges with considerable soft tissue damage beneath the skin, the wound may require drainage. It is better to put in a small wick that permits exudation than to allow fluid to accumulate. Frequently such accumulation can be prevented by direct, suitably placed pressure on the wound. Direct pressure also serves to prevent edema of the wound edges, which may cause considerable tension on the sutures and finally disrupt them.

In suturing the wound, swelling and edema should be anticipated. Only enough sutures are used to obtain accurate wound approximation. This principle accounts for the emergency room aphorism that "the slicker the wound looks immediately after suture, the sloppier it looks the following day." This is not to imply that the repair should be careless but simply that one should not place multiple small, shallow sutures in an effort to obtain fine approximation since these will inevitably pull out as swelling ensues.

The wound should be carefully inspected daily over a period of several days since it is potentially infected and should be treated as such. If there is any suggestion of a collection of fluid in the wound, one or more stitches should be removed and the wound allowed to drain freely. The question of further participation in athletics before it has healed must depend entirely upon its location and extent. In many body areas the laceration can be adequately protected against both trauma and undue stretching of the skin and there is no reason why further participation cannot be permitted. Once there is evidence of any complication, more protection should be utilized and the inflamed wound must be treated by the usual measures of immobilization, warm wet dressings, antibiotics and general support. Careful primary attention to the lacerated wound will give very gratifying results. Antitetanic serum or tetanus toxoid should be given.

Puncture Wound

This condition has been defined as a wound by a penetrating object. The object may be small, as a splinter or nail, but even a rather broad object may penetrate through the skin, making a relatively small opening and continuing deeper into the soft tissues. This has the potentiality of a puncture wound and should be treated as such. Such wounds are not common in athletics but should be promptly and adequately treated when they do occur. The author recalls one instance during a track session when one of the participants was kneeling on one knee with the other thigh thrust forward when he received an errant javelin in his anterior thigh. This not only caused a puncture wound through the skin and ruptured the muscle mechanism but split the shaft of the femur.

Of first importance are the severity of the wound, the depth of the penetration and the possibility of underlying damage to the joints or bone, but particularly to the blood vessels or nerves. A penetrating wound over a joint should be assumed to have entered the joint without proof to the contrary since the potentialities of joint penetration are of major importance. A history is carefully taken as to the nature of the penetrating object, the depth of the penetration, whether or not it went through clothing, and whether the entering body was contaminated as in the case of the peg of a broken cleat or piece of wire or nail which happened to be on the playing field. It will not suffice to wash off the skin, apply protective dressing and "wait and see." It may be necessary to wait and see but this decision should be made only after careful history, thorough examination and some effort to explore the wound. If there is underlying damage which will require surgical repair, this repair should be done at once since the wound is potentially infected. Even a few hours delay will change it from a potentially to an actually infected wound. After that, definitive surgery is extremely hazardous.

Treatment.   After one has satisfied himself that there is no underlying damage, the wound itself is treated. The skin will often be puckered and discolored around the margin which indicates that the hole at one time was considerably larger than it is at the time of examination. The skin tends to stretch and tent inward under the pressure of the blow so that, when the point does penetrate the stretched skin, it may make a fairly large hole. When the skin returns to its normal tension this hole will shrink and appear minute. The importance of determining the nature of the object and the depth of penetration is obvious.

If the object was contaminated and penetrated deeply it will be wise to split the skin, examine the underlying tissue, clean out the sinus tract and then decide whether or not to carry out primary closure. Primary closure may be carried out if the wound has been treated promptly and satisfactorily lavaged. The use of a drain will depend upon the degree of damage and whether or not one expects continued oozing and collection of fluid. It is much better to let the fluids seep outside through a tissue drain than to accumulate in the wound to make an ideal medium for infection. Only if the wound seems minor, the penetrating object small and the depth not great is one justified in simply cleansing the skin and observing. If the decision is made to observe the wound, exactly that should be done—and frequently. It is not proper to wait until secondary symptoms demand attention, for by this time a definite infection will be developing. (For tetanus serum see below.)

Blisters

Mechanical.   Blisters on the skin may occur under varying circumstances, the most common being friction from an ill-fitting shoe or a wrinkle in the sock. Another frequent source is irritation by adhesive tape or by friction between the tape and skin due to the fact that the tape was poorly applied, has been under undue tension or that the individual has perspired and so separated the tape from

Figure 25.　　Cross section drawing of the vicinity of the first metatarsal head, showing the heavy epidermis of callus with a blister lying between this and the underlying dermis. A needle has been inserted to draw out the fluid. (Needle inserted away from the blister margin, through intact skin.)

the skin in certain areas while it remains adherent to the skin in others. In any event the resulting traction on the skin tends to separate its superficial layers from the underlying dermis, the area fills with exudate and the blister forms. While the blister itself may be a relatively simple and apparently minor ailment, its location may be such as to make it a problem of some magnitude. A blister on the back of the heel, for example, may handicap the player throughout the season. Extensive vesiculation under the adhesive tape may render it impossible to use adhesive in that particular area of the body and so vital protection may have to be discontinued with resultant injury to the unprotected joint or ligament beneath.

Another disabling area of vesiculation is the sole of the foot where it is not uncommon to have a blister directly under the first toe or first metatarsal head. This is particularly common in the track man who runs in light shoes but with a very pointed spike so that he may get direct pressure in a single area of the sole. This constant sliding of the skin on itself results in blistering. The skin of the sole is thick and a very deep blister under the skin (Fig. 25) may go unrecognized and be treated as a simple contusion. I have seen such a blister enlarge until it separated a large portion of the calloused skin under the forefoot. This condition manifestly is not compatible with competition.

The best treatment of blisters is PREVENTION. Carefully fitted shoes and clean, wrinkle-free socks are extremely important. If strapping or wrapping is used it should be carefully placed and its location changed if it begins to irritate the skin. Careful preparation of the skin before application of adhesive will often prevent irritation either by reaction to the tape or by partial slipping of the tape on the skin. A simple wrinkle in the tape in a weight-bearing area of the body may cause prompt blistering beneath it. If an irritated area develops which appears to be the prelude to a blister, careful protection should be used either by a very thin smooth tape applied directly to the skin or by soft padding to prevent friction between the skin and equipment. An ounce of prevention is certainly worth a pound of cure here.

Once a blister develops, proper TREATMENT is of considerable importance. Here again the location of the lesion makes some difference in the type of treatment instituted. If the blister is located in an area where there ordinarily is no friction, as the thigh or calf, the top of the blister may be removed, the area carefully cleansed and the resultant abraded area treated appropriately (with benzoin spray, for instance). This management, however, is not practicable for a blister caused by pressure from a shoe or another piece of equipment. In this instance it is quite important to protect the skin over the blister. The blister should be treated by passing a hypodermic needle through the adjacent skin and into the blister to drain the fluid and relieve the pressure. This is particularly applicable on the plantar surface of the foot so that some of the callus can be preserved until such time as the floor of the blister develops some resistance of its own. Once the roof of the blister is broken it is well to trim it all away and treat the floor by benzoin solution, proper protection, etc. The ragged edges of the top of the blister not only irritate the lesion further but serve to form peripheral pockets containing infected fluid.

Chemical. Chemical blistering is not frequent since the marking of fields by lime is no longer common practice. It does have the added complication of irritation of the surrounding skin and should be treated by protection by bland emollients much as in a thermal burn. The *thermal burn* has no particular application to athletic injuries but occasionally occurs as a result of carelessly applied physical therapeutic measures and as such may be extremely distressing. The burn from the ultraviolet machine is of course similar to sunburn and should be treated as such. Injuries from the infrared or electric heating pad and various types of hot packs are true thermal burns and may cause vesiculation, but usually remain a local reaction. These direct heat applications usually cause sufficient pain that the treatment is stopped before the burn is severe. The result is usually first degree or at the worst a mild second degree burn with only moderate vesiculation. The deep electrical burns caused by diathermy or other inductive agents may be extremely severe. A diathermy burn should be very carefully investigated to determine whether or not the damage is limited to the skin. It may well be so since ofttimes the burn is secondary to the condensation of fluid between the applicator and the skin, thus it actually is from hot water. If it is a true electrical burn the deep tissues may indeed be burned more severely than the skin. An electrical therapeutic appliance is no plaything and its indiscriminate use by untrained personnel should be frowned upon. The patient should be instructed not to put too much faith in the dials of the machine, and he should be told to report the slightest discomfort since it is neither safe nor desirable to have the heat reach the level of discomfort to the part being treated.

Skin Infections

Skin infections secondary to direct trauma are ofttimes the bane of the training room since they may start in one player and spread like wildfire through the whole squad. Any skin infection however superficial should be very carefully washed, the surrounding skin cleansed, protective dressing applied and great care taken not to reinfect the skin by use of dirty clothing. It is obvious that once suppuration occurs the pimple or boil should be opened under aseptic technique and the area of surrounding skin protected by careful cleansing with antiseptic solution and protective dressing. The dressing should be destroyed and not indiscriminately tossed to the floor. Many of the so-called eczemas are indeed skin infections and the affected player's clothes should be isolated from the remainder of the squad.

Fungus infections are particularly distressing and are prone to develop under adhesive tape applied to the feet. Occasionally on removal of the tape the whole plantar integument will peel off as a result of extensive fungus undermining. Application of proper fungicidal measures will clear up the local lesion quite adequately. The big danger is that casual handling of the socks, contamination of the floor and common shower stalls will spread the fungus from the player who is relatively immune to his own fungus to his neighbor who has no resistance to this particular organism. While it may be an entirely latent infection in one player his locker mate may develop a virulent infection. Ordinary rules of cleanliness, soap and water, clean socks, some type of bath shoes, will help to minimize this problem. If it becomes epidemic in a given situation, special measures will be necessary to sterilize the shower stalls, locker room floors, etc. Enteric drugs are promising.

Tetanus Prevention

The problem of tetanus is very important in the athletic program in spite of its great rarity. It is one condition in which prevention is almost completely effective and treatment is relatively ineffective, therefore little justification exists for not employing preventive techniques.

Toxoid. Ideally, every athlete should have tetanus toxoid injections prior to his participation in sports. These injections have been well proven, were adopted by the armed forces and have been extremely effective in eliminating the danger of tetanus from questionable wounds. There is ordinarily no reaction to toxoid injections and it would be entirely feasible at the beginning of the school year to insist on them for each athlete. If the patient has had toxoid within the year one can relax about the ordinary skin involvement. If he sustains a particularly virulent type of puncture wound, as by a rusty nail, injection of a booster dose of toxoid can be given at that time with no danger of reaction and with complete effectiveness since tetanus develops rather slowly and the toxoid booster can develop the antibodies much more rapidly than the organism develops its toxin.

Antitetanus Serum. If the player has not had toxoid and he has any type of a wound with undermining of the skin, it is imperative that he have antitetanic serum. If there is the least question about his needing it, he needs it! A precaution of utmost importance is to check the individual for sensitivity. The fact that he has previously taken antitetanic serum without reaction is not pertinent at all since this very injection to which he had no reaction may indeed have been the one that sensitized him. Once the wound has occurred it is too late to start the active immunity of tetanus toxoid. If active immunity has previously been instituted by toxoid injection, the toxoid booster will be better than antitetanic serum since the resulting active protection is much longer lasting than the neutralizing effect of the antitetanic serum. Serum reaction may be delayed.

STRAIN

Strain may be defined as damage to a tendon or muscle occasioned by overuse or overstress. It is important that we distinguish between strain and sprain, apply-

ing the former term to muscle and tendon and the latter to ligament. Much confusion can thus be averted. Strain of a tendon could obviously consist of anything
from minor irritation to near complete avulsion of the tendon from its attachment
or within its substance. Strain of a muscle includes those cases of overuse and overstretching short of an actual muscle rupture, either from forcible avulsion or from
a direct blow.

Simple Strain

In the ordinary strain there is no appreciable hemorrhage, the pathologic
changes being confined to a low grade inflammatory reaction with swelling and
edema and some disruption of the adjacent fibers. Diagnosis will depend upon
testing of the function of the muscle involved and seeking the location of the pain.
This will be relatively easy early and becomes very difficult as the whole muscle
goes into spasm. Careful localization of the injury is important if one intends to
use local measures, which may be of considerable value in many cases.

The exact location and function of the unit involved has a great deal to do
with the importance of treatment. For example, in the football player strain of the
hamstrings or of the quadriceps or of the calf may be completely disabling. In the
baseball player strain of the muscles of the throwing arm may wholly prevent participation at his usual position. The many complications of simple strain will be
discussed in later sections and these are, of course, the most important factors in
the decision as to the further participation of the injured player.

In essence, *treatment* consists in relieving the acute condition by injection
of a local anesthetic followed by a corticoid, use of local heat, and protection
against any movement which causes pain. The amount of protection applied must
vary with the degree of damage so that in some cases all that is necessary is to
limit the patient's activity while in others it may be essential to prevent all stress
by immobilization either of the patient or the part. The criterion for the amount of
protection is pain. Function should be resumed just as soon as possible but it must
be pain-free. The man with a strain of the hamstrings may well exercise his leg in
the whirlpool in the very early stages, whereas to get out and run would impede
his recovery. One is constantly torn between the desire to rehabilitate the muscle by
active use and the knowledge that overuse will cause recurrence. A strain has a
marked tendency to recur. It takes an extremely farsighted physician or trainer to
regulate the activities to that fine point which will restore the player at the earliest
possible moment.

Violent Strain; Musculotendinous Injury

Those injuries to the musculotendinous unit caused by a single, violent injury
may be of any degree. The tendon may be torn from the bone or pulled apart. The
musculotendinous junction may be ruptured or the muscle itself may tear. These
injuries result from either violent contraction of the muscle against resistance as
when the sprinter comes out of the blocks, or from violent overstretching of the
muscle while it is forcibly contracted as when the arm is forcibly extended from
a flexed position, with the biceps taut. Certain areas of the body are particularly
prone to these injuries, particularly the hamstrings, the biceps brachii and the
plantaris.

Treatment.   One should take extreme care in a musculotendinous injury to determine if possible whether there has been a complete disruption of the unit. If there has been and it is recognized early, immediate surgical repair is extremely gratifying. Later surgical repair may be impossible. If the injury is less than complete an attempt should be made to evaluate the degree of the tear and treat it accordingly. This will fall into the categories of rupture of muscle fibers with hematoma, strain of the attachment of the tendon to the bone, and partial separation of tendon from the muscle. Since one is going to treat each of these conditions by careful observation, physical therapy and protection, the speed of recovery will determine the length of time the protection should be carried out. Where the tendo achillis is partially torn from the soleus muscle, for example, local tenderness in this area with persistent spasm on active use of the soleus would be a danger signal pointing to the need for immobilization over a period sufficiently long to allow healing to take place (six to eight weeks). Actually, limited function of the muscle can be initiated before this time provided this function remains pain-free. As is the case in so many instances in the treatment of the athlete, it is extremely important to analyze the symptoms and determine the exact pathology at or near the time of the injury, since early treatment is highly satisfactory. Late treatment is at best a salvage procedure.

SPRAIN

Definition

A sprain may be defined as an injury to a ligament resulting from overstress which causes some degree of damage to the ligament fibers or their attachment. A ligament is a structure designed to prevent abnormal motion of a joint while permitting normal functional motion. Certain ligaments may bind two bones firmly together with relatively little motion, such as the tibiofibular syndesmosis which permits slight rotatory motion while preventing separation of the two bones. Other ligaments serve to reinforce a joint and permit a rather wide excursion of normal motion but prevent motion in an abnormal direction. Fundamentally, abnormal motion to a degree beyond the power of a ligament to withstand it will cause a sprain. This is to be contrasted with a direct blow over a ligament which may cause a contusion. As abnormal force is applied the ligament becomes tense and then gives way at one or the other of its attachments or at some point in the substance of the ligament (Fig. 26). If the attachment pulls loose with a fragment of bone, it is called a "sprain-fracture," but the mechanism is the same. The location of the damage will depend upon the weakest link in the chain of the ligament which may be within the ligament itself or at one of its attachments, possibly at the site of an area of previous damage. The extent of the damage depends upon the amount and duration of the force. If the abnormal force is arrested or terminated promptly, there may be little actual functional loss to the ligament and only a few of its fibers may be involved. In this instance there is localized hematoma formation with prompt deposit of fibrin in the hematoma. The fibrin is invaded by fibroblasts and as the reparative process proceeds the final termination is restoration of a normal ligament. If the damage is more severe so that there is actually more disrup-

tion of ligament fibers there may be considerable functional loss. Where the ligament is completely torn, all function is lost. In this case the findings will depend
upon the location of the tear. Ordinarily there will be relatively extensive hematoma
formation with swelling and edema. The process of repair will be much slower and
much less complete and will result in scar formation rather than restoration of
normal ligament.

Degree

For the purpose of this discussion sprain will be divided into three different
categories according to the severity of the injury.

Mild (Fig. 26, *A*).   This is a sprain in which a few fibers of a ligament
have been torn with some resultant hemorrhage into the ligament but with no

Figure 26.   Drawings illustrating various types of sprain.
A, Mild sprain, in which there is a little hematoma in a very localized area in the
ligament with only a few fibers separated.
B, Moderate sprain, a more severe tear of the ligament but with at least half of the fibers
remaining intact.
C, Severe sprain. Complete tear through the ligament with separation of the ends.
D, Sprain-fracture. The ligament is torn off bone with a fragment of bone.

actual functional loss. There is no demonstrable diminution in strength in the ligament. This is of considerable importance from the standpoint of treatment since
the factor of protection is not important. The ligament is not weakened.

Moderate (Fig. 26, *B*).   A moderate sprain is one in which some portion
of the ligament is torn and some degree of functional loss is present. The amount
of damage may vary from tearing of a relatively small portion of the ligament to
almost complete avulsion—from "mild" with no functional loss to "severe" with
complete functional loss of the ligament. The emphasis here must be on protection
since one may be unable to determine the actual extent of the damage. One would
not expect wide retraction of the torn ligament ends in a moderate sprain. Union
can therefore proceed in an orderly manner with replacement of fibrous scar by
ligament during the process of repair. If the damage is relatively severe, however,
there may be considerable permanent scar formation with resultant weakness in
this segment of the ligament. Obviously, protection here is mandatory to promote
efficient repair and prevent permanent weakness. "Once a sprain always a sprain"
is an euphemism not acceptable in the modern concept of therapy.

Severe (Fig. 26, *C*, *D*).   In severe sprain we predicate complete loss of
function of the ligament due to a force that either tears it completely away from
one or the other of its attachments or pulls it apart somewhere within its substance.
One must presume that there has been at some time wide separation of the ligament ends, else the tear would not have been complete. Since efficient repair is
dependent upon apposition of the torn ends of the ligament, it becomes vitally
important to replace the ligament ends in approximation. We have been able to
show experimentally that if the torn ends of the ligament are placed together the
tissues heal by ligament fiber which in many instances is stronger than the adjacent undamaged ligament. On the other hand, ligaments which heal across a gap
by scar formation never take on the characteristics of normal ligament.

It can be seen, therefore, that in mild sprain *treatment* is relatively unimportant and is designed mostly toward prevention of pain; and that in moderate sprain
the critical factor in treatment is protection in order to permit repair. On the other
hand, in severe or complete sprain the emphasis must be placed on reapposition of
the ligament ends in order to assure a ligament that not only heals in its normal
length but with its normal strength. It follows that diagnostic acumen is of great
importance in the management of ligament injuries since treatment depends upon
the nature of the lesion rather than upon the patient's progress following injury.

DISLOCATION

Dislocation may be defined as an actual displacement of the opposing contiguous surfaces making up a joint. This of necessity presumes loss of function of
some of the ligament structures of the joint since the ligaments are designed to
prevent displacement or abnormal motion. *Subluxation* is a partial dislocation. In
acute sprain when the ligament finally tears the joint subluxates either by a slipping
of the bone ends on themselves or by a separation of the bone ends. If the force
continues until the joint actually is disrupted there is a dislocation. This may be
spontaneously reduced or the bones may lock in the dislocated position (Fig. 27),
in either instance there is loss of function of the ligament.

It is possible to have a chronic dislocation without fresh damage to the liga-

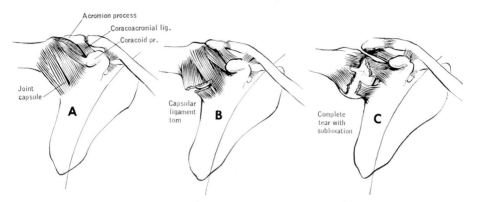

Figure 27.   Complete dislocation showing attendant ligament damage.

A, First stage of dislocation of the shoulder. The arm is externally rotated, abducted, tightening up the anterior and inferior capsular ligaments. The tuberosity hinges against the acromion.

B, Continuation of the force with the tuberosity locked firmly against the acromion. The ligament fibers tear antero-inferiorly and the head begins to subluxate.

C, Head subluxating downward and further away from the acromion. Complete rupture of the capsular ligaments.

ment. In this case one presupposes that the ligament has been previously torn or stretched to the point that dislocation of the joint occurs within the capacity of the surviving ligament. However, in acute dislocation or acute subluxation the ligament must tear. This is of considerable importance from the standpoint of treatment since if, in an acute dislocation, one visualizes a complete tear of one or more ligaments, he must certainly consider seriously the advisability of surgical repair.

Treatment.   Since dislocation is simply the end result of a severe sprain, it can be treated as such. Thus, protection is essential until the ligament has healed regardless of the method used to secure its repair. For example, if a shoulder dislocates it may readily be reduced either by a teammate, the coach or the physician. The fact that it remains out of joint 30 seconds or 30 days is no indication of the extent of ligament damage although it may have vast importance in the end result. Even if the joint dislocates and immediately reduces itself nonetheless there is ligament damage and treatment must be designed to further the repair of this tear. In some instances surgical repair will be advisable while in others it will not be necessary. In either event the importance of carrying out protection until the ligament completely heals cannot be overemphasized.

Dislocations as a class are vastly undertreated and as a result are notorious for poor end results. The dislocated finger may be promptly reduced, but, if the player continues to play or goes without medical care or without splinting of the finger, permanent disability of the involved joint almost inevitably results. Either a painful, swollen joint with restricted motion or a weak, relaxed joint with recurrent dislocation is often the consequence of a nonprotected dislocation. A minimum of six weeks is needed for a ligament to repair even under optimum circumstances.

TENOSYNOVITIS

Tenosynovitis may be defined as inflammation of the synovium surrounding a tendon. This inflammation is usually due to strain from unaccustomed overuse but may be due to a direct blow or to infection. The result is a reaction of the normally avascular synovium with increased blood supply, invasion by inflammatory cells, oversecretion of synovial fluid and increase in fibrin content causing so-called "sticky" adhesions between the tendon and its surrounding synovium. The exact manifestations vary greatly, depending upon the tendon involved, and will be considered in some detail under various headings. Actually the symptoms are those which would be expected to result from irritation on motion of the tendon. The first manifestation is pain on function which may progress to the point of constant pain even under rest. Crepitation is frequently present. As the tendon slides up and down it adheres to the synovium causing so-called "snowball crepitation," which can be felt by placing the fingers over the involved tendon while it slides up and down. As the condition progresses, the adherence between the tendon and synovium becomes more firm and may finally result in complete loss of the gliding capacity of the tendon within its sheath. This is particularly true in areas where there is a true tendon sheath (such as the long head of the biceps at the shoulder) and is not common where mesotendon is concerned as in the tendo achillis. *Treatment* is directed toward the pathology and the principles of treatment are rest, local heat and local injection. The specific treatment will vary according to the site of the condition.

Sequelae of Tenosynovitis

Under ordinary circumstances and with proper care, the tenosynovitis will subside completely and normal function results. In certain cases, however, either because of the severity of the condition or as the result of inadequate treatment or the anatomical characteristics of the area involved, complications may arise which may cause severe and permanent disability.

The first of two common sequelae of chronic tenosynovitis is *adhesive tenosynovitis*. As the name implies, the tendon and its surrounding sheath become bound in an inflammatory mass leading to actual adherence between the two which interferes with the normal gliding motion of the tendon (Fig. 28). This restriction of motion may be complete or only partial. The degree of disability will depend upon the location of the involved tendon. If it is in an area where there is a true sheath, such adherence will prevent motion completely and the tendon loses its function in regard to this particular area. On the other hand, if it is in an area not constricted by a true sheath the adherence may simply result in traction strain and possibly some restriction of function rather than complete loss. Treatment for true adhesive tenosynovitis is difficult since if the adhesions are trimmed away they may promptly re-form. However, resection of the sheath or transferring the tendon to a less constricted area may be effective remedies.

The second common sequela is *constrictive tenosynovitis* caused by thickening of the walls of the sheath with resultant narrowness of its lumen. This frequently occurs in an area where more than one tendon passes through the same tunnel or sheath. In such an instance the tendon itself is not adherent to the sheath but the sheath is so tight that the tendon will not slide through it. This may start as an initial snapping such as a trigger finger and may terminate in complete loss of gliding power of the tendon through this tunnel. Whereas adhesive tenosynovitis is difficult to treat adequately, this constricting type is readily relieved by

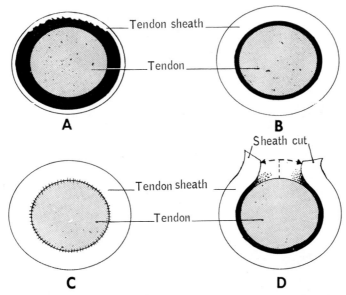

Figure 28.   Tenosynovitis. *A*, Drawing showing the tendon lying in the sheath with some irritation of the inner wall of the sheath. *B*, Same area, showing the tendon sheath and underlying tendon both swollen and the sheath very tight. *C*, Same area, showing the sheath and tendon adherent to each other. *D*, The area after sectioning of the sheath and releasing of the pressure.

simply enlarging the tunnel surgically by resection of a part of the sheath. These conditions will be discussed in some detail in relationship to specific areas in the body.

BURSITIS

Bursitis may be defined as an inflammatory reaction within a bursa. This may vary in degree from very mild irritative synovitis with discomfort to suppurative bursitis with actual abscess formation. A bursa is specifically designed to facilitate motion between contiguous layers of the human body, and the athlete with his extremes of motion is particularly prone to bursal involvement resulting from repetitive local trauma due to tissue friction or from direct blows.

The examples of bursitis are legion. The bursae most frequently damaged by direct trauma are the prepatellar lying between the patella and the skin (Fig. 29) and the olecranon between the olecranon process of the ulna and the skin. The trauma is usually a repeated one resulting in synovial irritation with thickening of synovium and formation of excess fluid. A large sac of synovial fluid is contained within the bursa. By virtue of the increased tension in the bursa, additional direct trauma tends to further distend its walls until the bursa may reach an amazing size. *Treatment* is directed toward prevention of repeated injury and reduction of the irritation within the bursa. Aspiration of fluid, local injection of corticoids, protection against direct trauma and application of a pressure bandage to appose the walls of the sac are in order. If the condition becomes chronic and the synovitis is persistent, surgical removal of the bursa may become necessary.

Patella

Prepatellar
bursa

Superficial and
deep infrapatellar
bursae

Figure 29. Drawing showing the patellar bursae.

Bursitis caused by friction between moving parts is exemplified by that occurring in the bursa beneath the internal hamstrings tendon at the knee. Here the principal manifestation of bursitis will be pain on motion of the knee, tenderness over the bursa and local inflammatory reaction. Aspiration will be of little value but local injection may reduce the inflammation. *Treatment* must consist in preventing the motion that is causing the inflammation rather than protecting it against direct trauma. Local injection of a long-acting anesthetic agent plus a corticoid together with application of local heat and a protective splint is of value. Here again it is important to continue protection until healing is complete since recurrence is very likely if the activity that originally caused the inflammation is resumed earlier.

SYNOVIAL HERNIA

Another condition involving the tendon sheath and sometimes the joint is the synovial hernia or so-called *ganglion*. This condition as a rule results from a defect in the fibrous sheath of the joint or tendon that permits a segment of underlying synovium to herniate through it. In the athlete it usually follows a mild sprain although it may also be degenerative in nature. The irritation accompanying this herniation results in continued secretion of fluid so that the sac gradually fills up and enlarges. In some instances it may reach an amazing size.

As a rule the synovial hernia will appear as a small, discrete, sometimes extremely hard nodule lying directly over the tendon or the joint capsule. It is often impossible to tell whether the primary involvement is tendon or joint. The consistency of the tumor may vary from that of bone to that of a soft, fluctuant, obviously liquid mass. This difference in consistency is more apparent than real and is due to the degree of tension within the sac since the sac uniformly will be found to contain a clear, gelatinous, viscous fluid which is blood-tinged only following aspiration or recent trauma. Certain areas of the body have a particular predilection for synovial hernia, notably the wrist.

The *differential diagnosis* is that of the tumor mass and is not unduly difficult. Synovial hernia may be confused with a dislocated bone such as the semilunar at the wrist. It must be distinguished from a neoplasm. Its general location, the lack of local symptoms, the consistency—all are definite diagnostic leads. The mass will ordinarily be translucent to transillumination but this may on occasion be extremely difficult to demonstrate by this procedure owing to the unfavorable location. Pain is not a notable factor. The complaint usually is that of a sprain of an adjacent joint. There may be pain and aching on overuse. Frequently extremes of motion may cause considerable discomfort particularly if the protrusion is recent and rather tight.

Treatment of a synovial hernia is essentially surgical. Although these masses do tend to come and go and so may respond to periods of splinting and protection or snug wrapping, these measures do not usually solve the problem. They merely postpone it. I have, however, known of many cases in which the ganglion has spontaneously regressed and to my knowledge never recurred. When it is symptomatic enough that it is interfering with athletic activity it should be removed. In surgical excision great care must be taken to remove the whole mass. The defect in the capsule or sheath must be repaired since recurrence is very likely after incomplete removal. The prevalent habit of making a ½ inch incision and popping the mass out like a cyst is really no more effective than the time-honored method of beating it with the edge of a book and is doomed to failure. I well recall a romance that was blighted when I temporarily cured a ganglion over the dorsum of the lady's foot by a sharp blow with the edge of a frying pan.

Aspiration followed by injection of corticoids has been recommended. In my experience this has been unsatisfactory. However, it may serve to postpone definitive treatment until a more suitable time. To the athlete such a time is at the termination of his season of activity. Under these circumstances the joint should be carefully protected against overstrain. There is no objection to adequate strapping and continued participation provided this can be made pain-free. Following successful surgical removal, rehabilitation should be as careful as following any joint surgery and protective strapping should be used throughout the remainder of the season since there is some weakness of the joint inherent in this condition.

FRACTURE

There is nothing particularly unique in the *treatment* of fractures of the athlete. The general principles previously mentioned must be constantly born in mind, for while one should always attempt to get the best result in the quickest time with a minimum of interference of activity, this becomes particularly pertinent in the athlete. By and large, a definite fracture is usually well and adequately treated, since the injury is severe enough to make the diagnosis obvious. The use of x-ray examination is so universal now that the ordinary fracture is recognized early.

Certain exceptions to the above statement will be discussed in detail under proper headings. I would like to mention specifically fracture of the navicular at the wrist, "march" fracture of the metatarsals (Fig. 30), and fatigue fracture of the fibula (Fig. 23). These conditions are all too frequently overlooked because the

Figure 30. Typical "march" fracture in a young athlete. Notice complete absence of any fracture line as such. Uneventful healing.

immediate symptoms may be rather chronic in nature. Invaluable time is lost while the crippled athlete believes he has a strain or a sprain. The ideal time for treatment has frequently passed when the condition is finally rcognized.

Another type of fracture that may easily be overlooked is the avulsion fracture. The athlete is subject to sudden spurts of violent activity which may forcibly avulse a fragment of bone either at a tendon or a muscle attachment (Fig. 31). The condition is primarily one of muscle or tendon injury, the bone fragment being incidental. Its treatment should be that of the primary condition. Neglect or oversight may cause long periods of chronic disability. This is particularly true since the fracture is very prone to calcification or ossification of the accompanying hematoma.

The optimal treatment of fractures depends upon prompt and definitive diagnosis. Since these patients are in good health and in splendid physical condition one may almost always use the best method of treatment without that compromise necessitated by the patient's poor condition which is so often necessary in regular practice. Hence, we are more prone to carry out open reduction of the various fractures where indicated, not only because the general condition of the patient will permit it but because by firm internal fixation we are ofttimes able to start rehabilitation at once. We may even be able to avoid entirely external fixation involving the adjacent joints.

Rehabilitation. The great importance of maintaining the athlete in good physical condition, if he intends to resume his athletic activity in the near future, must be borne in mind. If we presume in the case of a certain fracture that the patient will be able to resume athletic activity in four weeks, he will be wholly unable to do this if he has not in the meantime continued his rigorous training. For example, a minimal fracture of a malleolus without displacement may require fixation in a cast for four weeks. Throughout this period of time the patient should be actively exercising his opposite extremity and his upper extremities. He should keep up exercises vigorous enough to maintain his endurance to some extent and keep on his training diet in order to avoid gaining weight. It is important also that the muscles of the involved extremity should be actively exercised. In this instance the boot cast itself can serve as a weight to permit exercise of the quadriceps, hamstrings, hip, abdomen and back. It is not so commonly recognized that by isotonic contractions of the muscles within the cast he may also keep the muscles of the lower leg and foot in tone.

Again depending upon the location of the fracture, it may be possible to apply protective splints or a protective dressing in such a way that he can resume competition. With judicious application of proper equipment participation, even in football, may be permitted.

It can be seen that the whole success of such a program depends upon prompt, definitive diagnosis so that healing may progress rapidly and efficiently. Adequate protection must be maintained to minimize irritation at the fracture line which may result in overcalcification or delayed union. A prompt return to athletic competition will be hastened by early diagnosis, accurate repositioning, firm fixation, either internal or external, continuing rehabilitation and protective dressing. The doctor who is capable of treating fractures should have sufficient ingenuity to devise a specific program for each definite condition.

This book will make no attempt to cover the whole field of fractures but some that are more common to athletes will be discussed in considerable detail. An effort will be made to point out methods of treatment which have stood the test of time in regard to acceleration of physical activity following particular fractures.

Figure 31.   Fresh injury of the neck showing avulsion fracture of the tip of the seventh cervical spinous process.

OSTEOCHONDRITIS DISSECANS (OSTEOCHONDRAL FRACTURE)

Osteochondritis dissecans is a joint affection occurring most frequently in the knee. There is considerable disagreement concerning the exact etiology, some doctors claiming that the condition results from spontaneous ischemic necrosis due to faulty circulation in the epiphyseal vessels while others believe that it is due to trauma, with a fissure type fracture in the subchondral bone. As in so many conditions in which there is disagreement about the exact cause, it is probable that in certain instances more than one factor may be present. Thus, it may be that repeated trauma to the area will cause circulatory interference with infarction. In this case trauma precedes the ischemic necrosis. Or it may be that the necrosis develops spontaneously and the actual dislodging of the fragment may be due to trauma superimposed on a pathological area.

In any event the pathology consists of the separation of a fragment of subchondral bone from the underlying matrix. This line of separation is filled with granulation tissue. The separated bone necroses because of poor circulation and in effect becomes a sequestrum. Since the articular cartilage over this fragment is nourished primarily by the synovial fluid, the cartilage does not at this stage necrose but remains intact. In fact, the whole cycle of separation, necrosis and regeneration may occur without any defect in the articular cartilage and may terminate in spontaneous healing of the condition. On the other hand, if enough of the fragment is absorbed to permit it to depress into the crater in the epiphyseal bone, fissuring of the cartilage and ultimate separation may occur. It may be that in some cases trauma is the factor that ultimately breaks the fragment loose. So in some

Figure 32.   Osteochondritis dissecans. A, Note the fragment on the medial femoral condyle, not detached. B, Five months later the mass is resolving with no treatment.

Figure 33.   Osteochondritis dissecans with free fragment. On removal, this fragment was found to be attached to a portion of the posterior cruciate ligament.

cases the fragment may never be separate and spontaneous recovery ensues. In other cases the fragment may become entirely free in the joint and act as a foreign body. The age incidence coincides with the age of active athletics, namely, adolescence and early adulthood. Thus, this condition is frequently seen in athletes. There is no preventive measure of any value.

The condition may be completely asymptomatic and be discovered only by incidental x-rays. More commonly there will be discomfort in the joint, sometimes accompanied by effusion with symptoms of internal derangement. This may go on until there is actually locking of the joint if the fragment becomes free or if a flap of cartilage turns up and interposes between the articular surfaces. Many patients will present themselves with the complaint of chronic nonspecific joint pain with very few localizing symptoms.

The *management* varies from no treatment to operative excision of the fragment and will be discussed in detail under the various joint categories. In general it may be said that, in the very young, treatment should be conservative since many cases will show spontaneous regression (Fig. 32) if the part is protected from weight bearing. In a non-weight-bearing joint, surgery is less frequently required than in a weight-bearing joint. If the fragment completely separates (Fig. 33) or forms a flap interfering with motion of a joint, surgical treatment is mandatory with removal of the fragment and trimming off of the cartilaginous margins of the crater. Further measures will depend upon the extent and location of the lesion since function, particularly weight bearing, may need to be restricted. Drilling of the sclerotic crater may help reconstitution of the cartilage.

MUSCLE CRAMPING

Muscle spasm or cramping is a very frequent complaint in the athlete. I am sure that there are many causes for this condition. I am equally sure that there are many things which are called muscle spasm or cramping which are due to some other pathologic state. Actually, the etiology and the pathology seem to be inextricably confused. Many common injuries will cause spasm of the muscle. Some of the more common are a blow to the muscle causing slight infiltration of blood, and overstretch of the muscle causing rupture of some of the fibers and strain by overcontraction of the muscle against resistance. Each of these causes the same type of injury to the muscle unit.

Frequently the muscle cramp or spasm appears to be an entity in itself. One of the most common and dramatic examples is the severe cramping that occurs in the calf of the apparently normal athlete. While going at full speed he suddenly gets a violent contraction of the calf which pulls the foot down into equinus and causes severe cramping pain. Indeed, this may come on when actual exertion is at a minimum, at least in respect to any overuse or overstretching. There are several causes of this condition, some remediable and some not. There appears to be no doubt that reduction of the quantity of salt by excessive perspiration will cause a condition in which the muscles of the body are quite subject to cramping. Changes in temperature, sudden chilling or even sudden overheating may also be responsible. Dietary considerations are sometimes important. Many of these factors can be obviated in an adequate training program. Such metabolic causes will require more emphasis on prevention than on cure.

In another category are those cases in which there is definite local impairment of circulation to the part, as when the cuff of the pants is too tight around the calf or the calf muscle has been strapped circumferentially in such a way as to interfere with its blood supply. There is no actual pathologic change in the muscle other than rapid build-up of muscle waste products and diminution of oxygen supply. Overfatigue may cause cramping for much the same reasons that constriction does.

Ruling out all these potential causes for cramping, there still remains a group of cases in which there is no specifically recognizable cause for the condition. In most instances the player has had no preliminary symptoms, the muscle jumps into intractable spasm and the player is rendered helpless both by the pain and by the restriction of motion. Examination will elicit nothing other than the contracted muscle. The muscle is not particularly tender. There is no swelling or edema. One should suspect muscle spasm when sudden severe pain occurs in any muscular area of the body. This is particularly prevalent in the neck, in the back, in the hamstrings and calf. The fact that the cramping is common in weight-bearing portions of the anatomy but relatively infrequent in the upper extremities may be of some significance.

Treatment is usually simple and in the majority of instances can be administered by the player himself. His immediate instinct is to apply local pressure to the spastic muscle and to try to force it through a normal range of motion. The player will sit on the ground and grab his calf firmly with one hand while he dorsiflexes his foot with the other—an expedient that is often amazingly effective. The cramp may be released by simple contraction of the opposing muscle so that if there is a cramp in one flank, stretching the muscle by leaning to the opposite side will frequently relieve the tension.

If the player needs help in relaxing his spasm, the same principles apply. Steady, even, firm but atraumatic local pressure will often give dramatic relief. So also will simple stretching of the muscle. The combination of the two appears to be even more effective. One should constantly bear in mind that he is trying to restore only a normal range of motion; he must not overstretch the muscle. In the contracted hamstring, the knee should be extended but forceful straight leg raising should not be carried out. If the calf is involved, the foot should be pushed up to 90 degrees but not forced into extreme dorsal flexion. For this reason these manipulations should be carefully controlled. Passive manipulation should be applied steadily and smoothly with no jerk or swing. To apply massive force with leverage against a muscle in spasm may result in rupture of the muscle fibers or even avulsion of the tendon in which case a relatively simple condition is replaced by one much more serious. I know of no place in the treatment of any acute injury where this type of excessive manipulative force is desirable. It certainly is not desirable in the treatment of muscle spasm.

The same thing can be said about massage. Massage directed toward restoring circulation to the muscle is quite acceptable whereas deep kneading or pounding or pummeling of a muscle that is already insufficiently supplied with metabolites can result only in harm. As the muscle spasm relaxes, relatively gentle massage toward the direction of the venous flow may be useful. The muscle may be tapped gently from side to side by the two hands with a rolling manipulation of the muscle between the two palms. Usually this cramp is relatively short-lived and the player may continue to compete although the condition is quite prone to recur within the immediate future. If the cramping is more persistent, it will require further treatment. This consists of rest of the part and application of local heat. This can be done by whirlpool baths, warm packs, infrared or diathermy or in fact any heat modality. Inductive heat appears to be more effective than radiant heat. Massage is valuable in restoring circulation to the muscle.

A patient who has had persistent muscle spasm may have residual soreness and aching in the muscle and during this period he should avoid forceful activity. A carefully planned regimen of physical therapy with gradually increasing resistive exercises within his tolerance and short of pain-producing stimuli should be carried out. It may well be that these persistent symptoms following cramp are actually due to ruptured muscle fibers with edema and blood infiltration and should be treated as such. The duration of treatment will depend upon the symptoms. We cannot agree that the best treatment for torn muscle fibers with hematoma into the muscles is immediate active use in spite of pain and muscle spasm.

PHLEBITIS

Phlebitis is not a common condition in the athlete, at least as a definite clinical entity. There is, of course, a certain amount of phlebitis accompanying contusions, sprains or strains but this is a secondary local reaction and is quite amenable to the measures taken for relief of the specific injury. In the treatment of any local inflammatory condition one should be on the alert to detect signs of phlebitis. This is particularly pertinent in the lower extremities where the saphenous vein is quite susceptible to inflammation. The symptoms of developing phlebitis may be lost in the symptoms of the original lesion. If the phlebitis is local and of little consequence, rest of the part and support by a snugly fitting elastic bandage may suffice.

If it is more generalized and there is considerable febrile reaction, anticoagulant therapy should be instituted. This will require hospitalization. The main factor here is to be on the alert for developing phlebitis so that it can be treated before it becomes a problem.

LYMPHADENITIS AND LYMPHANGITIS

Lymphadenitis and lymphangitis frequently accompany infection and are particularly prevalent following abrasions of the hand and infection around the feet such as ingrown toenail or severe athlete's foot. The involvement of the lymph system is due to the drainage from the infection. The symptoms are increasing pain in the local lesion followed by appearance of red streaks extending toward the neighboring lymph glands (lymphangitis). If one is familiar with the distribution of the lymph system he will not expect to find glands at the back of the knee involved in an infection in an area of the foot that drains directly to the groin. These red streaks will have local heat and tenderness but are not particularly painful. Soreness will develop in the regional lymph glands which may become swollen and inflamed (lymphadenitis). Only occasionally will they go on to suppuration.

Treatment. The development of lymphadenitis demands more adequate treatment to the local lesion such as adequate drainage of the infection, elevation of the part and local heat. Antibiotics should be used and one of the broad-spectrum type will usually be adequate. If it is possible to get a culture and determine which antibiotic is most effective, this should be done. This will require 24 to 48 hours and the antibiotic therapy should not be postponed while awaiting a report from the laboratory. If the local lesion is handled well, the secondary involvement of the lymph system will usually promptly subside. Needless to say, active athletics should not be permitted during the period of inflammation, not only to protect the affected player but also to protect his fellows from contamination. This player should not participate in athletics until the condition has entirely subsided and there is no longer inflammation in the glands.

NERVE INJURY

Contusion

Fortunately, the nervous system is not too commonly involved in injuries to the athlete since the player is usually in excellent condition with strong muscles to protect the nerve from overstress. In only a few areas of the body are the nerves particularly exposed to trauma and these will be considered in the discussion of specific areas. The peripheral nerves most frequently involved are the ulnar nerve at the elbow, the peroneal nerve behind the fibular head, the radial nerve in the midarm and the axillary nerve at the shoulder. The injury is usually from a direct blow on the nerve causing a contusion. There is an immediate "shocking" sensation followed by numbness and pain. The condition may be entirely transient. The player may "shake it off" in a few minutes and be none the worse for the experience. If the injury is more severe there will be persistent aching pain along the distribution of the nerve, the result of swelling and edema and congestion within the nerve and nerve sheath. The treatment of this degree of contusion should depend upon the area involved and the severity of the symptoms. In general, as long as the symptoms are relatively acute, the part should be protected against overuse. By all means the nerve should be protected against further contusion.

In the isolated case there may be paralysis of the muscles supplied by the nerve. This may be immediate, due to direct damage to the nerve fibers. In this instance, one should seriously consider whether the nerve may actually have been crushed by the blow. Usually, the early symptoms of numbness, aching and pain will be followed by disability of the muscle involved which may progress to complete loss of function. If the peroneal is involved, there will be a foot drop. If it is the ulnar nerve, there will be weakness and loss of function of the intrinsic muscles of the hand. There may be hypesthesia or sensory loss throughout the sensory distribution of these mixed nerves. As long as this weakness or paralysis continues, the muscle should be supported by cast or brace. Physical therapy should be instituted to encourage return of function in the muscles. Recovery is almost always complete and usually is fairly rapid. The need for further protection after recovery from the paralysis will depend upon the condition of the muscle. The muscle should be protected as long as it is weak. Its strength should be improved by appropriate physical therapy.

Stress

Another type of injury to the nervous system is caused by overstretch of the nerve, for example, overstretching of the peroneal nerve after rupture of the lateral collateral ligaments of the knee. A recent case was seen eight months following an injury in which the patient "sprained" the lateral ligament of the knee. Examination revealed peroneal paralysis with positive Tinel sign just above the head of the fibula. There was instability of the lateral collateral ligament. Exploration revealed a badly scarred peroneal nerve, tightly bound down with scar from the torn lateral collateral ligament. The nerve was carefully dissected out with separation of the fibers entirely across the 1½ inch scarred-in area. The lateral collateral ligament was advanced on its femoral attachment. The patient was in splints for eight weeks and wore a drop-foot brace most of the time for one year. At the end of this period he had active but not complete dorsiflexion with complete recovery from his sensory paralysis except for a little hypesthesia over the top of the foot. His knee was stable. It required three months before he got any return and over a year before it was complete. He is now a football scholarship college player.

In such a case the severity of the ligament injury may screen the nerve condition so that it is not recognized until later. The symptoms will vary with the severity of the injury. If there is a complete avulsion of the nerve, there will be immediate and complete loss of function whereas if the nerve is stretched but not torn there will be hemorrhage and shock to the fibers but function will be more slowly and less completely lost. Whenever there has been complete loss of function of a nerve, one must decide whether or not surgical exploration is justified. The examining physician is responsible for the early detection of these injuries. Any statement by the patient about numbness, weakness or loss of motion should be carefully investigated. It is very important to determine the function of the nerve before definitive treatment is undertaken. A classical example is the dislocated elbow. If one discovers some hours, days or even weeks later that there is paralysis of the median nerve, it may be impossible for him to determine definitely whether this injury was athletic or iatrogenic. It is of particular importance to outline carefully any sensory loss since its diminution or increase in such an area may well be the determining factor in selecting the proper treatment.

Treatment. From the surgical standpoint, one should be quite conservative in treatment of an injury to the nerve. In a great majority of these cases gradual recovery will take place as the weeks go by. Such recovery will ordinarily be well advanced at the end of three months if it is likely to be complete. On the other hand, late surgical suture of the nerve may be quite successful and one can afford to delay exploration for a reasonable period of time (three or four months). Most surgeons would agree that if nerve repair is to be done, it should be done within the first six months if at all possible. I should like to repeat that a well regulated, faithfully adhered-to physical therapy program is of extreme importance. This serves to prevent deformity by contracture of the muscles during the period of complete paralysis and serves to build up the strength of the muscles as the nerve function returns.

The subject of nerve involvement in conditions of the neck and spine includes some rather special problems and will be discussed in detail under these headings.

PART III

The Treatment of Injuries in Specific Areas

CHAPTER

5

Craniocerebral
Injuries in Athletics

By HARRY WILKINS, M.D.

INTRODUCTION

INJURIES TO THE HEAD in athletic events, like injuries to other portions of the body, take on special interest with today's emphasis on youth fitness and on outdoor living. This is also true of spectator events related to various organized and unorganized competitive activities in the athletic field. Physicians must accept the responsibility of handling, at least to some degree, injuries to the head which occur in their vicinity. One might prefer that specialists in the various fields involved with the care of injured persons handle these problems; nevertheless, each individual physician has an obligation to keep abreast of up-to-date methods not only in prevention of death but also in prevention of irreparable damage to the brain caused by even a brief delay in the application of proper therapeutic measures. An understanding of the principles involved in handling the problem of head injury may prevent loss of life but more often is effective in minimizing tissue damage within the cranial cavity.

A variable degree of danger is to be found in most athletic events. In some, such as football, direct body contact or the blow from falling and striking the ground may constitute the chief danger. In baseball, to be struck by a pitched ball or by a bat produces forces that may produce damage of a particular type such as a comminuted, depressed fracture. The javelin and discus exposes the participant to possible penetrating wounds of the skull. Boxing is an especially dangerous sport and from time to time a fatal intracranial hemorrhage is reported even in professional bouts. Recently a nationally known baseball player was reported to have been injured while playing golf. He was struck on the forehead by a golf ball and dropped to the ground where he lay perfectly still. He was thought by his companions to have been killed. Fortunately, he responded promptly and his recovery was complete. Injuries from a heavier object such as the shot may either seriously damage the skull or, without skull fracture, produce serious damage to the brain of the so-called closed injury type. This year in our own practice three instances of head injury in youngsters of grade school level have been treated, two in which the injury was inflicted by a thrown ball and one in which the blow was from a bat. In basketball, tennis and ice skating the danger arises from falling. The rapidly moving head comes to an abrupt stop against the playing surface, causing either fracture of the skull or damage by contusion or hemorrhage without fracture. These may be combined to produce an even more complex problem.

Prevention of injuries to the head is a potent factor in athletics. This is accomplished best by a combination of effort on the part of the director or coach, the trainers and with the advice of the physician and cooperation of the parents. This spring a statewide approach was made along these lines when the Department of Postgraduate Training at the Oklahoma Medical Center arranged for a day-long session for coaches, trainers and physicians at which time outstanding men in various fields participated in a joint program. A panel made up of specialists was present to comment on the respective responsibilities of each in lessening the morbidity and fatality among injured athletes.

The growing importance of this subject in medical postgraduate education is further manifest by the presentation made by Dr. Richard C. Schneider,[1] University of Michigan neurosugeon, at the Wisconsin State Medical Society Meeting for 1961, held in Milwaukee. He presented statistics relating to the death of 14 players from injury to the brain or spinal cord occurring in 1959 as recorded by the Serious Injuries and Fatalities Committee of the American Football Coaches Association. Actually there were 208 fatalities from either head or cervical cord injury reported to this group in the period from 1947 through 1959. Additional efforts by physicians to further the cause of prevention and care of the injured athlete were made this spring when a panel spoke before the Committee on Trauma of the American College of Surgeons in May, 1961. Another meeting of this type was held in St. Louis late in August, 1961.

As physicians we should be alert and willing to lend a hand in this cause, by proper understanding of the principles involved and by taking prompt action in applying proper measures when confronted with a person injured in an athletic event. It is to be considered an emergency and must be treated as such. The aid of the specialist may be necessary in some instances but more often the problem can be handled by practitioners in the locality in which the injury occurs. The physician should, therefore, place himself in the position of the spectator, who in attending an athletic event, is suddenly called upon to care for a person suffering obvious damage to the head or who, because of loss of consciousness, raises the question, "Is this the result of craniocerebral injury?" A quick evaluation of the individual's general state may give the proper answer, but more often the observation of symptoms as they develop over a period of time, coupled with signs that may be present if one will take the trouble to look for them, is necessary. A review of the over-all problem of diagnosis is, therefore, being presented, and an effort will be made to correlate the symptoms, signs and treatment.

In head injuries the damage to the brain itself is of far more importance than damage to the cranium; in fact, in athletic events many of the serious injuries occur without fracture of the skull. The importance of fundamental factors involved warrant discussions of anatomy, physiology and pathology as they relate to specific injuries and to the problem as a whole.

PREVENTION

Experience is the best preventive. This is immediately evident when one considers the infrequency of serious injury in the professional football league or professional major baseball leagues. The beginner must be taught how to avoid injury by the coach or director of the particular athletic event which he is sponsoring. Revision of equipment has played a definite role in reducing the number of serious injuries to the head but even the present day equipment can be improved upon if suggestions made by Schneider[1] are carried out. In certain activities, such as the trampoline, participants should be denied the use of such equipment until they have been properly instructed in the safety measures that are necessary. Last but not least is the insistence on withdrawal from competition of any person who is known to be ill or who has not had proper sleep. Potent drugs contribute to injury by dulling the judgment of the player in protecting himself as well as other participants. Their use must be condemned.

ANATOMICAL CONSIDERATIONS

The mobility of the head and its relationship to the remainder of the body by virtue of the cervical portion of the vertebral column contribute to its vulnerability to injury. The scalp is a sensitive, protective coating for the skull and in severe skull injuries may play a major role in avoiding damage from infection as well as in protecting the brain from loss of substance in open comminuted fractures. The direction from which the blood supply is furnished, coupled with extensive collateral arterial supply, contributes to better healing of wounds by primary intent. Fractures of the skull, when simple linear lines are noted in the x-ray, may take on significance only when the fractures are seen to cross grooves or canals of important blood channels, especially those of the middle meningeal arteries. Fracture lines that enter one of the paranasal sinuses or cross the petrous portion of the temporal bone are of special importance when accompanied by the loss of cerebrospinal fluid from the nose or ear.

The division of the cranial cavity by certain prominent structures is an important factor in the mechanical effects of the injury. Each structure may contribute to subsequent complications as the brain shifts by compression, by massive clot or from cerebral swelling. Botterell[2] has called attention to damage to the tip of temporal lobes when the brain is forced forward, over and against the temporosphenoidal ridge. The brain stem and cerebellar hemispheres may be damaged by contact with the clivus and the petrous ridges. The slant of these structures lessens the direct contusing effect. The intact tentorium aids in preventing the movement that is damaging to the relationship of the frontotemporal structure to the temporo-sphenoidal ridge. The falx and tentorium on the one hand serve to limit the motion that places stress on traversing veins but may themselves prove to be a hazard when cerebral swelling or shift of structures from massive clot produces herniation beneath the falx and through the tentorial incisura. With herniation, important structures may be compromised by direct compression. Impaired circulation must be considered a greater hazard especially to the venous drainage from the midbrain and the basal ganglia. The occlusion or severe compromise of arterial circulation is especially dangerous. The posterior cerebral arteries pass backward and emerge from below the tentorium to reach the inferior surface of the temporo-occipital area. In doing so they are in contact with the thin margin of the tentorium and it is at this point that occlusion may occur to produce infarction of the inferior portion of the occipital lobe. The swelling associated with this process adds to local tissue destruction by hypoxia, if not relieved promptly.

The region of the foramen magnum is worthy of comment. If one looks from the foramen down into the upper cervical spinal canal he sees a gradually diminishing opening, like a funnel, lined with dura. This may produce tissue compression as the swollen herniating cerebellar tonsils tend to sink lower into the spinal canal. The interference with venous drainage as well as local compression affects the medulla and important cell clusters constituting the vital centers. This process, occurring from a space-occupying lesion such as a massive clot or as a result of massive brain swelling, may reach such a degree as to produce failure of vital functions, particularly of respiration. It may develop gradually and therefore give some warning sign by slowing the respiration or producing some irregularity. A similar sudden increase in medullary compression may occur with the rise of venous back pressure associated with vomiting or with straining in response to an enema. A similar phenomenon may occur if by spinal puncture one suddenly lowers the interspinal pressure below the level of the foramen. The rapid fall of pressure invites rapid progression of the pressure cone phenomenon, with sudden respiratory failure occurring either during the spinal puncture or within a period of hours.

I recall two instances in our own service where doctors not familiar with this fact had in the emergency room performed spinal puncture as a measure of evaluation of head injury. In one instance death occurred with the needle still in place. More often the process will occur a few hours after spinal puncture and, because of the delayed reaction, the operator may not realize that he has contributed to the fatality. The second case in this unpleasant experience occurred within a week of the first and, fortunately, the patient survived since there was sufficient warning to enable us to perform ventricular puncture for relief and proceed with the indicated definitive surgery at midnight. Needless to say, this experience occurring several years ago has been passed along from house officer group to house officer group and we have not had any repetitions.

CEREBRAL PHYSIOLOGY AND ITS ALTERATION BY INJURY

In the normal human being the functioning of the brain is rarely given much thought by physicians. It is necessary, however, to understand something of the normal physiological processes if we are to carry out proper evaluation of problems and apply treatment designed to give the best results. To gain this end, a simplified concept of processes in a single brain cell may serve to exemplify these points.

To function normally, a cell must have an adequate supply of oxygen. It must be sustained by proper nutrition. It must not be interfered with by compression from decreased room or from massive swelling within the brain. An inadequate supply of oxygen, whether due to faulty aeration of the blood in the lung or to decreased blood flow in shock, may produce irreparable damage. Impaired venous outflow fails to clear the products of cell metabolism. In a more general sense, this brings about intracellular, as well as intercellular, collection of fluid resulting in brain swelling and so disturbs the function of tissues involved.[3]

These facts demonstrate the absolute need for maintenance of a proper airway in the unconscious patient. Immediate clearing of the air pathways by one means or another, if they are obstructed, is imperative. If arrest of respiration prevails, artificial respiration is required. Complete evaluation of the patient's condition must await the establishment of a state of good aeration of the blood.

A proper arterial supply depends upon maintaining an adequate blood pressure. If there is massive loss of blood, prompt replacement of volume is needed. Excessive blood loss is infrequent and, fortunately, shock is not likely to occur with head injury. It is more apt to occur in the presence of complicating injuries to other portions of the body. Nevertheless, in contact activity the possibility of complicating injuries such as rupture of an abdominal viscus or fracture of a long bone must be kept in mind.

Compression from massive intracranial hemorrhage, whether intracerebral or subdural, is prone to make itself known by phenomena other than alterations in pulse rate, blood pressure changes and respiratory difficulties. These phenomena may occur in part after the passage of considerable time if the compressing lesion is not recognized and cared for through definitive surgical operative procedure.

Intracerebral clots, although space-occupying, are prone to give rise to focal phenomena in the unconscious patient as well as the patient who retains consciousness. These will be indicated by signs of impaired cerebral function, depending upon the location of the intracerebral hemorrhage. I am speaking here of massive subcortical clots which may occur in patients with or without fracture and which may be accompanied by acute subdural hematoma or in some instances even without evidence of subdural collection of blood.

Diffuse hemorrhage occurring in the midbrain and pons occasionally accompanies head injury. This generally is in patients with severe brain damage. It is especially prone to occur in the presence of unattended massive intracranial clots even though it may occur in epidural or subdural spaces.

There seems little doubt that compression of venous outflow from this area has a major role in producing diffuse small hemorrhages. From the physiological standpoint, the resulting phenomenon of profound loss of consciousness is outstanding. This may occur in cases of severe, diffuse contusion of the brain and be present from the outset. Marked loss of consciousness without other signs of intracranial hypertension should direct one's attention toward this area. There are apt to be additional physiological changes, the outstanding one being altered thermic control. Another important phenomenon is the increased oxygen requirement in the presence of hyperthermia, which is said to average approximately 7 per cent for each degree of temperature. One can readily comprehend how permanent damage may occur if the temperature ranges from 104° to 108°. Although patients have been known to survive temperatures of 108° for a short period of time if the underlying cause of disturbed physiology is corrected, rather serious residual changes are usually noted. These patients present the clinical picture of the postencephalitic syndrome which gradually improves, but never completely recovers.

A clinical phenomenon that may in time respond to proper treatment is *decerebrate rigidity*. As a rule the condition is bilateral but there may be some variations, with rigidity being more prominent and persistent on one side than the other. If not present from the outset, decerebrate rigidity points to the possibility of an otherwise unrecognized epidural hemorrhage or massive acute subdural hematoma. When present early in the post-traumatic period, it may be corrected by spinal fluid removal via spinal puncture. A favorable response is an encouraging finding and points to possible relief by emergency enlargement of the tentorial incisure by incising the tentorium to allow for normal escape of cerebrospinal fluid from the posterior fossa on its course to the supratentorial absorptive mechanism.

Disturbances in normal physiological responses of the *pupil* are highly important among the clinical signs of acute craniocerebral injury. It has long been recognized that the pupil is prone to be enlarged on the ipsilateral side of the massive intracranial clot, particularly in the epidural hemorrhage or an acute subdural hematoma. The enlargement may persist in chronic subdural hematoma but, fortunately, not so frequently. In general, dilatation of the pupil with contralateral motor pathway involvement will give a clue as to the presence or lateralization of a clot. Occasionally homolateral motor pathway signs may be found.[4]

The picture of impaired function due to space-occupying lesions such as massive clots, because of their nature, has a time element. Even rapid compression of the brain by *epidural hemorrhage* or arterial hemorrhage from any source will allow some time for evaluation if one is mindful of the possibility of its occurrence and diligently looks for altered signs of normal physiology to warn of its presence. The classical example is the epidural bleeding from rupture of the middle meningeal artery. This is particularly prone to occur in the case of the linear skull fracture that traverses the arterial groove in the floor of the middle fossa or more frequently at the lateral portion of the temporosphenoidal ridge where the vessel may pass through a deep channel or through a tunnel created by a bridged channel. The patient is apt to have a temporary loss of consciousness resulting from the commotion occurring at the moment of impact but from which rapid recovery is noted. He may appear quite all right within moments of the time of injury and continue so for some hours. With the progression of hemorrhage encroaching on the cranial cavity, altered consciousness is noted first in drowsiness. Along with this is an alteration in cardiac rate with the pulse slowing from the rapid rate of the athlete during participation in an event downward to a normal level and beyond this to actual *bradycardia*. As the process progresses, alteration in blood pressure assumes a typical pattern with systolic pressure rising more rapidly than the diastolic and in time creating a pulse pressure that steadily increases.

It has long been known to those interested in this problem that once the pulse pressure increases and the pulse rate decreases until it is below the level of pulse pressure, one has had warning that a phase of head injury has been reached in which time is of the essence. Apart from open comminuted fractures of the skull, this situation constitutes the only real indication for emergency surgical intervention in head injuries. By the time this change in pulse rate and pulse pressure has reached this stage, respiratory difficulties are prone to occur. First, there will be a slowing, then an irregularity and finally cessation of respiration. I have known of an instance in which a general surgeon, mindful of his responsibilities and realizing the lack of time to obtain help from a specialist or time to transport the patient to a neurosurgical center, prepared for emergency craniotomy believing that he was dealing with an epidural hemorrhage. As the patient was being taken to the operating room, respiration ceased and she was given artificial respiration. The epidural clot was rapidly exposed by subtemporal decompression and the patient's respiratory rate was restored and shortly became normal. After evacuation of the clot and control of bleeding from the middle meningeal artery, the patient was responding in a perfectly normal, conscious manner in a matter of a few hours and progressed on to complete recovery. I have often referred to this surgeon's experience in pointing out the need for the individual physician to suspect this type of lesion, watch carefully for signs of its development and then have the courage to act. The opportunity will not arise often but each head injury patient must be suspected of having this type of lesion until sufficient time for observation of progressive symptoms of intracranial hemorrhage proves the contrary.

Hemorrhage from rupture of an intracranial aneurysm will rarely coincide with acute trauma in athletic events. Rupture of intracranial aneurysm may, however, take place at any time and might, therefore, be considered when dealing with trauma in athletic events. One is less apt to see progression of the compression syndrome in this type of lesion and confuse the picture with epidural hemorrhage since bleeding is apt to come promptly under control through natural processes. As time progresses following such bleeding, meningeal signs will predominate in the majority of instances.

In the chronic hemorrhagic lesions, i.e., *subdural hematoma* and *intracerebral hematoma*, an understanding of the physical process involved is helpful to the clinician. The hemorrhage is usually venous in origin although lesser arteries may contribute to the intracerebral clots. Hemorrhage from rupture of an aneurysm coincidental to athletic activity may erode adjacent brain tissue to produce a space-occupying clot. In all of these lesions, hemorrhage is controlled by one or more natural factors. Why, then, should the symptoms develop days or weeks later? With time and the disintegration of the clot, a neomembrane is being formed. This being semipermeable, osmosis increases the volume of this mass, gradually producing effects that result in definite, or at times subtle, symptoms.[5] Another characteristic is that of variability of symptoms from hour to hour, advancing and receding out of keeping with pressure signs due to tumor. As mentioned previously, inequality of the pupil without other evidence of occulomotor nerve impairment is present in a high percentage of patients with hematoma. A word of caution is warranted. Examine the patient in a subdued light. On numerous occasions I have observed that a slight inequality is missed by using bright light, causing sufficient response to overcome the deficit and equalize the pupillary aperture.

DIAGNOSIS AND TREATMENT

An attempt will be made to correlate the symptoms, signs and treatment by presenting in sequence the steps to be taken in handling the injured athlete. In every instance of such injury, one must at once consider the possibility that the patient may have severe brain damage, although this is rare. On the other hand, the athlete may not have sustained severe damage at the moment of impact but is a potential candidate for fatal complications from infection as in the case of compound fracture or fracture into a sinus or compression from massive clot in rupture of a middle meningeal artery. When a player is down on the field, has fallen on the basketball court, has been struck by a baseball or a bat, the immediate responsibility rests with the coach, trainer and teammates. An efficient trainer or his assistant will have been observing the play on the field. Rawlinson[6] has stated that, by watching every play, he may get a clue as to the type of injury occurring. If a teammate sees that an athlete is down on the field, it is his duty to watch and assist with this player's care while awaiting the trainer who is allowed to go onto the field. In many instances a physician assigned to the team is on the sideline bench and may go on the field to see the patient.

EMERGENCY PROBLEMS

Brief Loss of Consciousness

If there is loss of consciousness, it should be noted whether the patient is breathing. If he is not, artificial respiration must be administered. This should not be delayed until the patient is moved from the field but should be started immediately to avoid even a brief time of complete anoxia. In the majority of instances, the injured person will resume breathing and can at this point be removed from the field by stretcher. The one whose loss of consciousness is not accompanied by respiratory failure may maintain good pulse and recover consciousness rather promptly. It is this type of injury that has carried the often used name "concussion." This does not indicate actual damage to the brain but simply indicates there has been a momentary lapse of consciousness without evidence of actual organic injury.

If there is a lapse of only a matter of seconds followed by a correct response to questions pertaining to current events and by ability to maintain his balance and to use all four extremities, the player may be allowed to resume play. In the event his teammates observe in him a lack of understanding of signals or failure in properly carrying them out, he must be replaced until observation over a period of several minutes reveals that he has recovered completely. The player who is unconscious for more than a minute or two should be withdrawn from the game. He may, if able, be allowed to remain on the bench but should be observed closely for defects in his behavior which may be interpreted as manifestations of progressive signs of actual brain injury. During this initial period immediately after the injury, damage to covering structures may be found even on cursory examination. If there is bleeding from a scalp wound or if blood is escaping from the ear, nose or throat, he should by all means be transported to the hospital for observation particularly if the loss of blood seems to come from the nasal passage or from the ears. Blood loss from laceration of the scalp requires immediate control by application of pressure to the major vessels supplying the area until a proper compression dressing can be applied.

Shock

During this period immediately after injury, evidence of marked pallor, rapid respiration and reduction of pulse pressure at the wrist all suggest the presence of shock. Shock is an infrequent phenomenon in the case of brain damage. It should call attention to the possibility of an associated injury, possibly an obvious one such as fracture of a long bone. In the absence of obvious signs of injury that would tend to produce shock, the possibility of associated damage to the abdominal viscera must take precedence over the injury to the head. In this unconscious patient, care must be exercised to maintain an open airway and to remove secretions and blood from the nasopharynx. The patient should be placed with the head lower than the remainder of the body with the legs elevated moderately. He should be turned into a lateral position with the mouth and nasopharynx dependent. In this way secretions will not be aspirated to add further insult by obstructing the airway. The patient in shock is truly an emergency problem. Considering whether or not the brain has been damaged or whether the patient is simply unconscious from the decreased blood supply requires time and close observation. The maintenance of a clear airway and the measures taken to sustain the circulation do more toward preventing additional brain damage than any other steps that can be taken. We have not had occasion to see an athlete with combined head injury and ruptured abdominal viscus but where such a problem exists, rapid preparation for exploration and management of the damaged viscus with replacement of blood loss is imperative in bringing the patient through this critical stage without irreparable and widespread brain cell damage. Once the cause of the shock has been eliminated and his condition has stabilized, then appropriate measures for handling the head injury problem may be carried out. These will be taken up later.

Fracture of the Skull

The family members, lay friends and the press will press one for a report as to the presence of fracture of the skull. Clarification of this point by obtaining stereoscopic lateral and postero-anterior views of the skull by x-ray is desirable even in the patient with visibly comminuted, depressed fracture or with open fracture. Still, it is a diagnostic step that can await application of the more urgent supportive measures and response to treatment from shock. This study should be done either by the use of a portable x-ray machine or of a unit in the modern surgical suite. As an aid to operative treatment, this is warranted in each surgically treated patient requiring emergency care.

Massive Intracranial Hemorrhage

Now to return to the athlete who following injury remains unconscious. He must be hospitalized and treated by supportive measures with close observation, repeated neurological examinations to evaluate the progress of improvement or to show increased signs of brain damage. Compression of the brain from massive intracranial hemorrhage will most often produce a rather classical group of symptoms. This is true whether there is a brief period of unconsciousness followed by lucid interval or a period in which consciousness is lost and the lucid interval does not appear. Observation for the degree of responsiveness is important. One person may be able, although slightly unconscious, to arouse in response to spoken commands. Painful stimuli may be applied to an extremity producing no response whatever in deep unconsciousness while in the lightly unconscious patient a withdrawal or purposeful movement of the extremity is elicited. If bilateral testing shows no response, then more painful stimuli may be applied. I find that as a rule pressure exerted upward just medial to the lobe of the ear causes considerable pain without damaging any structures. Bilateral application of such a pressure may not only cause a response either by groaning or general movement but may reveal a weakness of one side or the other so long as the stimulus is applied equally to the right and left. This is often a valuable clue toward recognition of the side on which the lesion may be developing.

The condition of the pupils is a helpful guide. Bilaterally constricted pupils suggest diffuse brain damage—particularly damage low in the brain stem. At higher levels the same may occur except for the region of the third nerve nucleus. It would appear that through impaired sympathetic function the pupillary constriction may take place. Bilateral dilatation of pupils with deepening coma is a serious sign and even gives warning of near terminal conditions so far as the functions within the brain stem are concerned. The unilateral dilatation of a pupil not only suggests that the patient is suffering from a massive clot but aids in lateralization since these lesions almost without exception occur on the homolateral side. When this phenomenon is accompanied by increased tone of muscles in the opposite arm and leg, the sign takes on greater significance.

A check of blood pressure, pulse and respiration at frequent intervals is the next most reliable course of observation. As intracranial pressure develops rapidly, an increase in blood pressure occurs with the systolic pressure rising more rapidly than the diastolic. With increase in the pulse pressure, the pulse rate will tend to decrease progressively and, on reaching a figure lower than the pulse pressure, will point to grave danger of subsequent respiratory involvement.

Bilateral Perforator and Burr Exploration.   More often there is at first a retardation of the respiration which may then become irregular and present the typical Cheyne-Stokes type of breathing. This is the patient who must be treated as an emergency and preparation for bilateral perforator and burr exploration is advisable. One may have sufficient lateralizing signs to warrant unilateral exploration but the possibility of hemorrhage occurring bilaterally warrants in most instances the additional brief time that it would require to prepare an exploratory burr opening on the opposite side. If the presence of EPIDURAL CLOT is verified with perforator and burr openings in the temporofrontal region, the incision may be extended to allow the added exposure of the subtemporal decompression. The fascia and muscle is split from the zygomatic arch upward to a point just short of the superior attachment of the temporal muscle. Following retraction of the muscle, the perforator and burr openings can be enlarged with the rongeur. A clot arising from the middle meningeal artery is found to be extradural and should be removed rapidly, using the suction and a special instrument such as bayonet with cups. This clot is likely to be of currant jelly consistency and tends to be somewhat adherent to the underlying dura, particularly along the vessel near the site of rupture. As a rule, the site of bleeding from the middle meningeal vessel will come into view as the clot is removed. One must keep in mind the probability that the artery may need to be exposed at the foramen spinosum where it can be occluded by electro-coagulation, by placing a ligature about the vessel and severing the artery superior to the ligature or by wedging a bit of bone wax and cotton into the foramen and pressing it firmly in place. I recall that Dr. Ernest Sachs[7] was prone to use a small peg of wood, orris root, shaped to plug the foramen. The wooden peg was forced into the foramen until it was flush with the surrounding floor of the middle fossa.

A massive intracranial clot which may resemble to some extent the above type of arterial hemorrhage is that of ACUTE SUBDURAL HEMORRHAGE. This occurs when there is actual contusion and laceration of the brain along with damage to a sizeable branch of the middle cerebral artery. The above described phenomenon of brain compression is apt to be less rapid and has in our experience more often been associated with a convulsive attack than has epidural hemorrhage. The surgical approach is the same as for the epidural hemorrhage but on finding the dura in place, somewhat distended and bluish in color, incision of the dura permits extrusion of the currant jelly clot. This is far more serious and difficult to handle because of the likelihood of more widespread passage of blood over the convexity and because of the associated damage to the brain tissue itself. The tip of the temporal lobe and undersurface of the frontal lobe at the temporosphenoidal wing is particularly vulnerable to laceration and contusion which produces acute subdural hematoma.[8] In addition to removal of the clot insofar as it is possible to reach the bounds of the clot over the convexity, one must also remove the destroyed brain tissue. The control of hemorrhage in this area is best accomplished by some means other than coagulation since occlusion of one or more of the major branches of the middle cerebral artery is certain to produce marked residual motor pathway deficit. Realizing that with puncture of an artery for angiograms, bleeding comparable to that of a large cerebral vessel may respond to light pressure applied at the site of the leak, we have tended to apply gelfoam or, better still, a small muscle stamp supported by gelfoam to control a sizeable arterial leak. I find this has worked quite satisfactorily and believe we have decreased some of the postoperative deficit that would come from attempts at control of hemorrhage by application of clips, by ligation of the vessel or by electrocoagulation.

As in the case of the epidural hemorrhage, there is no need to open the dura. In fact, venous ooze from the dural surface and from the bone may be controlled by distending the dura by gentle injection of saline into the underlying subarachnoid space in preparation for closure of the wound. The wound should be closed in layers, suturing the muscle separately. It should not be included in the fascial closure since this will prevent the muscle from moving during contraction. If hemostasis has been satisfactory, there is no need for drainage. In acute subdural hemorrhage, after the clot and the damaged brain tissue have been removed, the dura is left open to the full extent of the temporal bone defect. Having the advantage of subtemporal decompression outweighs any disadvantage in having the dura open.

In the patient who has sustained a serious, diffuse contusion of the brain with profound loss of consciousness, the tendency toward *hyperthermia* and *decerebrate rigidity* has always raised the question of massive intracranial clot. Occasionally, however, this condition of decerebrate rigidity may have developed early following the injury and would, therefore, not be in keeping with the compression of the brain that one observes in the presence of a massive clot. The bilaterality of symptoms also tends to point to some process of more diffuse type. In 1939, we observed a patient presenting this group of symptoms and signs. Feeling that she was rapidly approaching death, we resorted to a spinal puncture to check the possible response to lowering the intracranial pressure by removal of fluid. One would be in error to resort to spinal puncture in a suspected case of marked intracranial pressure from massive clot or from diffuse brain swelling. I would advise against its use in the presence of any symptoms of severe brain damage including those of decerebrate rigidity. Fortunately, in this particularly desperate situation the patient relaxed so remarkably from this procedure that some process other than diffuse damage throughout the midbrain was considered to be present.

One could postulate that with enlargement of the midbrain by swelling, the subarachnoid pathways at the tentorial level had been obstructed and that to enlarge the tentorial incisura by incising the tentorium might have some merit. A right subtemporal decompression will permit on ventricle puncture the observation that the lateral ventricle is not enlarged. Only a small amount of fluid escapes from the compressed ventricle. The temporal lobe can be retracted and on exposure of the superior surface of the tentorium and its incision lateral to the free margin, a surprising amount of cerebrospinal fluid will be allowed to escape through this incision from beneath the tentorium. On removal of the fluid, the brain should be quite relaxed and should pulsate freely. The incision may be carried from this point 2.5 cm. lateral to the free margin along a transverse course to the free margin about midway between the petrous ridge and the junction of the tentorium with the falx. One may encounter a traversing vein between the cerebellar hemisphere and the tentorium or a fairly broad venous channel within the tentorium itself. There is also a small venous channel near the free margin of the tentorium and with coagulation of those points and removal of the fluid as it wells into the wound, the available space will be surprising. An excess of cerebrospinal fluid in the subtentorial level may have escaped through the aqueduct and the fourth ventricle but have failed to reach the convexity, which is the point of absorption, owing to the constriction at the tentorial level. This patient will improve, the high temperature subside and the patient gradually recover except for some possible residual symptoms as in the syndrome of the postencephalitic patient.

Laceration of the Scalp

A laceration of the scalp or a compound, comminuted depressed fracture also warrants emergency surgery. All scalp lacerations should be treated as soon as the patient's condition has stabilized and evaluation has shown lack of symptoms or signs pointing toward massive intracranial clot. In laceration without fracture or in linear fracture without depression, the repair should be carried out employing proper surgical technique. This involves shaving the area widely about the site of the laceration and careful cleansing of the wound followed by excision of the wound margins to remove any debris which might be retained within the ragged margins. Undercutting the scalp to permit sufficient mobilization and the approximation of the galeal layer with interrupted nonabsorbable suture seems most acceptable. A separate layer of interrupted sutures is used to approximate the skin edges. This will allow removal of the stitches within 24 hours and prompt healing of the wound with minimal scarring. We have utilized a strip of sterile cellophane placed directly over the line of suture to prevent adherence of gauze to the wound margins. If there is loss of scalp due to the bruising type of blow, some revision of the wound may be required to permit primary closure. There is considerable latitude in this phase of repair of the scalp. In rare instances actual plastic maneuvers requiring transfer of scalp from an adjacent undamaged area and utilization of split thickness graft to cover the denuded area may be necessary.

Comminuted Depressed Fracture

In cases of comminuted, depressed bone, the approach is made just as above in handling the laceration of the scalp. The fragments of bone are gently removed and preserved in a saline bath to be used in closing the defect in the skull. When the fragments have been removed, evaluation of the subjacent damage can be carried out. If the dura remains intact but is bluish from subdural clot, the dura should be opened and the clot removed by suction and irrigation. If the brain is lacerated the divitalized or pulpified tissue is removed by a combination of irrigation with saline and suction until the obviously destroyed tissue is cleared away. One may then control bleeding by electrocoagulation and the use of gelfoam and then close the dura without drainage. In the event there has been loss of dura, one may utilize gelfoam or polyethylene film to cover the cortex out beyond the margins of the dural defect. I prefer to complete the closure over this membrane by splitting the dura and turning the outer layer as a patch to cover the defect or by removing pericranial tissue from the point adjacent to the fracture in order to complete the closure of the dura. Bone fragments are washed thoroughly, trimmed to remove any adherent debris and to remove spicules of bone. These fragments are then used to form a mosaic, filling the bone defect on the level with the surrounding convexity. The scalp closure is then carried out as in the repair of lacerations of the scalp. Occasionally the depressed fragments will be so severely contaminated as to contraindicate their replacement and only in this circumstance does one seem warranted in closing without covering the bone defect. It is far more hazardous to utilize a bone substitute in a recently compounded injury than it is to insert a substitute at a subsequent operative procedure some months after complete healing has taken place.

LATER PROBLEMS

Treatment Measures

With the above emergency problems cared for we can return our attention to the patient who has sustained loss of consciousness but has failed to recover promptly as the patient with mild head injury would have been apt to do. The unconscious patient must have his nasopharynx and tracheae cleared of secretions. He must be given a maintenance quantity of fluid. He must either be catheterized or be fitted with an external condom-like connection to care for the incontinence. A frequent change of position aids in the care of the respiratory problem while preventing damage to the skin from constant pressure over a bony prominence. Antibiotics are used when indicated for urinary tract infection, respiratory infection and for wound infection if one should be so unfortunate as to have one of these complications.

Control of the temperature in severe head injuries is frequently a problem. With diffuse brain damage, particularly with involvement of the midbrain areas, hyperthermia occurs as a serious complication. This is detected by frequent check of temperature and can be controlled by measures that will improve the circulation and by the application of external cooling by the thermal blanket. The utilization of aspirin in 10 to 15 grain doses every four to six hours for temperatures of 102° or above has been found quite helpful along with the application of external cooling. One should not forget the help afforded by the colonic flush, using cool water. At any point during the care of the head injury patient, oxygen may be required, not only to relieve conditions of poor aeration of blood in the lung and for the cases of shock and low pressure but also in the presence of high fever. We prefer giving this by nasal catheter or a similar arrangement in preference to the use of the oxygen tent, as the use of the tent impedes attention to the patient's needs and the maintenance of close observation of the vital functions. Intermittent use of positive pressure insufflator (Bennett, Bird, Haliburton) which operates from the pressure from the oxygen cylinder has proved of help in obtaining complete aeration of the lungs. The addition of Aleviare aids in clearing mucus from the bronchial tree by direct action and by inducing cough.

Fluids and Nutrients. In the patient with prolonged loss of consciousness, it is necessary to maintain along with an adequate supply of fluid something of nutrient value until such time as the patient is able to take food orally. In the beginning there is generally an advantage in administering fluid intravenously, a person of average adult size requiring a minimum of 2000 cc. of fluid per 24 hours. If there is vomiting or sweating, electrolyte requirements must be met. As a rule 500 cc. of 5 per cent glucose in saline and 1500 cc. of 5 per cent glucose in water will maintain the fluid in satisfactory electrolyte balance. There are instances in which the electrolyte balance becomes a problem and may require substances other than chlorides. If within a few days from the time of injury the individual has stabilized and has not been found to be suffering from massive intracranial clot and if vomiting has subsided, the maintenance of fluid and nutrition may be handled by introduction of a plastic stomach tube through the nostril. This will permit the administration of fluids and of liquid nourishment.

Making the Patient Comfortable. Through this period of care for the person who has persistent loss of consciousness, numerous problems may arise. First, there is the question of restlessness and necessity for sedatives. It is a good principle to use as little sedation as possible. Although unresponsive and unconscious, the individual may be quite susceptible to annoying stimuli such as noises and especially to painful stimuli. Morphine and narcotics that tend to depress the respiration are contraindicated. If the patient has a progressively increasing disturbance, the ever present danger is that of respiratory failure and death.

The distress from other injuries may be relieved by proper splinting of the fractures in the extremities, by attention to discomfort from overdistention of the bladder, by alleviation of distress from remaining in one position too long. Annoying, noisy environment should be eliminated by correcting the problem at hand. The patient may in addition require some sedation and this is best done by the use of pain-relieving medicine of the less depressing type. Aspirin as a rectal suppository can be used to good effect. In those not relieved by this simple measure, I prefer to use small to moderate doses of codeine unless symptoms of sensitivity to this drug develop. Sparine or Vespirin can be used in small to moderate doses but one should avoid giving tranquilizers, barbiturates or medication that is found to depress respiration or which appears to stimulate and aggravate the patient rather than to afford relief.

Chronic Subdural Hemorrhage

Repeated neurological evaluation should be made at frequent intervals in the acute case and at less frequent intervals as time elapses. It is by this means that one can evaluate progressive symptoms of chronic subdural clots, the variations in brain swelling and the symptoms and signs of subarachnoid bleeding. It is well to remember that subdural hemorrhage, although space-occupying, is one lesion that may reach considerable size without giving rise to papilledema. A progressive increase in somnolence after some days of loss of consciousness may be the only warning of the presence of a chronic subdural hematoma. Of course, if there are inequalities of pupils that did not exist earlier, convulsions, or unilateral motor pathway signs such as increased muscle tone and paresis, the probability of a subdural clot demands especially careful evaluation of neurological signs. An increase in reflex activity associated with decreased abdominal reflex and positive motor signs such as Hoffmann sign in the upper extremity, Babinski and confirmatory signs in the lower extremities with an associated central type of facial weakness, all occurring on the same side, adds weight to the diagnosis. As a rule, these findings are contralateral to the side on which the pupil dilates. The presence of any one or more of these signs warrants the tentative diagnosis of subdural hematoma. It is better to suspect the possibility and even resort to burr exploration bilaterally with negative results than to fail to think of this complication of head injury and neglect or delay investigation for the clot until irreparable damage is done.

Chronic Intracerebral Hemorrhage

If the chronic clot is intracerebral, it will be apt to manifest itself by focal signs that are progressive but much less rapidly progressive than a complicating arterial thrombosis. The localizing signs may be subtle to the point of requiring angiography or ventriculography for exclusion of such a lesion or for accurately localizing the lesion in preparation for surgical intervention and evacuation of the clot. Early in the course of practice at the University of Oklahoma, I had occasion to see a faculty member from the University who fell while playing tennis. He was admitted to the University Hospital several days after the injury because of symptoms of increased intracranial pressure that were quite insidious in their onset and had not become evident for several days. He presented focal signs of left cerebellar deficit and on exploration was found to have a fairly large clot within the left cerebellar hemisphere which through the process of osmosis had gradually enlarged to obstruct the ventricular system and produce an internal hydrocephalus. Fortunately, his cerebellar signs were for the most part due to pressure of the lesion and evacuation of this clot permitted recovery of function to the point that he was quite successful in playing tennis after a few months of practice during his convalescent period.

Chronic Subarachnoid Hemorrhage and Aseptic Meningitis

One of the complications of head injury is the response to subarachnoid bleeding. Blood will spread throughout the ventricular system with severe damage to the brain but more often will escape into the subarchnoid space to spread throughout the spinal and cranial subarachnoid space. This gives rise to certain symptoms that are in keeping with meningeal inflammation. One must, therefore, be mindful of the need for differential diagnosis between true purulent meningitis and aseptic meningitis resulting from liberation of elements of hemoglobin into the subarachnoid fluid. This is particularly important if there has been loss of cerebrospinal fluid by injury extending into the paranasal sinuses or if there is escape of blood-stained spinal fluid from the external auditory canal in fractures involving the petrous ridge. In the presence of cerebrospinal leak from the nose or ear, spinal puncture is contraindicated unless rather definite evidence of purulent meningitis is present. Then a diagnostic puncture with direct smear and culture of the fluid while administering broad-spectrum antibiotics is the plan we have followed. When culture permits identification, sensitivity tests are requested as an aid to selection of the appropriate antibiotic. In the patient who develops photophobia and stiff neck and positive meningeal signs such as Kernig and Brudzinski within 48 to 72 hours after head injury, we are inclined to favor the diagnosis of subarachnoid hemorrhage resulting in aseptic meningitis.

In aseptic meningitis the pulse is slow in proportion to the temperature and the temperature is prone to be low grade rather than the septic, spiking high temperature of purulent meningitis. Vagal stimulation by the chemicals released by breakdown of red cells in the spinal fluid may account for the slow pulse. The leukocytosis in the peripheral blood is just as apt to run high in the case of aseptic meningitis as in septic meningitis.

Because of the clinical evidence of improvement in the patient's condition in cases that I have been privileged to follow, I feel warranted in removing spinal fluid to verify the diagnosis of subarachnoid bleeding. Daily punctures removing 15 to 20 cc. of fluid seems to mobilize the fluid and to speed up improvement of symptoms. Examination of the removed fluid reveals increasing xanthochromia to a maximum, then a gradual decrease until the fluid becomes clear. An increase in white blood cells in the spinal fluid is to be expected and, just as in septic meningitis, the early predominant cell type is the polymorphonuclear cell. Smear and culture to exclude bacterial invasion is important. As a rule three to six spinal punctures at intervals of 24 to 48 hours will suffice to see a patient through the more disturbing signs of meningeal involvement and will aid materially in the comfort of the patient if he is conscious and able to appreciate improvement. In the unconscious patient, decrease in restlessness, improved pulse rate and lowering of the temperature have been observed sufficiently often to convince me that this is a helpful therapeutic measure. That this is not accepted by some[8, 9] does not warrant abandoning it.

Control of Cerebral Swelling

The problem of controlling cerebral swelling is one that has given rise to much controversy. We must recognize that brain swelling is a major factor involved in injury to the brain. It can be controlled to some extent by proper clearing of airways to maintain a good oxygen supply and by the delivery of this supply to the brain by maintaining adequate circulation. Even with these steps, however, there are instances in which additional help may be gained by dehydration. This must not be overdone since damage to tissues can take place in the dehydrated state just as in the state of compression from brain swelling. I do not agree with the concept of withholding fluid. I insist that an adequate basic fluid supply must be maintained. I believe that a basic 24 hour requirement is 2000 cc. with some increase in this amount with the febrile state, with vomiting or with loss by excessive sweating. We have made use of concentrated glucose in years gone by, administering 50 cc. of 50 per cent solution for rather prompt effect in mobilizing fluid from body tissues by withdrawing it to the blood stream. This has certain drawbacks and must be supplemented by more continuous, less dramatic measures. I refer to the rectal use of a concentrated solution of magnesium sulfate (saturated solution, 50 per cent), given in doses of 4 to 6 ounces to the average adult and with directions that it be retained for a period of 15 to 20 minutes and that it be removed by siphon if not expelled within 30 minutes. We have no fear of toxic effects from the absorption of magnesium sulfate if the above precaution is employed. This can be repeated every four to six hours and generally within a period of 24 to 48 hours may be markedly reduced or discontinued if the patient has shown improvement. It is effective in relieving the distress of intracranial pressure as demonstrated in its use in the conscious patient who is experiencing headache. In the unconscious patient the lessened irritability also manifests some benefit from this approach. This can be discontinued and resumed again if the patient's responses are not improving or if there should be regression of consciousness. It is well to keep in mind throughout the period of the use of this measure that even in the presence of an expanding lesion such as subdural hematoma the measures for dehydration may be effective up to a point. For this reason, careful observation of the neurological signs is imperative and must guide one in the decision to continue with the conservative program or to investigate by burr openings or by ventriculography. The diagnosis must be clarified when clinical improvement is not progressive and reasonably rapid. That the matter of using methods of dehydration in the treatment of brain injury remains controversial is evident in the writings of Fay,[10] Evans[8] and Bragdon.[11]

In recent years a number of pertinent improvements in the management of various aspects of brain damage have been introduced. Outstanding among these is the utilization of urea, which has been shown to be quite effective in reducing fluid volume intracranially by increasing the urinary output.[12] Urea is available in crystalline form in 40 and 90 gram containers. It must be mixed in solution of invert sugar and given in concentrations of 30 per cent. An indwelling catheter is mandatory in the unconscious patient. Over a period of more than 12 hours the use of 40 gram doses repeated at six to eight hour intervals should be adequate.

Utilization of gravity in improving venous outflow from the head is a worthwhile method in reducing the increase in intracranial pressure from cerebral swelling. If the arterial supply is adequate and if one can maintain clear upper respiratory pathways in a partially upright position, we find that the patient will progress more rapidly toward improvement with the head of the bed elevated by 15 to 20 inches. This position can be maintained with greater ease and will allow a shift from a right oblique to a left oblique position at intervals in order to lessen pulmonary stasis. The knee rest should be elevated moderately.

Control of Vomiting

Vomiting is often a disturbing symptom. It is dangerous not only from the standpoint of increasing the hazard of aspiration pneumonia but the act of vomiting by increasing venous back pressure gives rise to brief marked increase in intracranial pressure. This increase sometimes may cause the added pressure that will produce foraminal herniation particularly at the tentorial level. The use of Dramamine, Vespirin and Sparine depending on the patient's response to one or another of these drugs has proved quite helpful in lessening the tendency to vomit. Reduction of intracranial pressure aids in the control of nausea and vomiting.

Other Measures

It would seem superfluous to mention the need for administration of tetanus antitoxin or booster injection. Too often with everyone's attention focused on the patient's neurological problem, this important detail can easily be forgotten. It should be a rule every patient with a laceration of the scalp should have this protection.

During the past years the utilization of steroids in protection of brain tissue during the critical post-traumatic period has given us another potent therapeutic tool. Also, the protection of damaged cells by decreasing cellular metabolism has been lately re-emphasized. Sachs[7] made use of cracked ice heaped over the patient protected by a rubber sheet in controlling thermal disorders occurring following surgical procdures for tumor. Now hypothermia in a much more controllable form is being used in head injury problems.[13] This is a useful addition to our armamentarium for the treatment of the severely damaged brain. These latter two measures are potent, dangerous when used without attention to minute details and must be varied on change in condition, even of slight degree. For these reasons their use must be limited to facilities having a properly organized, trained staff.

Rehabilitation

The management of the patient who has sustained serious brain injury does not cease with the recovery from the immediate loss of consciousness and life-threatening conditions. It is necessary that rehabilitation take place in an orderly manner. With encouragement offered by members of the family and the personnel caring for the seriously injured patient, a far better and more complete rehabilitation is possible.

REFERENCES

1. Schneider, R. C.: Serious and fatal football injuries involving the head and spinal cord. J.A.M.A. 177:362-267, 1961.
2. Botterell, E. H.: Disruption of frontal and temporal lobes as a cause of secondary coma

following head injury. Paper read at the meeting of the Harvey Cushing Society, November 14, 1947.

3. Evans, J. P. and Schienker, I. M.: Post-traumatic cerebral edema. J. Neurosurg. 2:306-314, 1945.

4. Rand, C. W.: Significance of dilated pupil on homolateral hemiplegic side in cases of intracranial hemorrhage following head injuries. Report of seven cases. Arch. Surg. 18: 1176-1189, 1929.

5. Gardner, W. J.: Traumatic subdural hematoma with particular reference to the latent interval. Arch. Neurol. & Psychiat. 27:847-858, 1932.

6. Rawlinson, Kenneth: Modern athletic training. Englewood Cliffs, N. J., Prentice-Hall, Inc., 1961.

7. Sachs, Ernest: The care of the neurosurgical patient. St. Louis, C. V. Mosby Co., 1944.

8. Evans, J. P.: Acute head injury. Springfield, Ill., Charles C Thomas, 1950.

9. Sprong, K.: Disappearance of blood from cerebrospinal fluid in traumatic subarachnoid hemorrhage: Ineffectiveness of repeated lumbar punctures. Surg. Gynec. & Obst. 58:705-710.

10. Fay, Temple: The treatment of acute and chronic cases of cerebral trauma by methods of dehydration. Am. Surg. 101:76-132, 1935.

11. Bragdon, F. H.: Alterations observed in craniocerebral injuries following the use of dehydrating agents. Research Publ. Assoc. Nervous and Mental Disease 24:545-561, 1943.

12. Javid, Manucher: Urea in intracranial surgery. J. Neurosurgery 18:51-57, 1961.

13. Lazarthes, G. and Compan L.: Hypothermia in the treatment of craniocerebral traumatism. J. Neurosurg. 15:162-167, 1958.

6

Injuries of
the Face

ANATOMICAL CONSIDERATIONS

A BRIEF DISCUSSION of some of the anatomical characteristics of the face is pertinent since they relate specifically to the type of injury to be expected and the treatment recommended. Practically the entire face is subcutaneous. The skin extending from the hair line above to the neck below is stretched over subcutaneous bone with relatively few areas protected by any intervening structure. In the upper face, the hard bone of the skull is separated from the skin only by the very thin muscles of the scalp and the aponeurosis connecting these muscles. The bony structures of this portion of the face are entirely immobile and serve as protection for the brain. At the supraorbital margins, the layers of the cranium separate to form the frontal sinus which may be of almost any size. The characteristic "beetling brow" does not necessarily imply any change in contour of the cranial cavity but rather a large frontal sinus. This portion of the face is essentially part of the skull. Moving laterally from the midline in front, one finds the temporal fossae filled with the fanlike temporal muscles. The muscle layer here is considerably thicker than directly in front. The supraorbital nerves pass out of the orbital cavity through the supraorbital foramen at the junction of the inner and middle one-third of the superior orbital margin and pass subcutaneously up over the forehead. The essential injury in this area is contusion and its complications rather than strain or sprain.

The central portion of the face, that is, the area between the supraorbital

ridges and the bottom of the superior maxilla, presents a complicated maze of anatomical structures, some of which will be considered in more detail later in the
description of injuries to the various organs. The facial bones which in the infant
are separated by suture lines become fused relatively early but the very irregular
suture lines persist and may well be confused with fracture lines. The orbit, for
example, is a complete bony socket, open only anteriorly and posteriorly, yet is made
up of five or six different bones fitted together as in a jigsaw puzzle. The central
portion of the face also has no motion between its bony structures. However, it is
involved in motion of the lower jaw since many of the muscles attached to the
lower jaw have their origin on the fixed bones of the face. The lower portion of
the face, the mandibular portion, consists of the horseshoe-shaped mandible which
has bony contact with the rest of the skull only at the temporal articulations and
the teeth.

Injuries to the face are not nearly so frequent now as they have been in the
past. The football headgear and the various other helmets worn serve to protect not
only the skull but also the upper portion of the face. With the addition of a bar
of some type extending across the front of the face, the incidence of injuries to the
supraorbital ridge, the zygomatic process, the malar bone, the nose, the teeth and
jaw has been greatly reduced. Almost all of the professional and university teams
now require some sort of facial protection. Many of the high school and junior
schools are rapidly following suit (see Prevention of Injuries). I will not attempt
in this section to give the detailed treatment of each of the areas of the face but
rather will discuss those features of injuries which are likely to fall under the
aegis of the one treating athletic injuries.

LACERATION

The broad expanse of facial skin with underlying subcutaneous bone is subject
to contusion, abrasion and laceration more than any other type of injury. The
abrasion and laceration should be treated as elsewhere. One should bear in mind,
however, that an intervening aponeurotic layer is present between the skin and
bone on the forehead. It is important in laceration of the *forehead* or of the *scalp*
to determine whether the underlying muscle or galea has been damaged. Each
laceration should be carefully cleaned and the wound margins separated sufficiently
to explore the depths of the wound. There is no substitute for irrigation with
copious quantities of clean water. This is not necessarily sterile water. Running
water from the tap of the city water system is adequate and is always available.
If it is possible to hook up a tube or hose the procedure is simplified. Under hospital
conditions it is better to use sterile saline. It should be emphasized that it is the
force of the flowing water that cleans out the contaminants. If nothing else is available, an ordinary shower may be utilized in the preliminary cleansing.

Usually in athletics the wound is through the skin only and is in the nature
of a crushing, tearing injury rather than a direct cut. Such a wound extends deep
enough to expose but not damage the galea. It should be thoroughly cleansed and
hemostasis secured either by direct pressure or by injection of the skin edges with
procaine plus epinephrine. The use of procaine is advisable in any event since it will
make the repair of the wound much less painful. Once the skin edges are anes-

thetized they can be retracted gently and the area underneath investigated. Since the skin over the forehead is quite loose the defect in the underlying structures may be some distance above or below the split in the skin itself. The skin can be readily shifted and with a small curved forceps any underlying defect can be explored. If there is a defect in the galea, careful palpation will determine whether or not this extends downward to include the skull. Only after careful exploration of the wound should the skin be closed. Here, as anywhere in the face, it is extremely important to appose the skin edges accurately. Whether you are a believer in multiple, very small sutures or favor fewer but more widely spaced ones, the end result will depend greatly upon how accurately the edges of the skin are apposed. The skin cannot accommodate for overlapping or a vertical shift of its edges and a troublesome and unsightly ridge will remain if the original suture is sloppy. If the galea has been damaged and the wound can be thoroughly cleansed, the galea can be closed with one or two interrupted sutures. The wound should be carefully inspected daily for any accumulation of fluid under the skin or under the galea. This is a relatively silent area from the standpoint of sensitivity and a tremendous abscess may develop with relatively few symptoms. The abscess may spread under the skin or under the galea over the whole top of the head. Athletic participation may be permitted after a laceration of the area is carefully protected by a contact pad. A special foam rubber pad in the football helmet may be necessary. In other sports an appropriate protective pad may be molded to form a cup over the involved area.

Laceration of the *eyebrow* is a relatively common injury and requires the same treatment as indicated above. If the laceration is in the region of the supraorbital nerve, this nerve may be severed. In such an instance repair of the nerve should be carried out to avoid subsequent troublesome anesthesia, tenderness or itching on this side of the forehead.

In the *central portion* of the face laceration is also quite frequent and here again one must determine carefully whether or not there is damage to the underlying structures. This is quite obvious in lacerations about the eye. Lacerations about the face require meticulous handling and one must condemn the prevalent custom of rushing the player to the dressing room where someone places several stitches to close the wound with scant reference to either asepsis or accurate apposition. The emergency is not that great. If it is absolutely necessary for the player to compete throughout the remainder of the game, a suitable pad should be applied as a temporary expedient, with the definite understanding that a complete repair will be done at the earliest possible moment. Although this course is not recommended it certainly is better than to accept a less than perfect apposition of the wound edges. The definitive treatment should be carried out directly after the completion of the game and not the next day. If a delay of a few hours is unavoidable, the application of pressure and cold to the wound will help to control the swelling. By the next day it will be virtually impossible to carry out actual plastic closure of the laceration. Ideally, the suture should be done at once. It will never be as easy again. If the laceration is at all extensive it is preferable to anesthetize the wound edges, preferably by infiltration of procaine plus epinephrine as indicated above. It is particularly important that laceration of the *eyelids* receive very accurate closure in an effort to match up the skin creases. This is even more important if the laceration crosses the skin creases since an irregular scar will disfigure the eyelid and interfere with its motion.

So also laceration through the *alae of the nose* should be carefully closed, great care being taken to secure accurate apposition of the edges of the nostril. Similarly, laceration involving the *ear* requires accurate repositioning of the skin. In fact, there is no area of the face where meticulous handling is not essential. It is extremely distressing to have a scar across the face with one edge of the skin higher than the other. This is disfiguring in the female and very distressing to the male since it interferes with shaving. It also is often a source of unsightly ingrown hairs.

CONTUSION

By far the most common injury to the face is contusion. This may involve damage to the skin when it is caught between the hard, underlying bone and the force of the blow. The skin over the face is loose and an area of areolar tissue is present between it and the underlying structures. In the forehead there is an areolar space between the skin and the galea or the frontalis, offering ample room for local swelling with hematoma formation. A blow to the forehead is likely to be followed immediately by extensive swelling which may be diffuse, having the shape of an egg transected on its long axis, or local with simply a rounded area of local swelling. One should assure himself that there is no serious underlying pathology by close attention to the general symptoms of the patient as well as by local and general physical examination. Immediate application of cold and pressure will minimize the local swelling and may prevent to a great extent the infiltration of blood. It is debatable whether or not the local swelling should be aspirated. Very frequently the swelling is more in the nature of bloody edema than hematoma and in such an instance aspiration will be unrewarding. Only when the area feels distinctly fluctuant is aspiration indicated to expedite recovery. After the area is aspirated under careful aseptic precautions it should be infiltrated with hyaluronidase, then cold and pressure applied. The latter can be done quite simply by a circumferential wrap around the head. If it causes distressing headache after a few hours it is too tight and will need to be released and rewrapped. The ordinary elastic bandage makes a very adequate pressure bandage. If there are no complications there is no contraindication to athletic participation following such a contusion.

COMPLICATIONS OF CONTUSION

Injury to the Brain

The most critical complication of contusion of the forehead is injury to the brain and this has been discussed (Chap. 5). I believe it should be emphasized here, however, that if the patient has actually been knocked unconscious by such a blow he should be kept under very careful observation for at least 12 hours and resumption of athletic competition should not be permitted within that time. This is because of the danger of delayed intracranial hemorrhage or edema.

Fracture of the Skull

If the blow was so forceful as to fracture the skull, the patient should be immediately removed to a hospital and kept under constant observation. The most important consideration here is damage to the brain and this should take precedence over any attempt at correction of the deformity. There may be a fracture of the frontal bone which will involve the frontal sinus and not actually break into the cranial cavity. In such a case the deformity is usually minimal and requires no treatment. If the whole anterior wall of the frontal sinus is collapsed, advice should be sought from a competent otolaryngologist to determine whether or not the fragment should be elevated.

Supraorbital Nerve Damage

Contusion of the supraorbital ridge may cause damage to the supraorbital nerve as it passes over the ridge in the subcutaneous tissue. Expectant treatment is usually adopted here since in contusion the nerve is rarely severed and complete recovery follows. This is particularly true since this is a sensory nerve and tends to regenerate quite promptly.

Injury in the Vicinity of the Ear

Injury to the external ear is not common in amateur athletics. Professional prizefighters are frequently injured in this area but in the amateur ranks the athlete usually wears a protective pad. In football the ear is protected by the helmet.

In the simple contusion in which the ear is smashed against the mastoid, prompt care may often prevent seriously deforming sequelae. The ear should be carefully examined. Any hemorrhage between the perichondrium and cartilage should be aspirated under most aseptic conditions. If early hemorrhage is not present, an ice pack should be used to reduce the local edema. If edema persists and there appears to be fluid in the soft tissues which irons out the wrinkles and crevices of the ear, one might seriously consider release of the pressure of this fluid by multiple small incisions. These should be made under the most aseptic precautions since infection in this area may be serious.

A chronic infection may well supervene when contamination develops as a complication of the treatment of contusion and hematoma or when the initial injury breaks the skin. This causes local swelling and edema but has little or no systemic reaction. When the cartilage is involved there may be either dissecting infection along the perichondrium or an aseptic necrosis of the cartilage. This type of infection is very difficult to manage and the team physician would do well to seek specialized care from the plastic surgeon.

The resulting scar from contusion with infiltration of blood through the soft tissues results in some thickening of subcutaneous tissue and perichondrium so that each subsequent injury is more serious than the previous one and the final result is the well-known cauliflower ear which defies any very definitive treatment. Careful release of tissue tension by pressure bandage and application of ice are excellent preventive measures.

A laceration of the ear may occur from a sharp instrument. Much more common is the avulsion in which the ear is partially torn away. Such an injury occurs when the ear is forcibly pulled forward and the skin fold between the scalp and the ear is split. As the ear falls back into its normal position, this split may be completely concealed and infection may supervene because of contamination of the wound. Given a history of such an injury, a careful inspection of the ear should be made. If there is a laceration it should be carefully cleansed and sutured. Any tear in the external ear itself must be meticulously apposed, particularly if the auricular cartilage is torn, otherwise, an unsightly notch will appear at the suture line.

Injury to the *internal ear* is not frequent. The possible exception is the ruptured ear drum. The history of blow across the side of the head with pain, slight hemorrhage from the ear and a feeling of fullness in the ear demands investigation of the drum. These ruptures of the drum usually heal spontaneously but in the young athlete, if there is any question at all as to damage of the drum or inner or middle ear, the service of a competent otologist should be provided. Perhaps the most dangerous sequelae is infection.

Injury in the Vicinity of the Eye

Orbit. The orbit is anatomically constructed to give maximum protection to the eye. The supraorbital ridge above and infraorbital margin below, the malar bone on the outer side, the nasal bones on the inside, all serve to form a recess protecting the eye from a blow from anything other than a relatively small object. The elbow, knee or foot projected against the face will usually not reach the eye. A direct blow in this region results in the usual complications of contusion, namely, swelling and infiltration of fluids into the tissues to the extent that the eye may be promptly closed by edema of the lids and of the surrounding soft tissue. Very careful examination should be carried out to determine any underlying pathology. The eyelids should be carefully separated and the globe inspected. Meanwhile the patient is asked to roll his eye from side to side and up and down to permit visualization of the entire area of the sclera and cornea. The lid should be carefully examined for lacerations both along the folds of the lid and at the margins. If the injury is seen immediately, it may be relatively easy to palpate along the zygomatic arch and infraorbital margin to detect damage to the malar bone or zygoma. After swelling develops this becomes exceedingly difficult. One may be surprised after one or two weeks to discover that there has been a fracture of the orbit with displacement which was not previously recognized because of inadequacy of the early examination. If the injury seems severe and there is localized tenderness on the nose, the supraorbital ridge, the malar bone or the zygoma, special x-ray study should be carried out. These pictures are extremely difficult for the uninitiated to interpret. If there is any question, a competent radiologist or maxillofacial surgeon should be consulted.

If one is satisfied that there is no underlying complication he should proceed promptly to treatment. The most urgent measure in this early stage is an adequate ice pack. This should consist of crushed ice folded in soft cloth such as a towel rather than an ice bag. The ice bag is heavy, cumbersome and poorly tolerated by the patient. If the patient is to have an x-ray, an ice pack should be applied during the interim since time is of the essence. If the pack is carefully applied, it may be fastened in place by an elastic bandage and the patient made relatively comfortable.

Should the complication of fracture occur, the patient should be placed promptly under the care of the man who is to carry out the definitive treatment whether this be an ophthalmologist, an orthopedist or a maxillofacial surgeon. If there is any evidence whatever of injury to the eye, consultation should be sought with an ophthalmologist as promptly as possible since the vision of this eye may well be in the balance.

Cornea. The cornea is the most exposed portion of the eye. In sports, the most common injury is ABRASION of the cornea, either by an object such as the fingernail or by a rough, foreign body such as a piece of gravel. The patient will complain of pain, the feeling of roughness and irregularity even though the abrading agent is no longer present. If the foreign body is present but free it may be removed by a cotton applicator. If it is embedded, the services of an ophthalmologist are required for its removal. Lacrimation is an outstanding feature of abrasion. When it is present the eye should be very carefully examined since corneal abrasions may be extremely serious. The outer layer of the cornea will repair without scarring but, if the deep layer is involved, scarring will result. Always, when the seriousness of the injury is in doubt, ophthalmologic consultation is necessary. A blow on the cornea will on rare occasions cause an obviously serious injury.

For LACERATION of either the sclera or the cornea, prompt consultation should be sought. The main problem for the team physician is diagnosis. Careful study of the eye from all angles, having the patient roll the eye in all directions, should be carried out. In case of any doubt, a local anesthetic should be used to permit a more thorough examination.

The cornea may be damaged by CONTUSION although this is not common in sports. Its serious nature demands prompt consultation. In the presence of irritation or conjunctivitis from any of these injuries which appear to be minor, ophthalmic ointments will be of value, particularly those containing antibiotics.

Sclera. The sclera is the white supporting tunic of the eyeball surrounding the transparent cornea. The sclera is much more resistant to injury and much more capable of recovery than the cornea. Scarring is less important so that the consequences of injury to the sclera are not nearly so serious as those of the cornea.

The same general principles of management apply except that one has considerably more latitude since embedded foreign bodies may be removed by a cotton pledget or small forceps if the injury does not appear to be too severe. If there is a definite laceration, this should be seen by the ophthalmologist.

Globe. Contusion of the eye may damage the cornea, cause congestion and hemorrhage or, if forceful, rupture the globe. Rupture is obviously a serious injury that demands immediate consultation. Very often by the time the patient is seen, the eyelids are edematous and swollen. There is infiltration of blood and serum. The eye can be opened with extreme difficulty. One may be surprised as this swelling diminishes to find serious injury to the globe.

Other Injuries to the Eye. Other injuries to the eye will cause varying amounts of irritation with disturbance of vision, lacrimation, loss of accommodation, and loss of synchronous movements of the eyeball. Any of these symptoms demands ophthalmologic consultation.

Injury in the Vicinity of the Nose

Contusion of the nose presents many fascinating aspects, as has been recorded in song and story. However, it is not particularly funny to the recipient of the blow. Here again, careful attention to the possible complicating factors is most important. If the patient is seen before swelling occurs, a very adequate examination can be made digitally from the nasal bone to the infraorbital margin. A simple speculum and a flashlight will enable one to examine the inside of the nose fairly well in the early stages. Careful observation of the face may also reveal telltale deformity, particularly lateral deviation of the nose. I think it is of some advantage to have the patient look at himself in the mirror and also for the doctor to study the patient's physiognomy in the mirror. A tangential view of the nose is extremely important. With the patient lying supine the doctor can look across the forehead, down the bridge of the nose to the tip and observe a deviation which may not have been noticed otherwise. Palpation of the two nasal bones between the fingers will be rewarding since one can outline the exact area of pain on pressure. This may have some significance particularly if it is at the junction of the nasal bones with the frontal process or at their junction with each other in the midline. Careful palpation may determine a difference in the angle of the ridge of the nose. One side may seem flat and the other bulging. Sometimes actual crepitation can be felt. All this is much more effective if done early. In the later stages, swelling is very likely to be unilateral or at least worse on one side than the other and one will be convinced there is gross deformity of the nose when it is simply unilaterally increased swelling. X-ray study while important may be quite unsatisfactory. Tangential views of the nose may reveal variation of the angle of the bones with each other or possibly a defect or fracture line. Again, one must be very wary not to interpret a suture line as a fracture line.

If there appears to be a fracture of the nose, the patient should be promptly referred to a surgeon skilled in such cases. It will be his responsibility to decide upon the proper time for reduction of the fracture. It is unwise for the untrained physician to attempt reduction of the displaced nasal bones. The nose is an extremely prominent feature and may deviate from normal if the correction is imperfect. This crooked proboscis may haunt the unwary. Additionally, the internal mechanism of the nose with the intricate arrangement of the septum and various turbinates requires especial skill to prevent persistent intranasal symptoms.

Bleeding from the nose is a very common accompaniment of a blow, owing to the extremely copious blood supply of the nasal mucosa. Fortunately, bleeding from the nose is usually readily controlled without resorting to a major procedure. The patient should hold himself upright if possible rather than lie down or hold the head low. The nasal area should be covered with cold cloths or ice to constrict the vessels. Under ordinary circumstances if the patient is kept quiet, semi-erect and cold, bleeding promptly stops. If the bleeding is profuse and not easily arrested, careful packing of the anterior nares may reach the area of bleeding and control it. A tampon soaked in thrombin will be of help. It should be emphasized that the packing should not be forced deep into the nose or placed under pressure. Pressure is not required with this type of pack. If it becomes necessary to pack the posterior nares the equipment of the emergency room and the skill of one used to working in this area are required.

Nasal packing should not be left in place for a long time since it may force an infection backward through the cribriform plate and cause dangerous meningitis. Since the trauma of removing the pack will sometimes re-initiate the bleeding, various measures have been suggested to permit its easy removal. The pack may be inserted within a very thin film of rubber, packing the rubber ahead of the gauze so as to make a finger-like pouch. Vaseline gauze may be used. However, this method does lessen the effectiveness of the pack and gauze directly against the area, particularly if impregnated with thrombin, will be much more effective.

Injury in the Vicinity of the Malar Bone and Superior Maxilla

Contusion over the malar bones or superior maxilla extending back to the zygomatic arch may well cause a fracture in this area (Figs. 34 and 35). Fracture of the malar bone extends into the maxillary sinus. So too, on frequent occasions, does fracture of the superior maxilla and then it should be considered a compound fracture. A blow of sufficient severity will justify investigation to determine whether or not a fracture exists. Here again, as in the case of the nose and orbit, early examination is extremely rewarding since the next day the face will simply be a mass of tense, swollen edematous skin which prevents any pretense of adequate physical examination. Since the maxilla is important for attachment of the upper teeth and the zygoma and malar bone are concerned with protection and since all these bones are related with the orbit, the teeth and the mandible, careful attempt should be made to evaluate adequately any deformity. The maxillofacial surgeon should be consulted in case of serious injury. Expectant treatment should be carried out while awaiting consultation since it is of great importance to control the swelling.

Contusion around the mouth may cause damage to the teeth and this is usually accompanied by laceration of the lip. One should examine the inside of the lip since there may be an extensive laceration here that does not extend through the skin. A cursory examination of the teeth may fail to reveal the entire damage. A tooth that in breaking has included a portion of the alveolar process may not appear to be loose or broken. Direct pressure over each tooth will usually determine whether or not the attachment of that tooth is damaged. In many cases if a tooth is broken with a portion of the alveolar process, healing will occur if it is properly replaced and held whereas if it is overlooked a subsequent blow, although relatively minor, may knock the tooth completely out. Careful examination is the watchword here. A massive fracture of the face is uncommon in ordinary sports and if it occurs it should be readily recognized. The injury most likely to be overlooked is the one that seems relatively inconsequential.

A fractured alveolar process that includes one or more teeth should be very carefully reduced and held reduced by interdental wiring. In some instances simply wiring the upper teeth to a molded arch wire will be adequate. In others it may be necessary to wire the two jaws together. A good deal of expensive dental reparative work may be avoided by adequate early care in these cases. It is important to remember that any open wound about the mouth is subject to infection. Although the patient may be relatively immune to his own organisms, one cannot assume this to be the case. Any fracture of the alveolar process, into the sinus, into the nose or

Figure 34.   Fracture of zygomatic arch and malar bone bilaterally. Note the good view of
the nasal arch.

Figure 35.   Typical fracture of zygomatic arch on the left. Note normal arch on the right

into the mouth is compounded and should be considered an open fracture. Antibiotics are recommended and prompt attention must be given to any developing abscess. This applies to the lower as well as the upper jaw.

Injury in the Vicinity of the Lower Jaw

Dislocation of the Temporomandibular Joint. Such injuries are infrequent in the athlete, who is not subject to the forces that ordinarily cause them. In the ordinary process of mastication, the condyle of the mandible swings forward out of the cotyloid fossa and subluxates each time the mouth is opened. The force that causes dislocation is one that forces the mandible to open wider than its normal range on either or both sides. Dislocation may occur as the result of yawning, at which time the jaw is actively opened beyond its normal capacity and the condyle slips forward in front of the fossa and locks in this position. Conceivably it could be caused by forcible opening of the mouth but the immediate response of muscular resistance to this motion will usually prevent the dislocation. The dislocation usually occurs at a time when the muscles that pull the teeth into occlusion are relaxed in a synergistic manner as the muscles that open the jaw contract. An attempt to open the mouth widely, as to bite a large apple or to insert a billiard ball, may result in dislocation and locking of the temporomandibular joint. Once the condyle slips forward and locks, the muscle spasm intervenes and contraction of the masseter and temporals effectively locks the jaw in the dislocated position. This may be a habitual condition and result much as any habitual dislocation, either from an abnormally relaxed joint or from stretching of the capsule by repeated episodes of dislocation.

The dislocated jaw can be readily reduced if the patient can be made to relax. Before an attempt is made at reduction, the patient should be relaxed somewhat by sedation. In a cooperative patient, the operator's thumbs may be inserted onto the posterior inferior molars while the index fingers are locked under the point of the chin. Pressure downward on the thumb will unlock the condyles and rotatory pressure forward on the fingers will reduce the forward displacement. If the patient cannot relax, a light anesthetic may be necessary and will make the reduction easy. Forcible traumatic manipulation is neither necessary nor advisable.

If this has been the first episode, the jaw should be prevented from opening widely for a considerable period of time. Preliminary treatment by a Barton's bandage (Fig. 39) for a week or ten days will usually be adequate if the patient is cooperative enough to avoid over-opening of the jaw as in yawning. In recurrent habitual dislocation there probably is little value in temporary immobilization. I have seen many cases of habitual dislocation which were extremely distressing, particularly because of an almost irresistible impulse to yawn and so cause a recurrence. These cases have been relieved by wiring the teeth in apposition for four to six weeks. Threatening to wire the teeth together has in many instances been effective.

Fracture of the Mandible. The mandible is much more susceptible to damage than is the superior maxilla or the temporomandibular joint. Since fracture of the mandible is usually caused by a direct blow, a contusion may be the first thing that calls attention to the injury. Any contusion involving the mandible should be carefully examined. The entire inferior margin of the mandible is subcutaneous and by palpating carefully along the subcutaneous border one can determine areas of tenderness, areas of local swelling or any irregularity of this margin. If the injury is major, the fracture of the mandible may be quite obvious. The jaw will hang open, the lips may be badly swollen. There will be hemorrhage in the mouth where the gum is torn as the jaw fragments separate. These cases are readily diagnosed. Of greater difficulty is the case with little or minimal displacement. After careful observation and palpation the patient should be asked to open and close his mouth and to appose his teeth. Since most athletes with these injuries are young individuals, they usually have a complete set of molars. These should properly occlude without discomfort if there is no displacement. This is the best single test of the accuracy of reduction of any deformity following fracture. It is not advisable to attempt to produce motion at the fracture site. If motion is observed, however, it is quite obvious that a fracture is present. Roentgenographic examination in both anteroposterior and lateral planes should be made and should be carefully interpreted.

Fracture of the tooth-bearing area of the mandible is more readily determined than is fracture posteriorly where it may cross through the angle of the jaw (Fig. 36), through the condyle or through the condylar neck (Figs. 37 and 38). Here again, careful palpation is important. Have the patient open and close his jaw and observe whether or not the chin swings to one side or the other. Palpate the condyle as it comes forward out of the glenoid. Both of these signs are valuable. If the teeth appose properly and there is some question as to whether or not the jaw has been broken, a supportive bandage such as Barton's bandage (Fig. 39) should be applied to the mandible to hold it to the maxilla until a more detailed examination is made. If the mandibular fracture is undisplaced or can be readily reduced, interdental wiring to fasten the upper and lower teeth firmly together should be carried out. If perfect reduction cannot be obtained and one cannot be assured of perfect occlusion, consultation should be sought as early as

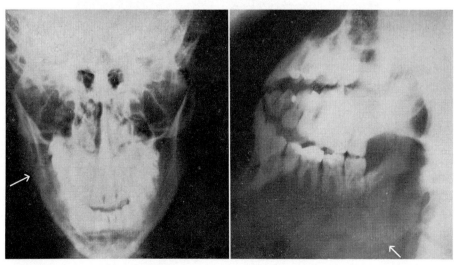

Figure 36. Incomplete fracture of angle of mandible on the right. This should be treated by immobilization of the jaw with interdental wiring.

Figure 37.   Fracture of the neck of the condyle on the right with fracture through the mandible on the same side. Whenever one fracture is shown in the mandible, search carefully for the second.

Figure 38.   Fracture of the condyle on the left, compared with the normal on the right.

Figure 39. Barton's bandage. A single turn. Many more turns make a firm, compact dressing.

possible. If there is any question about the occlusion, the patient's dentist may be able to provide a valuable hint as to any change in the position of the jaw. Frequently malocclusion predates the injury so it is wise to consult with the patient and with his parents to determine whether or not the patient previously had an overbite, underbite or irregular occlusion. I well recall spending an inordinate amount of time one humid Sunday morning in an attempt to get good occlusion in a man who had been more than slightly inebriated the night before. His truculence had been rewarded by a blow to the chin. In confiding to his wife that we were unable to get good occlusion she examined his mouth and said it had never been better than that. This proved to be the case. A little foreknowledge of this patient would have prevented a good deal of needless, painful and arduous manipulation.

The management of the patient with his teeth wired together can be difficult, particularly if he is a young and impatient athlete. Actually, it is more difficult when his teeth fit well than when they do not since it is easier for him to eat through the interstices of the teeth if they do not fit perfectly or if one is knocked out. We do not recommend knocking out a tooth to permit eating, however. It is important that the patient have adequate caloric and vitamin intake during the period when he cannot chew. Rich soups, whipped potatoes and gravy, and ground meat can be handled quite well. These will be very much more acceptable to the youth than a constant diet of malted milks and sweet drinks.

Interruption of Airway

One of the unusual complications of fracture of the face that occurs particularly in reference to the mandible but may also occur in the maxilla, is interruption of the airway. This complication is, of course, first in order of importance in any injury, taking priority over hemorrhage, contamination, unconsciousness or any other complication. The patient cannot long survive without adequate respiration. Occasionally in fractures of the superior maxilla edema may be severe enough in the back of the soft palate and in the throat to seriously interfere with respiration. It is the rule for nasal obstruction to occur in almost all of these injuries, hence breathing must be through the mouth. Swelling of the back of the tongue that presses the tongue against the pharynx is a very real hazard. Whoever is to care for the person with this type of injury should be warned of the urgency of an adequate airway. Holding the tongue forward by insertion of an anesthetist's airway is of value.

In fracture of the lower jaw, hemorrhage from the external maxillary artery may cause sufficient swelling at the base of the tongue and front of the neck to seriously interfere with breathing. While this is not common, it is extremely distressing when it occurs. At the Children's Hospital we had a case of fracture of the mandible that was accompanied by considerable bleeding. It was felt permissible to proceed with reduction of the fracture and apposition of the teeth by interdental wiring. In subsequent hours these measures compounded the problem rather than improved it. The swelling increased and a tracheotomy was necessary to permit breathing. Following this the surgeon had to tie off the carotid before the hemorrhage could be adequately controlled. It follows that any fracture of the mandible should be carefully observed and not left unattended until the critical period is past, that is, for 12 to 24 hours.

PENETRATING INJURIES

Occasionally there may be an injury to the face by a penetrating sharp object and the complications of such an injury, particularly injury to the eye, demand immediate hospitalization and definitive care. An injury to the *mouth* with damage to hard or soft palate or with severe intraoral bleeding may be easily overlooked. In case of any suspected penetrating wound, the patient should be questioned as to the nature of the injury and carefully examined to determine the depth of penetration and any possible damage to the underlying structures. Another area of the face that is rather frequently injured is the *tongue*. The most common injury of the tongue occurs when it is caught between the upper and lower teeth as the teeth are forcibly apposed in response to some external force. This is a painful injury but usually is not severe. If the laceration goes completely through the tongue it should be carefully sutured, apposing the edges exactly. Overlapping of the edges will give troublesome irregularity which may require the service of a plastic surgeon at a later date.

Injuries of the Shoulder Girdle

IN CONTRAST to the pelvis, which is a solid bony ring that provides great stability for transmitting the body weight from the trunk to the lower extremities, the shoulder girdle is a very loosely constructed, highly mobile mechanism of bones, muscles and ligaments designed to give great mobility to the upper extremity with only sufficient stability to provide a proper foundation for the muscular activity of the upper extremity (Fig. 40). The skeletal connection of the shoulder girdle to the trunk is extremely tenuous and consists only of the relatively insecure articulation of the inner end of the clavicle against the sternum and the first rib (Fig. 41). I will discuss only those details of anatomy that are needed to orient the reader in regard to the various areas of injury since a full anatomical study of this region would of necessity be voluminous.

Briefly, then, the *clavicle* acts as a strut or crane arm to prevent the shoulder from dropping forward across the chest. It is a rigid long bone with its inner end apposed to the sternum and its outer end apposed to the acromial process of the scapula. Thus it maintains a constant distance between the upper end of the arm and the midline of the chest. The shoulder may move forward, backward, upward or downward but so long as the clavicle maintains its integrity the shoulder will not approximate the midline. Thus, it may be seen that the clavicle has a vital role in shoulder function. The various muscles and ligaments about the thorax and neck tend to stabilize the clavicle in this position. Its function is well illustrated by the forward displacement of the shoulder which results when the clavicle is completely broken.

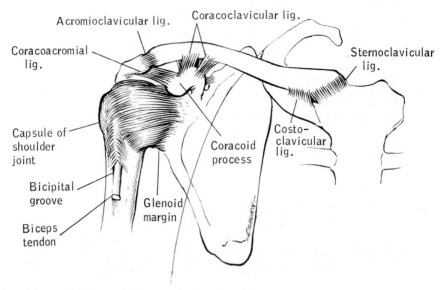

Figure 40.   Anatomical drawing showing the ligamentous structures about the shoulder girdle.

The *scapula* is a broad membranous bone designed primarily for muscle attachment (Fig. 41). It has no bony connection to the thorax. Its concave undersurface lies over the muscles of the posterolateral thoracic cage. On motions of the arm and shoulder, the scapula glides over the muscles of the chest wall through a wide range of motion which may be inward, outward, upward, downward, rotatory or any combination of these movements. Its range of motion is subject to the limitations of the clavicular strut and the excursion of the various muscles that control its motion. These muscles have both synergistic and antagonistic action which under normal circumstances permits very smooth movement of the scapula over the trunk. The scapula also serves for the origin of many of the muscles that move the arm. This motion of the arm may be carried out by various mechanisms. For example, the scapula may be fixed by synergistic contraction of antagonists and the arm then moves in relation to the rigid scapula. In this instance the muscles running from the scapula to the trunk are in tonic contraction and the muscles running from the scapula and trunk to the upper extremity move the upper extremity on this firm base. On the other hand, the muscles fixing the arm to the scapula may be fixed and the upper extremity is then moved by gliding of the scapula over the chest wall. Obviously, neither of these situations exists in the pure state under ordinary circumstances. Usually the movement is a synchronous one of the upper arm on the scapula and the scapula on the trunk. This makes for extremely smooth and coordinated action and permits precise motions of the upper extremity where controlled mobility is a good deal more important than stability. One of the early signs of a lesion about the shoulder girdle is a disturbance of this coordinated movement. Various clues may be obtained as to the character of the lesion by careful study of the motion of the arm and shoulder girdle, noting any disturbance of scapulohumeral rhythm.

There follows a discussion of various injuries to the shoulder in relation to specific areas. It should always be borne in mind, however, that the shoulder is an

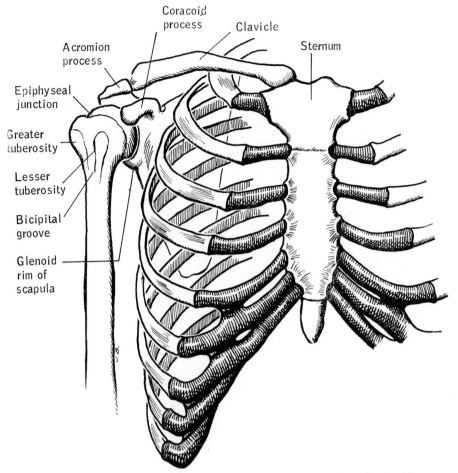

Coracoid
process

Clavicle

Acromion
process

Sternum

Epiphyseal
junction

Greater
tuberosity

Lesser
tuberosity

Bicipital
groove

Glenoid
rim of
scapula

Figure 41.   Anatomical drawing showing the bony structure about the shoulder.

extremely complex mechanism and that anything affecting one portion is bound to
have an effect on the other components of the girdle.

REGION OF THE STERNAL END OF THE CLAVICLE

ANATOMICAL CONSIDERATIONS

The integrity of the sternoclavicular joint is maintained by the ligamentous
structures that bind the inner end of the clavicle to the sternum and the first rib
(Fig. 42). There is little inherent bony stability in this articulation. Indeed, the
articulation is notably insecure. The inner end of the clavicle resting against the
oblique outer angle of the manubrium is in contact with not more than one-half of
the surface area of the end of the clavicle. It is secured by the *sternoclavicular* ligament, a circumferential band of capsular tissue passing from the head of the clavicle
to the sternum. This ligament serves to hold the clavicle against the sternum rather
than to hold it down. The major structure holding the inner end of the clavicle down
is the *costoclavicular* ligament. This is a rather broad band arising in the proximal

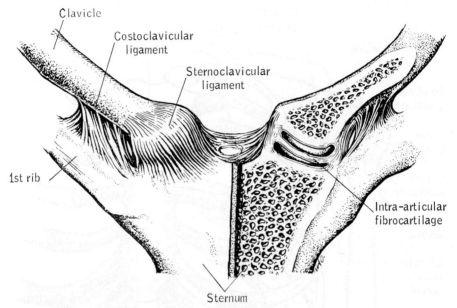

Figure 42.   Detail of inner end of the clavicle showing (left) the sternoclavicular area with ligaments intact, (right) cross section. (Redrawn from Spalteholtz, "Hand Atlas of Anatomy," published by J. B. Lippincott Co.)

one-fourth of the inferior margin of the clavicle and extending in an oblique manner downward and inward to attach to the first rib. This ligament is analogous to the coracoclavicular ligament at the outer end of the clavicle. These two ligaments together prevent the clavicle from displacing upward at either end.

It seems strange that this joint is not injured more frequently considering that it does have rotatory motion and has little anatomical security.

CONTUSION

Contusion in this area is not frequent since the athlete has been trained to protect the area of the anterior part of the neck and chest by tucking his chin down. In football the shoulder pads protect the area fairly adequately.

SPRAIN

The most common injury to the sternoclavicular joint is a sprain. The force applied to cause injury is one throwing the shoulder sharply forward. As the shoulder girdle moves forward and inward, force is applied along the long axis of the clavicle and the clavicle may be disrupted anywhere along its length. These forces on reaching the sternoclavicular joint tend to impel the inner end of the clavicle inward, upward and forward or the leverage may be such that it is inward, upward and backward. In either instance the major strain will be upon the costoclavicular ligament. If this gives way, the inner end of the clavicle slips upward and inward and this causes rupture of the sternoclavicular ligament. If the force is arrested after minimal damage, the result is a sprain of these ligaments. Stronger application of the force may rupture the sternoclavicular capsular ligaments while the costoclavicular ligaments remain relatively intact. In this case the inner end of the clavicle may snap in front of or behind the sternum and be held firmly in position by the intact costoclavicular ligament (Fig. 43, B). The treatment of this latter condition may be relatively simple if recognized early. Simple traction applied to the shoulder to pull it backward and outward with simultaneous direct pressure on the inner end of the clavicle will usually snap the bone back into place. If the costoclavicular ligament is intact a simple yoke or sling may be adequate for fixation.

If the driving force continues and the costoclavicular ligament is torn, dislocation or subluxation of the inner end of the clavicle takes place. In this instance the inner end of the clavicle is much more free and may ride upward over the sternum toward the midline (Fig. 43, C). Another modification of the same type of injury consists of a fracture-dislocation in which some part of the inferior portion of the inner end of the clavicle remains fixed by the ligament, whereas the upper portion of the clavicle breaks away and dislocates. This remaining fragment may include the whole costoclavicular attachment as well as the inferior portion of the head (Fig. 43, D). In this instance treatment is much more favorable since open reduc-

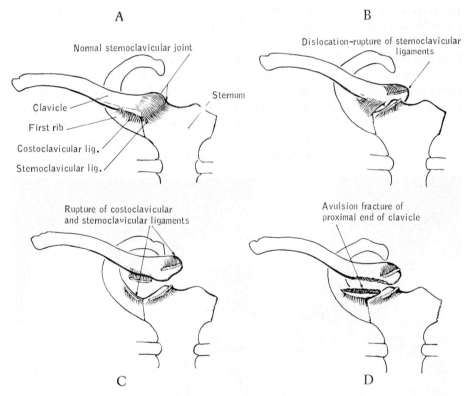

Figure 43.   A, Normal sternoclavicular joint. B, Dislocation with rupture of sterno clavicular ligaments. The end of the clavicle remains fixed behind the sternum. C, Similaı injury with rupture of both the costoclavicular and sternoclavicular ligament with the end of the clavicle free. D, Avulsion fracture of proximal end of clavicle with rupture of sternoclavicular ligament.

Figure 44. Fracture of inner end of clavicle on the right. Clinically, the patient, a boy, appeared to have sternoclavicular dislocation. His injury was actually a fracture-dislocation in that about the upper one-third of the inner end of the clavicle together with the shaft broke off from the lower two-thirds, which remained attached to the sternum and to the first rib. Repair was readily made by suture to the remaining fragment which simplified the procedure. The displacement was primarily forward so was not well revealed in the film. The x-rays show the patient facing backward.

tion and fixation of the distal portion of the clavicle to the unattached inferior segment are relatively simple. Careful internal fixation should result in complete recovery. Even if treatment for this condition is delayed it remains much more favorable since there is a firm base to which to attach the displaced portion of the clavicle. In this instance open operation and fixation should be recommended at any time and any stage of the injury. (See Figs. 44 and 45.)

The *treatment* of a sprain is the treatment of sprain in other areas. The local treatment is application of cold, then heat, compression, local injection and protection. Protection consists of immobilization of the shoulder or application of figure-of-8 yoke which tends to hold the shoulder girdle backward, combined with adhesive strapping of the local area. Strapping of the inner end of the clavicle is ineffective since it does not prevent the motion that causes stress on the ligament.

Figure 45. X-ray of the chest for lung disease revealed abnormality of the sternum. Clinical examination then revealed dislocation of the inner end of the clavicle, riding above and behind the sternum (left).

DISLOCATION

If the ligament tear is complete and the inner end of the clavicle dislocates, prompt reduction and operative repair of the ligaments will give very good results. Unfortunately, the condition is usually not recognized in its early stages and chronic upward displacement occurs (Fig. 46, A). This delay in diagnosis is contributed to by the fact that the deformity is not dramatic and that local swelling will obscure observation or palpation of the displacement. Added to this is the problem that good x-ray visualization is extremely difficult to obtain and errors in interpretation of the films are relatively common. The result is that several weeks will often have elapsed before persistence of discomfort after the swelling has subsided calls attention to the deformity and instability present. At this time it is difficult to treat.

Treatment.   Various measures designed for reconstruction of the costoclavicular ligament are not particularly successful, certainly not to the point where athletic participation should be encouraged after the procedure. It is unwise to fuse this joint because motion in the sternoclavicular joint occurs in almost any motion of the shoulder girdle. Usually one must be reconciled to accept the deformity and

Figure 46.   A, Showing original displacement of sternal end of clavicle. B, Removal of sternal end.

advise enough restriction of activity to minimize the discomfort. At this time local measures, such as corticoid injections, are palliative only. This is not to say that operative reconstruction should never be attempted. However, we usually reserve reconstruction for those cases marked by disabling pain as a result of the displacement. One of the most successful procedures to relieve pain in frank dislocation is resection of the inner end of the clavicle proximal to the costoclavicular attachment (Fig. 46, B). If the costoclavicular ligament is torn or redundant, an attempt should be made to reconstruct it.

REGION OF THE CLAVICULAR SHAFT

CONTUSION

The portion of the clavicle lying between the coracoclavicular ligament attachment, which coincides with the beginning of the distal flat portion of the clavicle, and the proximal expansion leading to the sternoclavicular joint is designated as the shaft of the clavicle. Since the clavicular shaft is subcutaneous it is subject to contusion, the skin and periosteum over the clavicle being impinged between the hard bone and the striking object. The injury is ordinarily readily recognizable because of local swelling. Hematoma formation may occur but it is not common in this area. Infiltration of blood into the skin and subcutaneous tissue usually occurs. Following a severe contusion the possibility of an injury to the underlying bone must always be considered. This can be settled fairly well by physical examination since fracture of the clavicle usually will result in considerable pain on any attempt to move the shoulder whereas simple contusion will not be painful on motion. Later, when there is diffuse swelling and blood infiltration, there may be pain on motion and the exact diagnosis will be more difficult. In case of doubt, x-ray will help to confirm the diagnosis.

There is nothing out of the ordinary about the *treatment* of contusion in this area. The usual measures are local injection, compression, cold and later heat. Simple contusion will require relatively little immobilization of the shoulder and by proper padding athletic participation may be continued. Continuation of pain on use of the shoulder should arouse suspicion of a greater injury and x-ray 10 to 14 days subsequent to the injury will often be enlightening even though early films have been negative. Incomplete fractures may be revealed by early callus formation or by signs of absorption at the fracture line.

FRACTURE

Fracture of the clavicle is a frequent athletic injury. It is much more likely to occur in the preadolescent or adolescent youngster than in the adult. In the adult, ligament injury either at the inner or outer end of the clavicle is more likely to occur than in the youngster. A detailed description of the various types of fracture of the clavicle will not be given here but a few generalities peculiar to athletic injury will be stated.

Treatment.   In the young individual, fracture of the clavicle is frequently green-stick in character and is as a rule relatively simple to treat. In a fracture of the clavicle in a patient under 10 or 12, open reduction is seldom indicated unless there is some complication. It is my belief that deformity should be corrected, that green-stick angulation should be reduced, that an attempt should be made to reduce the transverse fracture and that in the oblique or comminuted fracture in a child the shoulder should be held well back in order to prevent shortening of the bone. True enough, the youngster has great compensatory capacity and one may accept positions that would be intolerable in the adult. This should not be taken as an excuse for sloppy care and every effort should be made to restore the alignment and length of the clavicle to normal even though this requires anesthesia. The fracture will not ordinarily require open reduction since it is not necessary to have end-to-end apposition so long as length is reasonably well maintained. It should be emphasized that these statements apply to children and that the term "children" refers to bone age rather than to chronological age. The 13 year old girl with a fractured clavicle should be treated as an adult since her bone growth may well be

Figure 47.   *A,* Showing the fracture proximal to the coracoclavicular ligaments. Note particularly the upward riding of the proximal fragment and the normal relationship between the distal fragment and the scapula. It is virtually impossible to reduce and hold this fracture without internal fixation since the shoulder tends to fall downward and the proximal fragment to ride upward.

B, In this case fixation was intramedullary with the partially threaded pin left protruding under the skin proximally. This permits better motion of the shoulder than if the pin protrudes distally. The pin is removed after union is complete. The open epiphysis of the humerus indicates that the patient is an adolescent. Nonetheless, open reduction was indicated.

Figure 48.   Fracture at the junction of the outer and middle third of the clavicle proximal to the coracoclavicular ligament, held by intramedullary wire fixation. Comminuted butterfly fragments were held by two stainless steel wire loops. There was no damage to the ligaments of the shoulder.

almost completed. The husky six foot boy of 14 may have bones quite comparable to the average male of 16 or 17. One only deludes himself if he expects compensatory correction of a deformity in a person whose bone growth is relatively complete. I have no hesitation in advising open reduction of a fractured clavicle in a teenager if he is approaching the end of his growth period.

It should also be pointed out that an athlete does have certain important characteristics. In the first place, he is healthy and strong. In the second place, his skeletal structures must be restored to normal if possible. In the third place, healing time is vitally important. These factors must be considered in selecting the method of treatment of fracture of the shaft of the clavicle. My own preference in athletes of high school age or over is open reduction, with internal fixation by intramedullary pinning which is later removed (Fig. 47). This permits early mobility of the shoulder, prevents atrophy of muscle and stiffness of the joints. It does demand the ultimate in surgical technique and asepsis. One must have available a strong, healthy patient, intact uninfected skin, a qualified anesthetist, a first class surgical facility, proper tools and last but not least a capable surgeon. Lacking any one of these, conservative treatment is preferable.

On occasion comminution at the fracture site will make it advisable to support the intramedullary rod by wire sutures looped around the fragment. The wire sutures alone are usually not secure enough to permit the free use of the arm possible with the intramedullary rod (Fig. 48). In any event, the arm should be immobilized in a sling with a swathe (Fig. 49) for at least a couple of weeks to permit the local reaction to subside. The patient is encouraged to wear the sling alone for another two weeks and given permission to take it off ad lib. He should wear the sling while carrying out ordinary activities.

Figure 49.   Sling and swathe. General utility dressing for shoulder fixation. This does not give adequate support for acromioclavicular sprain or dislocation. It is ideal for more moderate injuries, for postoperative care, etc. Note the hand is supported in the triangular sling, yet is free for movement of the elbow and utilization of the fingers. The circular adhesive strip is double thickness and is placed over gauze to avoid irritating the skin of the chest wall. This circular swathe limits external rotation and abduction to any desired amount, depending upon its tightness.

REGION OF THE OUTER END OF THE CLAVICLE

ANATOMICAL CONSIDERATIONS

At the outer end of the clavicle an ingenious arrangement of bone and ligament promotes stability between the clavicle and scapula and prevents the clavicle from displacing upward but at the same time permits a wide range of motion of the upper extremity (Fig. 40). The outer end of the clavicle butts against the anteromedial aspect of the acromion and is firmly bound to the acromion by the *acromioclavicular* ligaments (capsular ligaments). A wedge-shaped fibrocartilaginous articular disc formed by a thickening of the anterosuperior part of the capsular ligament extends downward into the joint. It lies between the upper portion of the outer end of the clavicle and the acromion. This is sometimes referred to as the semilunar cartilage of the shoulder. The top of the shoulder presents a U-shaped bony subcutaneous surface, the anterior wing of the "U" beginning as the flat outer end of the clavicle, crossing the acromioclavicular joint and extending to the flat anterior process of the acromion which makes the bottom of the "U," directed laterally. The posterior wing of the "U" is the spine of the scapula which extends from the acromion transversely across the broadest portion of the scapula to blend into its vertebral border. This whole bony "U" is subcutaneous (Fig. 50).

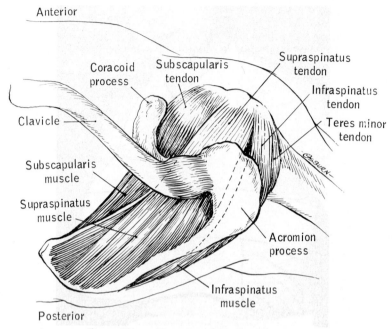

Figure 50.   Top view of the shoulder joint.

The acromioclavicular ligaments surround the joint but run in an almost horizontal direction in the anatomical position so that they are well designed to prevent
distraction of the two bones but are poorly designed to prevent upward displacement of the clavicle on the acromion. The ligaments between the clavicle and the
coracoid process of the scapula make up for this deficiency. The coracoid process
extends forward from the scapula much as a pointing finger crooked slightly laterally. It lies directly underneath the clavicle, being separated from it by approximately ½ inch. The long axes of the two bones are at right angles. The ligaments
arising along the superior surface of the coracoid twist approximately 90 degrees to
attach along the undersurface of the clavicle as a broad, flat band with different divisions, the trapezoid attaching most distally, the conoid proximally. Actually, these
are usually indistinguishable after an injury. These ligaments have a much more
vertical course than the acromioclavicular ligaments and effectively hold the clavicle
down to the scapula.

From the anterior portion of the coracoid the *coraco-acromial* ligament extends
upward and laterally to attach to the top of the acromion in front. This ligament
plays no part in acromioclavicular stability but actually serves to reinforce the
glenohumeral joint in front. The section of the clavicle from the conoid portion of
the coracoclavicular ligament to its distal end is called the *interligamentary* portion.
In this region it is a broad, flat bone with no medullary canal. Proximal to this the
clavicle becomes rounded and takes on the typical characteristics of a long bone.
The upper surfaces of the clavicle and the acromion together with the spine of the
scapula form the superior portion of the shoulder and are subcutaneous.

CONTUSION

The top of the shoulder is frequently contused. Because of the subcutaneous character of the bone there is often a subperiosteal hematoma and even more frequently rather severe damage to the skin. Contusion here is treated as in other areas. The major problem is to determine whether or not there is more serious injury to the underlying structures. One should locate accurately the area of contusion and by careful examination determine whether or not there is involvement of the acromioclavicular joint. In such a case the contusion may be entirely incidental.

SPRAIN-SUBLUXATION-DISLOCATION

Since there is no "built-in" bony stability between the acromion and clavicle, it follows that the entire integrity of this joint is maintained by ligamentous support. A sprain of these ligaments is caused by anything that forces the acromioclavicular joint through a range of motion beyond its normal capacity. Normally this joint has but little excursion. The acromioclavicular ligaments completely surrounding the joint permit only a certain degree of rocking motion but allow no actual flexion or extension.

Various forces may cause injury to the acromioclavicular joint. The most common is a downward blow against the outer end of the shoulder driving the acromion downward, the clavicle remaining upward. Another is traction on the arm pulling the shoulder away from the chest wall and causing true lateral displacement of the acromion. Neither of these, however, can adequately account for the instances of injury to this area caused by falling on the outstretched arm or on the point of the elbow. The football player is well protected by shoulder pads from a downward blow against the top of the shoulder. The sport most commonly involved in this type of force is polo where the horseman falls and lands on the unprotected point of the shoulder. I believe the mechanism causing the majority of these injuries in football is falling on the outstretched hand or flexed elbow with the arm flexed forward 90 degrees and in neutral lateral position. In this position the humerus drives against the glenoid and acromion, pushing them forcibly backward, and the clavicle remains forward so that stress is applied upon the acromioclavicular and also the coracoclavicular ligaments. This same mechanism could well cause an isolated injury to the acromioclavicular ligament by rotation of the scapula to permit the acromion to move backward while the coracoid either remains in normal relationship with the clavicle or actually rotates forward. As these various forces occur, stress is applied to the acromioclavicular ligament which permits a certain amount of upward displacement of the outer end of the clavicle. The tension is then taken on the coracoclavicular ligaments. Either of these may be injured to a variable degree.

Mild Ligament Sprain

In a mild sprain the force is contained before any real damage is done. There is moderate tearing of the fibers of the acromioclavicular or coracoclavicular ligament. In this case there is little or no disability of the shoulder. There is localized pain over the area of injury. This pain may be directly over the acromioclavicular joint or may be medial to the acromioclavicular joint just in front of the clavicle in the sulcus between the clavicle and the coracoid. In the well muscled individual this may be difficult to elicit by palpation. The differentiation between a mild sprain and a contusion is extremely difficult since a mild sprain does not entail any hypermobility and indeed ordinary motions of the shoulder girdle will elicit no pain.

Treatment here is relatively unimportant and indeed treatment of contusion and sprain may be quite similar, that is, local injection into the tender area, cold followed by heat, and the use of padding to protect from a blow rather than to restrict motion.

Moderate Ligament Sprain

In a moderate sprain of these ligaments we predicate relatively severe damage to the fibers of the ligament and in this case the symptoms will be more pronounced. Since there has been tearing of some of the ligament fibers there will be pain on forced motion of the shoulder even though there is no actual hypermobility of the clavicle on the acromion. In such a case we do not expect the clavicle to be riding high. There will be pain, swelling and tenderness, with the pain increased by an attempt to separate the acromion and clavicle by pulling on the arm. There is also pain on depressing the acromion in relation to the clavicle by pulling straight down on the arm with the arm against the side. This case can be distinguished from contusion by the severity of the symptoms and their aggravation when the ligament is placed under stress. Within a short time there will be local swelling at the joint which may simulate upward displacement of the clavicle.

Treatment of a moderate sprain of the acromioclavicular or coracoclavicular ligaments should be local and general. Local treatment is the same as for mild sprain; i.e., local injection of procaine plus hyaluronidase, application of cold followed by heat, pressure dressing in case of swelling. Protective treatment here is all-important since it is vital to prevent subsequent injury. One must visualize that a definite portion of the ligament is torn or avulsed and that the remaining portion is substantially weakened. If athletic participation is permitted in contact sports the next blow may well complete the tear.

It is important that the arm be strapped to the side in such a way as to push the arm upward and the clavicle downward. This can be done by various methods. One of the simplest and best for this type of injury is as follows. With the arm at the side and the elbow flexed to 90 degrees, the midpoint of a long strip of 3 inch tape is placed under the forearm about 2 inches distal to the elbow and carried forward up over the shoulder proximal to the acromioclavicular joint and then down the back, crossing toward the opposite side. The posterior portion of the long strip should go up the back of the arm, cross over the shoulder from back to front, then diagonally across the chest again medial to the acromioclavicular joint (Fig. 51, *A*). The dressing is completed by a circumferential strip of protective tape placed around the arm and the chest to hold the arm to the side (Fig. 51, *B*). These are the key straps of the dressing. The dressing is made more comfortable by suspending the forearm loosely in a choker type sling made of elastic stockinette around the wrist and behind the neck (Fig. 51, *C*). Additional adhesive strapping can be applied for compression directly over the shoulder if desirable. The principle

Figure 51. A, The vertical strip which holds the humerus upward and the clavicle downward. Note particularly the length of the strip since it extends from the waist line in the back to the waist line in front as a single strip. Note the leverage action as the hand and forearm drop downward at the waist, the short lever of the inner end of the ulna pushing the humerus upward.

B, The application of a tape swathe to hold the elbow to the side. This strip should not be tight. Before this strip is applied, a powdered ABD pad is placed in the axilla.

C, Choker sling of stockinette is added. This sling is loose and may be changed from the hand to the wrist or eliminated altogether as the patient wishes. Some of the details to note are the felt pads (here used with blue felt for contrast) to protect the skin at the pressure areas; also the felt pads within the stockinette back of the neck and under the hand.

Figure 52. Modification of dressing shown in Figure 51 which we often use post-operatively. In this instance the initial application is the pressure dressing over the wound and top of the shoulder using elastoplast. The second step is the application of a triangular sling carefully pinned around the elbow. Step 3 is the application of a swathe around the body to hold the arm to the side. The dressing is stabilized then by the vertical strip applied as in Figure 51, only over the dressing rather than over the skin.

of this support is that, as the weight of the forearm and hand drops distally, the lever fulcrum is at the broad band of the tape under the proximal forearm and the short posterior arm of the lever tends to thrust the humerus upward as the hand drops downward. There are obviously many modifications of this type of support and any one that effectively holds the clavicle down and the arm up is satisfactory (Fig. 52).

This type of support is continued a minimum of four weeks in order to permit the ligaments to unite and become relatively strong. It should be borne in mind that the simple force of the weight of the arm hanging at the side may be sufficient to distract the ligament ends. A period of rehabilitation will be required in order to mobilize the shoulder and improve the muscle tone in the upper extremity before participation in sports is advisable. Such a plan carefully followed will result in complete recovery from a rather severe sprain whereas if continued function is permitted the ligaments will gradually stretch and result in a loose acromioclavicular joint which is subject to either chronic disability or repeated injury.

Severe Ligament Sprain (Subluxation-Dislocation)

Severe ligament sprain is one in which one or more of the ligaments have been completely torn. It can be classified roughly into two categories: (1) complete tear of the acromioclavicular ligament with the coracoclavicular ligament intact and (2) a complete tear of the coracoclavicular and acromioclavicular ligaments.

Severe Sprain of the Acromioclavicular Ligament. It is possible for a complete tear of the acromioclavicular ligament to occur along with an incomplete tear of the coracoclavicular ligament. The force applied here is downward on the acromion and usually has an outward component so that the acromion is forced outward and downward away from the clavicle. This causes rupture of the horizontal fibers extending from the clavicle to the acromion. The resulting symptoms depend to some extent on the degree of injury to the coracoclavicular ligaments. If this is slight and largely of the distal component the symptoms will be those of moderate sprain, that is, local pain, swelling, and tenderness in the acromioclavicular joint. There will be pain on any effort to distract this joint or on downward pull on the arm or on manipulation of the shoulder toward wide abduction. There will frequently be a mild degree of instability between the outer end of the clavicle and acromion with the clavicle appearing to be slightly higher than the acromion. The space between the clavicle and acromion may well be widened in comparison to the normal or to the opposite shoulder. There will not be extensive upward riding of the clavicle in relation to the acromion. This cannot take place with intact coracoclavicular ligaments. One may visualize that there has been complete rupture of some of the fibers of the acromioclavicular ligament but that the scapula has rotated downward rather than displaced downward. The coracoclavicular ligament is still effective in holding the clavicle in its normal position in relation to the acromion.

TREATMENT of this type of acromioclavicular injury taxes the best judgment. Far too often the injury is treated by the so-called conservative method with resulting chronic relaxation of the acromioclavicular joint, arthritic changes and disability which may later require surgery. On the other hand, one hesitates to perform an open repair in the absence of upward displacement of the clavicle. Local treatment consists of the usual measures: aspiration, injection, cold then heat. The subluxation should be reduced by downward pressure on the clavicle and upward pressure on the arm. The temptation then is to maintain this reduction by external fixation and this is usually done by the method previously described (Fig. 51). That this is often ineffectual is indicated by the wide variety of methods suggested as improvements, i.e., support in a plaster jacket with straps over the clavicle in order to hold it down and various other lever actions designed to hold the acromion and clavicle together. In the final analysis I think surgical intervention is probably desirable in the majority of cases in the young athlete. If one can obtain complete reduction manually it would indicate there is no interposing tissue between the two bones. It is justifiable then to attempt skeletal fixation by pins through the acromion and into the clavicle without open reduction. Proper positioning of the pins is extremely difficult and this method is not for the uninitiated. However, the operator who has repeatedly inserted these pins at open reduction may be able to place two pins in a position adequate to hold the bones together. Some sort of threaded pin is desirable since it is important to prevent distraction of the acromion from the clavicle as well as to hold the clavicle down.

Complete Rupture of the Acromioclavicular and Coracoclavicular Ligaments. The second type of severe sprain presumes a complete rupture of both the acromioclavicular and coracoclavicular ligaments (Fig. 53). In this injury the local symptoms are more severe, there is more swelling, more tenderness, and pain is elicited on any manipulation of the shoulder. The characteristic finding, however, is marked

Figure 53. Complete acromioclavicular dislocation with obvious tearing of both ligaments. Note particularly the wide space between the coracoid and clavicle with the clavicle riding high above the acromion. The x-ray was made with the patient standing but with no weight.

Figure 54. Shows dramatically the upward displacement of the outer end of the clavicle in complete acromioclavicular dislocation. (From DePalma, "Fractures and Dislocations—An Atlas," Vol. 1, p. 227.)

upward riding of the outer end of the clavicle in relation to the scapula (Fig. 54). This may be quite obvious in clinical examination of the patient. When care is taken to examine him sitting up, if swelling is not severe the outer end of the clavicle can be felt and seen pushing up under the skin while the acromion remains downward. This finding may be completely obscured when the patient is lying supine but when he stands (Fig. 55), particularly with some weight in the hand, it becomes quite obvious. Comparable pictures of the two shoulders in the standing position will reveal the displacement. In this instance the displacement of the clavi-

Figure 55. A, With the patient supine, no dislocation is noted. B, Standing with 4 pounds suspended from the wrist. Note particularly the widening at the acromioclavicular joint and also difference in distance between the clavicle and coracoid. This is not as dramatic as Figure 53 but comparison with the supine position makes it quite obvious.

cle is primarily upward, whereas in the other type of subluxation the acromion pulls away from the outer end of the clavicle rather than downward. However, both types of displacement may well be present.

TREATMENT.   Although this dislocation is usually readily reduced, it is virtually impossible to hold reduction in a manner that will allow primary repair of the torn ligaments at their normal length. When one visualizes the pathologic changes this is readily apparent. In order for the clavicle to displace upward, the distance between the clavicle and coracoid must be increased (Fig. 53). The coracoclavicular and acromioclavicular ligaments are avulsed or torn and, unless the clavicle is held in the anatomical position until healing is complete, subluxation will inevitably recur and a painful, weak shoulder will be the result. For this reason it is my opinion that in the athlete a complete tear of these ligaments should be treated by surgical repair.

Again, we are faced with two alternatives. Once surgery has been decided upon, one must decide whether his operation should be designed merely to hold the clavicle in position or to repair the torn ligaments as well. It is my belief that if one is going to go to the trouble to carry out an open operation to fix the clavicle in position he should take advantage of this opportunity to appose and suture the torn ends of the coracoclavicular ligaments. In the ordinary case this can readily be accomplished since, after the skin is divided and the outer end of the clavicle is freed from its muscle attachments, the outer end may readily be displaced upward. Ready access can be had to the area of the injury between the clavicle and coracoid, and in most instances sutures can be placed in the coracoclavicular ligaments while the clavicle is displaced upward and can be tied after replacement of the clavicle and fixation in its normal position.

Figure 56.   Illustrating fixation across the acromioclavicular joint with two partially threaded pins. This is an old case as indicated by the calcification about the clavicle and it was felt advisable to resect ⅜ inch of the outer end of the clavicle. Wider resection than this is neither necessary nor desirable. Note the close approximation of the clavicle and coracoid. These pins should be removed after 8 to 10 weeks.

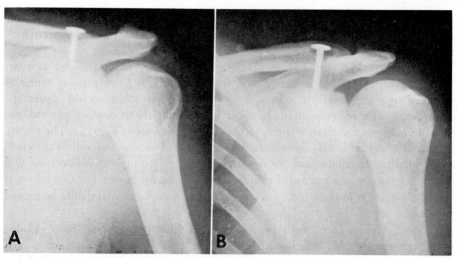

Figure 57.   Acromioclavicular dislocation treated by Bosworth screw. *A*, Postoperative picture. *B*, Follow-up picture showing marked reaction and absorption about the head of the screw. This type of fixation should be removed after healing.

Figure 58.   *A*, Showing fixation of outer end clavicle by braided silk through drill hole in clavicle. This is a late postoperative picture and is quite suggestive of erosion of the suture. *B*, Complete erosion through the clavicle with pathological fracture. *C*, After removal of the outer end of the clavicle.

Of vital importance following this operative procedure is firm fixation of the clavicle to the scapula. This can be done by various methods depending upon the choice of the surgeon. Basically the methods of fixation are either by transfixion of the acromion and clavicle or by fixation of the clavicle to the coracoid, or by both. The best method for fixing the clavicle to the acromion is the use of transfixion pins, preferably threaded at least in part, passing through the acromion across the joint and into the clavicle. It is necessary to use two pins since one may not give sufficient fixation (Fig. 56). If this is done, no fixation is needed between the coracoid and the clavicle other than the ligament repair.

Other methods of holding the coracoid and clavicle together are the Bosworth screw which transfixes the clavicle (Fig. 57) and extends into the coracoid, and suture around the coracoid and clavicle with fascia, braided silk or wire. There are some disadvantages in each method. My own preference is for acromioclavicular transfixion following suture of the coracoclavicular ligament, as previously described.

After threaded pin fixation is completed the acromioclavicular ligament should be carefully repaired. Strong internal fixation permits rapid mobilization of the shoulder joint and so shortens the period of disability. It is advisable for the arm to

Figure 59.   A, Acromioclavicular joint fixed by single nonthreaded pin. B. Migration of this pin—fortunately after healing of the ligaments. This could have been prevented by having a portion of the pin threaded. It is inadvisable to have the threaded part of the pin across the joint because it may break through the threaded area. Migration can also be prevented by bending the end of the pin.

be held in a sling for several weeks. This will permit active motion but protects against unguarded activity. Any type of metallic internal fixation should be removed after eight weeks. This includes the Bosworth screw which may work loose and break, the circumferential suture or wire which may erode through the clavicle (Fig. 58), and the transfixion pins which after a certain period may migrate (Fig. 59). Following successful repair with a good functional result, the patient may resume unlimited activity. It is wise for him to wear particularly well designed shoulder pads after such an injury. However, the best the shoulder pad can do is to protect the shoulder against a direct blow. It has no effect on forces which are transmitted through the arm.

CHRONIC LESIONS OF THE ACROMIOCLAVICULAR JOINT

A chronic irritative lesion of the acromioclavicular joint can be the consequence of repeated injuries which cause the acromion and clavicle to impinge forcibly (Fig. 60, A). Repeated minor sprains of the capsular ligament that result in thickening of the ligament and local swelling in the joint are another cause of this condition. It may go on to calcific deposits within the ligament or joint. There may be involvement of the intra-articular fibrocartilage, even with calcification or

Figure 60. *A,* Irritative lesion of the acromioclavicular joint with chronic arthritis. There appears to be some subluxation of the clavicle upward although the space between the coracoid and clavicle seems quite narrow. *B,* Shows resection of the outer end of the clavicle distal to the coracoclavicular ligaments.

Figure 61.   X-ray of the acromioclavicular joint showing calcification of the capsule and cartilage.

fragmentation of the cartilage (Fig. 61). The result is pain and tenderness particularly elicited by abduction of the arm as this movement forces the acromion and clavicle together.

TREATMENT.   This condition is basically a traumatic arthritis and may be treated as such by local heat, rest, injection of a long-acting local anesthetic and a corticoid preparation. It may be quite distressing since it is magnified by athletic activity such as throwing, falling on the outstretched hand or in fact any forceful activity of the shoulder girdle. If it does not respond adequately to nonsurgical treatment, surgery is justified. At this time the fibrocartilaginous disc should be removed and the joint carefully inspected. If there are definite irreversible changes in the articular cartilage it is wise to resect ½ or ¾ inch of the outer end of the clavicle (Fig. 60, B). Care should be taken to stay distal to the coracoclavicular ligament. This usually will give excellent results with essentially normal function of the shoulder.

FRACTURE

By "outer end of the clavicle" I am referring to that area lying distal to the coracoclavicular ligaments. This part of the clavicle is a broad, flat bone without a distinct medullary canal. The forces likely to cause a fracture of the clavicle in this area may be the same as those causing ligament injury. As the acromion is driven downward in relation to the clavicle the coracoclavicular as well as the acromioclavicular ligaments may remain intact and the bone will break proximal to the coracoclavicular ligaments. This will be a fracture of the shaft of the clavicle (Fig. 47), usually in the outer part of the middle third of the bone. In this instance the distal fragment will remain in normal relationship to the scapula while the proximal fragment rides upward. While this fracture is not actually one of the outer end of the clavicle, it does require mention here since it is virtually impossible to reduce and hold this fracture without some form of internal fixation. In the previous discussion of dislocation of the outer end of the clavicle, mention was made of the difficulty of holding the clavicle down in spite of the fact that its entire length was intact for the application of direct pressure downward. When the fracture is just proximal to the coracoclavicular ligaments the sharp distal end of the proximal fragment is not only short but it lies close to the neck and is not amenable to fixation by direct pressure. This type of fracture is best treated by intramedullary fixation following open reduction. To some extent these same principles apply to any fracture of the middle third of the clavicle but they are particularly pertinent as the ligamentous area is approached.

Another combination of forces may cause the fracture to be distal (Figs. 62 and 63) to the coracoclavicular ligaments and so be an *interligamentary* fracture. In this instance, as the acromion is driven downward the acromioclavicular ligaments remain intact but the coracoclavicular ligaments rupture. The fracture occurs within the flat distal portion of the clavicle. The distal fragment accompanies the acromion and is displaced downward; the proximal fragment displaces upward. The important consideration in this fracture as compared to the one previously described is that in the first instance the coracoclavicular ligaments remain intact and so the outer end of the clavicle remains securely fastened to the scapula. After reduction or internal fixation of the two fragments the acromioclavicular area is secure. In the instance under consideration the coracoclavicular ligaments are ruptured and fixation of the clavicle to the scapula is impaired.

This type of injury also requires open reduction, at which time some effort should be made to repair the coracoclavicular ligaments. The fracture line may be at any level between the two ligaments. If the distal fragment is small and involves only the outer 1 inch of the clavicle, it is preferable to remove the fragment, repair the coracoclavicular ligaments and thus shorten the healing period and diminish the probability of pain at the acromioclavicular joint following recovery. This is

Figure 62.   Comminuted fracture of the outer end of the clavicle in adult female. Note the distal portion is fragmented and remains intact to the acromion while the proximal just rides upward. There must be rupture of the coracoclavicular ligament.

Figure 63.   A, Anteroposterior view of outer end of the clavicle showing no evidence of injury. Clinical diagnosis of fracture led to vertical x-ray (B) which revealed interligamentary fracture.

particularly pertinent if a comminuted fracture involves the articular portion of the outer end of the clavicle. In many instances a small fragment will remain attached to the acromioclavicular ligament. This should by all means be removed. The surgeon must rely upon his good judgment as to whether in a given case it would be better to obtain bony fixation or to remove the fragments. As a rule of thumb, one might say that if he can obtain adequate surgical repair of the coracoclavicular ligaments there will be less necessity for bony union between the two fragments and thus the distal fragment might well be removed. Similarly, if the distal fragment is small or comminuted, bony security between the two fragments is not readily obtainable anyway and these fragments would be best removed. On the contrary, if ligament repair seems insecure the additional security of bony union in order to take advantage of the stability of the acromioclavicular ligament is important and one would prefer to leave the fragment in.

Interligamentary fractures may also be the result of a direct blow. In such a case the fracture line may be of any character. It may be comminuted, oblique, spiral or transverse, but is most frequently either oblique from above, downward and inward, or comminuted. Since both the acromioclavicular and coracoclavicular ligaments are intact, any extensive degree of displacement is unusual in this fracture by direct blow. Treatment in this instance will be by a sling with an adhesive strap placed under the elbow and around the distal end of the clavicle suitably padded with felt in order to maintain some direct pressure on the fractured area (Fig. 51).

It will thus be seen that from the standpoint of treatment it is quite important to distinguish between an interligamentary fracture by direct trauma of the bone and one caused by disrupting forces applied indirectly. In those caused by direct trauma, treatment requires only a relatively short period of external fixation whereas in the other types with ligament damage, open reduction is the treatment of choice. If open reduction for some reason cannot be carried out, then the same type of fixation should be used as was mentioned in relation to dislocations of the outer end of the clavicle, namely, the type of support that is designed to push the humerus upward and the clavicle downward (Fig. 51).

Rehabilitation is extremely important in these injuries and it will proceed much faster if there is good internal fixation of the bones. Needless to say, athletic

Figure 64.   Comminuted fracture of surgical neck of the humerus and greater
tuberosity without displacement. Note, however, avulsion fracture of the coracoid process which
was pulled off by the conjoined tendon of the short head of the biceps, coracobrachialis,
pectoralis minor. This was reduced and held by screw fixation, the whole shoulder then being
treated by sling only.

competition should not be permitted until healing is complete. In the case of torn
ligaments this will require six to eight weeks; in case of fractures somewhat longer
depending upon the progress of healing as checked by x-ray examination.

It should be remembered in any discussion of injuries about the shoulder that
the ligament attachments in tearing away may include a fragment of bone, the so-
called *avulsion* fractures. These should be treated basically as a ligament injury.
For example, the coracoid may be pulled off by the coracoclavicular ligament (Fig.
64), the small fragment of the proximal end of the clavicle may be torn off by the
sternoclavicular ligament, or a segment of the acromion or distal end of the clavicle
may be avulsed by the acromioclavicular ligament. In each instance the treatment
is basically that of ligament injury. In the majority of instances it is advisable to
remove the fragment unless it is large enough to allow its fixation to the parent
bone, in which case the additional stability gained by the fragment may be of considerable value. This is particularly pertinent at the inner end of the clavicle where
it is difficult to hold the clavicle down by ordinary suture through the ligament and
the firmly fixed proximal fragment may be utilized to fasten the clavicle down.

Fracture of the Acromion

Many of the same forces that fracture the outer end of the clavicle may also
fracture the acromial process. By far the most frequent force is direct trauma which
simply breaks off the end of the bone at any point distal to its attachment to the
body of the scapula through the spine of the scapula. These fractures are usually
without gross displacement and usually require little treatment in themselves. It is
important to recognize such a fracture. A fracture without displacement may not
be well visualized in the ordinary x-ray view and it may be necessary to take a vertical view through the distal end of the acromion to show it (Fig. 65). If there is
any question, repeated x-ray pictures are important. Many of these cases will be
diagnosed as a contusion and the fracture is recognized only after the "contusion"
has failed to heal within a reasonable period of time.

Figure 65.   Transverse fracture across the acromial process by direct downward force
against the acromion.

Treatment.   In the unusual case in which there is nonunion of the fracture
of the acromion, the distal fragment can usually be removed without serious disability to the shoulder if the deltoid muscle is sutured to the remaining stump.
Indeed, if the acute fracture involves as little as ½ inch of the distal end of the acromion, the best treatment will be excision of the fragment since healing will be much
more rapid and with much less likelihood of any residual complication.

Occasionally the acromion may be fractured by indirect force caused by
upward dislocation of the humerus against the acromial process (Fig. 66). This
usually is a major injury and will require specialized treatment. Frequently open
reduction is necessary because of the probability of soft tissue interposition preventing reduction of the dislocation. More frequently the force will cause subluxation
only. The fracture will be incomplete. Again treatment is dependent on recognition of the injury and requires some degree of protection of the arm against wide
abduction. If displacement is gross, open reduction is advisable. At operation the
fragment may be removed if small. If it is larger, open reduction and threaded wire
fixation may be carried out.

Figure 66.   Dislocation of the glenohumeral joint with fractured acromion. It is
unusual to get this picture since the dislocation is usually spontaneously reduced and the
severity of injury may well be overlooked.
(From McLaughlin, "Trauma," p. 263.)

REGION OF THE BODY OF THE SCAPULA

CONTUSION

The only area of the scapula that is commonly subject to contusion is its spine from the vertebral border to the tip of the acromion. This area is entirely subcutaneous and the skin may be severely contused between the underlying bone and the external blow. There may be a contusion of the bone. The diagnosis is readily made on the basis of the local reaction to the lesion with tenderness directly along the bone, usually sharply localized. Ordinary motions of the shoulder or scapula will not be painful in simple contusion. In case of a severe injury, x-ray visualization may be necessary to eliminate the possibility of a fracture of the spine of the scapula. It may be necessary to get tangential views in order to visualize the fracture line. In contact sports such as football, this area is very adequately protected by shoulder pads and so is infrequently hurt. *Treatment* is the application of cold, then heat, local injection and protective padding. With adequate padding, no interruption of participation in competitive sports need be expected from this type of injury.

The muscles overlying the scapula may be subject to contusion by a direct blow catching the muscle between the hard underlying bone and the striking force. This may be distinguished from other injuries by the localization of the tenderness plus pain on active contraction or passive stretching of the involved muscle. *Treatment* consists of cold, followed by heat, local injection and rest. It is unusual for calcification to occur following contusion of the muscles about the scapula.

STRAIN

The area of the scapula is quite subject to strain since the entire bone serves for the origin or insertion of many muscles. In many instances extremely powerful muscles may attach throughout a relatively small area (Fig. 67). Thus, it may be possible for the powerful latissimus dorsi muscle to avulse its attachment from the inferior angle. This may cause avulsion of the bone but more commonly a simple strain with rupture of some of the fibers at their attachment to the bone. A similar injury may occur at the superior angle of the scapula where the levator scapulae and rhomboideus minor may be subject to the same type of injury. Less frequently there may be injury in the region of the trapezius along the spine of the scapula or of the teres minor or triceps. Similarly, there may be damage to the rhomboideus major at its attachment along the vertebral border.

Acute Strain

All of these injuries are caused by violent muscle action and for this reason treatment must provide restriction of function of the muscle involved. In an acute injury *treatment* consists of local application of cold followed later by heat, injection of a local anesthetic plus hyaluronidase into the hematoma, and restriction of function of the muscle that has been damaged. The last can be carried out by placing the arm in a sling, which moderately restricts the activity of the arm. If the injury is severe, athletic competition is interdicted. Healing usually takes place without major definitive treatment. However, if a detectable fragment of bone is avulsed through an appreciable distance, one should seriously consider early removal of the fragment of bone and suture of the muscle to the fractured bed (Fig. 67). While this may seem a little radical in a situation in which spontaneous healing will probably take place, one must bear in mind that these situations involving actual separation of an avulsed fragment of bone frequently lead to nonunion with persistent pain. The athlete may better accept surgical treatment entailing a few weeks of early complete disability but offering the opportunity for more complete recovery rather than months or years of disability of a lower grade. This is particularly pertinent when one considers that the best nonsurgical treatment also should entail complete rest.

Chronic Strain

These same areas in the scapula may be involved in chronic irritative lesions with chronic strain of the various muscle attachments. In this situation ordinary

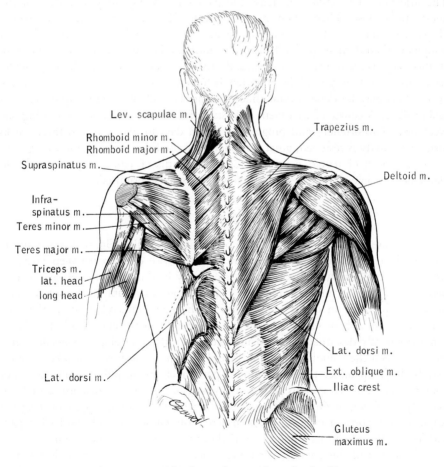

Figure 67.   Muscle attachments about the shoulder.

function of the muscle is usually pain-free. Violent exercise, particularly against resistance, causes recurrence of the symptoms of pain, muscle spasm and restriction of motion. This is the same type of chronic strain that may occur at the attachment of the tendo achillis or at the epicondyles of the elbow or in the hamstrings. *Treatment* may be extremely discouraging since resumption of forceful activity will often cause recurrence of symptoms. Fortunately, this is uncommon around the scapula. A period of complete rest together with repeated local injection of long-acting anesthetic plus a corticoid preparation may be rewarding if continued over a long enough period. Great care must be used that function is actually restricted to that tolerated by the muscle without increasing the irritation.

In the type of case just described the general plan of treatment would be as follows: Every effort is made to pin-point exactly the location of the lesion. This area is then injected with a local anesthetic. If this completely relieves the pain during the effective period of the anesthetic, one may feel confident that he has reached the area involved and may then proceed with local injection of a corticoid preparation. Following these measures, local inductive heat as by diathermy, microtherm or ultrasound should be utilized once or twice daily for 20 minutes. The injection may actually increase the pain immediately after the effect of the anesthetic is lost. There then may be 12 to 36 hours of acute exacerbation of pain, ofttimes to the extent that sedation is required. The pain and other symptoms should then gradually subside until marked improvement is obtained. If this improvement persists for several days but the symptoms then gradually recur, the injection should be repeated before the symptoms become too severe again. This may be done several times so long as gradual overall improvement is taking place. A course of treatment consists of four to six injections beginning one week apart (no oftener) and progressing to ten days to two weeks to three weeks apart. As activity is resumed, great care should be used that rehabilitation progresses below the level of irritative activity. Several months of pain-free activity should elapse before violent exercise of the involved muscle is permitted.

BURSITIS

There are many bursae around the body of the scapula (Fig. 68), since bursae are found in any area where friction would otherwise develop between layers of tissue. One can readily appreciate their frequency in this area of excessive motion between the various muscles attaching to the scapula. Probably the most constant bursa, except those in direct relationship to the glenohumeral joint, is that one lying between the body of the scapula and the muscles of the chest wall. This bursa is not frequently described anatomically and may indeed develop as a result of irritation between the scapula and the muscles following some type of injury. A bursa may be high up under the supraspinous portion of the scapula or may be lower lying beneath the infraspinous part. Symptoms of bursitis in this area are related particularly to motion of the scapula against the chest wall so that approximating the scapulae posteriorly or crossing the arm across the chest anteriorly will elicit pain and frequently, when this motion is carried out under tension, crepitation.

Treatment of this condition is by rest, heat and local injection. It is easier to get a needle into the area under the scapula with the scapula rotated forward. A

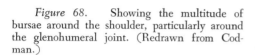

Figure 68.   Showing the multitude of bursae around the shoulder, particularly around the glenohumeral joint. (Redrawn from Codman.)

test of the accuracy of the localization of the injection is the prompt relief of pain which continues while the local anesthetic is effective.

FRACTURE

Fracture of the body of the scapula is not a common athletic injury because of the protection given the bone by overlying and underlying cushions of muscle. Usually, only a violent force will cause fracture. Mention was made earlier of avulsion injury and fracture of the spine of the scapula. The body of the scapula can be fractured by muscle contraction but this is extremely unusual. Symptoms will be those of a severe contusion and the diagnosis must be made by x-ray visualization.

Treatment.   Reduction of a fracture of the body of the scapula (Figs. 69 and 70) is rarely necessary. In fact, it is virtually impossible to reduce the fragments short of open operation. Since the body of the scapula is primarily for muscle attachments the only indication for internal fixation of the fragments would be their actual overlapping with a resulting roughness of the undersurface of the bone, extreme enough to interfere with motion of the scapula over the chest wall. This rarely occurs and I have never seen it as a result of athletic injury.

Treatment, therefore, is local, consisting of aspiration and injection of the hematoma, early cold followed by heat, and protection against extremes of motion. It is probably advisable to use a firm compression bandage from 24 to 48 hours, strapping the scapula snugly against the chest wall. The arm is then suspended in a sling (Fig. 52). This retentive dressing should be removed after 7 to 14 days and motion of the shoulder and scapula encouraged within the limits of pain. It should be emphasized that it is inadvisable to immobilize the shoulder for more than a few days. The protective sling which is utilized will permit pendulum exercises which should gradually increase both in range and frequency as the pain and tenderness subside. Active function will return promptly but it may be many months before forceful use of the extremity is pain-free.

Figure 69.   Comminuted fracture of scapula caused by fall on the outer aspect of the shoulder. Humeral head drove against the glenoid, fracturing the neck with comminuted fracture lines extending throughout the body of the scapula. No treatment is required other than support.

Figure 70.   Fractured scapula caused by a direct fall on the blade of the scapula. Comminuted fracture without displacement. The patient was a very thin, poorly muscled individual.

REGION OF THE SHOULDER JOINT (GLENOHUMERAL JOINT)

ANATOMICAL CONSIDERATIONS

The functional anatomy of the shoulder joint defies brief description. The student is referred to the classic book "The Shoulder" by E. A. Codman, whose narrative description of the functional motion of the shoulder joint in 1934 has not been improved upon. Only a few essentials of functional anatomy can be touched upon here.

The shoulder is an extremely complex joint owing to the fact that not only the glenohumeral joint itself but the structures making up the foundation for the glenohumeral joint are extremely mobile, so that many of the muscles and indeed even the ligaments may have separate functions under different circumstances. In describing motions of the shoulder, one had best proceed from the base of the anatomical position with the arm at the side, the palm facing forward and the scapula snugly against the chest wall (Figs. 40 and 41). Structurally, the joint is a modified ball and socket without bony stability. Whereas the acetabulum is designed to give maximum stability to the hip and yet maintain some degree of motion, the shoulder joint sacrifices stability for extreme mobility.

The glenohumeral joint itself consists of a small, shallow, saucer-like structure on the neck of the scapula (glenoid fossa) (Fig. 40) and the head of the humerus. The humeral head rests against the glenoid and is so much larger than the glenoid that the latter serves not so much as a receptacle for the head as it does as a base against which the head may be stabilized in its circumduction motions. The capsule of the joint is somewhat redundant but is reinforced in front by capsular thickenings which give some degree of stability anteriorly. These bands, which consist of the superomedial and inferior glenohumeral ligaments, are tight when the humerus is placed in external rotation and abduction. It can be appreciated that, from the standpoint of ligament stability, they are not sufficient to hold the head against the glenoid but simply tend to prevent anterior displacement as the head rotates into abduction-external rotation.

These deficiencies in ligament structure are counterbalanced by the muscles of the rotator cuff (Fig. 71). These muscles pass from the scapula anteriorly, superiorly and posteriorly over the humeral head, attaching around the periphery of the head to the greater tuberosity. Together they form sort of a hood (Fig. 50). By a tonic contraction of these muscles the head is supported snugly against the glenoid (Fig. 72). The various tendons of the rotator cuff are indistinguishable as they reach their attachments and they form a continuous cuff around the neck of the humerus. In addition to these muscles, namely, the supraspinatus, infraspinatus and teres minor, anterior support is given by the extremely strong subscapularis tendon which passes directly in front of the humeral head in the anatomical position, covering approximately its inferior two-thirds (Fig. 73, B). These muscles acting individually cause rotation of the humeral head, the exact rotation depending upon the position from which the movement starts. From the anatomical position the subscapularis is an internal rotator. In a similar manner the teres minor supports the shoulder posteriorly and acts as an external rotator from the anatomical position.

While one is likely to think of the main function of the rotator cuff as being abduction and rotation of the arm, an equally essential function is that of holding the humeral head against the glenoid to permit abduction of the arm by the deltoid and other muscles without subluxation of the humeral head downward, since the socket of the glenoid is not sufficient to maintain stability (Fig. 72). Without the suspending action of the rotator cuff muscles, the head of the humerus would subluxate inferiorly as the arm is abducted. To further complicate the picture of the

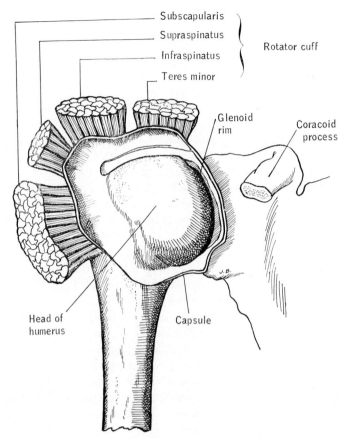

Figure 71. The rotator cuff, showing the relationships of the rotator cuff muscles with each other and with the capsules of the joint and the long head of the biceps which traverses between the subscapularis and supraspinatus. (Redrawn from Codman.)

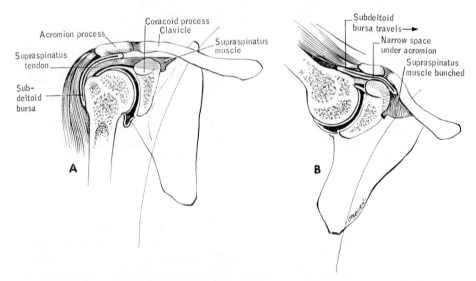

Figure 72. Sketch of relationships between the various components of the rotator cuff and the subacromial bursa. Note that the bursa underlies the acromion and the deltoid with more of it under the deltoid with the arm at the side.

A, Relationships with the arm at the side. *B,* With the arm widely abducted, showing "travel" of the bursa. Also narrow space for rotator cuff as it passes under acromion.

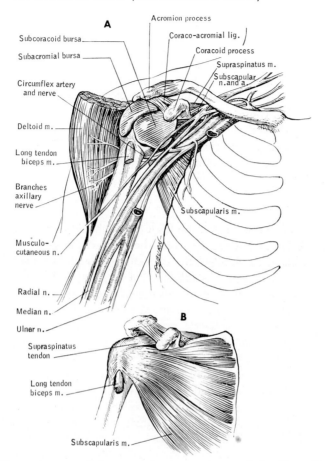

Acromion process

Subcoracoid bursa

Coraco-acromial lig.

Subacromial bursa

Coracoid process

Supraspinatus m.

Subscapular n. and a.

Circumflex artery and nerve

Deltoid m.

Long tendon biceps m.

Branches axillary nerve

Subscapularis m.

Musculo-cutaneous n.

Radial n.

Median n.

Ulner n.

Supraspinatus tendon

Long tendon biceps m.

Subscapularis m.

Figure 73.   Anatomical drawings of anterior region of shoulder with the anterior muscles removed.

A, With the subscapularis in situ showing the nerve supply to the deltoid muscle by the circumflex (axillary) nerve passing behind the humerus. Also, the relationships of the bursae.

B, Detail of the subscapularis and supraspinatus with the overlying structures removed. Note tendon of the long head of the biceps passing into the tunnel to become intracapsular.

tendons situated about the shoulder, the long head of the biceps passes through the bicipital groove or tunnel in front of the humeral head to pass over the head of the humerus, become intracapsular and finally reach its attachment at the top of the glenoid (Fig. 73).

This entire layer of muscle and tendon lies beneath the acromion. The more superficial covering of the shoulder joint consists of the bony acromial process which is reinforced in front by the coraco-acromial ligament to act as a roof over the medial part of the humeral head. The lateral continuation of this roof is the deltoid muscle which arises along the spine of the scapula, the acromion and the clavicle to extend down over the shoulder joint. Its fibers converge to their attachment at the deltoid tubercle about two-fifths of the way down the shaft of the humerus laterally. It can be seen that the shoulder joint proper is protected from external violence by the acromion and the deltoid.

CONTUSION

The most common contusion about the shoulder has already been described in the discussion of the acromion. The deltoid is subject to contusion, lying as it does in its exposed position over the humeral head. The deltoid is a thick resilient muscle and can stand considerable trauma. In competitive athletics it is protected well by shoulder pads so that contusion here is not common even in major trauma. The *treatment* is that of contusion anywhere else: cold, compression, heat, local aspiration, injection, rest. The duration of treatment depends upon the severity of the injury.

Axillary Nerve Damage

As the result of contusion over the front of the shoulder there may be damage to the axillary nerve. This nerve comes off the brachial plexus as a branch of the posterior cord at about the level of the coracoid process, leaves the posterior cord at a rather acute angle and proceeds sharply laterally and a little forward before it swings backward and continues laterally behind the shaft of the humerus. A direct blow striking just between the coracoid and the head of the humerus may contuse this nerve (Fig. 73).

The principal symptom of axillary nerve damage is a severe, numbing pain in the arm that causes the player to feel that the arm is useless. He may believe that his shoulder has been broken or that his arm has been "numbed." Examination at this time will reveal hypesthesia and reluctant function of the muscles of the upper arm. This rapidly disappears. Notable also is the inability to abduct the arm actively in the early stages. In a simple contusion this promptly clears and sometimes within a few minutes or at the most a few hours active function will reappear. Recovery is often so rapid that the player is able to return to the same game after a brief period of rest. In this instance one can visualize that the nerve has received a sufficient blow to cause temporary numbness, as when the ulnar nerve receives a blow at the elbow.

In the occasional case there will be persistent paralysis of the deltoid with an area of hypesthesia in the sensory distribution of the axillary nerve. If the patient is examined early, the findings will be basically negative, that is, there is no true paralysis of the hand or sensory loss, but the arm feels "asleep." There will usually be tenderness deep in front of the shoulder just lateral to the coracoid process. If the symptoms persist 24 to 48 hours the pattern of loss of function of the axillary nerve becomes clearer. Much more frequently there will be a period of apparent complete recovery with only occasional aching pain. This is followed by the onset of loss of function of the deltoid and development of anesthesia in the sensory distribution.

Treatment.   In the case marked by continuous and severe loss of function of the axillary nerve from the time of the accident, one is hard put to decide whether to recommend early exploration of the nerve or to wait for return of function. As a general rule, a period of watchful waiting is justified, the exact time depending upon the completeness of the loss or signs of possible recovery and function.

In the case that develops gradually over several weeks we may visualize a contusion and hematoma, with scar formation about the nerve that finally becomes constrictive. This lesion is usually incomplete but the weakness in the deltoid and loss of strength of abduction may be extremely distressing to the athlete. In many instances he is unable to raise his arm over his head. In other instances a complete paralysis of the nerve follows. I believe that if there is progressively increasing loss, exploration should not be delayed. In any event, I see little reason to wait beyond three months unless there is in the meantime some sign of improvement. During this period, physical therapeutic measures are of great value in maintaining the muscle tone and electrical stimulation of the deltoid is permissible on a professionally controlled basis. Care should be taken to prevent contracture of the shoulder with shortening of the adductors, with the result that the arm cannot be passively elevated.

At operation the axillary nerve should be exposed through the anterior incision if the blow has been frontal. By an approach along the deltopectoral interval and with reflection of the deltoid laterally, the brachial plexus may be exposed medial to the coracoid, the incision extending up under the clavicle. Access to this area is markedly facilitated by detaching the distal 1 inch of the coracoid and reflecting the biceps, coracobrachialis and pectoralis minor. The plexus can now be examined from the clavicle to the superior axillary fold.

Nerve operations in this area, and in fact in any other, require special technique and are not for the occasional surgeon. One practical approach to the problem is combined surgery by the orthopedist and neurosurgeon. This is an area frequently entered by the orthopedist during shoulder reconstruction. He may be better prepared for the exposure whereas the exact decision as to what to do with the nerve may require the specialized knowledge of the neurosurgeon. The author has participated in several such cases with good success. One patient had a neuroma just distal to the separation of the axillary nerve from the posterior cord. This was resected, the nerve repaired, good function returned. The player went on to a stellar career as a football player with no restriction of abduction of the shoulder. Two recent cases revealed rather minimal findings at operation but there were definite adhesions about the nerve that caused it to assume a more acute angle as it left the cord. This was aggravated by certain positions of the arm. In this instance the injury responded well to simple neurolysis and freeing of the adhesions. Several months may be needed for complete recovery.

It should be emphasized that the great majority of these cases are transient and probably of little true significance. Their recurrence may be avoided by an adjustment of the shoulder pad to protect this area a little more adequately. I believe the shoulder pad itself may often be the offender. As the arm is thrown up sharply and the shoulder pad comes forward its narrow edge is driven against the front of the shoulder, penetrates the sulcus between the muscles and reaches the nerve.

STRAIN

While contusion is a relatively minor problem about the shoulder, strain is an extremely major one. There may be some damage to the muscle or musculotendinous structures in any muscle that attaches at the shoulder. Since these muscles are many and the forces to which they are subject is legion, it is difficult to encompass this whole subject in a few short paragraphs.

The injury may be anything from a mild strain with some inflammation to complete avulsion of the tendon or of the tendon plus a fragment of bone. The symptoms will be similar but will vary considerably in degree. So, too, there is considerable difference between the type of symptoms in an acute and a chronic strain. These differences have been discussed at some length elsewhere.

Some grouping of the muscles involved will aid in the understanding of the pathologic changes present. The major internal rotators of the humerus are the subscapularis attaching to the lesser tuberosity, the latissimus dorsi and the teres major inserting into the internal lip of the intertubercular (bicipital) groove and the pectoralis major inserting at the outer lip of the intertubercular groove. Injuries to these attachments will be caused by forceful external rotation of the humerus against the resistance of these muscles or on active internal rotation of the humerus by their violent contraction. These muscles are opposed in external rotation by the muscles of the rotator cuff, particularly the infraspinatus, supraspinatus and teres minor. Both internal and external rotation are supported by the anterior and posterior fibers of the deltoid respectively.

The symptoms of an injury to these muscles are local tenderness at the site of their insertion, with pain elicited by active contraction or by passive stretching of the muscle involved. Thus, in an injury to the subscapularis, internal rotation of the arm against resistance or external rotation of the arm passively should cause pain in the same area, namely, over the lesser tuberosity.

Adduction of the arm is also carried out by many muscles. The internal and external rotators acting synchronously serve to adduct the arm against the chest wall. However, injury to the adductors of the arm is infrequent without some rotational component so that ordinarily adduction and internal rotation or adduction-external rotation will be the forces involved. The injury will probably be confined to either the internal or external rotators rather than to both.

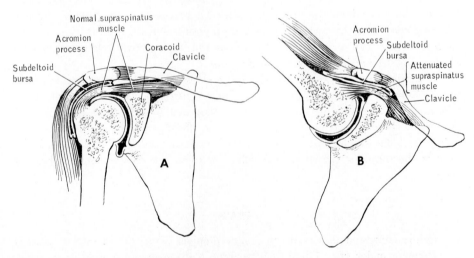

Figure 74.   Drawings demonstrating the attenuation of the supraspinatus as the arm is abducted.

In abduction of the shoulder the muscles of the rotator cuff fix the humerus against the glenoid and the deltoid raises the arm from the side (Fig. 74). True enough, the supraspinatus muscles have an abduction component but this is with a very short lever, and much more important than their ability to initiate abduction of the arm is their stabilization of the humeral head.

Lesions of the Rotator Cuff

Rotator cuff lesions are common in the adult, their frequency becoming greater as age advances. They are initiated by degenerative change in the tendons of the rotator cuff (Fig. 74). In the athlete such lesions are probably due mainly to attrition as the cuff passes under the acromial process. The isolated rupture of a portion of the cuff is an incident in the degenerative process and not the result of acute ligament or tendon rupture as in the case of the characteristic avulsions of the athlete. While in the adult the so-called "subdeltoid bursitis" is usually a sign of degenerative change in the rotator cuff, a true bursitis occurs in the young athlete, caused by a friction between the two walls of the subdeltoid bursa as they are impinged between the acromion and the cuff. This will be described later. The occasional case of calcification seen in the young athlete is probably in the bursa itself.

I do not recall having seen an acute rupture of the rotator cuff in the athlete unless it was accompanied by dislocation of the shoulder. Classical rotator cuff rupture, or supraspinatus rupture, is usually the result of active abduction of the arm against resistance and is not often a major injury. On the other hand, the acute rupture of the cuff seen in the combination of strain, sprain, subluxation and dislocation is due to a passive force with the humeral head forcibly jammed against the components of the cuff or with the elements of the cuff ruptured as the head dislocates and slips downward in relationship to the glenoid.

The rotator mechanism is subject to strain in the forceful motion of the shoulder in throwing or in tackling or wrestling. In such an injury the tenderness will be along the greater tuberosity and the pain will be in the shoulder or at the deltoid insertion. It may or may not be localized depending upon the promptness of examination, since the pain very rapidly becomes diffuse. There may be considerable difficulty in determining just what muscle action causes pain in the tendons of the rotator cuff and this condition is readily confused with subacromial bursitis. Actually, abduction of the shoulder, particularly against some resistance, will usually cause pain. If this strain is accompanied by some swelling and inflammatory reaction over the tendon it may well cause symptoms of accompanying bursitis.

Strain and Tenosynovitis of the Long Head of the Biceps

Another tendon quite subject to strain at the shoulder is the long head of the biceps (Fig. 73). This tendon passes through the tunnel formed by the intertubercular groove plus a thick fibrous roof so that the tendon is in effect in a sheath throughout an area of 1 to 2 inches in front of the humeral head. It passes through the groove, becomes intracapsular, and traverses the shoulder to attach on the superior lip of the glenoid above the humeral head. Motion of the shoulder with the elbow fixed, particularly in extension, causes this tendon to slide up and down forcibly through the groove. It may be subject to strain at its attachment to the glenoid but is more likely to develop tenosynovitis where is passes through the tunnel. The irritation of constant motion increases the inflammatory reaction until the tendon slides reluctantly through the tunnel and finally may cease to slide altogether. This tenosynovitis of the biceps tendon is extremely distressing from the standpoint of function of the shoulder since, with the restriction of motion and pain, many of the motions of the shoulder joint become quite limited. This is particularly true of abduction and external rotation so that rotation at the gleno-humeral joint becomes virtually impossible. Snap extension of the elbow increases this pain.

This condition may be diagnosed by localization of tenderness along the bicipital groove and by pain on rotation of the shoulder. The location of the tenderness moves with the humeral head as it rotates. There is pain on active contraction or passive stretching of tne biceps with its distal attachment fixed. A test for this motion is to extend the elbow and posteriorly flex the arm at the shoulder. This causes the tendon to slide through the groove. So also active function by pulling the arm forward across the chest with the forearm extended and with resistance against the hand will cause pain. In checking this motion one should be sure that the scapula does not simply rotate forward and so simulate glenohumeral motion while the motion is actually between the scapula and the chest wall.

Treatment of this condition is by local measures. The extremity should be put at rest. The tender area should be injected with local anesthetic and inductive heat utilized to reduce inflammatory reaction. If the condition is relatively chronic, injection of corticoid will ofttimes be quite effective. The same serial injections that are used in similar conditions elsewhere are effective here.

If the condition is intractable and does not respond to local treatment, surgical treatment may be highly successful. In this instance the shoulder is approached anteriorly, the bicipital groove is opened throughout its length, and the tendon is dislocated from the groove and detached from its glenoid attachment so that it no longer crosses the shoulder joint. It may then be replaced into the bicipital groove and sutured snugly into the groove or transferred to the short head of the biceps at the coracoid process. The latter procedure is somewhat more complicated but does serve to restore the function of the biceps in relation to the shoulder joint whereas, if the long head is attached into the humerus, the shoulder function of this particular muscle is lost. This does not seem to be of any material consequence and I prefer the simpler procedure, fixing the tendon firmly into the groove.

Tenosynovitis in the bicipital groove may go on to complete adherence of the tendon. This interdicts any extensive range of motion of the shoulder and one of two things occurs. Either the shoulder motion is restricted or the biceps ruptures proximal to the groove. In many instances there will be restriction of motion and then a sudden painful snap, after which it is noted that the shoulder motion is less restricted. This condition is not frequent in athletic injuries since it usually predicates some pre-existing degenerative change in the tendon itself. If it occurs it usually demands surgical treatment with removal of the remaining portion of the tendon from the glenohumeral joint and fixation of the proximal stump to the groove.

Biceps m.

Figure 75.   Showing biceps lesion; biceps bunching.

Acute Rupture of the Biceps Tendon

Acute rupture of the biceps tendon (Fig. 75) occurs as a result of forceful contraction of the biceps muscle or of forceful movement of the arm with the biceps muscle contracted. The injury may be avulsion of the tendon from the muscle belly or the tendon may rupture anywhere along its course or be pulled free from its attachment to the glenoid. The history is of immediate, sharp pain followed by tenderness along the course of the long head of the biceps. Diagnosis is made by having the patient contract the biceps with the arm abducted and externally rotated with the elbow at 90 degrees (Fig. 75). If the tear is complete it will be noted that the muscle belly moves toward the elbow as it contracts.

If acute rupture is diagnosed, the *treatment* is surgical. No attempt should be made to restore the attachment to the glenoid. The long head of the biceps should either be attached to the coracoid or fastened into the bicipital groove. Prompt recovery follows surgical treatment. Unrepaired rupture usually results in some weakness of the arm and frequently in pain, depending upon the location of the tear.

Subluxation of the Biceps Tendon

Another traumatic condition about the tendon of the biceps is a rupture or stretching of the fascial covering of the bicipital groove that permits the tendon to subluxate from the groove. This may occur as an acute injury. The predisposing factor for this condition is a congenitally shallow bicipital groove. The intertubercular groove may not only be shallow but may be broader than normal which permits the tendon to flatten out and slide back and forth within the groove itself (Fig. 76). The patient complains of a snap anteriorly in the shoulder with pain followed by residual soreness along the bicipital groove, elicited by the same motions that cause pain on tenosynovitis. Indeed, it may be indistinguishable from tenosynovitis. In the muscular athlete it is virtually impossible to palpate the subluxating tendon. If the condition becomes chronic as the result of a defect of

Figure 76.   *A,* Young lady with recurrent attacks of severe shoulder pain. Careful history elicited the fact that each attack started with a snap in front of the shoulder. Her findings were that of bicipital tendinitis during an attack. Between attacks she was completely relieved. Rotation of the arm at 90 degree abduction caused extreme pain. Her diffuse shoulder tenderness was localized at the bicipital groove. At surgery the shallow groove was noted with a redundant roof so that the tendon could slide out of the groove. The glenoid attachment was transferred to the bicipital groove with relief of symptoms.

B, A normal bicipital tunnel for comparison.

the roof of the groove with redundant tissue, a chronic synovitis usually occurs. On motion of the shoulder there is painful snapping as the tendon slips back and forth out of the groove, particularly on rotation of the arm. This condition also should be treated by surgical fixation of the tendon into the groove after detaching the tendon from the glenoid.

BURSITIS

Acute Subdeltoid Bursitis

The major bursae about the shoulder are the subacromial and the subscapular (Fig. 73). The subacromial bursa lies underneath the acromial process and extends out under the deltoid muscle to lie between the acromial process and deltoid and the humeral head and the rotator cuff. The bursa is separate and distinct from the glenohumeral joint. It has no connection with it but permits the tendons surrounding the humeral head to slide freely under the acromial process (Fig. 72). This bursa is frequently involved in injuries about the shoulder since any irritative lesion involving the rotator cuff will cause inflammatory reaction within the bursa so that the symptoms of bursitis may well obscure the primary lesion. Subdeltoid bursitis may be caused by excessive friction between the cuff and the acromion. As the irritation increases the thickness of the bursal lining, the pressure increases and the rolled-up synovium may form a fold that will at first snap as it slips under the glenoid (Fig. 77). Later it may check abduction at the point of impingement. The condition may also be caused by a direct blow over the shoulder which causes an inflammatory reaction that is aggravated by further motion. Primary subdeltoid bursitis is not common in the athlete. The bursitis is usually a secondary reaction so it behooves one to search for the primary lesion before instigating treatment.

Symptoms of acute subdeltoid bursitis are pain on motion of the shoulder, particularly abduction, tenderness over the tuberosity just distal to the acromial process, and pain on rotation of the shoulder, particularly internal rotation. Rotation forces the inflamed walls of the bursa into tight approximation so that manipulation of the arm into wide abduction as in the throwing motion or reaching behind the back will elicit major pain.

Treatment. Acute bursitis is treated by rest and local heat using wet packs, radiant lamp or diathermy. It will usually subside fairly rapidly. The condition is particularly annoying to the athlete and almost inevitably he will start active use of the shoulder before the inflammation has subsided. This results in renewed irritation of the bursa. It should be emphasized that comprehensive treatment of acute bursitis will prevent repeated recurrence of the acute bursitis or a resultant chronic synovitis, adhesions and a chronic subacromial bursitis.

Chronic Subdeltoid Bursitis

Chronic subacromial bursitis causes subacute or recurrent pain around the subacromial bursa. This may be due to chronic inflammation within the bursa itself but is much more likely to be due to irregularity of the bursal walls caused by adhesion between the two layers of the bursa or by irregularity and thickening of the rotator cuff which may be the result of a minor tear of the tendons. Symptoms of such a condition are pain on extremes of motion, particularly abduction, crepitation on rotation, and occasionally "snapping" of the shoulder when the roll of thickened synovium at the edge of the acromion finally snaps beneath it with a palpable painful click (Fig. 77).

In chronic bursitis the *treatment* is injection into the bursa of a local anesthetic and a corticoid in serial fashion. If this fails, surgical intervention should be carried out. The surgeon should be warned against excising the walls of the bursa if roughened surfaces are left to rub together. In case of an irregularity of the distal portion of the acromion, this portion may be excised. Indeed, up to 1 inch of the acromion may be excised in the presence of irreversible irregularity of the

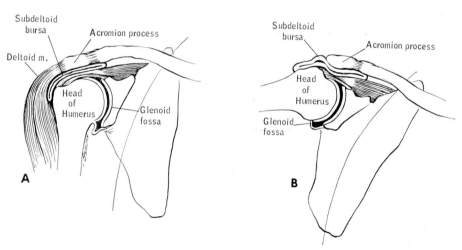

Figure 77.   Drawings of subdeltoid bursa rolled up and impinging against acromion.

Figure 78.   *A,* Retouched preoperative x-ray showing normal acromial process. *B,* After resection of the distal portion of the acromion which delays the impingement of the bursa under the acromial margin.

rotator cuff, with little resultant disability (Fig. 78). Occasionally the coraco-acromial ligament may be involved and it too should be excised if necessary.

Subscapularis Bursitis

The subscapularis bursa is a further extension of the sac surrounding the subscapularis tendon (Fig. 72). It usually has a direct connection with the joint. True bursitis here is not frequent. Usually there is more complicated involvement of the glenohumeral joint itself. There may, however, be a separate subcoracoid bursa which is a further extension of this same sac. Pain and tenderness in the area of the coracoid aggravated by external rotation of the arm against resistance or active internal rotation should make one suspect involvement in this area. Local treatment is of value. Physical therapy and local injection will usually give good relief.

Any of these bursae can give rise to prolonged disability. This is particularly true if the athlete is unwilling to rest the shoulder for a sufficient time to permit the inflammation to subside. Too early resumption of activity leads inevitably to recurrence of symptoms. Every time the symptoms recur they are more resistant to treatment. Finally irreversible disability ensues.

SPRAIN-SUBLUXATION-DISLOCATION

Sprain

It has been noted above that the ligaments or capsule contribute but little to the stability of the shoulder joint. The shoulder is pressed into the glenoid by the rotator cuff which consists of tendons. There is no inherent stability of the shoulder due to the capsular ligaments. As a result, sprain per se of the glenohumeral joint is a rather unusual occurrence and occurs basically in one direction. As the shoulder is abducted and externally rotated, tension is placed upon the anterior capsule with its ligament reinforcements (Fig. 79, A). The head tends to slide forward against the coraco-acromial ligament and against the capsule inferior to it. The coraco-acromial ligament, being an extremely strong structure, forces the head downward and the tension is caught on the anterior capsule and the capsular ligaments. As the abduction-external rotation force continues (as with the arm in the overhand throwing position), the capsular ligament may tear partially or completely (Fig. 79, B). This may occur at the attachment of the capsule along the labrum of the glenoid or indeed anywhere in the anterior capsule. If the tear is incomplete the shoulder does not subluxate or dislocate. The motion is arrested short of dislocation.

Diagnosis.   One of the symptoms of such a condition is pain at the time of the injury. The player will usually relate that his arm was forced backward and upward. For example, in an attempt to tackle another player as he runs by, the arm is carried forcibly backward and externally rotated (see Fig. 101). The pain is promptly relieved as the arm is placed at the side and there may be relatively little discomfort as long as the arm remains in this relaxed position. If the sprain is more severe there will be aching pain which is particularly aggravated by external rotation of the humerus. The player prefers to hold the arm to his side.

On examination there will be resistance to external rotation-abduction and pain on this motion. Marked muscle spasm of the adductors and internal rotators is stimulated by any attempt to externally rotate or abduct the arm. This motion will be more or less restricted depending upon the severity of the injury. On palpation there is tenderness in front of the shoulder joint, not along the bicipital groove but medial to it and down to the anterior portion of the humeral head and glenoid.

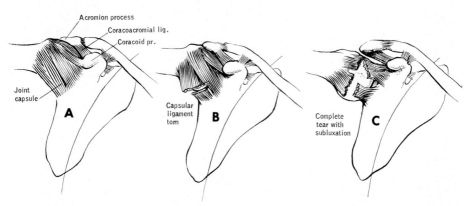

Figure 79.   Various degrees of sprain of the shoulder caused by abduction-external rotation.

A, Normal abduction-external rotation showing the anterior inferior portion of the capsule taut.

B, Forced external rotation combined with posterior flexion causes capsular tear.

C, Continuation of this motion rotates the anterior and inferior fibers to be superior and anterior respectively. The head emerges through the rent in the capsule and will dislocate if the movement continues.

This area may be difficult to palpate in the muscular athlete. Owing to the multiplicity of structures subject to injury in this area it may be extremely difficult to differentiate the condition from such things as a strain of the subscapularis attachment, strain of the rotator cuff, and involvement of the pectoralis major, all of which give similar symptoms.

Since the treatment is basically the same for all of these conditions the exact diagnosis may not be essential. However, there is one distinguishing characteristic. With a sprain of the ligament there should be no pain on active adduction or internal rotation of the shoulder within certain limits such as would be elicited with strain of the rotators or adductors. This is true particularly if the patient is examined early. Nevertheless, one infrequently can make a definitive diagnosis of strain of the glenohumeral joint.

Treatment. Since in sprain the capsule is completely relaxed with the arm in adduction and internal rotation, it is not necessary to immobilize the shoulder completely. Treatment should be by sling preferably worn under the shirt so that the arm is supported at the side and external rotation and abduction are prevented. A simple swathe over the chest and around the arm will accomplish the same result (Fig. 49). The patient should be instructed that any active use of the hand and forearm that does not cause discomfort is desirable. If the sprain is relatively severe, two or three weeks of protection in a sling may be necessary. In a less severe case, the wearing of a simple restraining chain (Fig. 80) may permit active participation in sports. A belt is placed around the chest, another around

Figure 80. Type of chain restraint popular with football players. Note the heavy leather strap around the waist not tight enough to interfere with respiration, and the wide leather band around the arm. In most instances now the chain between the two bands is replaced by a leather strap as indicated here. This does not prevent external rotation but does check abduction to some degree depending upon the tightness of the connecting strap.

the lower arm and the two are connected by a strap or chain of a length suitable to restrict abduction at the desired angle. This treatment is based on the fact that strain is not applied to this torn structure until the arm is in wide abduction and external rotation.

Anterior Subluxation

Subluxation of the shoulder is caused by the same basic mechanism that causes a sprain. This is particularly true of the anterior-inferior subluxation, which is the most frequent type of athletic injury to the shoulder. As the arm comes up into external rotation-abduction, the superior portion of the rotator cuff becomes posterior whereas the anterior inferior ligaments become anterior. In this position the humeral head is thrust forcibly against the glenohumeral ligaments in front using the rotator cuff as a sling around which the head rotates against the anterior capsule (Fig. 79, C). This causes a tearing of the anterior capsule and if this tearing is relatively complete the humeral head will actually subluxate forward and ride over the rim of the glenoid. The force being arrested, the movement reverses and the head promptly slips back into its normal position without ever having completely dislocated from the glenoid. It can readily be seen that this type of subluxation is actually a severe sprain that has caused disruption of the anterior capsule, since in a normal shoulder the head cannot slide over the glenoid rim without loss of integrity of some portion of the shoulder capsule. In the young adult this is almost always the anterior thickening of the capsule.

Symptoms.   The history is important in this condition. The history is of the arm being thrown up into external rotation and abduction and the feeling that the shoulder is slipping out of position, accompanied by severe pain in the anterior portion of the joint. Immediate relief is obtained as the arm slips back into neutral position and there may be very little discomfort so long as the arm is supported at the side. The symptoms will be identical to those of a sprain, only more severe. Any attempt at abduction-external rotation will cause muscle spasm and pain, and in many cases the feeling of imminent dislocation. The patient will often volunteer the statement that his shoulder has been out of joint and slipped back in. Indeed, it is often impossible to determine whether the injury has been a subluxation or a spontaneously reduced dislocation.

Treatment.   Treatment is based on the assumption that there is actual structural damage to the shoulder. I cannot overemphasize the importance of adequate treatment for subluxation or spontaneously reduced dislocation of the shoulder. This condition frequently occurs in the shoulder predisposed toward dislocation with flattening of the glenoid or a defect in the humeral head. It also occurs in an anatomically normal joint. If the torn ligaments are protected in the relaxed position there is every expectation that they will heal completely without undue lengthening. If constant irritation and stretching are permitted, the ligaments will heal not only with overlength but with scar rather than ligament structure, and potential weakness remains. This invites recurrence of subluxation, finally dislocation and often recurrent dislocation. External rotation-abduction of the arm must not be permitted during the healing period.

The treatment is basically the same as that for sprain, namely, fixation of the arm at the side in a sling with the arm either enclosed in the shirt or a circumferential swathe (Fig. 49). Meddlesome manipulation of the shoulder to determine the progress of the repair is to be condemned. Ligament structures heal slowly and the initial anastomosis between the torn ligament ends is extremely insecure. One single motion in external rotation-abduction will be enough to disrupt the infant union and successive motions constantly separate the edges. The patient, the coach, and indeed the physician must restrain their curiosity as to the progress of this repair and assume that short of three weeks there is no firm union and that it takes six weeks for union to be secure even under favorable circumstances. Careful treatment of this initial lesion will result in complete recovery. Unwise manipulation may result in a recurrent condition of the shoulder.

Inferior Subluxation

While the common subluxation of the shoulder is anterior, there is another type of subluxation of the humeral head which should be mentioned although it is not common in the athlete. I refer to the inferior subluxation in which the humeral head actually hangs out of the glenoid, the head riding over the inferior rim. This is of course a frequent occurrence in paralytic conditions of the shoulder and as a result of overheavy traction by a hanging cast. As such it is readily explained by the antecedent history and is not particularly related to athletic injuries. It is possible, however, to have acute subluxation of the shoulder as a result of injury to the rotator cuff. It is to be recalled that the rotator cuff suspends the head into the glenoid by the tonic action of the rotator muscles (Fig. 72). A rupture of any one of these muscles, as for example the supraspinatus or teres minor, will not result in any actual subluxation of the humeral head. However, if the whole rotator cuff is avulsed, the suspensory action of the cuff is lost and the humerus can be held in proper position only by strong contraction of the deltoid and other extrinsic muscles of the shoulder. This is a major injury and may have extremely distressing sequelae.

The writer recalls a recent case in which a young adult fell from a truck, his glove caught on the sideboard and his fall was sharply arrested by his arm held directly upward. His sudden suspension on his relaxed arm resulted in extreme pain and disability in the shoulder. His early examination and treatment were unfortunately superficial, consisting of application of a sling for a couple of weeks and then encouragement to return to work. At the time this patient was examined nine weeks after his injury, he wore a very snug sling with pressure under his elbow. He was extremely apprehensive on removal of the sling and when he was persuaded to permit his extrinsic muscles to relax he had pain in the shoulder and the feeling that the shoulder slipped out of place. Examination revealed a definite interval between the acromion and the head and it was possible to slip the head in and out of the shoulder joint inferiorly. This finding was confirmed both by examination and x-ray (Fig. 81). This patient was extremely apprehensive because he had learned that whenever he would relax the shoulder the head would fall out of joint. It would not actually dislocate but would subluxate inferiorly.

This patient's *treatment* was by open operation, at which time the whole rotator cuff was found to be detached and the whole area scarred in with resultant increase in length of the rotator cuff tendons. In the operation the entire cuff was pulled downward like a hood over the tuberosity and sutured there. This gave an extremely stable shoulder immediately. Snug support was continued six weeks to

Figure 81.　　Complete rupture of rotator cuff. *A,* Shoulder with the arm in sling. *B,* On removal of sling the head of the humerus subluxates over the glenoid rim.

prevent re-stress. The result was complete stability of the shoulder but considerable restriction of motion which could be attributed to the long immobilization—nine weeks preoperative, six weeks postoperative.

Admittedly this was an unusual injury but I believe it could have been diagnosed early by careful history and physical examination supported by x-ray. For this degree of subluxation I do not believe nonsurgical treatment is appropriate. However, if nonsurgical treatment is elected, the arm should be supported at the side with downward pressure on the clavicle and acromion and upward pressure on the humerus, in an effort to induce the rotator cuff to resume its normal position. The inadequacy of this becomes apparent when it is recognized this is a tendon avulsion and that the tone of the involved muscles, particularly as they go into spasm with the injury, will inevitably pull the tendon away from its attachment. The primary treatment should be surgical with repair of the rotator cuff down to the humerus.

A sprain or subluxation of the humeral head inferiorly BY ABDUCTION is possible, but infrequent. At the height of abduction the humeral head levers against the tip of the acromion and posterior portion of the head drives against the structures inferiorly (Fig. 82, *A*). This results in tearing of the capsule and ligament and if the

A   B

C   D

Figure 82.   Drawing illustrating various stages in the inferior sprain-subluxation-dislocation of the shoulder.

A, Arm in complete abduction with the scapula rotated, the tuberosity serving as a fulcrum for the acromion; stress is applied to the inferior glenohumeral ligaments.

B, The force continues, the ligaments rupture, the head subluxates.

C, As the force continues further the head goes into typical position of luxatio erecta and completely dislocates. The inferior capsule is completely torn.

D, After the arm drops back toward the anatomical position the head remains subglenoid or may slip further and become subcoracoid. (From DePalma, "Surgery of the Shoulder," J. B. Lippincott Co.)

tear is complete the humeral head may ride out on the inferior glenoid rim (Fig. 82, B). This is an extremely severe type of injury and if the force continues a complete inferior dislocation of the humerus results (Fig. 82, C). If the dislocation is not complete the arm drops promptly to the side and is resolutely held in place by the patient since he feels any attempt to abduct it will cause it to slip out of place. The history of the type of injury plus the fact that the tenderness is deep in the axilla up against the inferior portion of the humeral head will serve as a key to the diagnosis. Active abduction per se is not painful because if there is any strain on the internal structures, muscle spasm will force the arm to the side before the movement is extensive enough to be painful.

Treatment is by sling with the arm at the side. Since only complete abduction will put strain on this redundant inferior capsule, athletic participation may be allowed as soon as pain permits, provided that complete abduction of the arm is prevented. The degree of restriction of abduction necessary can be determined by steadily abducting the arm to the point where pain is elicited. Abduction beyond this point should be prevented by suitable apparatus. The familiar chain restraint with a wide band around the chest, a band around the arm and the two connected with a chain or strap is adequate (Fig. 80).

Posterior Subluxation

Posterior subluxation of the shoulder, meaning an incomplete posterior dislocation, presumably may occur (Fig. 83). The forces involved usually are direct backward thrust of the humerus with the arm forward flexed. This drives the head posteriorly from beneath the acromion. The posterior portion of the rotator cuff is in this instance damaged and the humeral head slides posteriorly. Owing to the muscular character of the posterior structures the subluxation is immediately reduced spontaneously and in my opinion its diagnosis with any degree of certainty is virtually impossible. The symptoms are those of strain of the posterior structures, pain on reproduction of the force causing dislocation so that with the humerus flexed forward and pushed backward there is a feeling of discomfort, and pain posteriorly in the shoulder. Attempts to internally rotate and flex the arm across the chest will also elicit pain. On examination tenderness is posterior and about the humeral head; indeed, the symptoms are identical with those of strain or partial avulsion of the external rotators of the shoulder.

Treatment.   Treatment is by immobilization with the arm at the side. Ordinary internal rotation to the extent of placing the forearm across the chest is not interdicted, particularly if it is not painful. If this results in painful strain posteriorly the arm may be immobilized at the side in a plaster spica with the arm in the anatomical position, the elbow flexed to 90 degrees and the forearm extended directly forward—a position similar to that used in certain fractures about the elbow. The duration of immobilization will depend upon the degree of symptoms and the amount of damage. The shoulder should be protected for about three weeks. It is an unusual force that causes this injury and is not likely to be recurrent. This explains the more rapid rehabilitation in this condition than in anterior subluxation

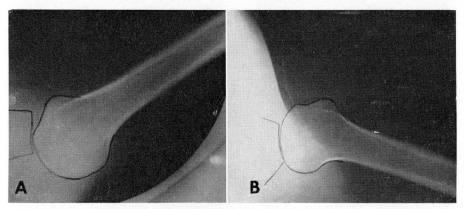

Figure 83.   Posterior subluxation of the shoulder, axillary view. *B,* The horizontal position. *A,* The arm swung forward toward the midline. As the head rotates it slips out of the glenoid posteriorly. This required posterior reconstruction of the capsule.

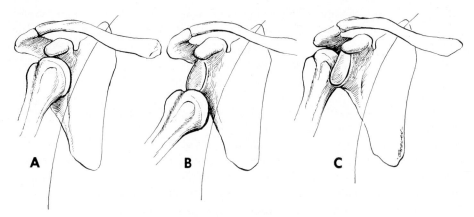

Figure 84.   Dislocations of the shoulder. *A*, Typical subcoracoid dislocation. *B*, Subglenoid
dislocation. *C*, Posterior dislocation.

where the position of external rotation-abduction is very frequent in athletic activities and so needs to be guarded against for a longer time.

Anterior Dislocation

Dislocation of the shoulder follows the loss of function of the restraining
structures about the shoulder and is caused by the same mechanism that causes the
subluxations described above. By far the most common type of dislocation of the
shoulder in young individuals of athletic age is the anterior-inferior (Fig. 84, *A*).
This is pure dislocation, unaccompanied by fracture, in young individuals. As age
advances the ligaments become firmer and the bone less strong so the dislocation
may be accompanied by avulsion fracture rather than a tear of the ligament itself.
In the young athlete it is almost always the ligament or muscle that gives way. As

Figure 85.   Subcoracoid dislocation of the shoulder, which is the classical anterior-inferior
dislocation; the head comes out in front and below.

the arm is forced into abduction and external rotation the humeral head is thrust against the anterior portion of the glenohumeral joint, the coraco-acromial ligament serves to force it downward and it then emerges anteriorly and inferiorly into the redundant area of the capsule which is protected by the glenohumeral ligaments (Fig. 40). These give way when they are torn from the glenoid labrum or because of avulsion of the labrum or actual disruption of the ligaments themselves. The head of the humerus slips over the glenoid rim, immediately slides forward to lodge between the rim of the glenoid and coracoid process, and the arm drops toward the side. This is the classical dislocation of the shoulder in young persons (Fig. 85). The damage to the ligament may be a transverse tear across the capsule and in addition the capsular reinforcements known as the glenohumeral ligaments may split with one passing above the humeral head and one below it. In some instances they actually grasp the humeral head in such a way as to impede reduction.

Symptoms.   While the diagnosis of the dislocated shoulder by appearance alone may be difficult in an extremely well muscled or heavy individual, it is usually easy. The acromion is prominent with a definite defect below it rather than the usual rounding out of the deltoid muscle (Fig. 86). The arm tends to be held away from the side and rotated slightly externally so that it is virtually impossible to move the forearm across the chest or abdomen in front of the body or to bring the elbow to the side. On examination the defect below the acromion is, in early cases, readily palpable and the roundness of the humeral head as it rests against the coracoid is also readily felt anteriorly. An attempt to manipulate the arm or to force the elbow to the side causes pain. The patient will usually permit some increase in abduction and external rotation but will resist adduction and internal rotation. At

Figure 86.   Photograph of subcoracoid dislocation of the shoulder. Note the prominent acromion, the arm held away from the side, the flat deltoid. (From McLaughlin, "Trauma," p. 246.)

the time of this examination a careful neurological examination should be made since not infrequently an injury to the brachial plexus occurs in dislocation of the shoulder. This possibility should be investigated before an attempt is made at reduction or one will wonder whether a later neurological deficit was caused by the injury itself or by the trauma of the reduction.

Treatment.   Anterior dislocation of the shoulder is an acute emergency and should be reduced as soon as adequate facilities are available. On occasion it may readily be reduced directly after the injury before pain and muscle spasm have developed. However, this is not to be attempted by the uninitiated since irreparable damage may be done to the bones or capsule and particularly to the nerve structures about the shoulder by unwise manipulation. Under no circumstances should force be used. The major obstacle to reduction is general spasm of the muscles about the shoulder, so that the humeral head is firmly fixed against the coracoid and under the glenoid rim. Any attempt to move it from this position will only increase the spasm. I cannot too severely condemn forcible manipulation of the shoulder, which will not accomplish the purpose of the reduction and simply increases spastic fixation.

The first prerequisite for reduction of the dislocation is complete relaxation of the shoulder. This may be possible without general anesthesia but once the dislocation has persisted beyond the first few minutes it becomes extremely difficult to obtain relaxation short of use of a general anesthetic. This is particularly true in the athlete who is very muscular, extremely apprehensive and is at the age where he has not yet developed sufficient equanimity to permit voluntary relaxation of these painful structures.

If the doctor sees the player at the time of his injury and is skilled in manipulation of the shoulder, he may attempt immediate reduction on the field without anesthesia. This is accomplished by laying the patient flat on his back on the ground, grasping his arm securely either by the wrist or with the elbow flexed and exerting direct traction distally. The traction should be gentle and not accompanied by any attempt at lateral motion (Fig. 87). In certain instances the humeral head will slip quietly into position. The time-honored method of placing the foot in the axilla is fraught with danger. Its only justification is to permit the operator to steady him-

Figure 87.   Reduction of the dislocated shoulder by steady, even pull on the arm in the supine position. The padded strap through the axilla is for mild countertraction and is often not necessary. This may be with or without anesthesia.

Figure 88.   A, The improper method. Note the foot is directly in the axilla, impinging the brachial plexus against the dislocated humeral head while the arm is levered over the foot. This can cause serious damage to the brachial plexus and is quite painful.

B, The proper position with the foot against the axillary wall for pressure while steady, even traction is made at about a 45 degree angle.

self, not to permit him to use excessive force or traction. The unshod foot is used and great care is taken not to put direct pressure against the humeral head (Fig. 88); rather, the foot should be more against the chest wall. Careless use of the foot in the axilla may well result in damage to the structures of the brachial plexus since they may be tightly caught against the humeral head.

If, after a reasonable trial of traction (60 seconds), the head does not reduce, the attempt should be abandoned. The player should be taken from the field to a place suitable for more adequate treatment. I believe he should be taken promptly to the infirmary or hospital, and x-rays made of the shoulder to confirm the diagnosis and to discover any accompanying bony abnormalities. Even if the dislocation is promptly reduced by traction, x-ray study should be made to eliminate the possibility of accompanying bony injury.

After the x-ray is made, a second and more comprehensive effort may be made to obtain reduction by simple traction. Detailed description of the various methods of reduction is not appropriate here, but a few deserve mention. The simplest one is to exert traction directly on the line of the trunk or possibly in slight abduction, with the patient flat on his back (Fig. 87). It must be emphasized that this traction must be pain-free or it will not accomplish its purpose. In another method the patient lies prone on the table with the involved arm hanging over the edge either

Figure 89.   Pendulant method of reduction without anesthesia. The weight must be suspended by the wrist, not grasped by the hand since complete relaxation is essential. The shoulder should swing free and the patient should be comfortable or else he will not relax.

with or without a weight suspended from the wrist (Fig. 89). Similar reduction may be carried out with the patient sitting with the arm hanging over the suitably padded back of a chair (Fig. 90). In all instances care must be taken that there is no pressure on the axillary structures. If these methods do not suffice for reduction, the patient should be given an anesthetic and an extremely atraumatic reduction

Figure 90.   Pendulant method of reduction without anesthesia. Note the pad in the axilla, the weight suspended from the wrist, not grasped by the hand.

carried out by the Kocher maneuver (Fig. 91) or by traction or by whatever careful manipulation will bring the head into proper relation with the glenoid. I cannot overemphasize the importance of atraumatic, careful, gentle manipulation. Force is not required to reduce the dislocated shoulder. Relaxation is imperative either with or without general anesthesia. Following reduction, x-ray examination should be made to confirm the position and again check for possible bony abnormalities or injuries.

Attendant fractures about the shoulder are not common in this age group. However, they may occur and as such will require definitive treatment. Avulsion of the greater or lesser tuberosity, fracture of the glenoid, fracture of the acromion, and involvement of the biceps tendon are complications that will demand the best care of the skilled orthopedist. If the shoulder does not readily and completely reduce, repeated attempts at manipulation are not justified.

The occasional damage to the nerves which accompanies injury to the brachial plexus may be the cause of considerable concern. In my opinion competent neurosurgical consultation is advisable in such cases of nerve injury. Ordinarily watchful waiting will be the treatment of choice, anticipating a gradual return of function since this damage is usually peripheral—a contusion to the nerve which will probably recover promptly. If recovery does not occur, exploration of the nerve is advisable and considerable judgment is required to determine the best time for it. Since recovery will occur in many cases without exploration, exploration is usually postponed several months. Once the indications are clear, however, it should be recommended and carried out without delay.

Following successful reduction the after-treatment consists of immobilization of the arm in a sling providing support under the elbow, with an added swathe around the chest in order to prevent abduction of the arm (Fig. 49). It should be emphasized that, for an acute complete dislocation to occur, there must be serious

Figure 91. The Kocher maneuver. *A,* Abduction-external rotation. *B,* Adduction-external rotation. *C,* The completed maneuver with internal rotation of the adducted arm.

damage to the ligaments and capsule of the joint. Thus, continued immobilization is required until they attain some degree of healing in direct apposition. The arm should be held in a sling for a minimum of three weeks and then mobilized only within the limits of pain. Active participation in sports without protection should not be permitted in less than six weeks. It is to be feared that this regimen is ordinarily not carried out. Following reduction, the player usually recovers promptly and within two weeks his arm feels very good to him. Overpersuasion may permit

Figure 92.   Typical exercises for reconstruction of shoulder muscles. (From Cave, "Fractures and Other Injuries," Year Book Publishers.)

him to participate, whereupon the dislocation promptly recurs. The patient should be encouraged to exercise within the limits of pain and the restriction of his dressing (Fig. 92). After three weeks of immobilization, rehabilitative measures may be stepped up sharply, particularly active motion against resistance to develop the muscles of the shoulder. Even during the time the arm is suspended in a sling and swathe, active use of the hand and the forearm and tonic contraction of the muscles about the upper arm and shoulder will permit the player to keep his arm in relatively good condition. It is extremely important that the musculature of the shoulder be in good condition before unprotected use of the arm is permitted since so much of the stability of the shoulder depends upon the strength of the muscles involved.

One need not fear restriction of motion as the result of immobilization of the arm at the side in this age group, although in the elderly this is an ever present danger.

Posterior Dislocation

Posterior dislocation of the shoulder is uncommon as an athletic injury. However, I have seen many late cases and the majority of them were unrecognized primarily. The cause is a direct driving force against the lower end of the humerus with the arm forward flexed. This force transmitted up the arm drives the head out posteriorly. No gross deformity of the shoulder is evident. The patient resists any motion of the shoulder and upon careful palpation less fullness of the humeral head in front and some increased fullness behind are felt. There is increased prominence of the coracoid. This is readily determined only very early since within a short time swelling about the shoulder from this extremely disabling injury will screen any visible physical findings. Motion of the shoulder is sharply restricted by muscle spasm. X-ray examination is extremely pertinent. In the late cases I have seen, x-rays had uniformly been taken but as uniformly misinterpreted. The pertinent finding in the x-ray is not any actual displacement of the humeral head backward, but rather, particularly in comparison with an x-ray of the other shoulder, an overlapping of the head of the humerus and glenoid (Fig. 84, C). This overlapping is not possible in a straight anteroposterior view of the normal shoulder and is extremely easy to overlook. It indicates that the humeral head is posterior to and slightly medial to its normal position so that the convexity of the humeral head does not fit against the concavity of the glenoid but appears medial to it (Figs. 93 and 94).

Treatment.   Reduction of the dislocation if seen early is by traction forward and pressure forward on the humeral head. The head usually will slip into place with an audible click. If the patient is seen later an anesthetic may be required. If he is seen very late the dislocation may be impossible to reduce. It is frequently accompanied by fracture of the posterior portion of the glenoid which may include as much as half of the entire glenoid. If this fragment does not replace into good position, surgical resection or internal fixation should be carried out. If the dislocation is seen late and is accompanied by this fracture, at open reduction it is necessary to remove the fragment and by suture replace the capsule to the remaining rim. If the fragment is large it should be replaced and supported by a bone graft.

Figure 93.   Anteroposterior x-ray of the shoulder showing posterior dislocation. To a casual glance no lesion is apparent. Careful inspection will reveal the head of the humerus medial to the glenoid convexity.

Figure 94.   Recurrent posterior dislocation of the shoulder. The vertical views demonstrate (*A*) the position with the head in the glenoid; (*B*) with it dislocated posteriorly.

Inferior Dislocation

Inferior dislocation of the shoulder occurs as the arm is forced into straight abduction. As the lateral part of the neck of the humerus impinges against the acromion the head is forced laterally against the inferior portion of the capsule and the capsular ligaments (Fig. 82). As the ligaments rupture or tear away from the lower glenoid margin the humeral head displaces laterally and slips downward over the inferior lip of the glenoid. As the arm is lowered to the side the head slides anteriorly and the dislocation becomes a subcoracoid dislocation (Figs. 82, D, and 85). The significance of this series of events is that the dislocation may be particularly resistant to any type of manipulative reduction other than straight traction. Indeed, many of the cases which reduce readily by straight traction in the long axis of the body may well be those in which the head has come out almost directly inferiorly. At the time of the examination it may be impossible to determine whether or not the head has come primarily forward or has gone directly inferiorly. Careful x-ray study should be made to determine the exact position of the head and whether there has been bony damage.

If the straight abduction force continues and the arm is forced over the head toward the midline of the body, a much more serious injury occurs. The humeral head is literally stripped of its attachments so that the capsule and rotator cuff have completely lost their integrity. In this instance the head locks in a position under the glenoid with the shaft of the humerus pointing directly upward so that the arm is held high over the head (*luxatio erecta*) (Fig. 95). I have never seen this

Figure 95.   Case of luxatio erecta. It is extremely unusual to get an x-ray in this position since ordinarily the arm drops back to the side and the dislocation becomes subcoracoid. This can be the termination of the situation described in Figure 82, C. (From McLaughlin, "Trauma." p. 262.)

occur as a result of an athletic injury. It is, of course, an extremely major injury. It is likely to be accompanied by nerve damage and will probably demand some sort of surgical intervention even if primary reduction can be obtained. In such an instance, repair of the rotator cuff may be indicated. This may well have been the injury to which I referred on page 158 of this chapter. In such a case there will be so much damage to the whole mechanism that the humeral head actually hangs out of the glenoid. At the time of the reduction of luxatio erecta, extreme care should be taken to avoid forceful manipulation since it may well add to the damage to the muscles, blood vessels and nerves. Under no circumstances should forcible reduction be attempted without anesthesia and under no circumstances should any force be used in repositioning the arm with the patient anesthetized.

Recurrent Dislocation

By far the most common recurrent dislocation of the shoulder is ANTERIOR dislocation. This occurs basically in two categories: first, a recurrent dislocation as the result of repeated episodes of acute traumatic dislocations in a normal shoulder, and second, a recurrent dislocation as the result of congenital deviations about the glenohumeral joint. It is of some importance to distinguish between these two conditions since the latter condition is likely to be bilateral and will demand surgical correction. If the deformity is severe enough, athletic competition should be interdicted.

The first variety, namely, that occurring because of repeated trauma, is usually the result of an acute injury, untreated or inadequately treated at the time of the first dislocation. The capsule fails to heal or heals too long and the next dislocation tears it a little bit more. With each successive dislocation, less force will be required for the dislocation and it reduces more easily. Finally the condition develops where the shoulder dislocates by simple abduction-external rotation without actual trauma. This type of case is readily amenable to surgical *treatment*. In some instances it may be improved by a long period of immobilization provided there have not been too many episodes of displacement. If, for example, it is the third episode and the shoulder has previously been inadequately immobilized, one might be justified in putting the arm at rest at the side for eight weeks, hoping that union and shortening of the ligament will occur. If this fails and if the recurrent episodes of subluxation or dislocation interfere with necessary activity, operative reconstruction of the shoulder can be carried out very successfully. I have operated upon many dislocations in this category and have yet to have had recurrence in an athlete. My personal preference is for a modification of the Putti-Platt procedure by combining it with the Bankhart type of local repair of the capsule to the glenoid rim if indicated.

In the second category, that of congenital malformations of the shoulder, reconstruction may be necessary and may be wholly successful (Figs. 96 and 97). In these cases dislocations may occur without any serious trauma. Study of the opposite shoulder should always be made.

Recurrent POSTERIOR dislocation of the shoulder is not frequently encountered since the primary condition itself is infrequent. I have personally seen more unreduced than recurrent posterior dislocations. One of the latter was in a swimmer who had the feeling his arm would subluxate at a certain point of his back stroke to the extent that it interfered markedly in the success of his swimming. Examina-

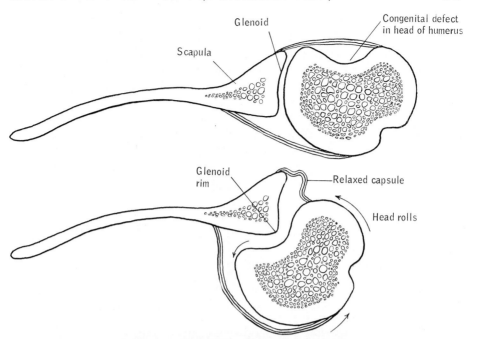

Glenoid

Scapula

Congenital defect
in head of humerus

Glenoid
rim

Relaxed capsule

Head rolls

Figure 96. Schematic drawing showing relaxation of the capsule as the glenoid rim drops into the congenital notch in the humeral head. This relaxation permits the head to slip out of the glenohumeral joint. (H. Osmond Clark, Journal of Bone & Joint Surgery, Vol. 30-B.)

Figure 97. X-ray showing congenital defect in the humeral head. As the flat portion of the head is opposed to the glenoid, the diameter of the head is markedly shortened and the capsule relaxed, predisposing to dislocation.

tion in these cases usually will not elicit pain and it is infrequently possible to demonstrate the subluxation clinically. One must depend almost entirely on the story of the patient that he has the feeling that the shoulder slips out posteriorly. Note carefully the position of the arm at which the head tends to slip. Ofttimes the history of falling on the outstretched arm or falling on the elbow with the arm forward will be a guide. In the case of the swimmer above mentioned, his arm was repaired posteriorly. I found a defect in the posterior capsule and was able to plicate it with good support, and he went on to be a champion Olympic swimmer with complete recovery from his instability.

FRACTURE

Fractures about the upper end of the humerus are not common in athletes and those that do occur are often the result of a dislocation of the shoulder, a frequent injury in this age group.

Avulsion Fracture

This uncommon type of fracture in athletes occurs about the glenohumeral area as a result of the traction of a tendon or ligament on a bony process as in dis-

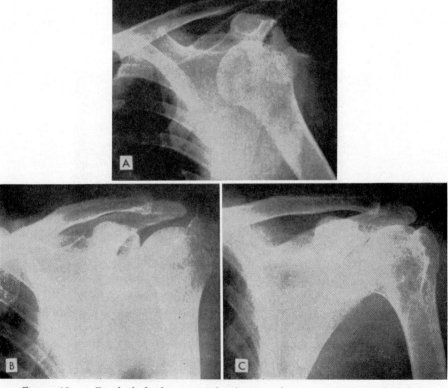

Figure 98.   Residual displacement of tuberosity fragment. *A,* Original dislocation. *B,* Following reduction by simple traction. *C,* Following cuff repair and reattachment of the tuberosity fragment. Result was excellent. (From McLaughlin, "Trauma," p. 252.)

location of the shoulder, which accounts for the majority of cases. The most frequent of the avulsion fractures involves the greater tuberosity.

Avulsion of the Greater Tuberosity.   In anterior dislocation of the shoulder as the arm rotates up and out and the humeral head slips forward, the extremely strong pull of the muscles of the rotator cuff may fix the tuberosity in situ. This results in separation of the tuberosity from the shaft. This may occur as an avulsion of the rotator cuff, an avulsion of a thin shell of bone, or an avulsion of the entire tuberosity (Fig. 98). The symptoms will be those of a severe injury to the shoulder. The dislocation may or may not have been spontaneously reduced but the player will usually relate that his shoulder has slipped out of the joint. It may have been reduced by a spectator or fellow player, or possibly the player's own motion will have reduced it spontaneously.

If the shoulder is dislocated, great care should be taken in the x-ray interpretation of the film made before and after reduction to rule out such a fracture. If spontaneous reduction has occurred, careful palpation will reveal tenderness over the greater tuberosity. There will be pain on an attempt to actively abduct or to externally rotate the arm. Given these findings, careful x-ray study should be made with the head in various positions of rotation since in some positions the fracture may seem to be reduced and in others it may appear to be displaced. The fracture in the tuberosity may be visualized well in some cases and poorly in others (Figs. 99 and 100).

TREATMENT.   If the fracture is an incomplete one and if the tuberosity remains in place in all positions of the humeral head, treatment may be nonsurgical. Simple immobilization of the arm in a sling will usually suffice. If this does not serve to relieve the pain, the addition of a swathe around the chest may do it. There is no need for a plaster spica in the ordinary case. If there is persistent displacement in any position of the humeral head, surgical intervention is desirable.

Figure 99.   A, X-ray showing avulsion of the greater tuberosity of the humerus. It does not reveal the displacement well but careful study will show that the top of the fragment is well above the rim of the head whereas in the reduction film it is replaced below the margin of the head.

B, Postreduction film.

Figure 100.   A, Avulsion fracture of tuberosity, the tuberosity remaining near its situs and
not elevated. B, Surgical treatment permitted solid union.

While healing in malposition may be acceptable in older people with sedentary habits, deformity of the head is not well tolerated by a person who has to use the arm in violent exercise, such as throwing or swinging a tennis racket or many of the other things required of the athlete. The tuberosity can be readily exposed by a muscle-splitting operation through the upper portion of the anterior third of the deltoid and fixation should be by suture, staple, screw, or whatever method seems best. If the entire tuberosity is detached, it should be replaced and held by internal fixation (Fig. 99, B). If a shell of bone has been torn away, this shell should be surgically excised and the tendon repaired to the avulsed bed. If extremely secure internal fixation of the fragment is not obtainable, removal of the fragment is advisable since rehabilitation progresses much more rapidly if healing is tendon to bone rather than bone to bone.

Following repair, rehabilitation will depend somewhat upon the security of the fixation. If fixation is very secure, either by a screw or a staple through a firm bony fragment or by adequate suture of the tendon through drill holes, motion can be started just as soon as the operative reaction subsides provided it does not include active abduction of the arm. If the arm is abducted against gravity the humeral head is forced against the glenoid and the rotator cuff takes up its function of suspending the head to prevent the slipping downward due to the leverage of the deltoid. This puts unusual stress on the tuberosity and must not be permitted. Pendulum movements against gravity, however, are acceptable on the first day (Fig. 92). Such active abduction-contraction with the arm at the side does not have the leverage disadvantage of abduction against gravity. It may be permitted up to 45 degrees and should not be against resistance until union is progressing well.

Avulsion of the Lesser Tuberosity.   Attached to the lesser tuberosity is the subscapularis muscle, a strong adductor and internal rotator. Violent external rotation and abduction of the arm against the resistance of the subscapularis may cause rupture of the subscapularis tendon or avulsion of the tuberosity. The history will usually be of violent and rapid external rotation of the arm as in attempting to tackle a player as he is going by (Fig. 101). The symptoms will be identical to those of sprain of the subscapularis tendon, with tenderness at the lesser tuberosity. There is pain on active internal rotation and on passive external rotation and/or abduction of the arm. Diagnosis of avulsion fracture must be made by x-ray. Here again one should try to determine whether the avulsion is complete or incomplete. It is necessary to take pictures in various positions of the arm and at various angles of the tube in order to demonstrate that the tuberosity is indeed firmly fixed in all positions. If it is separated, it will be pulled medially toward the coracoid. This is most readily demonstrated by x-ray with the arm abducted.

TREATMENT.　　Definitive treatment of this avulsion fracture is necessary in the young athlete. If separation of the fragment in any position of the humeral head can be demonstrated, surgical repair should be carried out. The same principles of fixation are used as noted above (greater tuberosity). If the fragment is large it may be secured by metallic fixation. If it is small, it should be removed and the tendon repaired to the bone. The latter procedure is probably the method of choice since it expedites the recovery. The approach is made by using the first stage of the Putti-Platt or Magnuson shoulder reconstruction. This approach is along the delto-pectoral groove. The deltoid attachment is reflected from the clavicle, after which the injured area is readily available. Following repair the arm should be immobilized at the side in a sling with a swathe around the chest. The duration of immobilization will depend upon the degree of fixation obtained. Four weeks should be the minimum and throughout this period active rehabilitation of the arm may be carried out short of abduction or external rotation.

Figure 101.　　Typical position causing avulsion of the subscapularis. The arm is forcefully externally rotated but not widely abducted.

Fracture by Direct Violence

In the young athlete the humeral head, which is strong and resilient at this age, is not frequently broken by direct trauma. If fracture does occur it is a stellate fracture, usually without displacement and hence very difficult to recognize. In fact, it may be recognized only by repeat films after two weeks which show absorption around the fissures. The history is of a direct blow as in a fall on the shoulder

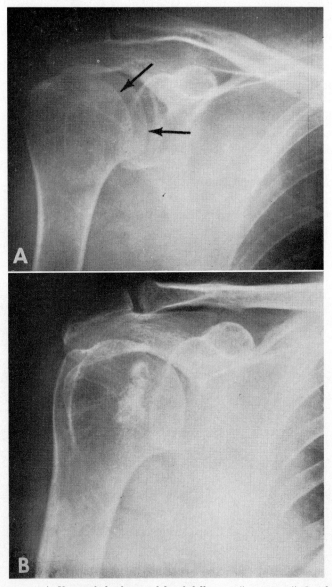

Figure 102.   *A,* X-ray of the humeral head following "contusion." Careful study will reveal two lines of periphery of the head, indicating a large segment of the head has been displaced.

B, The displacement reduced and bone bank bone packed into the defect. This is done by drill hole through the opposite side of the head. The fragment was driven back in position by an impactor.

or by a blunt object directly against the humeral head. The cartilage of the humeral head is somewhat less resilient than the other joints but there is no doubt that a direct blow to the head may cause chondral fracture either with fissuring of the cartilage or the actual dislodging of the fragments of cartilage. Fracture of the subchondral bone may lead to later chondromalacia of the bone or osteochondritis dissecans. None of these injuries is particularly disabling when it involves the head of the humerus. This is not a weight-bearing joint and there is a relatively small proportion of the head in contact with the glenoid at any one time. A little irregularity is well tolerated. By the time the fracture is recognized, the necessity for any immobilization will probably be past since the only immobilization indicated would be to suspend the arm in a sling and encourage motion within the limits of pain. In certain cases the humeral head may be pushed in much as one collapses one side of a ping-pong ball and probably by the same cause, that is, direct trauma over a relatively localized area. This may be caused by driving the ball of the humerus against the posterior lip of the glenoid or conceivably against the acromion.

This condition will have the same symptoms as contusion of the shoulder but they are more severe. Pain is out of proportion to that of ordinary contusion of the deltoid. Careful x-ray study with the head rotated in various positions will reveal the defect (Fig. 97). A posterior defect in such a position that the posterior edge of the glenoid may drop into it as the arm is abducted and externally rotated will predispose toward dislocation in identically the same manner as a congenital defect does.

Treatment. We have in at least one instance been able to reduce this deformity by drilling through the humeral head from the opposite side and actually pushing the cartilage upward by gently passing a punch through a drill hole made at the opposite side of the head. The defect was then packed with cancellous bone (Fig. 102). If the defect does not appear to be too severe, expectant treatment may be carried out and if subluxation occurs anterior plication may be done as in the repair of recurrent dislocation of the shoulder.

Fracture by Indirect Violence

This type of fracture is not common as a result of athletic endeavor but occasionally fractures through the surgical neck of the humerus will occur instead of a dislocation of the shoulder. In the adolescent this fracture may be through the proximal epiphysis (Fig. 103). In such a case the history of a violent injury followed by severe pain, localized swelling and tenderness together with resistance to any motion of the glenohumeral joint will suggest this serious injury. If the fracture is complete, x-ray will definitely confirm the diagnosis and appropriate measures can be carried out for treatment (Fig. 104). It should be borne in mind that if the injury involves epiphyses it is advisable to get as good reduction as may be obtained by atraumatic manipulation. If atraumaitc closed manipulation is unsatisfactory, open surgery should be carried out.

The chief diagnostic problem will arise with the incomplete fracture in which the displacement is slight. Here again x-ray will be confirmatory and treatment should be of the nonmeddlesome variety. It will be adequate to apply a sling with the arm to the side and to permit pendulant and pain-free movement from the beginning or at least as soon as the immediate reaction has subsided. Many weeks

Figure 103.   Fracture adjacent to proximal epiphysis of the humerus with only moderate
displacement. Treated by simple sling and swathe fixation.

Figure 104.   Fracture of the surgical
neck of the humerus without displacement.
Treated by sling without the necessity for
cast.

and months of rehabilitation may be spared if motion is initiated early in these
shoulder injuries.

Fracture of the Glenoid

Avulsion Fracture.   Avulsion fracture of the lip of the glenoid may occur
in combination with a complete or an incomplete dislocation of the shoulder either
anteriorly, posteriorly or inferiorly. In these instances the rim of the glenoid is
avulsed by the capsular attachment rather than broken off by the humeral head
since the humeral head is round and traverses the same arch as the glenoid. As the
head slides over the glenoid rim the capsule becomes very taut and may break off a

Figure 105.   Avulsion of antero-inferior margin of the glenoid in the course of a dislocation of the shoulder which was spontaneously reduced.

fragment of bone rather than separate. Thus, the anterior dislocation will pull off
the antero-inferior margin (Fig. 105), the posterior dislocation the posterior margin (Fig. 106), and the straight inferior dislocation (luxatio erecta) the inferior
margin of the glenoid. The true pathology is not so much fracture of the glenoid
as a capsular tear. In most instances nonsurgical treatment will suffice and either
bony or firm fibrous union will result. It is unusual for a single injury to cause
enough relaxation of the ligament or capsule to cause recurrent dislocation but repeated injuries may well do so, each one requiring less trauma than the one before.
If so, appropriate measures for the recurrent dislocation are in order. A reconstruction operation may be the answer if athletics are to be continued.

In the spontaneously reduced dislocation in which at the time of the examination the shoulder is in normal position, these glenoid marginal fractures will give
good insight into the degree of trauma. What may appear to be a simple sprain or
contusion may be revealed as a spontaneously reduced dislocation with attendant
damage to the capsule.

Another type of avulsion fracture about the glenoid which is peculiar to ath-

Figure 106.   Postoperative picture following reduction of old unreduced posterior disloca-tion. At operation the posterior margin of the glenoid was found to be displaced posteriorly.

letes is avulsion of a piece of bone by the triceps attachment along the inferior rim of the glenoid. Symptomatically there is pain on active stretching of the triceps muscle, and palpable tenderness along the inferior rim of the glenoid will usually be present. The fragment is difficult to visualize in the x-ray and may appear more as an area of calcification than as an avulsed fragment, particularly if the injury was recurrent in type (Fig. 107). Ordinarily, firm fibrous union will bind the frag-

Figure 107.   Fragmentation and calcification of the inferior lip of the glenoid following injury. This may have been from incomplete dislocation or from pull of the triceps tendon.

ment of the glenoid and there will be no residual symptoms. In the occasional case there will be pain on forcible use of the triceps. This is particularly likely in one who has to throw hard or use the arm in violent overhand motion as in tennis. In this case removal of the fragment of bone and re-suture of the tendon to the bed will result in relief of symptoms.

Following the acute injury a period of rest with local heat followed by active physical therapy will be of help in rehabilitation. It must be remembered that too early resumption of the violent activity that caused the original lesion will cause prompt recurrence. This accounts for the extremely poor results from treating shoulder lesions of this type in a baseball pitcher. Any change in his throwing habits

Figure 108. Series showing progress of calcification in the vicinity of the lower lip of the glenoid. This may well have been a partial avulsion of the triceps tendon with calcification and the resultant hematoma. (Rex Diveley, M.D., "Baseball Shoulder," J.A.M.A., Nov. 21, 1959.)

will usually result in loss of effectiveness and he soon resumes the same type of strain that hurt him in the first place.

Chronic irritation of the triceps attachment in this area may cause a deposition of calcium, which may be quite diffuse. It may be impossible in a chronic case to distinguish between the primary avulsion of a portion of the glenoid and deposits of calcium within the tendon of the triceps (Fig. 108). Since the treatment is identical, namely, physical therapy leading up to final surgical excision if it fails, the exact diagnosis probably is not too important.

Fracture by Direct Blow. The same force applied to the lateral side of the shoulder which may break the humeral head may also fracture the glenoid. This is a stellate fracture and in the athlete is usually without displacement. Gross displacement of the glenoid requires violent trauma. No treatment is necessary other than protection of the arm during the acute period by the application of a sling. The glenoid will tolerate a great degree of deformity with deep fissures in its surface without material interference with the function of the shoulder, since weight bearing is not involved.

A fracture of the glenoid may be caused by falling on the flexed elbow. In this case the humeral head may be driven forward or backward in such a way as to knock off a large portion of the anterior or posterior portion of the glenoid. In either case, if there is gross displacement of the anterior lip of more than 3/8 to 1/2 inch, the best treatment will be surgical replacement of the fragment (Fig. 105). If the posterior one-third of the glenoid is broken off, posterior subluxation or recurrent dislocation is likely to occur (Fig. 106). This deformity of the glenoid is easily corrected in a fresh fracture but is extremely difficult to correct following recurrent posterior dislocation. In the athlete such a fracture should be treated surgically using a posterior approach similar to that employed in recurrent posterior dislocation of the shoulder. When the rim of the glenoid is readily visualized extracapsularly, internal fixation may be utilized to restore the buttress. Similarly, in rupture of an anterior fragment that consists of as much as one-fourth of the glenoid, surgical repair should be carried out early.

Stellate fractures that simply enlarge the glenoid or increase its concavity will usually cause no disability.

Injuries of the Upper Arm

THIS CHAPTER will deal with the area between the shoulder and elbow joints and will not include discussion of either joint. *Anatomically* the arm consists of a single long bone relatively circular in cross section which is completely surrounded by muscles through which various vessels and nerves traverse from the shoulder to the lower arm. Injuries to this area are those peculiar to this anatomical type and are similar to those of the thigh.

CONTUSION

There is little subcutaneous bone in the upper arm since in all locations the skin is separated from the bone by an intervening layer or layers of muscle. This single exception is at the distal attachment of the deltoid to the lateral humerus. *Contusion of the skin*, therefore, is likely to be relatively benign and asymptomatic and to require little treatment. The structures lying between the skin and the bone, however, are quite subject to injury by contusion.

Contusion of Muscle

A direct blow over the biceps muscle in the front of the arm may well result in a contusion and hematoma of this muscle. However, this injury is neither frequent nor often disabling because of the thick muscle pad and the relatively smooth bone. Similarly, a direct blow over the triceps at the back of the arm may result in a painful, tender muscle but is not apt to present major complications.

In the presence of a contusion of the muscle, whatever its location, our first consideration is to rule out complications such as hemorrhage, nerve damage, and fracture of the underlying bone. If there is any suspicion of fracture an x-ray should be made. Careful examination of the muscle and tests of its function will usually reveal whether or not there has been a major rupture of the muscle fibers.

In the absence of any major complication, TREATMENT will vary depending upon the symptoms. If there is painful dysfunction I recommend the early application of a cold pack, wrapping the arm snugly with sheet wadding followed by an elastic bandage extending from the fingers to the axilla. More pressure should be applied in the vicinity of the contused area. The arm is then placed in a sling to put the involved muscle at rest. If the symptoms persist after several hours, the cold pack should be replaced by the application of local heat, using an electric pad, inductive heat or hot packs. Within a few days after the most acute symptoms subside, pain-free activity may be permitted. The whirlpool bath is a useful adjunct at this stage. The patient should be advised to use the arm strictly within the limits of pain. There is no place for massage or passive motion in the early treatment of a muscular contusion. Rehabilitation may progress parallel to the subsidence of symptoms. In this situation as in so many others in the athlete, too early and too extensive use of the involved muscle will only prolong the disability—a fact that needs repeated emphasis. Should a hematoma develop it is treated by aspiration, local injection and pressure bandage.

Contusion of Tendon and Bones (Blocker's Exostosis)

An injury of unusual significance is a *contusion of the middle third of the arm in the vicinity of and just anterior to the attachment of the deltoid muscle.* In this area the bone approximates the skin quite closely, particularly in the sulcus between the anterior distal portion of the deltoid and the belly of the biceps. This coincides with the area most frequently struck by the blocker as he throws his arm up to catch the impetus of the charging, opposing player. A direct blow by the hard headgear and, more particularly, repeated blows in this area will result in contusion of the tendon of the deltoid and of the periosteum of the humerus where the deltoid inserts. Adding to the vulnerability of this particular area is the fact that the anterior edge of the shoulder pad usually extends to about this level and the edge of the pad itself may well contribute to the damage rather than protect the area. The hemorrhage that occurs ordinarily is not extensive and, indeed, is not enough to be palpable as a hematoma. If this condition is recognized early it can be treated by adequate protection with a simple fiberboard pad which prevents recurrence of injury. Suitable measures such as local injection into the bruised area and early cold followed by heat will usually give prompt relief of the early lesion.

If the condition progresses and becomes chronic, a painful *periostitis* and *fibrositis* may develop. This is manifested by extreme tenderness just lateral to the belly of the biceps at the deltoid insertion. Treatment is by protection against further blows and local injection of a long-acting anesthetic and a corticoid preparation. Frequently dramatic improvement will result following such an injection. There is a definite tendency toward recurrence, however, and once this painful condition has developed, the player should be instructed to wear a suitable contact pad. This must be firmly fastened to the arm so that the pad itself does not slip around and cause further irritation.

Figure 109. Typical blocker's exostosis of humerus. A, Showing the early formation of bone having the appearance of myositis ossificans. Immature nature of the growth is indicated by irregular margins and relatively light deposit. B, The mature growth now appears as an exostosis firmly attached to the humerus with mature bone. C, Some months after removal. This mass did not recur because it was allowed to mature before it was disturbed surgically.

As a further sequence of this same condition, there is often spur formation along the bone (Fig. 109). This is not a true myositis ossificans but rather an irritative *exostosis* which arises from the bone and has all the characteristics of bone. It is not infiltrated through the muscle as is myositis ossificans. This exostosis extends anterolaterally, usually with a relatively sharp edge. It may become quite disabling owing to the pain of a direct blow. Once it reaches this stage it is not easily protected by a pad. The treatment of this condition is surgical excision, but it is extremely important that the growth be entirely mature before its removal is considered. The majority of these cases do not advance to this degree and if they are asymptomatic no treatment is indicated. The growth actually may appear and regress spontaneously (Fig. 110). If the mass is surgically removed during the stage of its formation it will recur. The author recently had a case in which the original lesion seemed quite mature and was readily removed. In a very few weeks there was development of a second exostosis above the level of the old lesion (Fig. 111). Although the main mass of bone seemed mature there was still a portion of it in the formative stage and the surgery simply triggered the formation of another spur. For a more complete discussion of myositis ossificans and exostosis, see the general discussion in Chapter 4, page 45, and the more specific discussion in Chapter 17, page 421. Whereas in myositis ossificans of the quadriceps active use appears to be the aggravating factor, in the described condition in the arm the exciting factor is repeated contusion. The patient can usually use his arm very well if he avoids a direct blow. The muscles themselves are not primarily involved since the mass usually lies in the plane between the deltoid and the biceps.

Figure 110.   A, Exostosis in front of the humerus two months after injury. The patient was advised that the growth was immature and should not be disturbed. B, Five months later the mass has regressed, matured, and is asymptomatic.

Figure 111.   Exostosis in front of humerus. A, The original lesion, matured, which was removed with no recurrence locally. B, Subsequent recurrence at a higher level without intervening injury.

Contusion of the Radial Nerve

As the radial nerve leaves the posterior cord and passes down the arm, it passes in a spiral fashion from superomedial to inferolateral, adjacent to the muscular spiral groove of the humerus. The nerve here is in closer relationship to the bone but is covered by the bellies of the triceps muscle. As it swings laterally just above the lateral epicondylar ridge, it becomes much more subcutaneous and is quite liable to contusion. A direct blow on the posterolateral arm may cause a serious lesion of the nerve. Usually it is accompanied by a shocking, tingling sensation extending to the radial portion of the hand, and the hand is "numbed."

There is no specific *treatment* for this condition other than that for contusion anywhere, i.e., early cold followed by heat and protection. If there is an actual radial palsy, suitable splinting should be applied to the wrist and hand to overcome the wrist drop and loss of extension of the fingers and thumb. Usually the involvement is not complete. Sensation may be impaired in the radial distribution but it is almost always present to some extent. Indeed, there may be complete motor loss with complete retention of sensation. Paresthesias are common. In such a case, early surgery is not advisable, but if the condition continues for three or four months without definite signs of improvement in voluntary motion, surgical intervention is indicated.

Usually the condition is one of constriction and edema rather than actual severance of the fibers, and may be relieved by appropriate neurolysis. At operation the nerve is carefully exposed and traced through the contused area. If it is bound down to the humerus or is caught in scar, it must be freed by meticulous atraumatic dissection. Any constrictions of the sheath are released. If the constriction is not too mature the sheath may be expanded by injecting saline into it and forcing the column of saline past the constriction. After the nerve is entirely free an effort should be made to suture the muscle layers so as to place an intervening muscle layer between the nerve and the bone. This condition is not frequent but is extremely distressing when it does occur.

STRAIN

Acute Strain

The muscles of the arm are subject to acute strain in excessive muscular activity. This strain may vary from a mild irritation of the tendon or muscle to a complete rupture. The tendinous strains will be discussed in conjunction with the adjacent joints. It may be difficult in some instances to distinguish between contusion of the muscle and acute strain or partial rupture. Frequently, indeed, the two may be simultaneous. That is, while the muscle is under a rather severe strain, it may receive a direct blow and the fibers may rupture. Clinically some distinction can be made between acute strain or muscle rupture and contusion since in strain function of the part is likely to more painful than palpation whereas in contusion the reverse is usually true. If a strain is suspected, for example in the biceps, the muscle should be carefully checked throughout its length and the exact area of tenderness to palpation determined. Palpation may also determine whether or not there is a defect in the muscle or some change in its shape. A test of function, particularly against resistance, will usually reveal a localizing point of pain, tenderness or separation.

Proper *treatment* should be instituted according to the findings. It is extremely important in strain that the muscle be protected from overuse or overstretch. It is therefore more vital to protect the arm in a sling or even a splint than it is to treat the condition locally. Optimum treatment is cold pack, later heat, compression and protection by splint. As the acute symptoms subside a more definitive diagnosis may be made and subsequent treatment determined. That is, if there appears to be a major defect in the muscle, more extensive treatment will be required than if the strain is minimal. If it can be determined that there is an actual rupture of the muscle or musculotendinous junction, surgical repair should definitely be considered. Since surgical repair is most successful if done early the importance of an early definitive diagnosis is apparent. The muscle most frequently damaged in the upper arm is the biceps, not only because it is more subject to a direct blow but also because the blow frequently will occur while the biceps is in strong contraction.

If the rupture is at the musculotendinous junction the same symptoms may be present as with rupture of the tendon except that the tenderness will be in the muscle rather than over the tendon. Tests for configuration of the biceps with the biceps in contraction may give a definite lead as to the completeness of the rupture (see Fig. 75, page 151). If this condition is to be treated nonsurgically or if the rupture is not complete, splinting should be continued at least three weeks and be followed by a sling which will restrict extension at the elbow. The patient should be cautioned not to contract the biceps against resistance. In the vast majority of the cases the rupture will be incomplete. The intact portion of the muscle protects the injured area and holds the torn fibers in relatively good apposition.

Chronic Strain

Chronic strain is much more likely to occur in a tendon and will be considered in our discussion of the adjacent joints. There may be a chronic strain of the musculotendinous junction or in the muscle itself which is evidenced by pain on overuse—either repetitive overuse or a single massive effort. This will differ from acute strain in that there will be no local signs of hemorrhage, swelling or separation of the muscle or tendon fibers. Instead, there is a feeling of strain on forced activity followed by stiffness and spasm of the muscle after a period of rest. The patient may go to sleep at night with only moderate soreness and awake in the morning with muscle spasm, stiffness and pain, much more severe than it had been the night before. The situation may develop in the baseball pitcher or the weight lifter or the javelin thrower.

The only real solution to this problem is rest and avoidance of the type of activity that caused the condition in the first place. This is quite disrupting to the young athlete and he frequently returns to his activity too soon and has prompt recurrence of his trouble. *Treatment,* therefore, should be local injection, local heat, protection against excessive use but not immobilization. Function should be encouraged but strictly within the limits of comfort. Since it is not necessary to use the upper extremity for weight bearing, the requisite inactivity can usually be accomplished without special apparatus. A sling may be required to remind the youth that strenuous activity is interdicted. The patient should be given a clear understanding of the rationale of the treatment. If this is comprehended a high degree of cooperation can be expected. The physician interested in the treatment of athletes should inform himself as to the anatomical characteristics of the muscles involved in the function of the arm and be prepared to guide the patient in the selection of those activities which he may continue and those which he should abandon. This is particularly pertinent as rehabilitation progresses and it becomes necessary to permit greater activity. If the strain is the result of a particular activity, as for example, baseball pitching, it may be found that the patient can tolerate some other field position before he can return to pitching since a somewhat different muscle activity is demanded of the pitcher than of the infielder, for example. So also, the pole vaulter might be permitted to participate in the hurdles or the high jump much sooner than he could his pole vaulting.

FRACTURE

Fracture of the humerus may occur but is not a common injury in athletic competition. In any injury that seems to be severe, x-ray examination should be made. In the shaft of the humerus the x-ray leaves little doubt as to whether or not there is a fracture. Fracture almost always causes some interference with function. The exception may be the greenstick fracture in the younger individual where the bone may be broken but the fragments are not disrupted. This can also be readily determined by x-ray visualization.

As with any injury in athletes, the goal of *treatment* must be complete recovery. One is, therefore, more justified in adopting definitive treatment than he would be in an older person. If a treatment can be utilized that will permit rehabilitation at a relatively early stage, this of course should be considered. Rehabilitation should be instituted as promptly as possible but participation in sports must not be allowed until the fracture is entirely healed and the muscles restored to normal size and tone. With an injury to the arm, it is usually entirely feasible to continue conditioning of the rest of the body and, indeed, of many portions of the arm itself during the actual healing period of the injury.

Injuries of
the Elbow

ANATOMICAL CONSIDERATIONS

THE ELBOW is a complicated joint consisting of three different articulations, those between the ulna and humerus, the radius and humerus and the radius and ulna. While it is primarily a hinge joint and so has motion in flexion and extension, it also participates in the rotatory motions of the forearm through the articulations of the radial head with the ulna and with the lower end of the humerus. The olecranon and coronoid process of the ulna form a deep socket (the olecranon fossa) which encircles the trochlea of the lower end of the humerus and provides a very stable joint. This joint permits only flexion and extension. The ulna does not rotate. On the other hand, the upper end of the radius makes a very unstable connection with the lower end of the humerus, the button-like head of the radius having a shallow depression with the same arc of curvature as the transverse arc of the capitellum of the humerus. On flexion and extension the head of the radius travels from the front to the back of the capitellum by simple gliding action. On rotation of the forearm the button of the radial head rotates through the shallow socket on the side of the ulna while its proximal end simply turns against the capitellum.

The integrity of the relationship between the head of the radius and the ulna and humerus depends entirely upon ligaments (Fig. 112). The radio-ulnar articulation is stabilized by the annular (orbicular) ligament which holds the head and the neck of the radius firmly against the radial fossa of the ulna. The stability of the radius and the lower end of the humerus is largely capsular in character, there being no collateral ligament extending from the outer side of the humerus to the head of the radius. A lateral ligament extends from the lateral epicondyle to a very firm connection with the annular ligament. Thus, the lateral integrity of this joint also depends upon the continuity of the annular ligament of the radius. On the medial side there are very strong ligaments extending from the medial epicondyle down to the medial surface of the coronoid and downward and backward to attach to the whole length of the olecranon from its proximal tip to the base of the coronoid process. The anterior part of this ligament is cordlike while the posterior part is shaped like a fan with the handle attached to the humerus. With the elbow in extension the anterior portion of the ligament becomes very tight while with the elbow in flexion the posterior part of the fan is tight. The capsule of the joint is relatively relaxed. There is no check ligament as such. Extension of the elbow is prevented as the olecranon process impinges against the olecranon fossa of the humerus. Flexion is checked by pressure of the muscles of the forearm and arm or by the coronoid process against the humerus. Rotation of the forearm is entirely dependent upon a smooth radial head with its outer circumference intact.

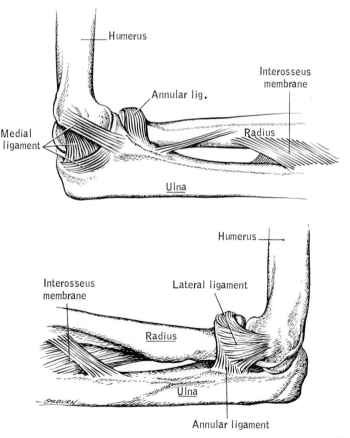

Figure 112.   Medial and lateral views of the elbow showing bony and ligamentous structures.

CONTUSION

There are several areas of subcutaneous bone at the elbow. The entire olecranon is subcutaneous as are the medial and lateral epicondyles and the supracondylar ridges. As might be expected in the circumstances, contusion is a common
injury in the elbow. Falling on the flexed elbow crushes the skin against the hard
bone of the olecranon and may result in severe contusion and abrasion or even
laceration over the point of the elbow. Since this area is relatively insensible the
injury is not especially painful; indeed, it may be overlooked. The area of the lateral
condyle and the radial head, however, is quite sensitive and a painful bruise here
may follow a direct blow to the side of the elbow—the medial side less often because
of its protected position. In contusion of any of these areas care should be taken to
determine whether there are other lesions. In cases of doubt, x-ray examination is
indicated.

In the uncomplicated contusion, *treatment* will depend upon the degree of
injury. Often none is required. If there is an accompanying hematoma, it should
be aspirated and local injection of hyaluronidase carried out. The area is then
wrapped in sheet wadding with the elbow as near a right angle as is comfortable
to the patient. A snug elastic bandage is wrapped over the arm from wrist to axilla.
In the early stages cold should be applied by ice pack. After 24 hours heat may be
used if necessary. An appropriate sling should be worn if an elastic bandage is used,
otherwise flexion and extension of the elbow against the tight bandage will simply
aggravate the contusion.

Contusion of the Ulnar Nerve

Contusion of the ulnar nerve is quite frequent because of its anatomical position at the elbow. As it traverses the inner side of the arm, it passes behind the
medial condyle through a tunnel, the floor of which is made up of the ulnar groove
of the humerus, the roof being a rather loose fibrous sheet. As the arm flexes and
extends, the nerve slides up and down in the ulnar groove. In this region the nerve
is subcutaneous and lies directly on the bone. Hence, a direct blow may damage the
nerve to a greater or lesser extent depending upon the strength and direction of
the force applied. The so-called "crazy bone" should have been named the "crazy
nerve" although certainly the bone does participate in the etiology of the syndrome.
A direct blow causes immediate severe pain with a shocking sensation extending
down to the ring and little fingers. This paresthesia is usually transient, disappearing after a few minutes or several hours depending upon the severity of the injury.

Under ordinary circumstances no permanent injury results from ulnar nerve
contusion, but occasionally there may be late sequelae. If the injury was sufficient
to cause bleeding into the nerve, adhesions may form within the nerve trunk itself
resulting in the development of ulnar palsy. The same effect may occur if the irritation is external to the nerve and there is constriction within the groove. In either
event the fibers are constricted, lose their elasticity and a progressively increasing
ulnar palsy results. The symptoms of delayed palsy consist of gradually increasing
numbness along the ulnar distribution of the forearm and hand which includes the
ulnar side of the lower forearm, the little finger, half of the ring finger and the

corresponding portion of the hand. The pain is ordinarily much more severe in the hand than at the elbow, although both may be quite painful. As the loss of nerve function continues there will be marked atrophy of the muscles of the hand. It should be recalled that a great majority of the intrinsic muscles of the hand are supplied by the ulnar nerve. One of the early symptoms is inability to adduct the little finger so as to place it against the ring finger. The metacarpal shafts will become more prominent because of intrinsic muscle atrophy. Contracture of the fingers will result as the condition progresses.

Definitive *treatment* in the early stages of ulnar palsy will usually prevent permanent disability. The condition is not ordinarily amenable to local injection and similar measures. If there is a definite palsy and the nerve appears to be constricted, treatment should be surgical. The skin is incised along the course of the nerve, which is then freed from the groove. Neurolysis is carried out to release the sheath and the nerve is transposed forward to pass in front of the condyle rather than behind it. If this operation has not been delayed too long, very good recovery can be expected.

Periosteal irritation may develop as a result of a direct blow over the subcutaneous bone. In this instance the bone remains tender and is very sensitive to pressure. This responds well to local injection of a long-acting anesthetic and corticoid and protection by adequate padding.

Contusion on the back of the arm over the triceps tendon may cause tenosynovitis in this area with resulting pain particularly on forced flexion of the elbow. As a rule this is not severe enough to cause impairment of triceps function. The usual measures prevail. Heat, rest and injection usually give prompt relief.

STRAIN

Musculotendinous strain about the elbow is quite frequent owing to the extremely forceful action required at the elbow joint in many sports. The powerful triceps muscle attaching to the olecranon is subject to strain anywhere from its attachment on the olecranon up to the musculotendinous junction. The symptoms consist of tenderness over the involved area, pain on forceful extension of the forearm against resistance and pain on complete flexion of the elbow. There may well be local heat if the condition is acute enough although this is not a diagnostic sign. Forceful active extension of the arm as in throwing will aggravate the condition.

Another common area of strain is in the biceps where it attaches below the neck of the radius. The biceps has a firm tendinous attachment to the radius and through the bicipital aponeurosis (lacertus fibrosus) to the fascia of the forearm. Strain may occur anywhere in this complex and indeed may be severe enough to tear the lacertus or to avulse the biceps from the radius. The ordinary signs of tendon rupture may be somewhat obscured, particularly if the radial attachment pulls off and the lacertus remains intact or if the lacertus pulls off and the radial attachment remains intact. Under these circumstances the shortening and bunching of the biceps which is so characteristic may not be present (Fig. 75, page 151). If there is complete rupture of the radial attachment it should be replaced surgically. This is true whether the attachment is torn from the muscle, torn in its substance or pulled off the bone. It is not necessary to repair the lacertus in the case of an independent injury. In fact, it is very infrequently torn since there is a certain amount of elasticity to its lateral attachment.

There may also be strain about the brachialis near its attachment to the ulna or of the anconeus or indeed of any of the muscles about the elbow. The symptoms will be those of disturbance of function of the particular muscle involved.

Epicondylitis (Tennis Elbow)

A type of involvement that is peculiar to the elbow develops along the medial and lateral epicondyles. The extensor-supinator muscles arise along the lateral epicondyle and the flexor-pronator muscles arise along the medial condyle, where they have an aponeurotic attachment. Either by contusion of the area or more commonly by strain, an irritation develops at the attachment of the aponeurosis to the bone that is quite characteristic. There is pain on the epicondyle which is aggravated by gripping. The pain extends down the corresponding group of the muscles, either medially or laterally, sometimes as far as the wrist. In the normal mechanism of clenching the fist one of the first phases of action is strong contraction of the carpal extensors in order to fix the wrist. If this did not occur the wrist would go into flexion and an ineffective fist result. This is exemplified by the hand in which there is radial paralysis. One is unable to make a fist, not because he cannot flex the fingers but because he cannot stabilize the wrist. So when the hand grasps an object, tension is placed on both the flexors and extensors of the wrist. Hence, simple gripping will cause pain whether the involvement be medial or lateral. On examination there is tenderness localized to the condyle or upward along the supracondylar ridge for a short distance. The tenderness may also extend down over the radial head but in the true epicondylitis the acute tenderness is directly on the condyle.

This condition may be extremely aggravating, particularly since it will often be chronic and recurrent and is increased by many activities of the forearm and hand. *Treatment* demands rest and in the severe case a splint that fixes the wrist in slight dorsiflexion and the elbow at 90 degrees may be needed. Local heat by diathermy, electric pad or whirlpool is useful. Dramatic results are often obtained by local injection, my preference being a long-acting local anesthetic plus a corticoid preparation. The needle should be inserted directly into the area of involvement with multiple puncture points. The anesthetic is injected until the tenderness is entirely relieved, after which the corticoid is injected into the same area. Following such an injection the pain may be much more severe for 12 to 24 hours but then subsides and the symptoms gradually improve until by the end of a few days they may be entirely gone. Should the symptoms then recur, a second or even a third or fourth injection may be necessary to obtain permanent relief. Throughout this period the patient must avoid the activities that caused the trouble. This frequently poses a problem since the activity that caused the condition may be an integral part of the regimen of this particular patient. Thus a pole vaulter may be unable to grasp his pole, a javelin player may be unable to snap his wrist or the baseball pitcher may have trouble gripping the ball or in sharply extending his elbow to throw. Hand shaking may be the offending activity and the resulting disability has been known to interfere with the activities of public figures. If nonsurgical measures fail the condition can ordinarily be relieved by detaching the muscles from the epicondyle and re-attaching them, thus eliminating the irritated area and permitting it to scar over.

While epicondylitis may follow a relatively acute strain it can also result from a chronic degenerative change by attrition of the aponeurotic fibers at the elbow. This occurs in certain types of athletics such as baseball pitching but it is not common in ordinary athletic pursuits, the acute sprain being the more likely cause. If there is degenerative change there may be calcification or even spur formation over the epicondyle. The patients present themselves complaining of an aching pain on the outer side of the elbow which is made more severe by active use of the forearm and hand.

This type of epicondylitis may seriously interfere with athletic competition, not so much because of pain at the elbow but because of restriction of use of the hand. The tender point should be protected by a contact pad. The patient should be warned to avoid gripping. Since this is extremely difficult in most sports it may be necessary to forbid participation for a period of several weeks.

The term "tennis elbow" is not entirely restricted to epicondylitis. Other conditions grouped under this category are radial head capsulitis and radiohumeral bursitis, for which see below.

SPRAIN

Since the elbow is a stable joint, ligament injury here is relatively uncommon. It is virtually impossible to sprain the elbow by excess flexion. In excessive extension, on the other hand, as the olecranon impinges against the back of the humerus, the continuing force drives the coronoid away from the trochlea of the humerus. This results in injury to the anterior portion of the collateral ligaments, particularly on the medial side. This injury may vary from a partial tear of little significance to complete rupture of the ligaments and capsule. As the force stops short of complete rupture, the elbow flexes, the tension is relaxed and there is no feeling of instability at the elbow joint because of its inherent bony stability and because of the fact that it does not require the degree of stability for weight bearing that is necessary at the knee.

The patient with such an injury will present himself with a history of hyperextension of the elbow and severe pain on the medial and sometimes the lateral side of the elbow which has been relieved by flexion so that he ordinarily will have his hand tucked into his shirt or his thumb hooked over his belt to prevent elbow extension. The symptoms at the time of the examination vary directly according to the severity of injury. Pain is not ordinarily a prominent factor. There will be localized tenderness at the site of the tear, either along the ulna on the medial side or along the epicondyle. There may also be pain along the lateral collateral ligaments at the site of the tear. Any attempt to extend the arm causes pain, and motion is stopped short of complete extension by muscle spasm. I have never seen a case in an athlete in which I could demonstrate excess motion indicating a complete tear.

The collateral ligaments may also be sprained by lateral motion. Forced abduction of the extended arm will damage the medial ligaments. Forced adduction will damage the lateral. Here again, instability is extremely infrequent and I find it very difficult to determine whether or not the rupture is complete unless there has been a complete dislocation of the elbow. Symptoms in the case of lateral stresses will be localized to the one side with the same findings as those for hyperextension, that is, tenderness along the site of the tear, local swelling, pain on attempt to reproduce the causative force.

Treatment of such a sprain is relatively simple. In the acute stage cold followed by heat and a protective sling will be adequate. Use of the extremity should be restricted for the first few days but unless the injury is quite symptomatic a splint is not necessary. As the acute symptoms subside, more motion may be permitted but always within the limits of pain for at least four weeks. At this time active unprotected function should be encouraged.

DISLOCATION

As the hyperextension force at the elbow continues, the olecranon remains fixed in the olecranon fossa, extension of the arm levers the coronoid completely around the trochlea, and the lower end of the humerus slides forward and downward to lodge against the anterior ulnar shaft distal to the coronoid (Fig. 113). At the same time the capitellum by virtue of rupture of the lateral collateral ligaments slides forward and downward so that it rests on the radial neck. There may be a lateral component of this dislocation so that the coronoid of the ulna may lie behind the capitellum rather than the trochlea (Fig. 114), in which instance the radial head is displaced laterally and does not appose the humerus.

Dislocation of the elbow cannot occur without rupture of the collateral ligaments. In many instances the force is relieved before this dislocation becomes complete and the elbow components slip back into their normal relationship. This subluxation or spontaneously reduced dislocation presumably has occurred whenever complete rupture of both collateral ligaments is diagnosed. The dislocated elbow

Figure 113.   Lateral x-ray of a dislocated elbow, showing the lower end of the humerus resting on the ulna in front of the coronoid. Note fragmentation of the coronoid.

has a rather typical deformity, with the olecranon prominent posteriorly and with the forearm extended slightly beyond a right angle. If the dislocation remains unreduced, immediate, extensive swelling occurs, rapidly obliterating the bony landmarks about the elbow.

The most pressing requirement on examination of such a patient is to determine the circulatory capacity to the hand since circulatory changes rapidly become irreversible. One should carefully determine the presence or absence of the radial pulse. Careful attention should be given to the capillary circulation of the nail beds. A second requirement is investigation of the possibility of involvement of the nerves. The nerve most likely to be involved is the median which is caught on the end of the humerus as the bone slides forward. Any interference with the nerve supply should be carefully determined. It is extremely important to record any neurological change *before* an attempt at reduction is made, else one may never know whether the nerve damage was immediate and was caused by the dislocation, or was caused by the trauma of reduction or developed later because of swelling and edema.

Treatment. A dislocated elbow is a surgical emergency. The result obtained from treatment of such an injury depends to a great extent upon the length of time the dislocation has been unreduced. If the arm is seen immediately after the injury (for instance on the playing field), one should take the time to investigate the circulation of the hand and to make a rough evaluation of the nerve supply. At this time, while the arm is numb and swelling has not taken place, it may be possible to reduce the deformity at once and without anesthesia. This must be done by the gentlest means since forceful manipulation will not only increase the muscle spasm and prevent reduction but may also cause severe damage to the nerve or blood supply which may have been spared at the time of injury. If the forearm is displaced laterally, usually to the radial side, the upper arm should be steadied by the doctor with one hand while with the other he grasps the forearm just below the elbow. By gentle manipulation the lateral deformity is usually easily corrected. Once this is accomplished the right arm of the operator must be shifted to grasp the wrist and steady, even traction applied along the long axis of the forearm as the elbow gradually moves toward extension. If this causes pain and spasm the attempt should be discontinued. If the patient can relax his muscles the elbow may slip easily into position. This may be facilitated by slight hyperextension of the forearm which permits the coronoid to slide under the trochlea whereupon the dislocation will be reduced as the forearm is gently flexed. If the emergency reduction is not successful or if the patient is not seen immediately, he should be moved to the nearest place where there are proper facilities for x-ray and anesthesia. X-ray examination before the reduction is highly desirable. This not only will provide some idea as to the exact location of the bones but also will demonstrate any accompanying fractures (Figs. 117 and 118).

Fractures frequently accompany dislocation of the elbow, the most common being those of the epicondyles, the coronoid and the radial head. The fractures are of either the avulsion or leverage type, and may greatly complicate the treatment of the dislocated elbow. The coronoid may be injured as it passes under the humerus by combination of muscle pull and direct impingement, the significance being that there may be avulsion of the anterior capsular ligaments and also of a portion of the brachialis attachment. Similarly the epicondyle may be avulsed by pull of the flexors or extensors. The medial epicondylar epiphysis is most frequently pulled off since it is the last epiphysis at the elbow to close. It may well be avulsed and the small button epiphysis be overlooked in its displaced position (Fig. 114). Many of these fractures require open reduction. If for any reason open reduction of the fracture is to be delayed beyond a very few hours the dislocation should be reduced at once—under anesthesia if necessary. It is extremely important that the dislocation be reduced at the earliest possible moment even if a second anesthetic will be required for later surgical replacement of a fragment. Prompt reduction of the dislocation will prevent excessive swelling in the soft tissues, excessive and long-continued stretching of the nerves or blood vessels, and other serious complications. The elbow invariably should be x-rayed following reduction *before application of a splint* (Fig. 114). I wish to emphasize this point, since it is very difficult to visualize by x-ray a small displaced fragment about the elbow through a plaster splint. If there is any doubt at all as to the relationship of the epicondyles or coronoid or radial head, similar x-rays should be made on the normal elbow and the two films carefully compared.

Following reduction of the dislocation one should again painstakingly assess the circulation of the hand. If possible the elbow should be fixed at 90 degrees by application of a splint. The circulation should again be evaluated in this position both before and after the application of the splint. Similarly, a check of nerve function should be carried out, although this must await recovery from the effects of the anesthetic. Then it should be done at the earliest possible moment since it is extremely important to know at what stage nerve symptoms develop. The decision as to the method of management of the nerve injury may depend wholly upon this knowledge. If there is sudden complete loss of function of the nerve at the time of the accident early repair is indicated, whereas if the onset is gradual a more con-

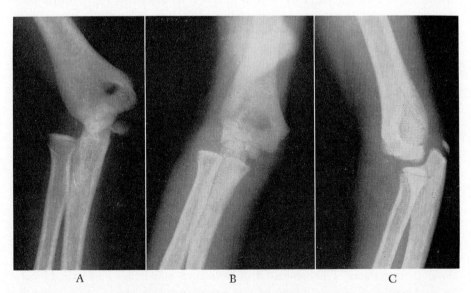

A   B   C

Figure 114.   A fracture-dislocation of the elbow in a child. *A,* Anteroposterior view before reduction. Note lateral displacement of the forearm in relation to arm. The medial epicondylar epiphysis is displaced with the ulna. *B,* Anteroposterior view before reduction. Note epicondylar epiphysis caught in joint. Also note the lateral displacement. *C,* Lateral view after reduction. Note epicondyle in joint.

servative attitude should be adopted. If the circulation is not intact with the elbow at 90 degrees the elbow should be extended to that position at which the circulation is satisfactory.

If there is evidence of arterial spasm with a white hand and absent radial pulse, an emergency situation exists that calls for immediate measures to restore the arterial circulation. A stellate ganglion block should be carried out. Vasodilator drugs should be given. Cold may be applied to the opposite hand. If such measures do not restore the arterial pulsation, the arm should be opened in the antecubital area and the artery identified and examined. Appropriate measures to restore circulation, such as stripping the artery if it is in spasm, repair or ligation if it is lacerated, are then carried out. These measures must not be delayed until irreversible changes take place in the hand. The hand is extremely vulnerable to circulatory disturbance. Simple loss of radial pulse does not mean arterial insufficiency. Loss of the pulse must be accompanied by signs of actual ischemia of the hand in order to justify exploration of the artery.

The duration of immobilization depends somewhat upon the degree of reaction in the elbow. Immobilization should be by anterior and posterior splints and not a solid cast (Fig. 115). There must be no constriction in the antecubital space. By the use of anterior-posterior splints the degree of tension in the forearm tissues can be readily assessed by palpation along the sides of the splint. The splints may be loosened if necessary and tightened as the swelling subsides. No attempt should be made to mobilize the arm until the swelling is well under control. If the case has been seen early and reduction carried out promptly there probably will not be excessive postreduction swelling. In such a case the arm should be immobilized in double splints for two weeks. At the end of two weeks if no pain and swelling are present in the elbow the anterior splint is removed and the posterior one continued. The posterior splint will permit a few degrees of flexion and extension and is worn for one more week, a total of three weeks. The arm is then placed in a sling which is to be worn another week. At the end of this time (four weeks) unrestricted active use of the arm can be permitted. Passive stretching has little place in the rehabilita-

Figure 115.   The anterior and posterior splint. *A,* Plaster splints carefully molded to the arm over sheet wadding. *B,* The dressing completed by application of gauze bandage.

Figure 116.   Calcification in the elbow capsule following dislocation.

tion of the elbow. There will be marked stiffness of the elbow following dislocation but motion should be complete after several months if meddlesome passive stretching is avoided.

Rehabilitation commences immediately by use of the fingers and thumb, setting of the muscles of the forearm, setting of the muscles of the upper arm, all within the limits of pain. As the course of treatment progresses to the use of the posterior splint alone, active flexion and extension of the elbow are permissible since this splint will "hinge" at the elbow. When the splint comes off, active use is encouraged, again within the limits of pain. Not before six weeks should forced motions be carried out. Any attempt to forcibly extend the elbow by passive stretching tends to delay the healing, increase the inflammatory reaction around the elbow and encourage calcium deposits. These deposits are not in the muscle in the nature of a myositis ossificans but are infiltrated throughout the capsule and ligaments of the joint (Fig. 116). Gravity is of great benefit in restoring extension and it may be acceptable to add to the effect of gravity by a lead wristlet (a pound or two). Little is gained by carrying a heavy weight, at least in the first six to eight weeks. A dislocated elbow is a serious injury and will require prolonged after-care. It should result in little or no permanent disability in the young athlete.

Calcification of the capsule of the elbow occurs not only with frank dislocation but with many lesser injuries of the ligament and capsule since this area is particularly prone to calcification. This often results in serious restriction of motion of the joint. Some of the most vulnerable areas are around the coronoid process of the humerus in the anterior capsule and the olecranon process of the humerus in the posterior capsule. Any calcification of either of these areas seriously restricts motion of the elbow. Calcification may also occur as a plaque of bone along the collateral ligaments where it not only restricts motion but may be quite painful on function.

Following dislocation or fracture-dislocation about the elbow, it is not unusual for calcification to surround the joint completely, causing serious disability. This tendency toward calcification should be recognized. Prompt care and rigorous management may tend to minimize this deposit. With adequate immobilization during the acute stage directly after the injury the extravasated blood is encouraged to absorb, thus minimizing calcification. Repeated manipulation at intervals of several days with resultant irritation tends to increase the calcification. A little later in the rehabilitation any attempt at forceful motion of the elbow stimulates calcification in the scar (see Fig. 19, page 46). These calcific deposits are not myositis ossificans since they do not occur in the muscle. Once the condition begins, treatment consists of immobilization and protection rather than manipulation. Nothing is gained by trying to prevent stiffness by manipulation once calcification is present. The temptation to remove the calcium surgically should be resisted for many months. It may ultimately be advisable to attempt excision of some calcific plaques but any attempt to do this before the growth is entirely mature and completely stable will only result in increased calcification. Indeed, the calcification may recur in any event.

FRACTURE-DISLOCATION

As has been mentioned above, fractures frequently accompany elbow dislocations. This is particularly true of those epiphyses which have not entirely closed. It is very common for the medial epicondylar epiphysis to be pulled off.

Epicondyles

The epicondyles serve for the attachment not only of the collateral ligaments of the elbow but also of strong muscles. All of these attachments are put under great stress during dislocation whether this dislocation be a straight forward dislocation of the humerus or has a lateral component. The bones carrying the attachments of the muscles are likely to be grossly displaced if the fracture is complete (Fig. 117).

Figure 117.   Spontaneously reduced dislocation of the elbow showing residual displacement of the medial epicondyle.

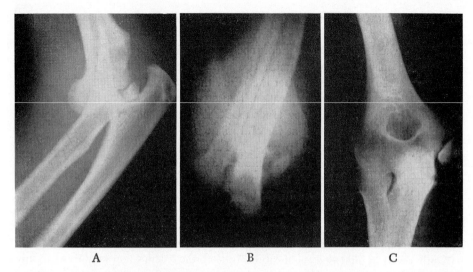

A   B   C

Figure 118.   Dislocated elbow with fracture of medial epicondyle. *A,* Showing dislocation with displacement of condyle into the joint. *B, C,* Showing reduction with poor position of the epicondyle.

Figure 119.   *A,* Avulsion of medial epicondyle. *B,* Replacement of condyle, held with nail. *C,* Late x-ray shows firm union.

Reduction of the elbow may catch the fragment within the joint (Fig. 114), and this may actually prevent complete reduction. X-ray examination as soon as possible after reduction of the dislocated elbow is imperative whether or not one was made before the reduction (Fig. 118). An avulsed condyle should be replaced surgically, even when the avulsion is simply of a muscle attachment with a small splinter of bone (Fig. 119) since firm fixation of this attachment will permit much more rapid motion and complete rehabilitation. The detached epicondyle tends to rotate because of the pull on its periphery so that it frequently presents its cortical surface toward the humerus and the fractured surface toward the skin (Fig. 120). Nonunion is quite common and growth disturbance inevitable when this occurs and is untreated (Fig. 121).

Figure 120.   A, Avulsion fracture of medial epicondyle with 90 degree rotation of the fragment. B, The fragment reduced and held with multiple Kirschner wires.

Figure 121.   A, Fracture of lateral condyle with growth retardation, causing marked cubitus valgus. B, Correction by osteotomy.

At operation the muscle or ligament attachment is carefully replaced with or without the fragment of bone. If the fragment is small it is better removed and the aponeurotic ligament fastened to the raw bone of the humerus. A larger fragment may be held in place by nail or screw or other suitable internal fixation (Figs. 119 and 120). Rehabilitative measures can proceed at about the same rate as if there had been no fracture, once internal fixation is secure. Any internal fixation should be removed after four to six weeks, particularly if it crosses the epiphyseal cartilage.

Ulnar Nerve Injury

The ulnar nerve is usually not injured in a posterior dislocation of the elbow. However, in a fracture involving the medial epicondyle, ulnar nerve injury occurs with some frequency. This again emphasizes the importance of careful evaluation of nerve injury prior to any manipulation or surgery. If there is evidence of ulnar nerve damage the nerve should be carefully examined at the time of the operation on the medial epicondyle. If there appears to be a possibility of its future involvement in scar, it should be transposed forward. On the other hand, if there is no sign of ulnar damage, it may be quite possible to replace the epicondyle without disturbing the nerve. The nerve must constantly be in the surgeon's consciousness, however, so that it is not inadvertently damaged either by the instruments or the internal fixation. Hence, it is desirable to locate the nerve early and to be sure of its integrity at the termination of the operation before the wound is closed. Following operation the function of the nerve should be determined at the earliest possible moment. If this is not done one may, upon the discovery of an ulnar palsy several days later, be unable to determine whether it was caused by a gradual constriction or later scar formation or by actual injury at operation. This may have a great deal of prognostic importance.

Coronoid Process

The coronoid may be broken off at the time of dislocation of the elbow (Fig. 122). If the fragment is small but somewhat displaced, it is best removed. If it comprises the major portion of the coronoid, its replacement may be necessary. This is a difficult procedure and should be postponed until the swelling of the elbow has subsided.

Figure 122.   Fracture-dislocation of the elbow. *A,* Fracture of radial head and fracture of the ulnar coronoid, with displacement. *B,* Resection of the radial head, replacement of the ulnar coronoid and fixation by screw.

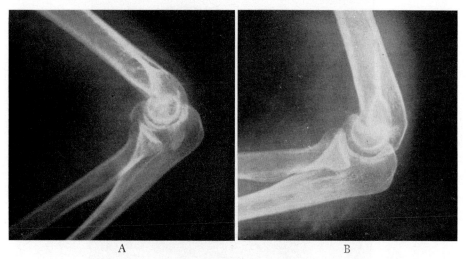

A   B

Figure 123.   *A,* Fracture of capitellum with separation of the fragments. This is the same
force that might break the radial head. *B,* Following open reduction.

Radial Head

At the time of dislocation of the elbow, the radial head is forcibly driven
against the lower end of the humerus and is frequently damaged. Indeed, many
complete fractures of the radial head have probably been accompanied by dislocation of the ulna which has reduced spontaneously. Treatment of a complete fracture of the radial head is almost always surgical since it is necessary that the head
be undistorted if normal rotation of the forearm is to be expected. Therefore, following a dislocation the head should be carefully examined roentgenologically (Fig.
122). A fragment that involves less than one-fourth of the entire circumference of
the radial head, particularly if it is on the lateral aspect of the head, may be
removed and the remaining intact head left in situ. One will often discover,
however, that there is also a comminuted fracture of the remaining portion of
the head as well as this small segment. These fractures are not avulsion fractures
since there is nothing attached to the rim of the radial head. They are caused by
direct force, hence there may be extensive chondral damage which does not show
on the film. There also may be damage to the cartilage of the capitellum of the
humerus (Fig. 123). These factors present another argument for early surgery in
fracture of the radial head in order that the nature of the lesion can be determined
and proper measures undertaken.

If there is a complete fracture of the radial head, particularly if it is comminuted in type, the head should be removed and the annular ligament carefully
repaired if it has been disrupted (Fig. 124). Most fractures through the radial neck
in adults should also be treated by excision of the radial head. Fractures occurring
in children before the upper radial epiphysis has closed should never be treated by
excision of the head, because of the disability following growth disturbances and
radial shortening. In these cases the head should carefully be replaced by open
reduction if manipulation fails, if there is angulation over 30 degrees or if there is
any lateral displacement.

Figure 124.   Fracture of radial head (A) with removal (B).

Figure 125.   Fracture-dislocation of elbow. The dislocation was reduced and the radial fragments allowed to remain. Subsequent picture (B) shows good healing of the radial head but with restriction of rotation, calcification of the medial capsule with restriction of flexion and extension, and pain. Radial head resection would have permitted earlier motion and better rehabilitation.

Olecranon

Almost all dislocations of the elbow are posterior. That is, the forearm moves posteriorly in relationship to the arm. This frequently has the lateral component indicated above. A true anterior dislocation of the elbow is virtually impossible without fracture either of the olecranon or the lower humerus. Anterior fracture-dislocation is a very serious injury usually resulting from force applied directly posteriorly (Fig. 126). The olecranon breaks, the triceps attachment holds the proximal fragments posteriorly, the lateral ligament gives way and the humerus moves backward into the fracture line. This same force may cause a fracture of the trochlea of the humerus or indeed of the entire distal end of the humerus. As the olecranon is driven into the distal end of the humerus it may act as a wedge and cause a condylar or T fracture. The radial head is not usually fractured in either of these instances since the forces applied do not put stress on it.

This injury must be treated surgically in order to obtain accurate replacement and firm internal fixation of the fragments. The exact type of fixation depends upon the circumstances. If the fragment is a single large block it may be held very well with a long intramedullary screw or pin. If the fragments are more comminuted a small plate may be needed. Some of the fragments or, indeed, all of the fragments may be removed with suture of the triceps tendon to the remaining olecranon (Fig. 127). One may remove a surprising amount of the olecranon process and not materially impair function of the elbow if the triceps is carefully repaired since the triceps sling gives sufficient stability. The elbow will tolerate considerably more roughness of the olecranon than the knee will of the patella because weight bearing is not involved. Open reduction following these injuries permits careful inspection of the cartilage, not only of the olecranon fossa but also of the humerus. The chondral fragments can be removed and the cartilage smoothed out with gratifying results.

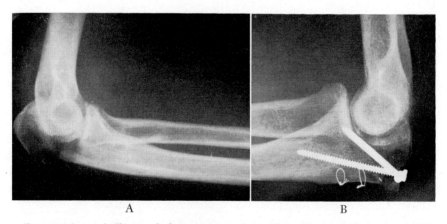

A   B

Figure 126.   A, Fractured olecranon at its base. This will require long intramedullary screw or pin for firm fixation. Treatment refused.

B, A similar case of fractured olecranon but with fractured coracoid. Note oblique screw transfixing olecranon and coronoid with longitudinal screw extending into the shaft. It is probably better to use a longer screw in the shaft but in a young individual good purchase can often be obtained without using intramedullary nail or screw.

Figure 127.   Fracture of olecranon after excision of broken tip and repair of tendon to olecranon.

The following steps are imperative in the treatment of complete dislocation of the elbow:

1. One must evaluate the circulation of the hand.
2. The nerve function of the hand must be determined.
3. Reduction must be completely atraumatic.
4. Careful x-ray study should be made after reduction before the splint is applied.
5. Appropriate treatment must be instituted for accompanying fractures about the elbow.
6. The elbow must be immobilized. It is not sufficient to simply use a sling.
7. Early forceful passive stretching of the elbow must not be carried out.
8. Patient, active rehabilitation will usually result in normal function.

FRACTURE

A complete discussion of fracture of the elbow, which is a large subject indeed, is not necessary here, the reader being referred to any standard text on treatment of fractures. However, there are certain peculiarities in the management of athletes with fracture about the elbow which should be emphasized.

A fracture of the elbow in a growing child is an extremely serious injury. The anatomical structure of the elbow is such that in children a supracondylar fracture, like a dislocation, may cause irreparable damage to the vessels or it may catch over the end of the bone with resulting impairment of the circulation. The fascia of the forearm is relatively inelastic and easily subject to intense swelling that

Figure 128.   Gangrene of the arm following a neglected fracture of the elbow. Amputation just below the shoulder was necessary.

results in irreparable damage to the forearm and hand (Fig. 128). Anyone who has seen or treated a case of Volkmann's contracture (Fig. 129) knows what a catastrophe it is. Of particular significance is the acute ischemia resulting from arterial spasm. This is contrasted sharply with the swelling of the hand resulting from venous congestion. The hand is cold, white and feels numb. There is no capillary pulse. This is an extreme emergency, and much more serious than ordinary congestion and swelling. It probably will not be relieved by ordinary measures such as straightening the elbow. It is obvious that any gross displacement at the fracture site should be completely reduced, particularly if there is anterior displacement. However, this condition may not be relieved by simple release of the pressure.

Figure 129.   Volkmann's contracture.

This syndrome demands immediate stellate ganglion block and emersion of the opposite hand in alternate ice and hot water. If such measures do not result in prompt restoration of circulation, the artery should be explored by incision in the antecubital fossa. The artery must be inspected and, if caught on a bony fragment, must be released. Ofttimes the artery is free but in spasm. Stripping of this artery will usually relieve the spasm and restore circulation. If the artery is lacerated or severed it must be repaired, replaced or ligated. Simple ligation will often relieve spasm and permit the collateral circulation to supply the distal area.

I know of no injury that requires more skill in management than the fractured elbow in a child. I make it an invariable rule in a child to x-ray both elbows and not try to remember or guess what the normal should be. By actually comparing one side with the other one can usually determine whether or not there is any displacement of fragments or disturbance of the normal relationships at the elbow.

Avulsion Fracture

In a previous section I have discussed fracture of the epicondyle in relation to dislocation. This same fracture may occur as an avulsion fracture by muscle violence without actual dislocation of the elbow. Not infrequently the medial epicondyle will be pulled off by the massive flexor pronator muscle contraction together with abduction stress on the forearm without acute dislocation of the elbow. This avulsion will be of the muscle and lateral ligament attachments at the elbow. Treatment is the same as previously indicated: accurate replacement and internal fixation with or without replacement of the fragment depending on its size and location.

It is possible for the olecranon to be avulsed by violent contraction of the triceps as the forearm is forcibly flexed, but this is unusual. If there is a complete fracture of the olecranon by such a force, the triceps attachment is of course disrupted. This should be repaired surgically regardless of the size of the fragment. If there is simply a "skin" of bone pulled off it should be treated exactly as tendon avulsion, namely, removal of the fragment and suture of the tendon to bone. If the fragment is larger it should be attached to the olecranon by internal fixation. The olecranon process makes up the trochlea fossa of the ulna and perfect positioning of the fragment is necessary to assure normal function. This cannot be obtained in the usual case by immobilization of the elbow in complete extension. Then, too, accurate and firm internal fixation permits rapid rehabilitation, whereas immobilization of the elbow in extension for a period long enough to permit the olecranon to unite will give rise to a great deal of difficulty in obtaining normal flexion later.

Direct contusion of the olecranon with the elbow flexed may result in fracture of the olecranon process. This may be comminuted and accompanied by anterior dislocation of the forearm on the humerus. This dislocation is usually spontaneously reduced before the patient is examined. Careful manipulation may determine whether or not there is instability of the ligaments in this direction. If this dislocation has been present, it greatly complicates the recovery. If the olecranon is broken it may be replaced and held by internal fixation. It may be necessary to remove some of the comminuted fragments in order to prevent overgrowth of callus. If the fragments are small and at the proximal tip they may be removed and the triceps sutured to the remaining olecranon.

BURSITIS

By far the most common bursal irritation at the elbow is of the olecranon bursa. This is the bursa lying between the skin and olecranon process to permit the skin to slide easily over the bony prominence (Fig. 130).

Acute Bursitis

Acute injury to the point of the elbow will usually result in hemorrhage into the olecranon bursa. The bursa distends with blood and there is synovial irritation. If this injury is seen early the blood may be aspirated, hyaluronidase injected and a pressure dressing applied. This will ordinarily relieve the condition although it may be necessary to aspirate more than once. More frequently, the condition does not receive early care since the symptoms and disability may not seem severe. The synovial irritation continues and a chronic bursitis ensues.

Occasionally following an injury or indeed without injury an infection occurs within the bursa and an acute suppurative bursitis ensues. The arm is hot, inflamed and red and the patient presents the ordinary signs of infection with malaise, fever, pain, restriction of motion, tenderness and swelling. If upon examination the bursa is found to be full of fluid this should be aspirated and a culture made. In the meantime the arm is immobilized in a sling and treated with continuous hot packs. An appropriate broad-spectrum antibiotic should be given in the hope that the acute inflammation will subside without the necessity for drainage. If the symptoms persist and aspiration does not relieve the effusion, the bursa should be drained surgically. Usually following acute inflammation and drainage the bursal walls become adherent and this automatically cures the bursitis. For the duration of the acute inflammation it is important that the arm be immobilized to avoid constant movement of the elbow. This is particularly true if an incision has been necessary. We advise an incision at either side of the bursa and the use of a through-and-through tissue drain which should be removed in a very few days as the inflammation subsides. Occasionally the infection will progress to spontaneous rupture of the bursa since

Olecranon bursitis

Figure 130.   Olecranon bursitis.

the skin over the back of the elbow is rather thin. The rupture usually occurs at the point of the olecranon and may leave a painful, adherent scar.

Much more frequently the bursitis is not suppurative. The bursa simply fills up with fluid under tension because of synovial irritation. This should be treated by aspiration followed by injection of a corticoid into the bursa and use of a pressure dressing. Repeated aspiration may be necessary but with proper treatment the acute bursitis will usually subside without apparent residual.

Chronic Bursitis

Since acute bursitis is frequently overlooked, minimized or undertreated, a chronic bursitis of the olecranon bursa is quite common. In this case the sac gradually enlarges, at times becoming quite tense with fluid. At other times the bursa is simply boggy and thick. Through the course of many weeks and months some of these bursae attain amazing size. The author has seen some as large as 7 inches long and 4 inches wide—a veritable bag of water dangling from the point of the elbow. When seen in the early stages these can often be relieved by aspiration, injection of a corticoid and pressure dressing, with the aspiration repeated at suitable intervals to prevent tension within the sac. Once the chronic bursitis is well established, surgical excision is usually the only means of obtaining permanent relief. Cartilaginous, or occasionally calcific, nodules may develop in the floor of the bursa which are readily palpable beneath the skin. They may become quite tender to pressure, giving rise to severe discomfort particularly when one rests his weight on the elbow. Surgical excision is simple since easy access can be obtained to this area. It is important to remove all of the bursa. Tacking the redundant skin to the underlying tissue may serve to prevent reaccumulation of fluid in the space and hence recurrence of the bursitis.

Radiohumeral Bursitis

Radiohumeral bursitis is frequently called "tennis elbow" and confused with epicondylitis. The radiohumeral bursa lies directly under the aponeurosis and as it passes over the radial head it permits the aponeurosis to slide freely over the humeral condyle and the radial capsule. Gripping will cause pressure on this area and so will cause pain simply by tensing the aponeurosis over the bursa, if the latter is inflamed. There usually is not sufficient bursal fluid to cause fluctuation. On examination the tenderness is localized over the radial head rather than over the epicondyle.

This condition responds well to local treatment with injection of a long-acting local anesthetic and a corticoid followed by elimination of the movements that cause pain. Indeed, it responds very well to the same therapy that relieves an epicondylitis.

OSTEOCHONDROSES

Osteochondritis dissecans is not common in the elbow except in certain avocations. The baseball pitcher, for example, is very prone to injury of the articular cartilage with resulting "joint mice," pitting of the cartilage, etc. X-ray diagnosis of osteochrondritis dissecans in articular cartilage at the elbow is difficult. Usually

Figure 131.   Excessive calcification following dislocation of elbow treated by early active use.

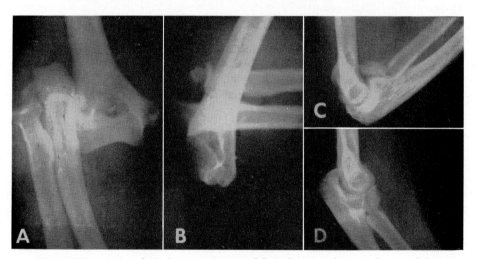

Figure 132.   A and B, Anteroposterior and lateral views of severe fracture-dislocation of the elbow, fracture of radial head and ulnar coronoid. C, Radial head removed. Remaining coronoid caused extensive calcification. D, Same as C, in extension, showing range of motion.

it is not seen until the fragment becomes detached. Indeed, it appears that the deposits may be largely in the nature of concretions formed within the joint as the result of chrondral tags and synovial irritation. While these occasionally will reach an amazing size (Fig. 131), they are usually very small and give trouble simply by being impinged between the olecranon and the back of the humerus (Fig. 133). Surgical removal is quite successful although repetition of the same activity that caused them to form may cause recurrence. At the time of removal the joint should be carefully explored and any suspicious areas of loose cartilage carefully

A   B

Figure 133.   X-ray of right (A) and left (B) elbow of professional football player who had gradually increasing disability culminating in sharp restriction of motion of the right elbow after he fell on his elbow. This is a chronic traumatic bilateral arthritis which markedly improved by surgical removal of the foreign bodies and spurs. No other joints were involved.

trimmed away. The joint should be thoroughly lavaged to wash out small rice bodies. If the foreign bodies appear to be the result of chronic synovitis the elbow can be treated by the usual measures of injection, local heat and protection. In chronic synovitis extensive effusion in the elbow is not common. The capsule is not redundant and is not prone to distend as it does in other joints during acute inflammation. Complete avoidance of the forceful action that caused this condition may be necessary to prevent prompt recurrence.

Injuries of
the Forearm

ANATOMICAL CONSIDERATIONS

WHILE to a large extent injuries to the forearm concern function of the wrist and hand, there are certain anatomical considerations in the forearm proper that merit review (Fig. 134). Whereas in the upper arm there is a single bone surrounded by a mass of muscle, the forearm contains two bones with the rather complex interrelated movements that were described in the chapter on the elbow. The ulna, being large at the elbow and small at the wrist, serves to give good stability between the humerus and the forearm. This humero-ulnar articulation permits motion in only one plane, flexion and extension. The ulna is fixed to the humerus and does not rotate so that the position of the entire shaft of the ulna is constant in relationship to the upper arm. At the lower forearm the radius is the larger bone and it alone articulates with the carpus. The radiocarpal joint is of the ball and socket type which permits motion in any direction. The range of motion permitted is due to ligamentous limitations rather than any bony block. The axial relationship of the radius to the carpus and hand is constant in the sense that there is little rotary motion between the carpus and the radius. Pronation-supination of the hand occurs by the rolling of the radius and carpus as a unit around the axis of the fixed ulna.

While the two bones of the forearm are essentially parallel to each other, the radius arches enough to allow considerable space between it and the ulna in the middle third whereas they are in contact at the proximal and the distal radio-ulnar

217

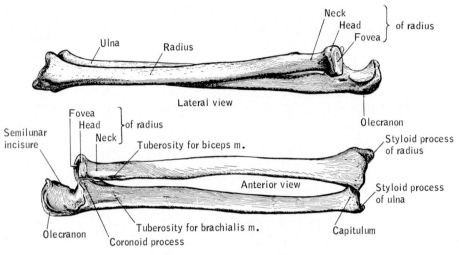

Figure 134.   The anatomy of forearm.

joints. The integrity of these two joints is entirely ligamentous. Each joint consists of a small saucer-like bed for the radial head at the upper end of the ulna and a small fossa for the ulna on the lower radius. The two bones are firmly bound together by the interosseous membrane. The fibers of this membrane are so interdigitated and decussated as to permit rotation of the radius over the ulna while maintaining constant tension of some of their fibers. The upper end of the radius is firmly fastened to the ulna by the orbicular ligament. At the distal end the ulna is bound to the radius by a similar arrangement so that these ligaments give considerable inherent stability to the two joints. On either side of the interosseous membrane lie the blood vessels and nerves. An extremely intricate complex of muscles attach along the shafts of the two bones. The synergistic action of these muscles carries out all the complicated motions of the wrist and hand, each of the muscles having a somewhat different function depending upon the relative position of the hand and the forearm and arm.

This is not the place for a more detailed discussion of the anatomy of the forearm. The reader is urged to consult a good atlas of anatomy, and he is bound to be amazed by the ingenuity with which the function of the hand is assured. The entire dorsal surface of the ulna is subcutaneous so that from the tip of the olecranon to the ulnar styloid the bone can readily be palpated beneath the skin. The only subcutaneous areas on the radius are at its proximal and distal extremities.

CONTUSION

The forearm is very subject to contusion because of the substantial area of subcutaneous bone. This is doubly true since the forearm is toward the distal extremity of the most active member of the body and so often comes in violent contact with an opposing player or an obstacle. Hence, a contusion may result from a fall on the olecranon process with the elbow flexed or from a direct blow against the subcutaneous shaft of the ulna.

Contusion of the Skin

In either of the above instances the result is damage to the skin with typical excoriation, pain, local swelling and hematoma. The most frequent complications which may arise are olecranon bursitis at the elbow and a periostitis along the ulna. Ordinarily, contusion of the skin presents minimal disability and *treatment* should be largely of a local character: aspiration of the hematoma, injection of long-acting anesthetic, pressure dressing followed by application of cold in the early stages to be subsequently changed to heat. The area can be adequately protected by a pressure pad and usually contusion need not interfere with athletic participation. Chronic periostitis, if it results, may require more comprehensive treatment with injection of a corticoid and more extensive physical therapeutic measures.

Contusion Involving the Musculotendinous Structures

Of more consequence than contusion of the skin is contusion involving the musculotendinous structures. This is particularly pertinent in the lower forearm where the tendons become subcutaneous as they converge toward the carpal tunnel on the volar side and toward the extensor aponeurosis on the dorsal side of the wrist. In these circumstances the catching of a tendon and its sheath between the striking object and the underlying bone may well result in a serious and disabling *traumatic tenosynovitis*. In this condition there is a history of a direct blow followed by discomfort of a moderate degree. After 12 to 36 hours the pain increases and is particularly aggravated by motion of the part involved. For example, if the extensor carpi ulnaris tendon is involved there will be pain on dorsiflexion of the wrist against resistance, pain on passive palmar flexion of the wrist and pain on gripping. All of these activities are well nigh essential to athletic competition. If the tendon happens to be the long supinator the pain will be on function of this muscle, etc. It behooves one to make a careful analysis of the symptoms involved in order to determine what tendon is involved. Usually the pain will be well localized over the area of the contusion.

Treatment of a traumatic tenosynovitis demands rest of the involved tendon. It is completely futile to try to "work it out," or to use extensive physical therapy and at the same time encourage use. The part must be put at functional rest and the best criterion of the adequacy of immobilization is relief of pain. Painful motion should be eliminated. This may mean restriction of motion of the wrist either in rotation or flexion and extension and also interdiction of gripping. If a little time is taken to explain to the athlete the purpose of asking him not to exercise the part to the extent of causing pain, he can usually be permitted to exercise just short of the pain-producing movement and so continue his rehabilitation to some extent. Local treatment is of value and injection of the involved tendon sheath with local anesthetic and one of the corticoid preparations is worthwhile. It is, however, more successful in the chronic than in the acute stage. In the acute stage rest, local heat and protection will usually result in good recovery. Recovery is likely to be more complete following a tenosynovitis caused by contusion than one caused by strain. Very frequently a chronic tenosynovitis results. This will be discussed later under the proper heading.

Another complication of contusion is *fracture*. If the condition appears to be severe, the bone tenderness is acute, and function is painful, careful x-ray study should be made to rule out fracture.

Contusion higher in the forearm involving the belly of the muscle is similar in nature to muscular contusion anywhere and requires the same treatment, namely, aspiration, local injection, compression, cold followed by heat and protection against motion. However, contusion of the muscles of the forearm presents the additional problem in that the motions of these muscles are extremely complex and so may cause considerably more disability for a given degree of contusion than elsewhere in the body. Very early rehabilitative use of the fingers can nevertheless be permitted, always short of pain. Protection may consist simply in prevention of competition and careful instruction. For certain sports it is possible to support the wrist and so wrap the forearm that the injured muscle can be protected. This extensive wrapping should be carefully removed once competition is over to permit resumption of pain-free function.

STRAIN

Strain is a common problem in the forearm, where many tendons glide together in the same sheath or separately. Any one of these musculotendinous units may be subject to strain from overexertion caused by a single active contraction of the muscle against too much resistance, from overstretching of the musculotendinous unit or from chronic overuse of the unit. The unit may be damaged by the actual disruption of some of its fibers by stretching, by a single violent contraction of the muscle beyond its capacity, or by repeated contractions of the muscle beyond its fatigue quotient.

Acute Strain

In acute strain the symptoms are pain along the area of strain, usually at the musculotendinous junction or at the attachment of the tendon to the bone. At this stage, overstretching or active contraction of the unit will cause pain at the area of strain. As the condition continues a tenosynovitis develops with irritation between the tendon and its sheath or mesotendon. This results in hyperemia, local swelling, inflammation and exudation of fluid. As the tendon continues to slide within the irritated sheath, sticky adhesions result and the so-called "snowball" crepitation is elicited; i.e., with the finger over the tendon soft crepitation can be felt as the tendon slides up and down the sheath. This motion is painful and becomes increasingly so as use is continued. If the condition progresses, the tenosynovitis may become adhesive in which state the tendon refuses to slide and dense adhesions form between the tendon and sheath. In other circumstances the tendon itself thickens and becomes constricted by its sheath.

If the strain is in the muscle belly the pain will be muscular and more diffuse. This results either from congestion within the muscle or rupture of some of the muscle fibers, or both. In extreme cases the strain may be so severe that continued use may cause a rupture somewhere in the unit. This may be of the fibers of the muscle itself or at the origin of the muscle or the attachment of the tendon. Very careful analysis of the condition will permit one to determine the exact location and nature of injury and so suggest the treatment. Only by careful examination can one properly regulate the treatment of the condition since the treatment will vary from no specific treatment to surgical repair of the lacerated unit.

Treatment of the acute strain depends upon the severity of the condition and the exact unit involved. The principles of treatment are rest, local heat and protection. In the very early stage an ice pack and compression bandage may be used, particularly if hemorrhage within the muscle is suspected. Within a few hours cold should give way to local heat. Until the severity of the condition is determined it is wise to immobilize the forearm in a position that will relax the involved unit. If the muscles to the fingers are involved, immobilization should include the hand. A word of caution should be sounded against prolonged immobilization of the fingers. In the first place, the fingers do not tolerate immobilization well and the joints tend to stiffen very rapidly. In the second place, active unresisted motion of the fingers will put very little strain on the injured area, the exception being a case of acute tenosynovitis involving the tendons to the fingers themselves.

The strain and, indeed, the resulting tenosynovitis much more commonly involve the muscles to the wrist so that immobilization is adequate if it terminates at the distal palmar crease with the wrist placed in the slight cock-up position. Careful inspection of the forearm should be carried out at frequent intervals in order to determine the progress of the condition. As soon as unresisted movement of the wrist is pain-free, complete immobilization may be discontinued and protection substituted. In a strain of moderate severity this will usually be a week or ten days. If the condition has gone on to tenosynovitis, the treatment must be more prolonged and more intensive with absolute immobilization of the affected tendon and some sort of inductive heat which can be given through the splint. Once crepitation is detected, meddlesome testing should not be carried out for at least a week since repeated irritation only encourages adhesions and complete rest will permit resolution of the lesion. There is no place for local injection in the case of acute tenosynovitis. Only occasionally will there be sufficient fluid in the tendon sheath to justify aspiration.

Chronic Strain

Management of the chronic strain can be extremely difficult for the doctor and disheartening to the athlete. In the usual case the strain is caused by the very activity which the athlete wants to recommence and resumption will cause its recurrence. The condition should be managed by rest and local heat. Careful analysis of the cause of the strain may reveal some unusual habit or posture which can be altered to place less strain on the involved muscle. As in so many conditions, it is important that use of the muscle be held within the limits of discomfort and pain and that overuse be carefully avoided. In the management of chronic tenosynovitis the same general dicta apply. In this circumstance, however, local treatment is of considerable value and injection of a corticoid into the involved tendon sheath may speed up the recovery markedly. There are no areas in the forearm proper in which constricting tenosynovitis is a problem.

FRACTURE

The forearm is a common location for a fracture in the young individual, usually caused by a fall on the outstretched arm. Hence, in any instance following a fall in which there is severe pain with swelling and disability, fracture should be suspected. X-ray examination of the forearm is easy and should be carried out in case of any doubt. One common error in x-ray examination is to get anteroposterior and lateral views by simply rotating the hand on the film. This does not rotate the ulna and while it results in anteroposterior and lateral views of the radius, the ulna is shown in the same plane. The forearm epitomizes very well the rule that the adjacent joints should be visualized. In making an x-ray of the forearm the elbow and the wrist should be included. If there is any suspicion of epiphyseal separation or of some abnormality of the forearm, films of the opposite extremity should be taken for comparison.

A detailed discussion of the *treatment* of fractures of the forearm will not be given here since it is available in many good textbooks on fractures. A few points pertinent to the athlete should be mentioned, however.

Since the radius rotates around the ulna in pronation-supination of the forearm, one should be particularly careful to immobilize the elbow in case of fracture of the radius even at its distal end. An undisplaced fracture of the radius may become displaced by rotation of the forearm.

The so-called *"greenstick fracture,"* in which the forearm is bent and one cortex is broken and the other is intact, may trap the unwary. It is too easy to simply straighten the bone out and apply a splint or indeed a circular cast. Often as the fracture heals, however, the deformity recurs and on removing the splint marked bowing of the forearm bones is found (Fig. 135). This is particularly likely to happen if a solid cast is used since the cast becomes loose as the muscles atrophy and the swelling subsides. As a general rule, the greenstick fracture should be completely broken and this will usually require anesthesia. An exception is in the youngster in whom the dorsal cortex at the lower end of the forearm is buckled by a fracture equivalent to a Colles' fracture in the adult. The angulation can sometimes be straightened by a quick snap without anesthesia. Following fracture of the forearm the young athlete should wear some protection on this arm for several weeks.

Typical *Colles' fracture* is quite unusual in the athlete since ordinarily there will be a distal radial epiphyseal dislocation or fracture slightly higher in the forearm.

Subluxation of the distal radial epiphysis has considerable significance and requires careful handling in order to minimize the danger of growth disturbance. If the pain of the so-called "strained" wrist is actually at the lower end of the radius,

Figure 135.   A, Greenstick fracture of lower radius. B, Reduced and in splint without breaking the dorsal cortex. C, Recurrence of deformity in splint. This deformity may correct spontaneously since the child was only 7 years old and molding is already beginning. Surgery is not indicated.

Figure 136. "Sprain" of the wrist. Note the buckling of the dorsal cortex which indicates that this is the same injury shown in Figure 137 which was either spontaneously reduced or was incomplete to start with. No reduction necessary.

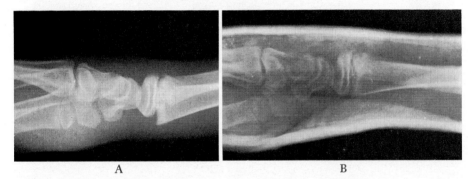

A   B

Figure 137. A, Epiphyseal dislocation of lower radius. Note the fragmentation of the dorsal cortex indicating that a part of the epiphysis is probably intact. Should premature closure occur in one portion of this epiphysis and not in another, deformity may occur.

B, Atraumatic but complete reduction gives some insurance against premature closure.

x-ray is mandatory. If the x-ray shows any abnormality in the epiphyseal plate, films of the opposite wrist should be made for careful comparison. Many times the so-called "sprained wrist" will actually be a slipping of the epiphysis (Fig. 136). In this instance the subluxation either was incomplete or was spontaneously reduced. In spite of normal appearing x-rays there will be persistent pain along the distal radial epiphyseal plate. Even if there is no displacement, the wrist should be immobilized until this tenderness disappears. If the epiphysis is displaced (Fig. 137) it should be reduced promptly and completely with as little trauma as possible. In any case of real or suspected damage to the epiphysis the parents should be warned of the possibility of growth disturbance with consequent radial shortening (Fig. 138). This does not often occur but may be quite deforming when it does. This same type of injury may result in a dislocation extending partially through the plate with a fracture extending up the radial shaft (Fig. 139). This also requires very careful reduction. Growth disturbance here may lead not only to overall shortening but to angulation, which is even more distressing than shortening. This case

Figure 138.   Radial shortening from epiphyseal disturbance following fracture of the lower radius. Note complete dislocation of the radio-ulnar joint, the ulna being distal to and behind the carpus. This was extremely disabling. Correction was carried out by shortening of the ulna and osteotomy of the radius.

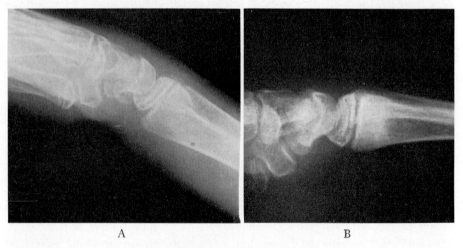

A   B

Figure 139.   A, Fracture-dislocation of lower epiphysis of the radius. Note the epiphyseal dislocation on the palmar two-thirds of the plate with fracture of the shaft dorsally. B, Early accurate repositioning will minimize the chances of epiphyseal disturbance and growth deformity.

should be very carefully followed and if angulation begins the viable part of the epiphysis should be closed to prevent increasing deformity.

Complete fractures of both bones of the forearm in the adolescent or adult are extremely difficult to reduce properly and hold in position by external means. One must bear in mind that in this category of patients one will wait in vain for correction of the deformity by natural forces. The beneficent effects of further growth which are so notable in the child will not be seen. Forearm fractures with displacement illustrate well the aphorism that fractures do not spontaneously improve in the splint. If the reduction looks bad before the splint is applied it is going to look worse when the splint is removed. There is no place for optimism in the management of a fracture in the athlete. Every effort must be made to restore the bones to their normal position. This is particularly true in the forearm where the interrelationships with the wrist and hand are extremely intricate.

CHAPTER

11

Injuries of
the Wrist

ANATOMICAL CONSIDERATIONS

THE WRIST covers the area from the distal end of the radius and ulna to the proximal end of the metacarpals (Figs. 140 and 141). This includes the eight carpal bones, the proximal articular surfaces of the metacarpals, the distal articular surface of the radius and the fibrocartilage at the distal end of the ulna. There is no articulation between the ulna and the carpus, the two being separated by a fibrocartilaginous disc which also separates the wrist joint proper from the distal radio-ulnar (Fig. 141A). The shallow concavity of the distal end of the radius is extended ulnarward by the articular disc which thus serves to broaden the carpal articulation. At the radiocarpal joint the proximal row of carpal bones together form a smooth convex surface that articulates with the concavity at the lower end of the radius.

The amazing complexities of the articulations of the carpal bones will not be discussed in detail here. It is important to recognize the relationships of these bones to one another and to the forearm and hand. The greater part of the motion at the wrist takes place between the carpals as a unit and the radius. However, there is a small amount of motion in each of the intercarpal joints. The navicular bone, the most radial of the proximal row, is long and boat-shaped and extends the furthest distally of this proximal row. In a transection through the wrist it will be noted that the capitate and to a less extent the hamate extend proximally into a concavity formed by the navicular, lunate and triquetrum. The two multangular

226

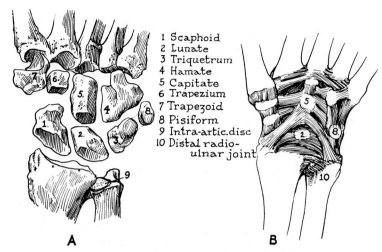

1 Scaphoid
2 Lunate
3 Triquetrum
4 Hamate
5 Capitate
6 Trapezium
7 Trapezoid
8 Pisiform
9 Intra-artic.disc
10 Distal radio-
      ulnar joint

A   B

Figure 140.   Structure of the wrist joint.

A, The bones of the carpal mechanism, opened on their volar surfaces, are irregular in size and shape but fit perfectly like the pieces of a jigsaw puzzle (after Grant).

B, Many strong ligaments hold the carpal bones firmly in place, connecting their volar surfaces to the radius, the metacarpals, and to each other.

The intra-articular disc separates the wrist joint from the distal radio-ulnar joint, and acts as a soft-part hinge upon which the radius swings around the ulnar head in supination and pronation. (From McLaughlin, "Trauma.")

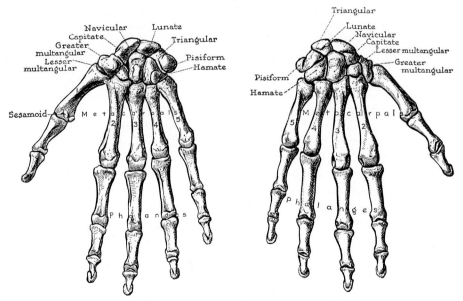

Figure 141.   Palmar and dorsal aspects of bones of the right wrist and hand. (From Anson, "Atlas of Human Anatomy.")

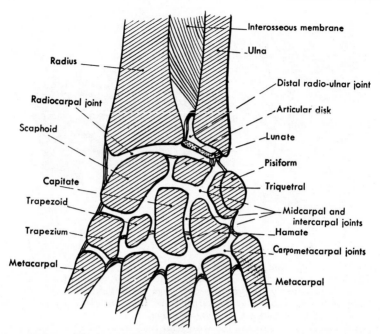

Figure 141A. The bones and the joint cavities of the wrist. Note that the radiocarpal and inferior radio-ulnar joint cavities are separate and distinct; that the midcarpal joint is continuous with the intercarpal joints between both the proximal and distal rows of the carpals; and that the carpometacarpal joints, except for that of the thumb, are continuous with the intermetacarpal joints and with the distal parts of the intercarpal joints, but have no communication with the midcarpal joint. (From Hollinshead "Functional Anatomy.")

bones are relatively short. Thus, the navicular extends across the two rows of the carpals, its distal portion actually extending more than halfway down the length of the capitate, a fact which makes it particularly vulnerable to injury on forceful motion through the midcarpal joint.

The entire lower end of the forearm, metacarpals and carpals are firmly bound together by the volar carpal ligaments which make a dense impenetrable ligamentous mass on the palmar surface of the wrist. Dorsally the ligaments are much weaker. These ligaments, and particularly the radial and the ulnar collateral ligaments, have various main conponents. The pisiform bone actually lies within the tendon of the flexor carpi ulnaris so that in effect the flexor carpi ulnaris attaches to the pisiform and in turn to the rest of the carpus through the strong ligaments extending from the pisiform to the metacarpals and to the hamate. Injury to the pisiform, therefore, is in a somewhat different category than injury to the other carpal bones.

In addition to the strong ligaments that bind these bones together there is a heavy band called the volar carpal ligament which extends from the greater multangular bone across to the hook of the hamate. By virtue of this ligamentous strap the volar carpal tunnel is formed, three sides of which are made up by the carpal bones themselves, the roof by the ligament (Fig. 142). Through this tunnel pass the flexor tendons to the fingers together with the median nerve. This sets the stage for the carpal tunnel syndrome. While the carpal bones are not in a true sense sub-

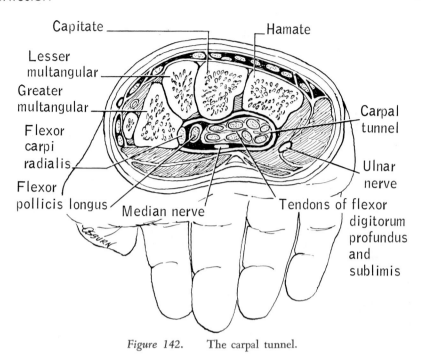

Figure 142.   The carpal tunnel.

cutaneous, they are covered only by ligaments, tendons, blood vessels and nerves, there being no muscular pad in the vicinity of the wrist.

CONTUSION

Contusion of the wrist is a frequent occurrence. It is not usually due to a fall but rather to a direct blow by the knee or headgear or foot when the outstretched hand is lying on the ground. Owing to the multiplicity of tendons in the wrist, the resulting injury is much more likely to involve them than the skin or bone. Hence, at the time of such an injury the wrist should be carefully examined for associated injury to the underlying structures. If the contusion seems severe, x-rays should be taken not only in the anteroposterior and lateral but in the right and left oblique planes. The carpal bones are not frequently fractured by a direct blow unless the crushing injury is especially severe. Tendon injury is quite common from contusion and, if overlooked or minimized, may progress to a chronic tenosynovitis with all its attendant disability.

Treatment.   Contusion of the wrist is treated by the usual measures according to its severity. If there is any doubt as to underlying injury to either tendon or bone a splint should be applied. If there is no involvement of the radio-ulnar joint, the splint may be limited to the forearm. A good test for the adequacy of the splint is to rotate the forearm through a complete arc of pronation-supination. If this causes pain the splint should go above the elbow. In the early stage the splint may be incorporated into the compression bandage and an ice pack used. Ordinarily the contusion is not too severe and an elastic bandage wrapped over a protective pad will be adequate, the more extensive treatment being reserved for the complications.

Laceration also will be found fairly commonly in the wrist although not as frequently as in the hand. This will be discussed in some detail in the section on the hand.

STRAIN

The general treatment of strain in this area was discussed in the section on the forearm. Since there are no muscles in the wrist proper, muscular strain does not occur here. However, this area is particularly vulnerable to tenosynovitis. The tenosynovitis may be the result of contusion of the tendon sheath, the tendon being caught between a blunt object and the hard bone, or it may be caused by a single violent muscular contraction against resistance or by violent passive motion. The most common cause for tenosynovitis in the wrist, however, is chronic overuse. With the multiplicity of tendons tenosynovitis may become a highly complicated problem. It will require the usual type of treatment, namely, local injection, rest, heat and protection as indicated above.

Tendon Rupture

Each of the many tendon attachments in the region of the wrist is subject to strain, those particularly vulnerable being the flexors and extensors of the wrist. The same forces that cause tenosynovitis may rupture some of the tendon fibers at their attachment. Usually the force is a violent passive motion rather than an active contraction of the muscle. The history is of a fall with resultant pain at the site of the attachment of the tendon. The injury may easily be confused with contusion of the wrist or sprain or carpal fracture, the significant finding being pain on active contraction of the muscle involved. Thus, if the extensor carpi radialis is avulsed from its carpal attachment, active dorsiflexion of the wrist against resistance will cause pain. This is not ordinarily the case in a sprain or a fracture. It is important to determine if possible the degree of injury. The detachment is usually not complete.

Treatment.   To relieve pain the wrist should be immobilized in the position in which the involved tendon is relaxed. If this tendon is an extensor the wrist is put in the cock-up position. If it is the flexor, the wrist is placed in flexion. This immobilization, which is most readily accomplished by plaster splints, must continue until the healing is complete, after which the wrist is carefully protected for the remainder of the playing season against the particular motion that caused the injury.

If the condition becomes chronic and there is persistent tenderness at the site of the tendon attachment and discomfort on active use of the muscle, local treatment is of some value. In these instances we advise injection of the area with a long-acting local anesthetic followed by a corticoid preparation. A test of the effectiveness of the injection is that the pain and tenderness must be completely relieved following the anesthetic injection. This will indicate that the condition has been correctly located. It should be remembered that many of these tendons have extensive insertions, particularly into the ligaments at the wrist and at the bases of the metacarpals. Following complete relief of pain and tenderness by anesthetic injection a corticoid is injected into the same area. In the chronic condition it is not necessary to immobilize the wrist completely but the patient should be warned against any activity that causes discomfort. Some sort of wrist wrapping or strapping is advisable. Since the wrist flexors and extensors are tight whenever the fingers are made into a tight fist, forceful gripping should be discontinued during the treatment period, particularly if it causes discomfort. X-ray study should be carried out in any such condition involving the wrist. Occasionally a small flake of bone caused by avulsion of the tendon fibers if visualized in the x-ray will permit localization of the injury.

If the detachment is complete, it should be repaired surgically.

Certain peculiar characteristics of the wrist predispose to the pathological entities now to be described.

de Quervain's Disease (Constrictive Tenosynovitis)

As the tendons to the thumb cross over the lower end of the radius on its radial aspect, they pass through tunnels made up of grooves on the lower end of the radius and a fibrous retinaculum forming the roof. In particular, the long abductor and short extensor of the thumb pass directly over the styloid process of the radius and multiple tendons of the abductor pass through the same sheath. This sheath is directly subcutaneous. Tenosynovitis in this area is quite common, usually as a result of overuse of the wrist and thumb. These tendons slide through the tunnel not only in movements of the thumb but on movements of the wrist with the thumb fixed. As the condition progresses, the tendon tends to swell and the sheath to thicken and a situation arises analogous to "trigger finger" so that, while one tendon slides through the groove, another one hangs and doubles up. In the early stages it may then slip through the constriction with a palpable click (Fig. 143).

During the early stage of this condition use of the wrist is increasingly painful. An actual swelling appears over the styloid of the radius which on palpation is very firm and tender. At this stage the tendons will slide through the tunnel although with discomfort. A good test for this condition is to grasp the flexed thumb with the fingers, thus fixing the thumb flexion. Then adduct the wrist. This will cause severe pain in the area of the constriction since by this maneuver all the tendons are forced through the tunnel at the same time. The condition may progress until no motion of these tendons through the tunnel is possible.

If the condition is diagnosed in the early stage, *treatment* consists in immobili-

Figure 143. Stenosis of the two tendons in one osseofibrous canal. (K. L. Loomis, Journal of Bone and Joint Surgery, Vol. 33-A, 1951.)

zation of the wrist including the thumb if motion of the thumb is painful. Injection of the tender area with a long-acting local anesthetic and a corticoid may have some value. Care should be taken not to perforate the tendons themselves with the needle since this may increase the swelling. Local heat is a useful adjunct and if treatment is carried out promptly the condition should subside. Once it establishes itself it is very prone to recur.

Fortunately, surgical treatment is extremely effective. Through a small transverse skin incision across the radial styloid, the thickened tunnel can be visualized and its roof carefully divided. It may be necessary to unroof more than one compartment in a well established case, since the adjacent compartments frequently become involved. Attention must be called to possible variations in the insertion of the abductor pollicis longus tendon (Fig. 144). The best procedure is to actu-

Figure 144.   Variations in the insertion of the abductor pollicis longus tendon, associated with stenosing tenosynovitis. (T. Lacey II, H. L. Goldstein and C. E. Tobin, Journal of Bone and Joint Surgery, Vol. 33-A).

ally resect the entire roof of the tunnel rather than to split it since the condition may recur as the separated edges heal. A few days of immobilization after the operation will suffice and recovery is usually prompt and complete.

Carpal Tunnel Syndrome

The carpal tunnel syndrome develops from the unusual relationships on the volar aspect of the wrist, where the eight flexor tendons of the fingers pass through the constricted confines of the carpal tunnel (Fig. 142). Included in their mass is the median nerve. The median nerve is the most vulnerable and compressible of the structures at this location and so is the innocent bystander which bears the brunt of the damage. The syndrome may be initiated by direct trauma, such as a fall on the outstretched hand, which causes swelling and thickening of the volar carpal ligament. It may be initiated by tenosynovitis of the flexor tendons. It is not an infrequent complication of an injury such as a Colles' fracture or indeed fracture of any of the carpal bones.

The essential ingredient of the carpal tunnel syndrome is either swelling of the structures within the tunnel or constriction of the tunnel, or both. Under these circumstances pressure on the median nerve is evidenced first by tingling in the distribution of the median nerve at the tips of the fingers. The unwary physician may be deluded into believing that the involvement is in the fingers or in the nerve higher up in the arm. The characteristic distribution in the long and index fingers should lead one to suspect this condition. Careful examination then will elicit tenderness to deep pressure on the volar ligament which may increase the pain and paresthesia in the median distribution. Atrophy of the thenar muscles is a late manifestation. The condition should be diagnosed long before this occurs.

Treatment.   If the syndrome is diagnosed early, immobilization of the wrist may give relief since it accomplishes two things. In the first place it puts the swollen parts at rest and thus permits subsidence of the inflammation. In the second place it prevents the tendons from sliding up and down over the nerve. If the condition does not respond promptly to conservative treatment or if it shows signs of progression it should be treated surgically. Surgical treatment is highly successful but in this area it is not for the uninitiated. The transverse carpal ligament is exposed and resected (Fig. 144A). If there is definite constriction of the median nerve a saline neurolysis, accomplished by inserting a small needle into the nerve sheath above the constriction and forcing saline within the sheath to stretch it at the constricted area, is advisable. This is probably less traumatic than mechanical neurolysis carried out by splitting the sheath by sharp dissection. If irreversible changes of the nerve have not occurred, recovery will be complete.

Strain or Fracture of the Pisiform Bone

Anatomically the pisiform does not actually make up a part of the carpal joints Basically it lies within the tendon of the flexor carpi ulnaris but it has a small articulation with the hamate and this attachment, continuing down to the carpus through the ligament, connects the pisiform to the carpus. Forcible strain on the flexor carpi ulnaris tendon may cause injury here quite similar to that of injury around the

Figure 144A.   Carpal tunnel syndrome, classical. Constriction of the palmar carpal ligament. Note the palmar carpal ligament has been resected and reflected with the retractor.

patella. The tendon may be avulsed from the pisiform (Fig. 145). The pisiform may be pulled loose from its attachments or may actually break. The injury commonly occurs from a fall on the outstretched hand when the wrist is in dorsiflexion and the tendon is stretched tight. Tenderness along the palmar aspect of the hand and often sharply localized over the pisiform bone should lead one to suspect pisiform damage. On careful examination the flexor carpi ulnaris tendon can be palpated to its attachment in the bone and determination made of the exact loca-

Figure 145.   Avulsion of the pisiform by the flexor carpi ulnaris tendon. Fragment removed and tendon repaired to the carpus.

tion of the lesion. Both dorsiflexion of the wrist with radial deviation and active contraction of the flexor carpi ulnaris will cause pain. X-ray examination may or may not reveal involvement of the bone.

Treatment. The condition is treated as a strain. If rupture is complete (very unusual) the pisiform should be removed and the tendon repaired. If the condition is treated as a contusion the progress of recovery will be disappointing since constant re-injury by use of the involved muscle may prolong and even prevent recovery. In a chronic injury in this region calcification within the tendon is quite prone to occur, the result of a chronic tendinitis with degenerative change or of calcific growth within the hematoma.

Injury of the Triangular Cartilage

The fibrocartilaginous extension of the radiocarpal joint lying between the ulna and the carpus is subject to injury in sprains or fractures about the lower end of the forearm. The symptoms are of tenderness and pain not on the ulnar styloid but in the sulcus between the ulna and carpus. This is particularly elicited by lateral motion of the wrist, either by impingement as the wrist is pulled into adduction or by distraction as it is pulled into radial flexion. Rupture of the fibers of this ligamentous and cartilaginous structure may result in hemorrhage and degeneration. Calcification is a late manifestation of this same condition.

Treatment. During the acute phase this condition will ordinarily respond well to immobilization although it is quite prone to recur. In the chronic stage local injection into the cartilage of an anesthetic plus a corticoid may give considerable relief. If relief cannot be obtained the cartilage may be excised including the calcified area. Care should be taken not to damage the ulnar collateral ligament. If the ulnar collateral ligament is damaged it should be adequately repaired since a large part of the stability of the wrist depends upon the integrity of this structure.

Dislocation of the Extensor Carpi Ulnaris Tendon

This tendon lies in a groove along the medial side of the distal ulna. Dislocation is manifested by a feeling of slipping as the wrist is rotated, and by pain in the area. Attempts to hold the extensor in the groove are not often successful. The condition will usually become symptom-free except for the slipping and requires no particular treatment.

GANGLION

Ganglion, which has been previously discussed (page 64), has a predilection for the dorsum of the wrist, where it often causes disability particularly on forceful use. There is lively controversy as to the exact cause of the growth, many believing it to be a degenerative change and others considering it a synovial herniation either from the carpal joints or from one of the tendon sheaths. It probably arises from a variety of causes. In the wrist it usually presents itself as a soft, fluctuant, non-tender mass distal to the dorsal carpal ligament. It may protrude between any of the various tendons of the back of the hand but seems to be most common directly over the capitate. The condition seems to follow chronic strain or chronic sprain of the wrist but in many instances there is no history of trauma. It must be differ-

entiated from an effusion within the tendon sheath and from other types of soft
tissue tumor. Sometimes amazingly firm, it may feel like a cartilaginous or bony mass
under the skin. The mass is usually movable but not freely so since it has a firm
underlying attachment. Effusion in a tendon sheath is infrequent on the back of
the wrist and it is ordinarily not as firm as a ganglion and is more linear. In the case
of the firm tumor x-ray examination should be made to rule out possible bone
involvement.

   Treatment.   A ganglion may spontaneously regress and disappear altogether, or it may disappear and then reappear. The time-honored methods of break·
ing the sac and of aspiration will usually fail. I have not had satisfactory results
from the injection of corticoid, as has been reported by others. If the mass is trouble
some, causes pain or is too unsightly, it should be removed surgically. The success
of surgical removal depends upon adequate repair of whatever defect is found.
Sometimes the tumor can be dissected out intact. In still other instances it will be
diffuse so that the presenting part is comparable to the top of an iceberg in that
the mass covers a good deal of the posterior carpus beneath the tendons. If the ligaments are split or if there is a defect in the capsule of the wrist, careful suture is
necessary after removal of the ganglion. If there is a pedicle communicating to the
tendon or carpal joints, as is often the case, it should be carefully closed. After
removal of a ganglion the hand is immobilized in a cock-up wrist splint for at least
three weeks. True enough, this may result in some restriction of motion of the
wrist which may persist for several weeks but in my experience recurrence is much
less likely if the wrist is protected during the healing period.

   Ganglion may occur on the palmar aspect of the wrist or on the flexor tendons
to the fingers. Treatment is the same whatever the location.

SPRAIN-SUBLUXATION-FRACTURE-DISLOCATION

   Since by our definition *sprain* is a ligament injury, it is relatively uncommon
in the wrist. Most of the so-called "sprains"—and the diagnosis is a frequent one—are
not sprains at all but are strains of the tendon attachments or injuries to the bone.
The ligaments of the wrist permit a large amount of motion in the radiocarpal joint
but very little motion in the intercarpal joints. The massive ligaments on the volar
aspect of the wrist are so strong that in hyperextension the injury is more likely to be
a fracture of the carpal bones which may be incomplete or a contusion of the articular surfaces or possibly chondral fracture, rather than a tearing of the ligaments. It is
felt by some that in hyperextension there may be actual slipping of one row of carpals on the other which permits damage to the dorsal carpal ligaments although this
is rather difficult to demonstrate. Suffice it to say that in the very common dorsiflexion injury of the wrist, the damage is usually on the dorsal aspect. One should
therefore be very wary of the diagnosis of sprain of the wrist, i.e., ligament damage,
in the common dorsiflexion injury. On dorsal flexion of the wrist pain is more
frequent over the back of the wrist and forearm than over the front although the
greatest stress on the ligament would appear to have been on the volar side. If there
is tenderness over the carpus, careful x-ray study should be made and the carpal
bones closely studied both as to their position and condition.

   If the x-ray study is negative, as it usually is, and a diagnosis of "sprain" is made, the TREATMENT is by immobilization with the wrist in slight dorsiflexion for two or three weeks, unless the symptoms completely subside before this time, and by physical therapy. If facilities permit, the splints may be removed for daily treatment always within the limits of pain-free motion. When athletic participation is permitted the wrist should be carefully strapped to prevent re-injury since these conditions tend to be quite chronic. At the end of the period of immobilization further x-ray study should be carried out since linear fractures through the carpal bones may well be revealed in this second picture when they did not show in the first. The common carpal fracture is through the navicular at its midpoint since the navicular takes a good deal of stress of the wrist, whether it be in dorsiflexion or palmar flexion, because of its position bridging the two rows of carpals.

Subluxation and dislocation may accompany ligament injury and in the wrist they have some peculiar characteristics. Dislocation of the radiocarpal joint is extremely uncommon although it has happened as a result of violent action. A complete carpal dislocation is also uncommon and is obviously a serious injury. Both of these conditions present manifest deformity and disability, hence are readily diagnosed and ordinarily receive good treatment. The diagnosis of the exact dislocation through the carpus offers great difficulty, but careful x-ray study of the normal as well as the injured wrist in several positions will cut down the margin of error. It is particularly important that these conditions be diagnosed early since, as with most dislocations, the longer the dislocation remains unreduced the greater will be the likelihood of recurrence and of permanent residual disability. So in the presence of major swelling, pain and particularly deformity of the wrist prompt definitive treatment must be sought if there is any question as to the extent of injury or the perfection of reduction.

Dislocation of the Lunate (Semilunar Bone)

The most common dislocation in the wrist is of the lunate (Fig. 146). The shape of this bone lying between the massive capitate and the lower end of the radius makes it particularly prone to volar dislocation since the bone is narrow in its dorsal portion and quite wide at its volar margin. Forceful compression of the lunate against the capitate by dorsiflexion of the wrist slips this bone forward much in the manner of an apple seed pinched between the fingers (Fig. 146, B). The dorsal carpal ligament, which is attached to the lunate, gives way and the lunate slips forward, its convex proximal surface lodging along the undersurface of the

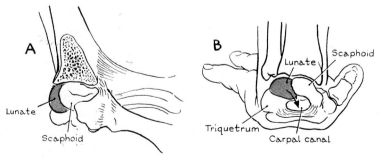

Figure 146.   Drawing showing dislocated lunate. (From McLaughlin, "Trauma.")

Figure 147.   Dislocated carpal lunate. The patient fell forcibly on the outstretched arm and another player fell over him. Note (A) the complete forward displacement of the lunate in relation to the carpus. B, Anteroposterior view shows the fracture of the styloid of the radius and styloid of ulna. The carpal dislocation was overlooked in treating the radius and ulna. It was recognized later and the lunate was removed with consequent disability.

capitate. If the dislocation is more pronounced the bone may be completely extruded from the space and may locate almost anywhere on the volar surface of the carpus. If the disrupting force is relatively mild the subluxation or dislocation may reduce spontaneously, but the damage to the dorsal carpal ligament will remain. Indeed, this may be the mechanism of sprains of the wrist in which the force is dorsal flexion but the ligament injured is actually on the side that is not overstretched.

It is extremely easy to overlook a dislocation of the lunate (Fig. 147). Clinically, the wrist will be painful. It will be tender on the dorsum just distal to the lower end of the radius. Brawny swelling will usually prevent palpation of the space where the lunate should be. On the palmar aspect of the wrist, particularly if it is examined early, there is a palpable thickened area under the flexor tendons, quite unlike the corresponding area, on the opposite wrist. Motion may not be acutely painful if the lunate is not locked under the volar ligaments; if the lunate is locked, motion may be completely prevented. In such a case careful x-ray study will reveal the deformity, particularly if the film is compared to a similar one of the opposite wrist.

Occasionally the displacement will be accompanied by neurological symptoms since the extruded lunate tends to compress the carpal tunnel. Frequently there will be paresthesia and pain in the median distribution of the hand, i.e., the first and second fingers, but in the acute injury these are easily overlooked because of the pain. It has been aptly said that the sprained wrist accompanied by symptoms of involvement of the median nerve in the hand is an indication of lunate dislocation. (Fig. 146, B.)

Treatment of these cases is often casual until late complications call attention to the diagnosis. By that time successful treatment will be virtually impossible. If the diagnosis can be made early, manipulative treatment is highly successful. Under complete anesthesia, straight traction combined with moderate dorsiflexion of the wrist open up the space from which the lunate was displaced and direct pressure against the lunate on the volar surface of the wrist will slip it into position. Once the bone is reduced the wrist should be moderately flexed. This tends to close the space again and maintain the proper position. Following reduction the wrist is protected by splinting in semiflexion for three weeks. It should then be moved into a neutral position for the fourth week. After this it is protected against dorsiflexion for several more weeks, particularly if athletic competition is to be permitted. It should be emphasized that closed reduction should be prompt if it is to be successful. If the bone is going to reduce at all, it will reduce by gentle manipulation. Force is neither necessary nor advisable. If closed reduction fails, open reduction should be carried out.

In far too many cases the diagnosis is not made early and the patients present themselves several days or several weeks after the injury. Closed reduction should not be attempted after the lapse of more than a week since then it is virtually impossible to open the space and reduce the bone. Even if the dislocation is reduced it is with so much attendant trauma that necrosis is inevitable. Open operation is relatively successful if carried out within the first few weeks. Afterward removal of the bone is probably more desirable than an attempt to force the lunate into its normal position. As is true in other dislocations, the longer the lunate remains dislocated, the greater is the likelihood of circulatory changes. For this reason many surgeons advise removal of the bone if it has remained dislocated more than two or three weeks. However, this does not give a normal wrist and I believe that in the athlete one should attempt reduction of the bone even if this means it later must be removed because of avascular necrosis. As might be expected, a dorsal incision is much to be preferred, and for two pertinent reasons. In the first place, considerable damage may be done to the remaining blood supply if the bone is dissected out from the front since the only remaining attachment to the lunate is the volar ligament. Secondly, it is necessary to traverse very vital structures on the volar aspect of the wrist in order to reach the dislocated bone. Dorsal exposure, while it may present some difficulties in actually reaching the bone, will be much less traumatic from both standpoints. In the very late case in which a firm decision has been made to remove the bone, a volar incision should be made. I cannot emphasize too strongly that the principal peril in these wrist injuries is that the true diagnosis will be overlooked and hence the ideal opportunity for definitive treatment will be lost. Any of the other carpal bones may be dislocated although this is quite uncommon.

Perilunar Dislocation

In dislocation of the lunate this bone dislocates both in relation to the radius and to the carpus so that there is a true dislocation of the lunate alone. In the so-called perilunar dislocation (Fig. 148) the lunate remains with the radius, and the

Figure 148.   Perilunar dislocation. Note that the lunate has remained with the radius while the rest of the carpus is dislocated dorsally. This case is unusual in that the navicular is intact. Frequently the proximal half of the navicular remains with the lunate, the remainder of the bone dislocating with the rest of the carpus. The "1" on the dome of the greater multangular in B should appose "2" on the concavity of the lunate as in view C.

carpus dislocates on the lunate and radius. This is almost never a pure dislocation. Usually the navicular bone either dislocates and the whole bone remains with the radius and the lunate or more commonly the navicular fractures at its vulnerable waist and its proximal fragment remains with the lunate and the radius. There are many possible combinations; for example, the entire proximal row of carpal bones may remain with the radius and the dislocation be intercarpal, or any combination of these bones may remain with the radius.

   Treatment.   This is an extremely serious type of fracture-dislocation and bodes ill for normal function of the wrist. For this reason this type of dislocation should be handled by the specialist. It is extremely important not only to get a perfect reduction but to maintain it. This dislocation is notably unstable because of the extensive damage to the carpal ligaments. Each of the carpal bones must fit exactly against the other if function is to be normal. Even if reduction of the displacement is obtained, one still must deal with the fracture so that the overall problem becomes very complicated. Time is of the very essence since the dislocation rapidly becomes irreducible because of massive fibrosis through the wrist. Should this occur, wrist fusion is practically the only procedure offering some salvage of function of the wrist.

   Chronic arthritic changes are common in these fracture-dislocations even under the most favorable circumstances. It behooves one to be precisely analytical in his studies of these obviously serious injuries to the wrist. X-ray diagnosis of a fracture-dislocation through the carpus is difficult and only by very careful study, with x-ray comparison of the injured wrist and the normal one, can one have a reasonable hope of success. One should be particularly suspicious in the sprain that is slow to recover or of the wrist that feels thick from front to back. For this reason no wrist injury should be treated for a long period of time without repeated careful observation

Figure 149. Radiocarpal dislocation. End result of a serious injury to the wrist. There was a fracture of the radial styloid which was reduced and held by a transfixion screw. The dislocation of the entire carpus on the lower end of the radius was not held reduced. Wrist fusion was the only solution to this painful wrist.

Figure 150. Fracture of hamate caused by forcible dorsiflexion and ulnar deviation of the wrist. At operation for removal of these fragments there was found to be very extensive ligament damage to the carpus indicating that the patient had had a carpometacarpal dislocation which had spontaneously reduced.

since the deformity, which may be obscured by swelling, may become quite evident once the swelling has been reduced.

Dislocation of the Navicular

A rather unusual injury of the carpus is dislocation of the navicular. This injury is much more readily determined by x-ray study since the radial-carpal relationship is more obviously disturbed than in the lunate dislocation. It is unusual for this dislocation to occur as an isolated injury; it is frequently the residual of an incompletely reduced perilunar or intercarpal dislocation.

Treatment. If the dislocation is seen and recognized early it may be reduced by manipulation. The wrist is placed in complete ulnar flexion to open up the space between the styloid of the radius and carpus, after which the navicular may be rotated in position by direct pressure of the fingers. It must be obvious that this can be much more readily accomplished early than late. As with most dislocations, the longer the navicular remains displaced the more likelihood there is of an aseptic necrosis of the bone. If the dislocation is recognized after several weeks, an attempt at open reduction may be carried out. If to obtain open reduction the navicular will have to be forced into position or held in position by forcible radial flexion of the wrist it may be advisable instead to remove it. However, if there seems to be some possibility of restoration of the circulation to the bone, reduction can be tried and fusion of the wrist or excision of the navicular done at a later operation if the first procedure fails.

Sprain-Fracture

Avulsion of the ligament from the bone results in a sprain-fracture. Careful x-ray study made in various positions may reveal the flake of bone lifted up from one of the carpals or from the lower radius or the ulnar styloid. As a general rule, sprain-fractures require longer for union than simple sprain. In some instances painful nonunion may develop between the flake of bone and the parent bone. In such a case it may be necessary to remove the fragment surgically and suture the tendon to its original bed.

Avulsion of the Ulnar Styloid

The styloid process of the ulna may be pulled off by the ulnar collateral ligament. This is in reality an injury to the ulnar collateral ligament and should be treated as such. It usually will heal with fibrous union without instability. If instability does occur, or if the area is painful on function, the styloid should be removed and the ligament sutured to the lower end of the ulna.

Avulsion of the Radial Styloid

The styloid process of the radius is not as vulnerable as is the styloid of the ulna, nor are its ligament attachments as strong. Usually a force that will break the styloid of the radius will either tear the radiocarpal ligament or break the lower end of the radius. A sharp ulnar flexion of the wrist with little or no dorsal component may cause avulsion of the radial styloid (Fig. 151). In such a case the symptoms will be those of sprain. There will be pain on ulnar deviation of the wrist but little pain on flexion and extension. The tenderness will be at the tip of

Figure 151.   *A,* Fracture of the styloid of the radius; presumably the fragment was pulled off
   by the lateral ligament. *B,* Note perfect union one month following screw fixation.

the styloid just at the base of the thumb. Careful examination will distinguish between tenderness over the navicular or over the base of the metacarpal of the thumb
and that over the radial styloid. These areas are all subcutaneous and can be readily
palpated. In palpating the dorsal surface of the radius one may be misled into believing that the condition is a sprain since the tenderness will be lateral rather than
dorsal. Any injury of this severity merits x-ray films taken in anteroposterior,
lateral and oblique planes. Careful study of the films will be necessary to reveal the
precise nature of the lesion. A very small fragment, hardly recognizable in the
x-ray, should be treated as a carpal sprain. On the other hand, a significant amount
of the styloid may be pulled away (Fig. 151). Poorly planned x-ray films may fail
to reveal the displacement.

   Treatment.   Since this fracture involves the articular surface of the radiocarpal joint, it is subject to the same prerequisites of treatment as are articular fractures elsewhere. The fragment must be perfectly reduced and firmly held until union
is secure or it must be removed and the ligament sutured to the radius. If the fragment is as substantial as in Figure 151, where it involves roughly two-fifths of the
articular surface, it should be replaced. The main problem is recognition of the
nature of the injury. It will be futile to try to replace the fragment and maintain
fixation by any bizarre position of the wrist. Internal fixation is an absolute
necessity.

FRACTURE

Fracture of the Navicular

   For reasons previously mentioned, the most common carpal fracture is of the
navicular. The fact that the navicular bridges the intercarpal joint, that it is directly

A   B

Figure 152. Acute fracture through the waist of the carpal navicular (*A*). Treated by plaster cast with solid union four months later (*B*).

impinged upon by the lower radius on dorsiflexion and radial deviation of the wrist, and that it has a rather narrow waist all contribute to this injury (Figs. 152, 153). The force is usually hyperextension as by falling on the outstretched hand—a force similar to that causing lunate dislocation or Colles' fracture. Following such an injury there will be pain through the wrist, not at the lower end of the radius but just distal to it. Careful x-ray study may well be negative. The diagnosis of sprain

Figure 153. *A,* Avulsion fracture of the carpal navicular by traction on the radiocarpal ligament. *B,* Solid union four months later following cast immobilization.

of the wrist is acceptable here if one is prepared to treat the sprain adequately, that is, by immobilization of the wrist for two or three weeks. At the end of two weeks the wrist should be re-x-rayed, care being taken to get oblique views. Frequently a fracture line will be revealed in this second x-ray. If the x-ray in two weeks is negative and symptoms still persist after four or five weeks, films should again be made with the wrist in various positions since the assumption must be that there is a fracture of the navicular until it can definitely be ruled out.

The *treatment of an undisplaced fracture* of the navicular is immobilization for a period long enough to permit the fracture to heal completely. This will be many weeks or months. The progress of union should be checked by x-ray. The original dressing should be anterior and posterior splints extending from the proximal interphalangeal joint to below the elbow with the wrist in slight dorsal flexion. The first phalanx of the thumb is included. This type of fixation is continued for a variable time depending upon the amount of swelling. If there is little reaction in the hand and no danger of constriction a solid cast may be applied at the first visit. In the presence of considerable swelling, however, plaster splints with some compression are used instead, the cast being postponed until the size of the wrist has somewhat stabilized. In any event immobilization should be early and complete, with the hand in the grasping position. No bizarre position of the wrist is either necessary or desirable. Since complete immobilization is important (Fig. 154) the

Figure 154.   Classical fracture through the waist of the navicular showing fibrous healing with spur formation following inadequate immobilization.

gauntlet cast should be changed if it becomes loose, as it usually does. This may require a change of cast every two or three weeks, at which time the x-ray check of the progress of union should be made. When union appears to be secure across the fracture line, as revealed in a good oblique x-ray picture, the gauntlet may be supplanted by a leather wristlet or adhesive strapping. If athletic competition is to be permitted, dorsiflexion of the wrist must be prevented by an adequate support. In the fracture without displacement it may not be necessary to immobilize the thumb. My own practice is to include the base of the thumb to the metacarpophalangeal joint and thus permit phalangeal but not metacarpal motion.

In a complete fracture and particularly in fracture with displacement or instability the type of immobilization described will not be adequate. The management of such a fracture requires the utmost in skill and judgment. If there is displacement an attempt may be made by manipulation to reduce the fragments. The hand is checked in radial deviation or in ulnar deviation, flexion or extension, to determine what position makes the fragments the most stable. It is my own opinion that such a fracture should be treated by operation to obtain perfect reduction and held with transfixion screw or pins. By this method immobilization can be assured at the fracture site although at the expense of some further sacrifice of circulation to the fragments. If the fracture line is actually unstable so that in various positions the fragments can be shown to move on each other, it is extremely unlikely that simple immobilization of the wrist will prevent motion. Indeed, immobilization of the wrist does not prevent rotation of the forearm and in rotation of the forearm there is inevitably some torsion at the radiocarpal joint.

Following operation the same treatment should be carried out as for a fracture without displacement. The after-care of such a fracture requires sound judgment. There seems little justification for continuing immobilization for many months if union does not appear to be progressing or if the fragment has become sclerotic or cystic. True enough, prolonged immobilization has in some cases finally resulted in bony union, but in my experience these are few and far between. The displaced fracture that has been unrecognized and is discovered after several weeks is also probably doomed to nonunion. In the x-ray study as the union or nonunion develops, decision must be made in each case on whether to continue immobilization or recommend some other type of treatment. If union is not at least proceeding satisfactorily after three or four months I would advise removal of the external fixation to allow function of the wrist.

Many of these ununited fractures are entirely pain-free and allow remarkably good wrist function (Fig. 155). If this is the case surgery is not advisable since any type of open reduction and grafting for delayed union or nonunion has a high percentage of failure. If symptoms persist and are disabling (Fig. 156) then one must consider the various possibilities for treatment of nonunion. I know of no treatment that can promise a normal wrist and the choice is a very difficult one. One must depend to a large extent upon the nature and condition of the navicular bone. If there is carpal arthritis and particularly arthritis of the radiocarpal joint, solid union of the navicular will not relieve the symptoms (Figs. 157 and 158). If the fracture is central and the bone fragments are relatively viable, bone grafting

Figure 155.   Longstanding nonunion of the carpal navicular fracture which occurred in football. Patient is now 60 with advanced degenerative arthritis of the radiocarpal joint and sclerosis of the adjacent margins of the fragments.

Figure 156.   Untreated fractured navicular with resultant cystic changes and considerable disability. This type of case is not amenable to bone grafting. The salvage procedure here would probably be radial styloidectomy although this would not completely relieve the symptoms.

Figure 157.   *A,* Unrecognized fracture through the waist of the carpal navicular which has gone on to union but with marked narrowing of the joint space and radiocarpal arthritis. This house painter was unable to work.

B, His symptoms were ameliorated by radial styloidectomy.

Figure 158.   *A,* Fracture of middle third of navicular with nonunion and bone spurring on navicular and radial styloid. *B,* Treated by excision of the radial styloid and bone graft with navicular pegs. Solid union. Good clinical result.

Figure 159.   A, Compression fracture of the body of the navicular caused by sharp radial flexion of the wrist so that the bone is impinged between the radial styloid and triquetrum.

B, This painful injury was relieved by removal of the fragment. Athletics resumed. If recognized early, this condition should be treated by immobilization with the wrist in ulnar flexion so that the carpal capsule will tend to pull the fragment back into position.

should be attempted and is frequently successful (Fig. 157). Since following this procedure there often will be chondral damage around the fracture site, it is advisable to remove the styloid of the radius (Figs. 157 and 158) so that the fracture line does not articulate across the lower end of the radius. Indeed, if the arthritis is localized to this area, a radial styloidectomy may be the treatment of choice either with or without grafting of the navicular. If, on the other hand, one fragment is small or there is comminution of one or the other fragment, these fragments should be removed (Fig. 159). Indeed, this probably should be done as a primary procedure in such a case. Because of the very poor prognosis in nonunion, it is extremely important that these fractures be diagnosed early since treatment of the acute fracture is highly successful while treatment of the nonunion is very unsatisfactory.

Should one be allowed to participate in sports following a fracture of the navicular? Most teams will not allow a member to wear a plaster cast; therefore, he should not be allowed to participate during the period in which union may still be expected. If injury has occurred in spring practice and several months have elapsed and union is not expected, should the patient be allowed to participate? I have permitted this where it seemed that nonunion was inevitable and there was no justification for further immobilization. I recall one player who "sprained" his wrist in spring practice. The navicular fracture was revealed after several weeks and he was treated by immobilization throughout the summer without union and was permitted to play the following season wearing a suitable leather gauntlet. At the end of the season, bone grafting was carried out (Fig. 160). Whether or not this is justifiable I think depends upon the drive of the particular patient and the importance to him of his participation.

Figure 160.   *A,* Fractured navicular through the waist as an acute injury. This was immobilized in plaster for four months (*B*) with no bony union. The patient was allowed to play football with the arm carefully protected in a brace and at the end of the season radial styloidectomy with peg grafts of the navicular was carried out with solid union (*C*). Arrow indicates well preserved radial navicular joint space.

Compression Fracture

Since the carpus is made up entirely of cancellous bone and since it is subject to compression forces such as a fall on the clenched fist or on the outstretched hand, it would seem that compression fractures of the carpal bones should be frequent. The fact that they are so rarely diagnosed does not necessarily mean they rarely occur. I am sure that many of the so-called sprains of the wrist which improve with that tardiness which is so aggravating to the athlete may well be compression fractures of the carpals. Diagnosis is virtually impossible by early x-ray. Later x-rays which might be expected to show some atrophy or condensation of bone are extremely difficult to interpret because many of the bones are superimposed. Clinically the diagnosis of compression fracture is also difficult since the ordinary findings of this fracture are quite confusing at the wrist. Local tenderness is present whether the injury is a sprain or a fracture. Pain on forced motion is also likely in either. The unusual fact that many of the "sprains" of the dorsum of the wrist are caused by dorsiflexion forces may give a clue. It is possible that many of these dorsal flexion "sprains" may actually be compression or chondral fractures of one or the other carpal bones.

No specific *treatment* is required for the acute condition other than rest and protection. Since this is also the treatment for a sprain, one does not err in applying protective support to any wrist injury provided he first assures himself that no condition is present that requires more definitive treatment. A compression fracture will heal much more slowly than the ordinary sprain. If the symptoms are persistent over a long period of time one may be unable to decide whether the lesion is a compression fracture, a synovitis or some type of chondral damage. Since all will require basically the same treatment, namely, protection against the motion that causes the pain, a definitive diagnosis may be academic except that the prognosis may be somewhat more grave in one condition than the others. The wrist should be protected against painful motion progressively by splint, by a leather wristlet, by adhesive strapping and finally elastic wrapping. Only thus may we

Figure 161.   Classical Kienböck's disease (osteochondritis of the lunate), old, in which the bone involuted incompletely leaving a sclerosed, deformed bone causing painful carpal function. The symptoms were relieved somewhat by removal of the carpal lunate. Early recognition of this osteochondritis and immobilization would have prevented this poor result.

minimize the tendency for occurrence of chronic arthritis, which can be extremely serious in the carpus where there are so many interrelated joints. In the final analysis, the treatment for persistent chronic arthritis is fusion of the wrist. The intervening treatment should be physical therapy, local injection and other measures ordinarily employed for chronic traumatic arthritis elsewhere.

Kienböck's Disease.   The so-called Kienböck's disease (Fig. 161), which is a late involvement of the lunate, may well be the result of compression fracture of this bone. The disease is variously called osteitis, osteochondritis or malacia of the lunate and is most common in the adolescent. In this condition there is definite involvement of the lunate with bony changes, the bone going through various stages, i.e., atrophy followed by sclerosis and later decalcification, often with fragmentation resulting in marked change in shape of the bone. The deformity may be prevented by early recognition and protection. Should a youth with an osteochondritis of the lunate be permitted to participate in sports? Certainly he should not during the early stage. He should never play unless there is adequate protection applied in the nature of a gauntlet cast or a reinforced wrist and forearm splint. The period of resolution of this bone may require a couple of years. The same condition may involve the other carpal bones and requires the same treatment.

Chondral Fracture

Almost the same can be said about chondral or osteochondral fracture as has been said above about compression fracture. It seems inevitable that there will be serious damage to the cartilage of the carpus in many injuries of the wrist. These cannot be visualized by x-ray in the early stages. The late changes to be expected are those so often associated with chronic arthritis, namely, irregularity of the joint cartilage, narrowing of the joint space, painful motion and tenderness to pressure. If actual fragments of cartilage loose in the carpal joints could be recognized early, surgical excision would be the treatment of choice. They are, however almost impossible to diagnose unless the fracture includes a small portion of bone. Many of the wrists that show small "flakes" of bone are very likely to have a rather large chondral fragment. I feel sure that if one would analyze the injury carefully and come to this conclusion, the final result would be markedly improved by early removal of this fragment. The mild chondral injury goes on to a good recovery. The moderate ones leave aching pain and pain on forced motion. The severe ones terminate in intercarpal arthritis.

SUMMARY

From the foregoing comment the conclusion is inevitable that successful treatment of the carpal injury can be expected only when one takes the pains to analyze the injury carefully. Diligent evaluation of the forces applied will be extremely rewarding. Precise clinical study with location of tender points by using the rubber end of a pencil may enable one to pinpoint the lesion. A painstaking study of the effect of the various directions of motion will give invaluable aid. In short, the treatment must depend upon a very careful and exact analysis of the condition one is treating. Only by such methods can one avoid the embarrassment and humiliation of realizing that he is dependent upon Father Time for his diagnosis. This is often to the extreme detriment of his patient.

Injuries of
the Hand

ANATOMICAL CONSIDERATIONS

THE HAND is an amazingly intricate mechanism and represents the prime raison d'etre of the upper extremity. The shoulder, arm, forearm and wrist are designed to permit efficient function of the multitudinous mechanisms of the hand by increasing the leverage action and permitting activity at a distance from the trunk. No attempt will be made to discuss in detail the entire mechanics of the hand. The author strongly urges every doctor to become familiar with the structures of this ingenious machine. Certainly no one is justified in attempting treatment of any serious injury to the hand unless he is fully cognizant of the functional anatomy of the area. It is far better to apply a protective dressing and splint and transport the injured player to some location where his injury can be adequately handled than to attempt emergency repair of any serious injury. This is not to condone delay in the management of an injury but simply to emphasize the fact that the peril of injudicious treatment is greater than that of reasonable delay.

The five metacarpal bones articulate proximally with the distal row of the carpals, each presenting a differently shaped proximal articular surface depending upon its relationship with the carpal bones (Fig. 162).* The four finger metacarpals articulate with each other. The second, third, fourth and fifth metacarpals and the carpus are intimately and firmly bound together by capsular ligaments. Indeed,

* It is not practicable to include in this book many illustrations of the anatomy of the hand. The reader is referred to the excellent illustrations in Anson or Grant.

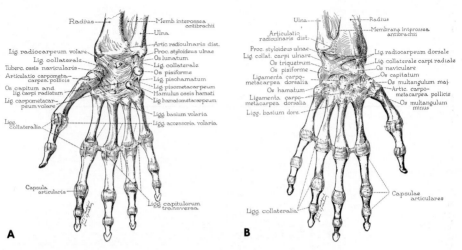

Figure 162.   Bones and joints of the distal forearm, wrist and hand. *A,* Palmar (ventral) aspect. *B,* Dorsal aspect. (From Anson, "Atlas of Human Anatomy.")

it is impossible to distinguish between the various capsular ligaments extending from the lower end of the radius to the bases of the metacarpals. They have various fibrous thickenings and interdigitations but the whole carpus and metacarpals are bound to the forearm by a continuous fibrous mass. The proximal ends of the meta-carpals are essentially concave to fit onto the convex surfaces of the carpal bones but they are irregularly so and present various ridges and facets. The metacarpal of the thumb is separated from the other metacarpal bones and articulates with the greater multangular at about a 45 degree angle to the other metacarpals. This articulation is roughly saddle-shaped to conform to the convexity of the distal end of the greater multangular. This joint has a separate capsule and is capable of much more motion than the other metacarpocarpal joints. As a matter of fact, there is relatively little motion between the carpus and other metacarpals. The greater portion of wrist motion is in the radiocarpal joint and the whole wrist and hand move as a unit on the radiocarpal joint which has ball-and-socket motion. Further extensions of the intermetacarpal ligaments along the metacarpal shafts of the second to the fifth metacarpal bind these bones together. These thicken again to form the transverse capsular ligaments which hold the metacarpal heads together. The bases are bound extremely firmly and have little motion. The heads, on the other hand, are much more loosely contained and have considerable motion each on the other.

So, it will be seen that the metacarpals are bound together at both ends, being firmly bound on the proximal end while the distal end is loose enough to permit some volar and dorsal motion. There is actually little capacity for separation of the metacarpal heads. The round distal extremity of the metacarpal forms a single condyle which is convex in two directions, permitting the shallow concave fossa at the base of the proximal phalanx to rotate around the metacarpal head with a physiological gliding motion but a functional hinge effect. The convexity from side to side permits this same phalanx to adduct and abduct, and indeed each of the fingers has some power of circumduction although this is of much greater range in the second and fifth than in the third and fourth. The capsular ligaments hold these joints firmly in position, their lateral thickenings forming the collateral ligaments.

The interphalangeal joints differ from the metacarpophalangeal joints in that their convexity is only in the one plane so that the only motion possible in the interphalangeal joints is flexion and extension. These joints also have lateral thickenings forming the collateral ligaments. It should be noted that these ligaments are tight with the finger in flexion rather than in extension. The thumb acts as an independent unit from the fingers although the anatomical characteristics are similar in that there are two hinge joints, one the distal interphalangeal joint and the other between the proximal phalanx and the first metacarpal. The same anatomical condition which is present in the metacarpophalangeal joints of the fingers is present in the metacarpocarpal joint of the thumb. The interphalangeal joints permit only flexion and extension with a slight lateral component in the proximal interphalangeal joint.

So much for the skeletal part of the organ. By far the more intricate part of the hand is the extremely ingenious array of long and short muscles to permit various combinations of motion (Figs. 163 to 166). Only a few of these details will be mentioned here. As has been mentioned in our discussion of the wrist, the long flexor tendons to the fingers converge to pass through the carpal tunnel and then separate to go to the fingers. The fascia over the carpal tunnel continues down as the palmar aponeurosis and forms a very firm fascial covering between the tendons, blood

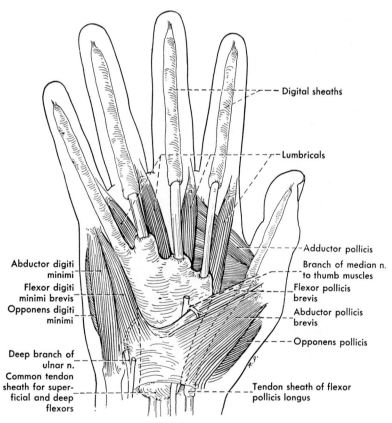

Figure 163.   Short muscles of the thumb and little finger, and flexor tendon sheaths of the hand. (From Hollinshead, "Functional Anatomy.")

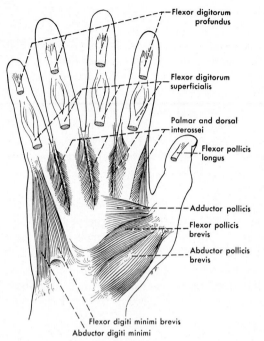

Figure 164.   The flexors of the interphalangeal and metacarpophalangeal joints. Note that each joint has its own special flexor or flexors. (From Hollinshead, "Functional Anatomy.")

Figure 165.   The flexor tendons on a finger, anterior and lateral views. (From Hollinshead, "Functional Anatomy.")

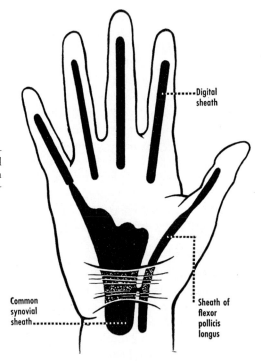

Figure 166. Diagram of a common arrangement of the synovial sheaths of the flexor tendons. (From Gardner, Gray & O'Rahilly, "Anatomy.")

vessels and nerves and the skin of the palm. The skin of the palm is very firmly fixed to this aponeurosis, flexion of the palm being permitted by flexor creases and fixed folds in the skin. This palmar fascia extends out onto the fingers as far as the distal phalanx, so that all of the skin from the tip of the fingers back into the wrist is firmly fixed to the underlying structures on the palmar side.

On the dorsal side of the skin is loose and thin and not bound down to the underlying structures. The subcutaneous areas of the hand are the dorsal surface of the metacarpals and to a considerable extent the dorsum of all the phalanges. In fact, it can be said that the whole dorsum of the hand has very little tissue between the bone and the skin, the exception being areas where the extensor tendons intervene. On the volar aspect the flexor tendons extend down into the fingers, being held by pulleys at each of the flexor creases so that they do not bow across the hand as the fingers are flexed. The whole area between the metacarpal bones is filled with the various interossei and lumbricales which serve to give adduction and abduction to the fingers and contribute to various other combinations of motion. The blood vessels and nerves are well protected on the palmar aspect as they extend down to pass along the medial and lateral side of each finger toward the volar aspect.

Other anatomical characteristics will be noted from time to time in the discussion of the various types of injuries.

CONTUSION AND ABRASION

The hand is very much exposed to contusion. The fact that it is the most distal part of the most active member of the body makes it extremely susceptible to damage. Many of its functions actually depend upon the hand getting into areas where it may be contused. The athlete is not ordinarily exposed to crushing type injuries such as the tremendously crunching effect of the punch press. The most common contusions of the hand in the athlete come from direct impact such as the foot on the outstretched hand with the fingers extended or by a blow of the fist against an opposing blunt object with the fingers closed. Very often these will result in a combination of an abrasion and contusion or a contusion and laceration.

Although the hand, and particularly the back of the hand, is particularly prone to rapid swelling, hematomata are not common. The blood on the back of the hand is much more likely to infiltrate up and down under the loose skin than it is to collect in a localized pool. On the palmar surface of the hand there is not room for excessive hematoma formation because of the very nature of the tightly closed spaces. The bleeding is usually in the form of extravasation of blood through the tissues rather than collection into a pool. If a hematoma can be demonstrated it should be treated by aspiration and pressure bandage under strict surgical asepsis.

The Dorsum of the Hand

The skin over the back of the hand is so loose that it swells rapidly but is not subject to hematoma formation between the skin and underlying fascia. Certain complications do occur from contusion which should be thought of, particularly if the contusion appears to be of rather serious import. Nerve damage is not likely from direct contusion because the major nerves lie on the volar aspect and are well protected. The tendons, however, lie subcutaneously and may be caught between the underlying bone and the contusing object. So, too, if the fist is clenched and the knuckle forcibly driven against a hard object there may be chondral damage to the end of the metacarpal, there may be damage to the extensor tendon as it passes over the metacarpal head, or there may be a fracture or infraction of the bone.

These areas, which are mainly subcutaneous, are quite available for careful physical examination. One can frequently determine whether or not there is fracture of the underlying bone by simple palpation along with careful manipulation. Motion of the fingers should be carefully checked to determine whether there is any loss of tendon function. Nerve function should also be carefully checked. This can be quickly done and may save many headaches later. If the contusion seems quite severe with local tenderness, pain and swelling, an x-ray should be made and carefully studied. Provided the x-ray is negative or if it is necessary for some reason to delay taking the picture, *early treatment* of the contusion should be initiated by a very careful cleansing of the skin with soap and water. The athlete is likely to be in an area where there is dirt, dust or various other contaminants and these may be ground into open cuts or abraded areas. The cleansing is better done at once than at a later time. Copious amounts of running water with bland soap are greatly to be preferred to alcohol or various antiseptics. There is no necessity for painting the part with antiseptic provided it can be carefully cleaned with soap. Following such cleansing the area can be protected by an unguent, a thin Vaseline strip being appropriate. Some may prefer an antibiotic ointment and I see no objection to this if inquiry is made as to any possible sensitivity. Once the skin has been carefully cleaned, attention must be given to the underlying condition. It is best treated by a firm pressure dressing with mechanic's waste or similar soft material placed over the contused area and snugly wrapped in place with an elastic bandage. An ice pack is then applied. Careful inspection of the hand is carried out after 12 hours and if the swelling is under control the ice may be discontinued. It is inadvisable to use heat for the first 36 hours.

Subsequent treatment will depend upon the extent of the contusion. If the area remains swollen, edematous and painful and particularly if there is pain on motion of the fingers, particularly active extension, one should protect the hand much longer because of the possibility of tenosynovitis which may be quite crippling and may last for many weeks. If function of the fingers remains pain-free, a rigid protective dressing may be applied over the back of the hand and snugly held in place by an elastic bandage. Participation in sports may be continued, always provided that function of the fingers is pain-free. Careful re-examination from time to time will detect any possible later complication such as involvement of the intrinsic muscles of the hand, localized phlebitis, lymphangitis, etc.

The Palm

A particularly distressing injury to the hand is a contusion in the palm in which there is damage to the intrinsic muscles. This occurs most commonly at the base of the hand in the thenar and hypothenar eminences where the intrinsic muscles to the thumb and to the little finger are involved. This injury is of the "stone bruise" type which may require considerable time to subside. The palmar portion of the hand is a relatively closed space and any localized swelling here can be quite distressing. I have previously mentioned carpal tenosynovitis. Contusion directly over the transverse ligament may give rise to the tunnel syndrome. Contusion of the distal part of the palm may cause severe tenderness over the metacarpal heads so that gripping over a hard object such as the golf club or tennis racket may be quite painful. This condition may be quite disabling. If these conditions persist, later treatment may be necessary consisting of local injection of a long-acting anesthetic and a corticoid preparation. Physical therapy, particularly with the heat modalities, is appropriate here.

The Fingers

The fingers are also subject to contusion and painful injuries may result. One should mention injuries to the fingernail or to the palmar space of the distal phalanx. Often the two are combined. In the distal phalanx of the fingers and thumb the skin is firmly bound to the bone on the palmar aspect by fibrous septa which in effect make multiple closed spaces. These prevent the skin from sliding which would interfere with picking up objects between thumb and fingers. On the back of the distal phalanx is the nail which is very closely apposed to the bone, being separated only by the nail bed. Contusion here is likely to cause hemorrhage into the closed spaces either under the fingernail or in the tip of the phalanx. As the hematoma develops, it causes pressure symptoms and a throbbing pressure-type pain that is extremely distressing. Immediate *treatment* for such a condition is application of cold, the hand being held in ice water or placed directly in crushed ice. If swelling subsides early enough, the severe symptoms may be prevented. Should blood accumulate under the nail at this early stage, it is advisable to drill through the nail to permit the blood to be evacuated. Needless to say, this should be done under aseptic technique since infection in this space is of extremely serious consequence. Every-

Figure 167.   Tuft fracture, lateral (*A*) and anteroposterior (*B*) views. Note swelling of
the tip of the finger.

one has his preferred method of drilling the nail. My own preference is to drill
carefully through with a convex type knife blade such as No. 10 Bard-Parker, which
will drill through the nail without pressure. However, there are many suitable ways
to open this space. After the bleeding stops the cold may be discontinued but heat
should not be instituted for 48 hours. A protective splint will usually give considerable relief.

This contusion of the tip of the finger may be complicated by fracture of the
tuft of the phalanx. This requires no particular treatment but is an indication of the
severity of the injury. Frequently this tuft does not go on to bony union but fibrous
union appears to be adequate (Fig. 167).

Various complications are seen in this condition, making a careful examination
of the area mandatory. In order to clean it thoroughly it is usually necessary to anesthetize the finger by injecting procaine into either side at its base. Once the finger
is insensitive and the pain is gone, a much more definitive examination can be carried out. The nail should be carefully studied. Frequently, the root of the nail has
slipped out from under the eponychial fold and its proximal end lies on top of the
skin. In this case enough of the proximal end of the nail should be cut away to
permit the nail to fall back again onto the nail bed. The finger is then dressed carefully with a Vaseline strip and a splint is applied with moderate pressure. This nail
will need to be carefully protected in the athlete. In many instances the root will
not fasten down to the nail bed and protection will be needed until the new nail
grows out under it. It is my practice to clip off the old nail just distal to the advanc-

ing edge of the new nail (Fig. 168). These injuries to the fingers are often lightly treated and all too often result in various deformities which may be quite painful in the very sensitive area at the end of the finger. I cannot overemphasize the importance of cleanliness in treating these injuries.

Infection of the Finger Tip. In spite of the greatest care, and in other cases because of inadequate care, infection of the finger tip may intervene in management of these injuries. If there has been a considerable amount of soft tissue contamination, a broad-spectrum antibiotic should be given immediately following the injury. The wound should be carefully inspected from time to time for signs of local infection. This is particularly pertinent if there is relief of pain for a period and then recurrence of insistent, throbbing, boring pain which is a characteristic of tension in a closed space. Should infection develop it is imperative to initiate drainage. On the other hand, one should not lightly open up these spaces if infection is not actually present. As a general rule, infection will develop only after an interval of time. That is, the initial symptoms will subside, the fingers will appear to be doing well, then recurrent pain will dominate the picture. Under these circumstances one is justified in assuming that infection is present.

If there is involvement of the nail, a portion of the involved nail may be lifted up and trimmed away to permit release of the fluids collected beneath it. If the

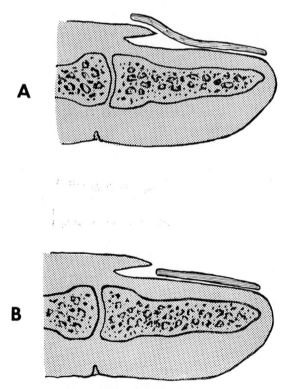

Figure 168. Lateral drawing of tip of finger showing (*A*) the nail avulsed from its root and lying on top of the skin on dorsum of the finger and (*B*) proximal end of nail cut off to permit the nail to fall back into the nail bed.

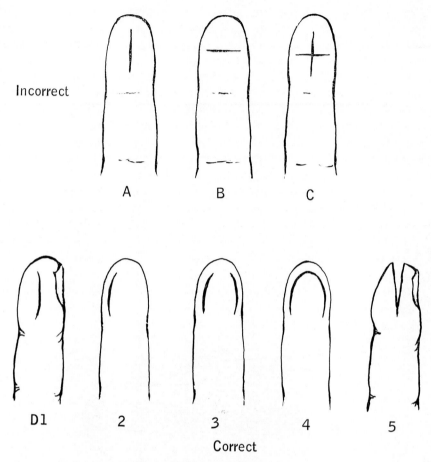

Figure 169.   Drawings showing various incisions.
WRONG: *A,* Vertical incision along ball of finger. *B,* Transverse incision along ball of finger. *C,* Cruciate incision over ball of finger.
RIGHT: *D,* These incisions are all segments of circumferential incisions. *1, 2, 3,* Lateral incisions on either side, connected with small drain. *4, 5,* The two lateral incisions connected to make the circumferential incision.

infection is in the pulp of the finger (Fig. 169), this space should be opened. Incision should never be mode over the ball of the finger (Fig. 169, *A*), neither in a linear fashion nor transverse (Fig. 169, *B*). The so-called "fish-mouth" incision is usually not necessary since the lateral components alone will suffice. It is better to make an incision along the lateral side of the distal phalanx and frequently along each lateral side (Fig. 169, *D3,4*). An instrument is passed from one incision through to the other to be sure that the space between the bone and pulp of the finger is adequately drained. If through-and-through tissue drain is used, it should be removed not more than 48 hours later. It is probably preferable although considerably more difficult to insert a small drain from either side of the finger. Great care should be taken in the placing of the drain so that it does not act as a plug rather than a drain. For this reason Vaseline strips, iodoform strips, etc., are probably inadvisable here. Many times these simply block the drainage. Very frequently as the strip is removed after a day or two there is a general exudation of fluid or pus, indicating a damming up effect of the drain which was inserted for the opposite purpose. One should be very careful to avoid mutilating incisions anywhere in the hand. They are not often necessary and may cause painful adherent scars and considerable loss of function. We have recently seen a case in which the infection of the tip of the finger was untreated for several days. On removal of the dressing the abscess was found to point directly in the middle of the ball of the finger with complete destruction of the skin here. Needless to say, this wound drained at this spot. All that was done in this instance was to lift off the dead skin, permit the pus to drain out and then establish drainage laterally hoping that the center wound would close with minimal scar formation.

There is no place on an athletic team for a player with an infected hand. His dressing should not be changed in the dressing room or training room since spread of his infection through other members of the team may be disastrous. This applies as well to any infection elsewhere. If a player has an abrasion that is contaminated and draining pus, he should be barred from the dressing room until the purulent stage has passed. The hand should be treated with warm saline dressings. After the suppuration has cleared, the abraded area should be carefully protected with unguent and a suitable dressing. Even at this stage the player should be warned not to peel his dressing off and throw it on the floor or in the shower or any other place where it can contaminate the room.

Infection About the Fingernail.   Although not strictly in the realm of an athletic injury, this subject should be considered here since it is a frequent involvement of the athlete. Indeed, it may often follow relatively minor injuries about the nail with impingement of the paronychial fold against the side of the nail.

Simple contusion of the nail or along the side of the nail may cause some abrasion or laceration of the skin. An inflammatory reaction about the nail results, with the familiar picture of a red, inflamed, swollen nail fold. This may be an extremely distressing condition and materially handicaps the athlete, particularly if it is on the thumb or first or second finger. In the early stage it is best treated by local heat. It should be carefully explained to the player that adequate care in the early stage may well prevent considerable disability later. Soaking the area several times a day may prevent suppuration.

Suppuration, if it occurs, should be drained. The route of drainage is a moot question. If the involvement is close to the nail an instrument can be passed between the nail and paronychial fold and the nail gently lifted, permitting the pus to exude through this defect. This route of drainage has the advantage of not requiring a cut on the skin. It has the disadvantage that the nail fold tends to close down very readily on the nail and the abscess does not drain. If this occurs or if the infection seems to be away from the nail, a straight linear incision parallel to the nail edge will usually suffice for drainage. This incision can be carried down to the abscess. Local block of the finger is helpful. Occasionally ethyl chloride used locally will suffice. This incision will tend to gap open rather than to seal and drainage will be adequate. Hot soaks should be continued and the dressings applied should be sufficiently protective to prevent contamination of the finger from outside infection and to prevent the finger from being the source of contamination to the patient or to others.

An infection involving the base of the nail may be of more serious consequence since it tends to burrow under the proximal edge of the nail at the root and so form a subungual abscess. Prompt, adequate drainage must be carried out here, else the nail bed may be destroyed and permanent damage result. If the pus has actually elevated the proximal section of the nail (Fig. 168), this section of the nail should be removed to permit exposure of the nail bed at its root and prevent further undermining. As much of the nail should be removed at the proximal end as is undermined by the infection, otherwise the detached nail lying over the nail bed will serve to form a pocket of infection. Following complete drainage by resection of a portion of the root of the nail, this area must be carefully protected to prevent external contamination of the wound and spread of infection to other parts of the body. If the drainage has been carried out promptly there is every reason to expect regrowth of the nail. If drainage is delayed, destruction of the nail root and bed will lead to gross and often painful deformities.

LACERATION

Lacerations of the hand may have extremely serious consequences and should never be minimized. The laceration penetrates the skin with the finger in a certain position of flexion or extension. All too frequently when the cut is examined the finger may be in another position and superficial examination through the cut may reveal normal structures. It is dangerous to assume that the structures beneath are not involved unless the cut is carefully examined with the finger in various positions.

The first step in *treatment* of the lacerated hand is an assessment of the function of the part. This includes all of the motions of the involved area, both active and passive. One should then carefully check the nerve function, bearing in mind the distribution of the nerve which is likely to be injured. This check may be made without removing the dressing from the hand; in fact, there is no excuse for repeatedly removing the dressing to examine the hand if the laceration appears to be severe. As the player comes off the field a sterile dressing should be applied immediately and a firm pressure bandage wrapped around it. The player should then be taken to the infirmary or hospital where he is to be given definitive treatment. At that time and at that time only should the dressing be removed and the wound inspected. After the dressing has been carefully removed and the wound thoroughly inspected, determination should be made of the type of anesthesia indicated. If there is disturbance of tendon function, if there is loss of nerve function, if there appears to be any joint involvement, it probably is advisable to use a general anesthetic. An x-ray study should be made to determine any abnormality of the bony structures of the hand.

After these preliminary preparations the patient is taken to the operating room and given the appropriate anesthetic, either brachial block or general. Any definitive treatment is best carried out under tourniquet control. The dressing is removed and the surgeon, wearing sterile gloves, should carefully inspect the hand. This is not the time for a detailed examination of the wound itself. The next step is a thorough cleansing of the hand. A detergent is used to remove grease if necessary, otherwise soap and water are employed to cleanse the entire hand thoroughly, with particular attention to the area of the wound. The wound itself is thoroughly lavaged with running water. The hand is now redraped with sterile drapes, the medical team puts on new gowns and gloves and only then is the wound itself investigated. At this examination it should be possible to determine the degree of involvement of nerve or tendon. It may be that a tendon has been partially cut. This can be determined only by moving the finger through a full range of motion while inspecting the tendon throughout the area which could have been exposed to this wound. It is ordinarily not necessary to enlarge the wound widely simply for diagnostic purposes. If there is nerve damage, the wound should be enlarged enough to expose the nerve ends and permit nerve suture. If there is a combination of nerve and tendon damage, the tougher structures should be sutured first.

I will not attempt here to describe in full detail the repair of lacerated tendons but a few principles should be emphasized. As a general rule, it is not advisable to repair a tendon within a sheath. If it is determined that the laceration is within the sheath and it nevertheless seems advisable to repair the tendon, the sheath should be excised. It is never advisable to repair two tendons within the same sheath. If both the flexor profundus and sublimus have been severed within the same sheath, the sublimus should be sacrificed and the profundus alone repaired. Tendon as well as nerve suture in the hand is a highly specialized procedure and one should be thoroughly versed in the proper technique before he attempts even a simple repair. These injuries are not common in the athlete but when they do occur they are extremely important. The author knows of one instance in which an admirably fine job was done in suturing of one of the flexor tendons to the stump of the median nerve. Needless to say, the function of neither the tendon nor the nerve was restored. Following repair of the tendon or nerve, the extremity must be placed in the position that most relaxes the repaired structure and held there for at least three weeks to permit the early stages of repair to take place. After this, if the finger can be securely splinted with a dressing that is acceptable to the athletic authorities, participation in sports might be permitted.

Many of these injuries are locker room accidents such as thrusting the hand through a glass door and may indeed involve multiple tendons. One of our cases recently was in a young athlete who was in the hospital to have his knee cartilage removed. He attempted to close the transom type window over his bed by driving the heel of his hand against the glass. The glass broke and the jagged edges sectioned all the flexor tendons and median nerve at the level of the wrist. The only good thing about this accident was that he was in the proper locale to get early treatment. This could hardly be called an athletic injury although it certainly was an injury to an athlete. In this instance we were able to repair the tendons and the nerve since these tendons at this level were not within a sheath. Had the injury been deeper in the hand, repair would not have been possible to this extent and we would probably have elected to repair the profundus only.

A laceration in the athlete that has particular connotations is the *lacerated knuckle* caused by striking the human tooth. This illustrates very well several of the important factors in the treatment of lacerations. For example, it is a contaminated wound and should be treated as such by meticulous cleansing of the part. Again, the extensor tendon, which is part of the capsule of the metacarpophalangeal joint, is cut with the finger flexed. When it is examined with the finger in extension, the laceration of the tendon has now traveled considerably proximal to the cut in the skin and may be completely overlooked. To treat such a wound as a casual "barked" knuckle is to court disaster. In the first place, infection from human bite is one of the most difficult infections to treat. In the second place there will remain not only a defect in the capsule but also irregularity of the metacarpophalangeal joint. In this instance the proper treatment is to carefully retract the wound edges, thoroughly lavage the wound, clip away any obvious dead tissue, being very penurious about sacrificing tissue, and then examine the tendon carefully by flexing the finger. If necessary the wound may be enlarged to permit careful suture of the tendon. When the skin is to be closed the contused, devitalized edge may be trimmed away in a very minimal fashion. It is important to get well demarcated skin edges. The wound may be closed without drainage but must be watched very carefully—and the patient as well—for any developing infection. One should give a prophylactic broad-spectrum antibiotic in any case. If infection is imminent or actually develops, the skin edges should be opened to permit drainage.

PUNCTURE WOUND

Puncture wounds of the hand are infrequent in athletes, although common enough generally. A wound in the hand by a sharp cleat is almost always a laceration since the skin in the dorsum of the hand tears as the cleat hits it and skids. Puncture wounds may be caused by contaminants on the playing field or by sharp projecting points on the player's equipment. After a puncture wound, particularly on the palmar side, the hand should be carefully checked for disturbance of nerve or tendon function. If this function remains intact, the wound should be treated expectantly, that is, the surrounding area thoroughly cleaned, sterile dressing applied and the wound regularly observed. If any sign of deep-seated infection appears, adequate drainage must be provided immediately since infection within the closed spaces of the hand can be extremely severe and may lead to a crippling degree of disability. The player should be instructed that if he experiences general symptoms such as fever or malaise or that if he has aching or throbbing in the hand he should report at once for a careful examination to determine the severity of the involvement. In the extremely early stage there may be considerable deep soreness. This should not be confused with infection since infection is unlikely to develop for several days. Here once more is illustrated the extreme value of careful primary examination. If this examination elicits no particular soreness through the hand, of much more significance will be any soreness developing after several days. One must be particularly careful in the hand to avoid an iatrogenic lesion. An uncautious scalpel or scissors may readily spread the infection into the tendon sheath or palmar space, or may actually sever a nerve or vessel. It is axiomatic that any puncture wound requires tetanus antitoxin or toxoid. It probably also requires a broad-spectrum antibiotic. (See tetanus antitoxin, page 56.)

In any penetrating wound one must always suspect the presence of foreign material, particularly glass. Clothing or similar material is not frequently carried into the tissues of the hand.

STRAIN (MUSCULOTENDINOUS INJURIES)

With the vast complex of musculotendinous units in the hand it is obvious that strain will occur with great frequency. There are two basic categories of these musculotendinous units: the long flexors and the long extensors which are entirely tendinous in the hand and the intrinsic muscles wherein the entire musculo-tendinous unit is contained within the hand itself.

Strain in the hand is due to two primary causes. One is excessive overuse against resistance and the second is overstretching of the unit beyond its normal extensile range. In the intrinsic muscles of the hand the former cause is by far the most common and usually consists in repeated use beyond the total capacity of the unit rather than a single excessive contraction. This is not a common injury in athletic competition but may occur in such sports as gymnastics or certain sports requiring constant gripping such as rowing or tennis or golf. The initial symptoms will be cramping and fatigue of the muscles involved, with pain on function against resistance. If the activity is discontinued at this stage, recovery is prompt and with-out residual. Continuation of overuse may result in persistent muscle spasm or even contracture. Tenosynovitis as such is not common in the intrinsic muscles of the hand since the tendons have very short excursion and ordinarily do not become irritated from overuse.

Strain in the long musculotendinous units may be manifested in the forearm near the musculotendinous junction and has been discussed (page 230). It may also reveal itself as a tenosynovitis in the palm or more distally in the fingers. There may also be irritation at the attachment of the tendon to the phalanx. Irritation or strain of the attachment of the wrist flexors and extensors as they reach the base of the metacarpals may give symptoms in this area. These conditions, which result from overuse, must be treated primarily by rest. Rest is the one essential ingredient for recovery. Other modes of treatment that may accelerate recovery are the use of local heat, particularly the penetrating modalities, and the local injection of an anesthetic and a corticoid. These are of considerable value if the irritation is specifi-cally within the sheath or tendinous attachment or even at the musculotendinous junction. Injection is much more successful if the condition is quite local. A local spot of discomfort over the dorsum of the base of the second metacarpal with tender-ness on pressure and pain on dorsiflexion of the wrist against resistance may be interpreted as strain of the attachment of the extensor carpi radialis, and local injec-tion of this area will give prompt and ofttimes permanent relief, always provided that the etiological factor is eliminated. To relieve such a case, the hand and wrist should be supported by a forearm splint with the wrist in dorsal flexion. When competition is resumed, the wrist should be taped. Keeping in mind that the cause is overuse rather than overstretch, one must be careful to avoid active use of the muscle. Hence, a serious involvement of the carpal flexors or extensors will pretty well interdict athletics.

Whereas strain of the short flexors is most often within the muscle and is due primarily to overuse, long flexor involvement may well be in the tendon unit and is frequently due to overstretch, particularly against resistance. For example, a wrist that is forcibly dorsiflexed with the wrist flexors contracted may suffer strain of its flexors. This strain may be anything from a slight separation of some of the fibers in the musculotendinous junction or at the attachment of the tendon in the hand, to a complete avulsion. Symptomatically there will be pain at the site of involve-ment, pain on active contraction of the muscle, pain on passive stretching of the muscle. If the rupture is complete, there will be loss of function of the muscle. There may be bunching up of the muscle as it contracts with the distal end of the tendon pulling free, so that the muscle may actually shorten but the wrist not flex. If it can be determined that the tendon is avulsed, surgical treatment is indicated and the tendon should be sutured to its attachment. Much more frequently the strain is partial and the treatment in this instance will be protection, first against overstretch, second against overuse. This protection must be continued a sufficient time to permit the strength of the tendon to be restored. With only slight involvement, little or no immobilization will be needed, whereas if there was extensive tearing, protection must be carried out for several weeks. One can usually assess the degree of involvement by the rate of subsidence of symptoms and so regulate the degree and extent of immobilization. If there is irritation within the tendon sheath of these long flexors, the part must be immobilized. Injection of a steroid into the tendon sheath is of considerable value together with physical therapy. Function should be resumed very slowly here, else there will be prompt recurrence of symptoms. Although it is difficult to elicit in the hand, snowball crepitation can sometimes be felt along the tendon sheath in this condition. If felt, it is diagnostic.

SPRAIN-SUBLUXATION-DISLOCATION

It should be emphasized again that injuries to the components of the hand are extremely serious from the functional point of view. One must always bear in mind that almost the whole function of the upper extremity rests in the capability of the fingers and thumb. In spite of this fact, injuries to the hand proper are often considered minor injuries and all too frequently the treatment they receive could be classified as minor too. Since there is a considerable difference functionally and anatomically between the thumb and the remaining fingers, or more accurately between the first ray and the remaining rays of the hand, they should be discussed under separate headings.

Thumb Ray

Carpometacarpal Joint.   Since the thumb is the opposing member of the group, it of necessity must have more mobility. The carpometacarpal joint is extremely mobile, its action in effect being that of a universal joint so that it moves in all directions: flexion and extension, adduction and abduction, circumduction and rotation. For this to occur the stability of the joint must be maintained almost entirely by ligaments since there is no bony restriction to any particular motion. Forced motion in any direction beyond the strength of the ligament support will cause a sprain which may be mild, moderate or severe. If the force is continued, a subluxation or dislocation will occur. For example, forceful wide abduction of the thumb produces hyperextension of the carpometacarpal joint, which throws a strain on the anterior portion of the capsule. If the force is arrested, the injury may be mild or moderate and a sprain results. If it continues the injury will be severe and the base may dislocate as it passes out through a rent in the capsule with the thumb actually bent backward over the wrist, due to complete disruption of the anterior structures of the joint. Similarly, the dorsal capsule may be injured by hyperflexion. The foolish habit of grasping the thumb within the fingers and then striking a blow with the clenched fist will tend to rotate the base of the metacarpal dorsally and rupture the dorsal ligaments. Subluxation is more likely to occur here than dislocation, although disruption of the capsule may be complete. There may be sprain of the medial components, less frequently of the lateral.

Treatment will vary according to the severity of injury. Mild sprain of the carpometacarpal joint is extremely common and manifests itself by pain around the joint, tenderness to pressure over the area, and pain on reproduction of the motion that caused the injury. Within a few hours the area of the base of the thumb will be swollen, edematous and almost any motion will cause pain. Treatment should be directed toward protection of the joint against stress until the healing is complete. If the injury is mild, simple adhesive strapping will suffice to prevent overstretch. If the injury is moderate to severe, the joint should be immobilized by plaster fixation in a position such as would be assumed by grasping a 3-inch ball. It is not necessary to immobilize the fingers but the splint should include the hand and wrist and the thumb as far as the middle of the proximal phalanx. The duration of the immobilization will vary with the severity of the injury. As a general rule, the cast should be left on about three weeks and then the thumb should be protected against strain by adequate taping for the next three weeks. Later the thumb should be protected during contact sports if the ligament rupture was complete.

If there is subluxation or instability of this joint, great care must be taken to immobilize the joint in its normal relationship. If the subluxation cannot be reduced and held by simple plaster fixation, traction should be applied. In these cases immobilization will be considerably longer since at least six weeks are needed for the ligament and capsule to unite firmly even under most favorable circumstances.

Simple dislocation of this joint is not a frequent injury. If the force is sufficient to disrupt it, a fracture-dislocation will occur, the so-called Bennett fracture (Figs. 178 and 179), which leaves a smaller or lesser portion of the end of the metacarpal fixed to the anterior capsular ligaments while the remaining portion dislocates (see page 279). It may be that a frank dislocation does occur and that it is reduced promptly and at the time it is seen by the physician there is no deformity. If dislocation occurs and persists, it should be reduced by traction along the long axis of the thumb with gradual abduction while local pressure is placed on the dorsal aspect of the proximal end of the phalanx to force the metacarpal back into its normal carpal relationship. If it is unstable in this position, some form of internal fixation is advisable since it is extremely difficult to hold it by plaster alone. While the thumb is held manually a transfixion pin may be drilled through the base of the bone and into the adjacent carpal or into the adjacent second metacarpal (Fig. 173). Ideally it probably would be better at this time to open the dorsal aspect of the joint and repair the ligament. I have not done this frequently enough to warrant an opinion on its merits. The fact that one so often sees a hypermobile, painful and even subluxating joint following this injury would suggest that some improvement in treatment is indicated. The usual error is of inadequate immobilization rather than inadequate reduction. After Bennett fracture or dislocation of the thumb, the athlete should wear supportive strapping (Fig. 170) for the rest of the season.

Treatment of the chronic sprain is difficult since continued participation in sports causes frequent re-injury. The first requirement is an adequate support that is tolerable to the patient and yet protects the joint. Adhesive strapping is not dependable since it requires someone to apply it and frequently it is not applied

Figure 170.   Basket weave strapping of thumb. (Courtesy of Rawlinson, "Modern Athletic Training," © 1961 by Prentice-Hall, Inc.)

properly. An injury may occur while the strapping is off. A little slip-on protector that fits around the wrist can be devised by the brace maker and is quite effective. At the time of the acute episode of a chronic sprain, local injection of a corticoid into the joint is quite effective and the usual physical therapeutic measures will help.

   Metacarpophalangeal Joint.   The metacarpophalangeal joint of the thumb (Fig. 171, A) permits motion primarily in flexion and extension. However, there is an element of adduction and abduction permitted by the convex concave lateral curvature of the head of the metacarpal and base of the phalanx. The collateral ligaments definitely restrict adduction and abduction. This joint is extremely vulnerable to sprain since, as the thumb is abducted, the metacarpal becomes fixed and the force applied to the end of the thumb is directed right against the metacarpophalangeal joint. The lateral stress may be either toward adduction or abduction and the sprain is to the collateral ligaments. The force may be in straight extension and the sprain is on the anterior capsule. If the force is limited, the resultant injury is of low grade and no instability results. If the force continues, subluxation occurs as the result of tearing of the ligament involved (Fig. 171, B). Thus, if the force is abduction, the medial collateral ligament will tear, the phalanx and metacarpal will separate and the joint will open up on the medial side. As soon as the force is released the thumb falls back into its normal position and reveals no obvious abnormality. The pain will be along the medial side of the joint and, as with sprains elsewhere, in the final analysis the determination of the degree of lateral instability is of utmost importance. If the force involved is hyperextension, the anterior capsule tears (Fig. 171, C), the phalanx moves backward over the metacarpal head, the metacarpal head thrusts forward through the anterior capsule. Here again, if the force is relieved, the joint may slip back into position and be spontaneously reduced.

   A sprain to this area may cause chronic disability for months or years or even permanently. I suspect that inadequate treatment of the first injury is mainly responsible for this—treatment that permitted the ligaments and capsule to heal with redundancy. Thus recurrent subluxation is easily produced. Many baseball players,

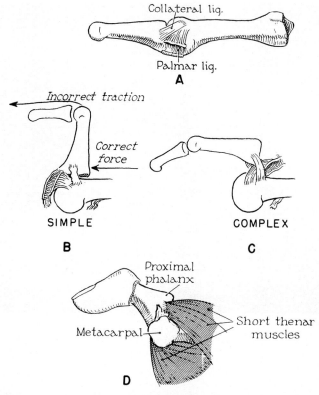

Figure 171.   Simple and complex metacarpophalangeal dislocation.

A, The volar aspect of a metacarpophalangeal joint capsule is reinforced with a palmar ligament or fibrocartilage.

B, In a simple dislocation the phalanx is hyperextended and the palmar ligament hangs like a curtain over the metacarpal head. Traction may pivot the phalanx on the intact collateral ligaments and interpose the palmar ligament between the bones. The phalanx should be pushed into place.

C, The finger is not hyperextended on, but more nearly parallel to, the metacarpal in a complex dislocation. The volar joint capsule and palmar ligament are interposed, and usually prevent reduction by manipulation.

D, In the metacarpophalangeal joint of the thumb the short thenar muscles augment the pivot force predisposing to complex dislocation. (From McLaughlin, "Trauma.")

particularly catchers, have such an involvement and the least hyperextension of the thumb or flexion of the thumb across the palm will cause recurrence of the painful, swollen joint. The thumb should be immobilized for at least three weeks if the injury seems severe and then protected for several more weeks by very comprehensive strapping that will permit only a minimum of motion in the metacarpophalangeal joint but that leaves the distal phalanx relatively free. The degree of immobilization and duration of protection will depend upon the response to treatment. So long as the interphalangeal joints are given motion relatively early (within three weeks), one need not fear prolonged immobilization. I have yet to see an instance of restriction of motion in this metacarpophalangeal joint that could be attributed to overlong immobilization. Protection of the joint in the young individual is particularly important. One has only to experience a recurrent or chronic

Figure 172.   Lateral ligament injury of the metacarpophalangeal joint of the thumb, avulsing the corner of the proximal end of the phalanx. This is really a ligament injury and requires repair either by pinning the fragment or removing the fragment and repairing the ligament.

sprain of this joint to appreciate the seriousness of the resulting handicap to the budding athlete.

In the case of a complete dislocation, the mere fact that the dislocation reaches the doctor unreduced is a warning signal. Under ordinary circumstances this dislocation will reduce spontaneously. If it does not do it at once or if it does not do it spontaneously, almost certainly the injured person himself will have grabbed the thumb and pulled it into position, ofttimes with the eager help of one of his teammates. Hence, if the dislocation will reduce by simple traction and manual manipu-

Figure 173.   *A,* Fracture-dislocation of first metacarpal on the trapezium by a force similar to that causing a Bennett fracture. *B,* Excellent postoperative fixation is obtained in this case by transfixion through the metacarpal base into the base of the adjacent metacarpal.

lation, it will be reduced already before the doctor sees it. If this dislocation is seen almost immediately, one is justified in attempting an atraumatic manipulation without anesthesia. The traction should be in the long axis of the deformed thumb, whatever its position. Direct distal pressure of the operator's thumb against the base of the metacarpal will slide it into position as the phalanx is flexed (Fig. 171, B). This dislocation cannot be reduced by traction along the long axis of the forearm (Fig. 171, C) since this simply locks the dislocation in position.

If the complete dislocation does not readily reduce by such methods, one should consider an open reduction on the assumption that the metacarpal head is caught in the rent in the capsule or between the two flexor tendons (Figs. 171, C, and 174). The hand should be prepared as for surgery, the anesthetic given and a second attempt made to reduce the dislocation under anesthesia. If it does not reduce promptly with minimal stress, force should not be used since this only damages the periarticular structures. Open operation should be carried out at once. It should be emphasized here as in all dislocations that time is of the essence and one must not wait days or even long hours before final reduction is carried out.

If the injury is moderate or if deformity is spontaneously reduced, the thumb should be treated by immobilization of the joint, plaster splints being my preference, the splints in this instance going out beyond the interphalangeal joint, extending back to the wrist and down onto the thenar eminence. It is not essential to immobilize the wrist. After the splint is applied, motion of the thumb itself should not increase the discomfort. If it does, the wrist should be included until the muscle spasm has subsided, possibly a week. After a week or so in splints a thumb spica cast may be used to complete three weeks of immobilization. Since the ligaments are not securely healed at this stage the thumb should be carefully taped to prevent the motion that puts stress on the involved ligament. This should continue at least three additional weeks. After this the thumb must be taped during athletic participation until all tenderness is gone (three or four weeks longer).

Interphalangeal Joint.   Sprain of the interphalangeal joint is not nearly as frequent as sprain of the other two joints of the thumb, the leverage factor being

Figure 174.   Complete dislocation of metacarpophalangeal joint of thumb. This could be reduced only by open reduction since the flexor tendons were looped around the metacarpal head.

such that more strain is applied to either of the latter by a given force than to the interphalangeal joint. Lateral motion of the distal phalanx will tear the opposing collateral ligament and the pain will be on the opposite side of the thumb from the applied force. Since the interphalangeal joint is a hinge joint, there is no appreciable lateral motion and the joint should be carefully checked for lateral instability. If there is instability or if a small fragment of bone is revealed in the x-ray, one must assume that the collateral ligament has been avulsed or torn and the protection should be correspondingly longer (Fig. 172). If one could diagnose with certainty a tear of the collateral ligament, primary repair of the ligament would probably be the treatment of choice. All too frequently, the instability is not recognized until several weeks later when swelling, pain and disability persist and one notices the phalanx is deviating to the opposite side. At this time one may belatedly discover instability of the collateral ligament. Reconstruction is then necessary rather than repair, and is correspondingly more difficult and less successful. In the treatment of injury to the interphalangeal joint immobilization is indicated for at least three weeks if the injury is relatively severe.

Finger Rays

Metacarpal Area.   The areas where sprain may occur are at the carpometacarpal, the metacarpophalangeal and the interphalangeal joints. Sprain at the BASE OF THE METACARPAL is not common. This whole area is firmly bound together by the dorsal and palmar ligaments of the wrist and hand so that they are firmly adherent not only to each other but to the carpus. There is but little lateral motion in these joints and lateral stresses are not readily applied. The sprain is much more likely to involve the wrist than it is the carpometacarpal joint since the same force puts tension on both areas and the wrist is much more vulnerable than is the carpometacarpal joint.

At the DISTAL END OF THE METACARPALS, the joints are in effect universal joints permitting flexion and extension, adduction and abduction, and circumduction. Extremes of these motions may cause a sprain of the capsular ligaments. The ones most likely to be involved in this are the index and little fingers since either one may be forcibly abducted away from the hand whereas it is much more difficult to abduct the other two fingers to the degree necessary to damage the capsular ligaments.

The most common injury is damage to the ligament holding the metacarpal heads together. The same force that pulls the fingers apart may tear the ligament binding the metacarpal heads together and this may occur at any space. That is, the long and ring fingers may be forcibly separated and so tear the ligament between the third and fourth metacarpals. This is much more likely to occur than tear of the capsular ligament of the metacarpophalangeal joint. This injury is readily overlooked. It is usually minimized but may result in weeks or months of disability of the hand and, indeed, may lead to chronic sprain with repeated re-injury and resultant disability. This injury is readily identified if the hand is examined with the condition in mind since simple separation of the two involved fingers will cause severe pain. The most common areas are between the fourth and fifth metacarpals and between the second and third. Treatment is relatively simple. If the hand is dressed in such a manner as to hold the fingers together, free motion can be per-

mitted to the phalanges and actually athletic competition can be continued if
fixation is firm enough to prevent separation of the metacarpal heads. Protection
should be continued full time for at least three weeks and when there is stress it
should be continued for another three weeks. This injury is not particularly disabling and essentially free function of the hand can be carried out so long as the protective dressing is worn.

The only force likely to cause a sprain of the metacarpophalangeal joint is
hyperextension. In this instance the anterior capsule becomes tight. As the force
continues, this capsule may tear. This may be of slight degree or may be complete
avulsion leading to dislocation. This may involve a single finger or more than one.
Symptomatically, any sprain involving the metacarpals will present tenderness at
the area of the tear and pain will be caused by reproduction of the motion that
caused the injury.

Sprain of the carpometacarpal joint may be severe enough to cause actual dislocation. This is quite infrequent and is readily recognized as a very serious injury
which demands definitive care in expert hands. Dislocation of the distal end of the
metacarpal at the metacarpophalangeal joint occurs as a result of the same hyperextension that causes sprain of the anterior capsule. As the force continues, the proximal phalanx moves backward over the metacarpal. The metacarpal head is thrust
forward, the anterior capsule tears and the phalanx dislocates onto the back of the
metacarpal and stands at a 90 degree angle to the metacarpal (Figs. 171 B, and
174). As mentioned previously, it is quite unlikely that this dislocation is seen in its
pure state. Almost inevitably someone has attempted to straighten the finger. If this
attempt has been made by simply flexing the phalanx, this will usually result in sliding the phalanx back along the dorsum of the metacarpal and impinging a flap of
capsule between the phalanx and metacarpal head (Fig. 171, C). Such manipulation is to be condemned and should not be done by the physician who attempts
reduction.

If the deformity is of the right angle variety, reduction can frequently be
accomplished by pressure distally along the base of the phalanx in the direction of
the long axis of the metacarpal while the finger is maintained in hyperextension
(Fig. 171, B). This permits the base of the phalanx to slide over the metacarpal
head and, as it resumes its normal position in relation to the metacarpal head, flexion
of the finger will reduce the dislocation. An attempt may be made to carry out
this manipulation without anesthesia provided the dislocation is seen very early and
also provided that there has been no traumatic attempt to carry out reduction earlier.

If the dislocation presents with the finger and metacarpal parallel but with
the phalanx resting on the back of the metacarpal neck, it is quite unlikely that it
can be reduced without anesthesia (Fig. 171, C). It is our practice in such an
instance to be prepared for surgery at the time the anesthetic is given since it may
be impossible to reduce the dislocation even under anesthesia. Under anesthesia,
traction may be placed on the phalanx along the axis of the metacarpal. Ofttimes
this will successfully reduce the dislocation. If it does not, the phalanx may be
very carefully hyperextended to the position of 90 degree angulation with the
metacarpal to place it back in the position it was in at the time of the dislocation.
This may remove the interposed tissue and permit classical reduction. If this cannot be done without undue force, it should not be continued and one should pro-

Figure 175. Taping for a sprained or dislocated finger. Flex the injured joints slightly. Using ½ inch adhesive tape apply a basketweave over the injured joint. Place a ⅛ inch thickness of soft sponge, felt or cotton between the fingers (optional) to prevent friction. With ½ inch tape, tape to an adjoining finger which will act as a splint. Leave the index finger free if possible. (Courtesy of Rawlinson, "Modern Athletic Training," © 1961 by Prentice-Hall, Inc.)

ceed to open reduction in order to disengage the interposed tissue and permit the metacarpal head to move backward under the phalanx. Following reduction, immobilization should be carried out for about two weeks but it is not necessary to immobilize the interphalangeal joints. Thus, rehabilitation can start at once.

Finger Area. Sprain of the interphalangeal joints may be caused by hyperextension of the joint which causes the anterior capsule to be torn or by excess lateral motion of this hinge joint. The interphalangeal joint has definite collateral ligaments. These ligaments are tight in flexion and relatively loose in extension. Lateral angulation of the phalanx will cause damage to the collateral ligament. This usually occurs with the involved joint in extension. A laceration of the collateral ligament may be an extremely painful injury and may result in disability if untreated. On the other hand, if it is immobilized this may also cause disability through stiffness. Careful examination of the finger will permit one to determine whether or not there is instability. If there is instability, the joint should be immobilized in extension with appropriate lateral deviation to close the joint on the involved side. This should be maintained for about two weeks. After that some motion may be permitted but flexion beyond 90 degrees should not be permitted for at least four weeks.

Sprain of the anterior capsule can be demonstrated by pain on an attempt to completely extend this joint. If the injury is severe, it may be possible to actually hyperextend the joint. In such an instance the joint should be immobilized in moderate flexion for a period of two or three weeks (Fig. 175). If there is no instability but pain alone, it should suffice to protect the finger a week or ten days and then permit motion, meanwhile warning the patient that he should not permit complete extension. If athletic competition is permitted, either in game or practice, the finger splint should be replaced during actual play for at least four weeks, since relatively minor repetition of the original injury may cause recurrence.

Dislocation of the interphalangeal joints is ordinarily caused by the same force that causes sprain of the anterior capsule. As the hyperextension continues, the anterior capsule tears, the head of the more proximal phalanx thrusts further through the palmar surface and may, indeed, come right on through the skin. Such an injury should be recognized as extremely serious (Fig. 176). It is frequently spontaneously reduced, particularly if incomplete. Even if the dislocation is complete, it will usually be reduced by the time one sees it if it is readily reducible. In the dislocations that do not reduce, the head of the phalanx is usually caught either in the capsule or in the flexor tendon in such a manner that it does not readily

Figure 176. Dislocation of proximal interphalangeal joint of the little finger. This dislocation usually entails severe injury to the collateral ligaments and is likely to heal with swollen, stiff joint or instability, or both.

reduce. If this is seen immediately after the injury, it may be reduced by manipulation. The first step in the manipulation is to reproduce the hyperextension to unlock it and then, by traction along the line of the dislocated phalanx, the base of the bone can be readily pushed down into contact with the head of the more proximal phalanx. If it does not reduce readily, procaine block may be quite adequate since muscle relaxation is not necessary here. If the dislocation is open, the wound is given a very thorough cleansing, using copious amounts of soap and water. The head is then reduced. If it is an early injury the skin edges are tacked together as a primary procedure.

Following any of these dislocations, the finger should be immobilized with the joint in some flexion (30 degrees) (Fig. 175). The finger should not be flexed to 90 degrees although this may seem to hold the dislocation more firmly. In this position the collateral ligaments are under undue tension and as healing occurs the ligaments are too long.

The dislocation may occur without actually tearing either or both collateral ligaments. After the finger is reduced, particularly if under anesthesia, careful check should be made to determine whether or not there is instability. If instability is present one should seriously consider repair of the collateral ligament. In many of these conditions there is redundancy of this ligament with migration of the more distal phalanx toward the opposite side, and a painful, unstable, afunctional joint may result.

The same components are present in dislocation of the interphalangeal joint as are present in dislocation of the knee, for example. It is a serious injury and may well result in permanent disability, particularly if treatment is casual (Fig. 177). One

Figure 177.   Old dislocation of proximal interphalangeal joint of ring finger with unstable, painful, swollen joint and limitation of flexion and extension. Note ulnar deviation of middle phalanx. Early ligament repair might have prevented this disabling condition.

should study the x-ray carefully, particularly after reduction, since it may provide evidence of an avulsion of the ligament or possibly a fracture of one of the margins of the phalangeal base.

FRACTURE

Thumb Ray

Metacarpal Area.   The same forces that produce dislocation of the thumb may also cause fracture. One of the most frequent fractures of the thumb is the Bennett fracture which is in reality a dislocation of the carpometacarpal joint with avulsion fracture of some portion of the medial proximal margin of the base of the metacarpal. The same force that will cause dislocation by direct force down the shaft of the metacarpal, such as a blow with the fist, drives the base of the metacarpal proximally and dorsally. Instead of the anterior capsule tearing, the bone breaks. Thus, the injury is not only a fracture of the metacarpal but also a tearing of the dorsal ligaments and capsule of the metacarpophalangeal joint. On examination the thumb appears foreshortened. It is thick at its base with prominence of the base of the shaft of the metacarpal. Traction-abduction readily reduces the deformity and one may suspect a simple dislocation. On relaxing the traction, the deformity promptly recurs. X-ray reveals the injury (Fig. 178).

In my opinion traction and abduction with pressure against the base of the phalanx will not adequately hold this fracture and are unnecessarily cumbersome. If traction is elected, skeletal traction should be used either through the distal end

Figure 178.   A, Bennett fracture. This fracture is completely unstable. B, This fracture is best fixed by internal fixation. This particular wire is not well placed but did hold.

Figure 179.   Bennett fracture.

A, The Bennett fracture is produced by a blow against the dorsal surface of the clenched thumb. The small inner triangular fragment articulates normally; the remainder of the metacarpal subluxates, due to muscle pull.

B, Maintenance of reduction requires continuous traction, outward pressure against the distal and inward pressure against the proximal end of the thumb metacarpal. An excellent traction outrigger may be fashioned from a wire coat hanger.

(From McLaughlin, "Trauma.")

A   B

of the metacarpal or the shaft of the proximal phalanx (Fig. 179). The wrist must be flexed to the ulnar side, the thumb widely abducted with traction along its long axis. The cast is applied in this position, care being taken to place a felt pad at the pressure area on the base of the metacarpal. Elastic traction is then applied by an outrigger. The pull is along the long axis of the metacarpal. This position must be maintained for several weeks until union is fairly firm. The traction can then be removed but the cast must be replaced holding the thumb in abduction. It is notably difficult to hold this position and recurrence of deformity is frequent (Figs. 180 and 181).

My own preference is to carry out primary open reduction with internal fixation of the shaft of the bone to the fragment, either by transfixion threaded wire,

Figure 180.   *A*, Transverse fracture of base of thumb with displacement. *B*, Fixation in
wide abduction.

screw or wire loop. Following reduction of the dislocation, the dorsal capsule should
be repaired. The thumb can then be immobilized in a functional position, no bizarre
position being necessary to maintain correction. The interphalangeal joints can be
mobilized almost at once and, indeed, early motion can be permitted in the carpometacarpal joint if the internal fixation is relatively secure.

Fractures of the SHAFT of the metacarpal of the thumb and of the neck of the
metacarpal of the thumb are infrequent. If they do occur it is important to obtain
and maintain good position. The fracture of the middle of the shaft of the metacarpal will usually angulate dorsally and may be reduced by abduction of the thumb
and pressure over the fracture site. It may be held in this position by appropriate
plaster cast. If the position is not secure or does not hold, open reduction with internal fixation is the treatment of choice.

Figure 181.   Transverse, comminuted fracture of the base of the thumb, treated in traction.
Note dislocation of the carpophalangeal joint.

Phalanges.   Fractures of the PROXIMAL PHALANX of the thumb are not nearly as common as those of the remaining fingers. If complete, they are much more difficult to hold because of the extreme mobility of the normal thumb. Fixation should be with the thumb in flexion, both at the metacarpophalangeal and the interphalangeal joint. This may be maintained by a suitable plaster splint until swelling is stabilized. Then a plaster cast. It is imperative that good position be secured in order to preserve the function of the thumb. One must be particularly careful that there is no rotation of this phalanx. When the thumb is flexed and apposed, it should cross toward the base of the fifth metacarpal head, not toward the second. This permits apposition of the thumb to the various fingers. So-called mallet finger, or baseball finger, is unusual in the thumb and treatment is the same as in the remaining fingers. The same is true in fractures involving the interphalangeal joint and in crushing injuries of the tip of the distal phalanx.

Finger Rays

The subject of fracture of the metacarpals and phalanges is a voluminous one. The physician is referred to standard works on fractures or treatment of injuries to the hand for adequate detail. It is important here to review some of the details particularly pertinent to the athlete.

Metacarpals.   Fracture of the BASE OF THE METACARPAL (Fig. 182) occurs from a direct blow against the end of the metacarpal which transmits the force down the shaft as exemplified by the blow with the clenched fist. It may also be caused by a direct crushing force over the back of the hand as it rests on a solid surface. The metacarpal bases are so closely bound together that the fracture is not displaced. Diagnosis may be made by the history of the character of the injury and by the local findings. Tenderness will be extreme at the site of the break.

Figure 182.   Fracture of base of the metacarpal resulting from a blow with the clenched fist against the opponent's head. This comminuted type of fracture requires traction —in this instance straight traction—for reduction and fixation.

Direct pressure over the injured area is painful. Pain is elicited by tapping the end of the bone, the force being transmitted down the shaft of the metacarpal to the fracture site. Careful x-ray study is important since in many instances the fragments are impacted. This combined with the fact that the bones normally overlap may make x-ray interpretation difficult. One may be amazed to see after several weeks fractures that did not appear at all on the original x-ray. A particular effort should be made to note any possible dislocation. Since the palmar ligament is so much stronger than the dorsal, the force may drive the shaft backward, break off the anterior margin of the metacarpal and permit the shaft of the metacarpal and dorsal part of the proximal end to displace dorsally. This can be readily palpated immediately after the injury but is later concealed by swelling, edema and infiltration of blood. Very careful lateral x-ray views in several planes may be necessary to actually demonstrate this fracture. One may be chagrined after treating what appears to be contusion or sprain of the hand to find gross deformity of one of the bases, particularly the second or third metacarpal. On the other hand, if the injury is recognized early it may be reduced by traction. It may be difficult to maintain reduction by cast fixation only. Internal fixation is relatively simple since the bone may be transfixed to its neighbors after reduction without actually opening up the fracture site. At open reduction transfixion wires may be placed through the metacarpal and into the undisplaced proximal fragment. A little ingenuity will be well rewarded provided the diagnostic acuity has been sufficient to recognize this lesion. If the fracture is incomplete or without displacement, simple immobilization of the wrist and hand is adequate. It is not necessary to immobilize either the metacarpophalangeal joint or the interphalangeal joints. Protection should continue as long as the hand is symptomatic. The intrinsic stability here is such that in many circumstances immobilization may be discontinued within two weeks.

As the location of the injury moves distally to involve the METACARPAL SHAFT, it becomes more complicated in management. Many fractures of the third or fourth metacarpal, being surrounded on two sides by intact bone, may be without displacement and so require little or no treatment. Angulation of the shaft of the third or fourth metacarpal is not common (Fig. 183). If it occurs, it should be reduced by traction on the fingers, direct pressure over the fracture site and then transfixion of the shafts by Kirschner wire drilled across through the two adjacent and intact metacarpals above and below the fracture site. These can be cut off beneath the skin and virtually no external immobilization is required after the first few days. This internal fixation is more likely to be necessary in the oblique or transverse fracture (Fig. 184). The long spiral fracture ordinarily will maintain adequate position since a few millimeters of shortening of the bone will be of little consequence. When the fracture involves more than one metacarpal or when it involves the second or fifth, stability is much less secure. It has been my experience in the athlete that if there is a fracture with displacement in the shaft of either of these metacarpals, some sort of internal fixation is advisable. This is particularly true because fixation by plaster is extremely cumbersome and very often fails.

If plaster fixation is elected, the wrist should be dorsiflexed (Fig. 185). Direct pressure is applied over the angulated fracture site while traction is placed on the involved finger. If the fracture is unstable, skeletal traction may be necessary using any of the various methods such as a fish hook through the dorsal cortex of the

Figure 183.   Oblique, comminuted fracture of the shaft of fourth metacarpal, treated by manual traction and Kirschner wire transfixing two intact metacarpals. This is an excellent method.

Figure 184.   Spiral oblique fracture of middle of shaft of fourth metacarpal. Note that in the anteroposterior view the fracture line is not visible although the bone does look somewhat shorter. Because of the shortening, traction is indicated although the fracture will heal well without treatment.

Extensor diq. communis
Extensor expansion
Inteross.
Flexor diq. sublimis
A   Lumbrical
Flexor diq. profundus
B
C
Molded
plaster splint
D

Figure 185.   Fractures of the metacarpals.

A, Normal finger motors.

B, and C, The consistent deformity of metacarpal fractures resulting from muscle pull.

D, Correction of deformity requires pressure downward against the apex of the deformity, and upward under the metacarpal head. Pressure points by splint (arrows) must be watched closely for skin damage.

(From McLaughlin, "Trauma.")

proximal phalanx or transfixion traction through the proximal phalanx laterally. After the traction is applied and the fracture is reduced, a palmar splint should be applied with the wrist dorsiflexed, the metacarpophalangeal joint semiflexed and the proximal interphalangeal joint rather sharply flexed (90 degrees). This should be supported by a posterior splint plus a felt pressure pad over the fracture site which permits direct downward pressure against the angulated fracture site. This position is maintained by manual traction until the splint is hardened. After the plaster sets, some sort of outrigger must be applied to maintain traction on the involved finger. Bear in mind that this cannot be done with the fingers in extension but must be done with the fingers flexed.

I believe it is much more difficult to handle a metacarpal fracture by skeletal traction than it is by some form of internal fixation. Consequently if the fracture is not adequately supported by the cast alone without traction, I would abandon further efforts to hold it and would use internal fixation. Internal fixation is carried out with wire loops or a small plate or by transfixion of the fractured metacarpals to the intact ones. Another method is to use an intramedullary pin inserted into the distal end of the bone with the metacarpophalangeal joint in complete flexion (Fig. 186). In this latter method, since the pin traverses the metacarpal joint it should not be left in place more than three or four weeks.

It must be emphasized again that fracture of the metacarpals is a serious injury. If one intends to treat them, he should properly prepare himself by adequate study of the various factors involved not only in causing the deformity but in preventing its recurrence.

Fractures of the NECK OF THE METACARPAL are very common, the most frequent being of the fifth. They are often caused by the application of the knuckle of the clenched fist forcibly against someone's head as he ducks a blow to the face. The result is almost always a flexion deformity with the head rotated over the neck so that the head presents itself in the palm (Fig. 185, C). Examination of the metacarpal bone will show why forward rotation of the head causes such prominence in the palm of the hand. The head normally hooks forward to be much more prominent on the palmar than the dorsal surface. Forward angulation causes this normal prominence to be exaggerated. On examination this abnormality is readily palpable. This fracture is usually impacted but should not be left unreduced. It should be noted that there is usually more trouble with the third and fourth heads than with the others since they are less mobile and any gross displacement of the head into the palm will cause disability not only by impingement of the head but by pressure on the nerve and restriction of motion of the joint.

These fractures are usually readily reduced. Anesthesia is required. Under

Figure 186.   Fractured metacarpals from athletic injury. Reduction maintained by Kirschner wires. These wires transfix the metacarpal head and should be removed as soon as the union is solid enough. The finger should be immobilized until the wire is removed.

anesthesia it may be possible to manipulate the head by pressure of the surgeon's fingers over the shaft dorsally and pressure backward of his thumb against the head. Or it may be impacted so much that this simple manipulation is ineffective. In such a case the shaft of the proximal phalanx can be utilized to push the head dorsally on the metacarpal shaft after flexing the metacarpophalangeal joint to 90 degrees. One should not be deluded into believing he can flex the proximal phalanx into the palm, apply a pressure dressing and so reduce the fracture. The fracture must be disimpacted and reduced before any dressing is applied. Very frequently it may be held in a simple splint, maintaining the fingers in semiflexion (Fig. 185, D).

If the fracture seems unstable, it has been advocated that greater stability can be obtained by flexing the proximal phalanx to 90 degrees and splinting the finger in this position on the theory that pressure upward on the phalanx and downward on the back of the hand will hold this position. My experience with this method is not favorable. It is my belief that if the fracture will hold in this position, it will probably also be held securely by a splint in the functional position. It is virtually impossible to keep constant pressure on the back of the hand and on the distal end of the proximal phalanx in an active individual.

If the fracture is unstable my preference is to transfix it with a Kirschner wire going through the end of the knuckle and down the shaft of the metacarpal. This wire can be removed at the end of three weeks since this fracture stabilizes itself very rapidly. The more serious injuries of the hand involving multiple metacarpals with fractures and dislocation will require a great deal of skill and no effort should be spared to restore the function of the hand to normal.

Phalanges.   The PROXIMAL PHALANX is more commonly fractured than the other two phalanges. This is primarily due to the fact that the entire leverage of the fingers is brought to bear on the proximal phalanx while in the middle one there is a much shorter lever arm. Any of the phalanges may be fractured by a direct blow. This may be caused by the football cleat as the hand is stretched out on the hard ground or by catching the finger between two hard opposing objects such as the football helmet and the ground or the fiber pad on the pants or against a helmet or a shoe. This type of fracture from crushing injury is ordinarily stellate and without displacement. Whichever phalanx is involved, it may be treated by simple immobilization of the involved bone including the joint above and the one below, provided there is no rotating deformity.

The finger is not often broken by direct impact as in boxing since the flexed position tends to protect it from this force. The more serious fractures usually result from leverage action. In the proximal phalanx, this action is usually hyperextension of the fingers, the same force that causes dislocation of the proximal interphalangeal joint or the metacarpophalangeal joint.

At the BASE OF THE FINGER the injury may actually be a fracture-dislocation. As the phalanx slides backward over the metacarpal head the dorsal margin is broken off by direct impingement against the metacarpal or the palmar margin is pulled off by traction of the capsule. The dislocation in this instance is usually spontaneously reduced since the head does not tend to lock out of position. The result is that, when the player presents himself, he will have a painful, swollen, very tender metacarpophalangeal joint but without displacement. However, if the fractured fragment is large enough, instability results and the shaft

Figure 187. Transverse fracture and epiphyseal dislocation of the proximal phalanx of the fifth finger, treated by manipulation and splint. Solid union. No growth interference.

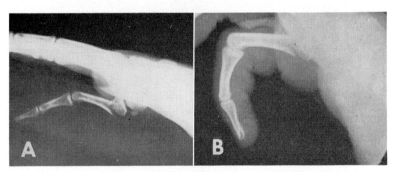

Figure 188. Fracture of the base of the proximal phalanx. *A,* Lateral view. Note the classical deformity. *B,* The finger is best held in the flexed position as illustrated. Traction is not necessary.

will subluxate. The tenderness will be at the base of the phalanx rather than over the metacarpal head. Careful x-ray examination will reveal the triangular shaped shadow of the fragmented bone. If the fragment is the posterior cortex, the metacarpophalangeal joint must be placed in extension in order to get apposition. If it is the palmar border, the finger should be placed in flexion. Following repositioning of the finger, careful x-ray study should be made to determine the exact alignment of this fragment. If it is not correctly positioned and held, the fracture should be treated by open reduction and pinning with a small threaded Kirschner wire. Since the joint surface is involved, the aphorism, "the nearer the joint, the more perfect the reduction must be," is pertinent.

This same type of fracture may occur on the lateral margins (Fig. 189) of the index or little finger as a result of forced abduction of the finger away from the midline. These injuries are in effect capsular or ligament injuries and should be treated as such.

Figure 189.   A, Avulsion fracture of the palmar lip of the proximal end of the middle phalanx as a result of hyperextension of the finger. This mild displacement requires no treatment other than fixation of the finger in a splint. B, Note the old baseball finger deformity in the distal phalanx and healed fracture of the dorsal lip of this phalanx.

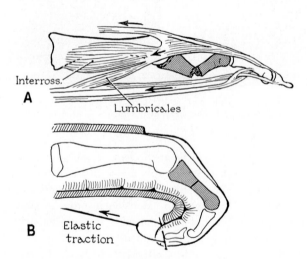

Figure 190.   Fractures of proximal phalanx.

A, All the muscle forces acting upon a fracture of the proximal phalanx collaborate to produce an angular deformity, apex forward.

B, Proximal phalanx fractures must be immobilized by well-fitting splints with the finger flexed. Unstable fractures may require supplemental traction.

(From McLaughlin, "Trauma.")

The same hyperextension force may fracture the SHAFT OF THE PROXIMAL PHALANX at any level, but most commonly through the middle third (Fig. 190). The fracture is transverse or oblique, and the distal fragment will angulate dorsally (Fig. 188). It may or may not be completely displaced. If the fracture is a stable fracture or can be made so, it may be supported in complete flexion of the finger by simple splint fixation. This applies particularly to the transverse fracture and more so to the transverse fracture where the fragment is angulated but not displaced. Careful manipulation will reduce the angulation and the fracture will be quite stable as the finger is held with all the interphalangeal joints and the metacarpophalangeal joint in complete flexion. It can be held in this position for about three weeks and then gently mobilized. In the young individual the resulting stiffness is not permanent. I have not found it necessary in these cases to use traction in the flexed position, preferring the following dressing (Fig. 191): The involved finger is joined to its immediate neighbor, i.e., if the ring finger is the one involved, I include the little finger; with the index finger, the long finger; with the long finger, the ring finger. This serves two purposes. It permits the fingers to be held in this position without strain and provides some stabilizing splint effect from the adjacent finger. After the finger is flexed a piece of adhesive tape is started over the metacarpal head, passed over the finger, down into the palm and up on the palmar surface of the hand and wrist. It is advisable to place a strip of sheet wadding between the two fingers and through the flexor creases of the fingers. This position when held by these two strips of tape will be quite secure. A strip of 1 inch tape is then passed from the back of the hand through the palm just proximal to the tip of the flexed fingers and back onto the dorsum of the hand. This serves to anchor the palmar strips. The whole is then included in a firm wrapping of gauze bandage. The fingers need not be flexed beyond the point of comfort and, if the hand is uncomfortable after the dressing is applied, it should be loosened sufficiently so that there is no feeling that the joints are overflexed. If the hand swells or the fingers feel numb, the tips should be carefully checked for circulation. This dressing may be buttressed if desirable by a plaster or plastic type splint which is about 2 inches wide and begins at the tips of the fingers and extends up over the dorsum of the hand. This will protect the hand against a direct blow on the injured area.

If the fracture is unstable, as will be the case in a comminuted or oblique

Figure 191. Drawing of the strapping described in the text. (Modified from Ochsner and DeBakey, "Christopher's Minor Surgery.")

Deformity of proximal phalanx

Tape

Reduction and immobilization

Sheet wadding

or spiral fracture, traction may be required to maintain the reduction (Fig. 190, B). There are many ways in which this traction can be applied. The finger should be in flexion. It is unwise to apply traction with the metacarpophalangeal joint extended. On the other hand, there is no particular objection to extension of the proximal interphalangeal joint. In my own practice, I prefer a plaster cast which includes the wrist and hand and goes down to the proximal interphalangeal joint on the palmar surface and to the metacarpal heads on the dorsal surface. The plaster should be molded so that the proximal joint can be flexed at least 45 degrees. An outrigger such as a bent piece of coat hanger wire can be incorporated into the back of the cast back of the fingers and flexed to the same angle as the proximal phalanges. Traction can then be applied to the finger distal to the proximal interphalangeal joint. This can be done by a small Kirschner wire passed through the base of the distal phalanx or a fishhook type wire drilled into the dorsum of the middle phalanx. Traction can be exerted by rubber bands. It is undesirable to include more than one finger in the traction but the splint should include an adjacent finger.

Open reduction of the fracture of the proximal phalanx is usually not necessary. It is neither desirable nor easy since internal fixation is very difficult to apply to this phalanx. It is not for the uninitiated. Intramedullary fixation can be carried out by passing the wire through the distal end of the proximal phalanx with the middle phalanx flexed at 90 degrees (Fig. 192). The finger must be supported with this joint flexed until the wire is removed since the wire will interfere with and cause irritation on motion. The wire may damage the proximal articular surface of the middle phalanx unless movement is prevented. There is not room in the finger for plate fixation without interference with tendon function. Any internal fixation that is used should be removed as promptly as stability will permit.

Fracture of the DISTAL END OF THE PROXIMAL PHALANX usually is a flexion fracture quite similar to fracture through the neck of the metacarpal. The distal end of phalanx is snubbed downward toward the palm with palmar angulation of the

Figure 192.   A, Fracture of proximal phalanx treated by Kirschner wire fixation. The middle third is treated by a wire through the proximal end of the metacarpal. B and C, Similar type of fracture with the wire through the distal end. This is the more acceptable of the two procedures.

distal fragment. This is usually a *transverse type* of fracture, often impacted. It can be readily reduced by hyperextension of the middle phalanx with pressure against the shaft of the proximal phalanx. The fragments will frequently move into position and be quite stable. In this instance the finger must be immobilized in complete extension in order to prevent occurrence of deformity. The pull on the anterior capsule of the joint by the extended middle phalanx will hold the head of the proximal phalanx in the proper position. The finger should not be maintained in this position more than two weeks since undue stiffness will result if held longer than this. At the end of two weeks, the finger should be slightly flexed and the splint continued.

My preference for a splint for the transverse type of fracture is carefully molded plaster applied as follows: A small splint about 1 inch wide and six layers thick is begun at the base of the finger on the palmar surface, passed over the end of the finger and back to the metacarpophalangeal joint. This is placed over a single layer of compacted sheet wadding. The splint should actually be applied with the finger in the position in which it is to be held so that the splint will not cause undue pressure such as might occur if it is applied before the finger is positioned. After the splint has set, a few circular turns of 1 inch gauze bandage may safely be applied from the base of the finger to the distal interphalangeal joint, leaving a gap at the tip of the finger covered only by gauze. This will permit the finger to be inspected for circulation. If this dressing is uncomfortable, it must be changed. Pressure necrosis can almost always be avoided by careful follow-up care since the finger should not be painful once the fragments are reduced.

"T" FRACTURE of the distal end of the proximal phalanx poses a more severe problem since it is quite unstable. Frequently the "T" fracture can be stabilized by careful reduction and transfixion across the condyles with a threaded Kirschner wire. It may then be treated as a stable fracture. The interphalangeal joint will not tolerate gross irregularity of the articular surface and open reduction should be resorted to if it is needed to secure good apposition. Rotation of the distal fragment is of extreme importance in fractures of the proximal phalanx. Rotation causes a concealed deformity which results in the finger flexing in the direction of the long axis of the forearm rather than toward the tubercle of the navicular. By way of explanation, as the fingers are flexed into the palm the long finger normally flexes directly downward toward the tubercle of the navicular. The index finger converges toward the midline as do the ring and little fingers so if a line is drawn down the axis of each flexed middle phalanx, these lines will converge at the wrist at the level of the navicular tubercle. Hence, any fixation of the finger should be in this axis rather than along the axis of its metacarpal. This is particularly true in the unstable fractures. The traction must be directed along this line. It is extremely distressing to have the fracture heal and have the fingers overlap as they flex because of failure to recognize the converging long axis of the flexed fingers.

MIDDLE PHALANX.   Fracture of the middle phalanx presents many of the same problems as those of the proximal. The fractures of the bases of the phalanges (Fig. 193) should be treated in the same way. In any fracture without displacement, a simple finger splint, preferably of aluminum, will be quite adequate to maintain the fingers in a semiflexed position of all the joints. It should be emphasized that

Figure 193.   Osteochondral fracture of interphalangeal joint revealed in
the oblique view (A), not apparent in the
anteroposterior view (B). The patient had
notable disability of this joint which was
only partially relieved by removing the
fragment as a later procedure.

the phalanges do not require long immobilization, for which there is no excuse since
it only invites stiffness.

In complete fractures of the middle phalanx that are unstable, the deformity
will vary considerably according to the location of the fracture because of the tendon attachments to this finger (Fig. 194, A). The extensor tendon has an attachment to the base of the phalanx whereas the flexor sublimis attaches to the middle
of the palmar surface of the phalanx. If the fracture lies between these two tendon
attachments, the distal fragment will go forward with the sublimis tendon; the
proximal fragment will be pulled backward by the extensor retinaculum. If the
fracture is transverse it may be stable after reduction. The finger may be splinted
in extension (not hyperextension) by simple plaster or aluminum splint. It should
be noted that the splint must be rigid and be so applied and maintained that it will
hold a constant position.

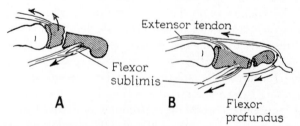

Figure 194.   Fractures of middle phalanx.
A, The small proximal fragment of a fracture of the middle phalanx proximal to the
sublimis insertion is extended by the central slip of the extensor mechanism. The distal fragment must be realigned with this uncontrollable fragment.
B, Both fragments of the middle phalanx are controllable when the fracture is distal to
the sublimis insertion. Immobilize in flexion.
(From McLaughlin, "Trauma.")

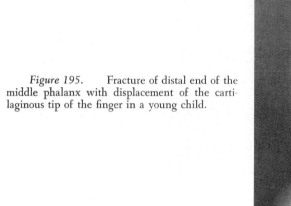

Figure 195.   Fracture of distal end of the middle phalanx with displacement of the cartilaginous tip of the finger in a young child.

In a fracture distal to the sublimus attachment (Figs. 194, B, and 195), the angulation of the proximal fragment is forward in the same manner as in the proximal phalanx and the same treatment will be necessary, that is, the maintenance of flexion of the fingers in all joints. This may be accomplished by the same apparatus as indicated for the proximal phalanx. If the fracture is comminuted or spiral and unstable, it should be treated by traction, in this instance with the splint extended slightly beyond the proximal interphalangeal joint and traction applied to the distal phalanx along the long axis of the middle phalanx which will ordinarily be at about 45 degrees of flexion from the extended position. This traction may be by Kirschner wire through the base of the distal phalanx, by pulp traction at the tip of the phalanx or through the nail. My own preference is a Kirschner wire through the distal phalanx. Once the fracture is fixed, careful x-ray study should be made to determine that the alignment is correct. I should emphasize particularly the importance of rotation in fracture of either proximal or distal phalanx. Rotation on the long axis of the finger will change the relationship of the interphalangeal joints with each other and present a quite obvious deformity after healing occurs (see Fig. 196).

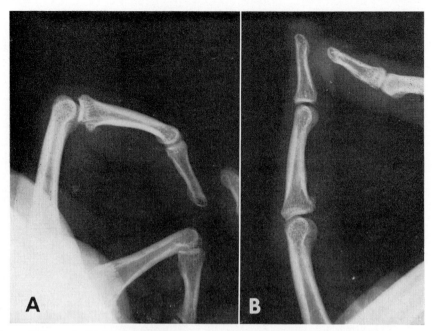

Figure 196.   A, Snubbing fracture of the anterior flange of the proximal end of the middle phalanx. B, Note reduction of the fragment by extension of the finger.

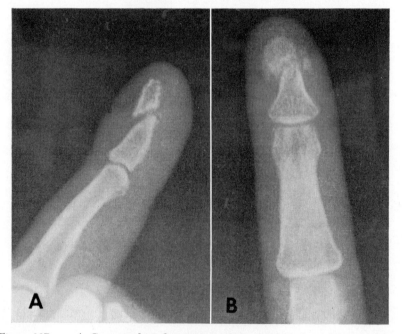

Figure 197.   A, Compound crushing injury of the distal phalanx. This was treated by simple dressing. The wound healed but the finger remained so painful that the patient was unable to work for four months. B, X-ray revealed malposition and nonunion. Treated by resection of the fragment with good recovery.

DISTAL PHALANX.   Fractures of the distal phalanx are almost always *crushing injuries* except for the avulsion fracture of the flexor or extensor tendons. This crushing injury may involve the tuft at the tip of the finger (Fig. 167) in which case the fracture itself is of much less significance than the crushing injury. It may involve the shaft or indeed extend back to involve the base and articular surface. Usually these fractures require no treatment other than the treatment of the soft tissue injury. However, the two distal phalanges of the finger should be immobilized by a metal splint in order to protect against direct blow or prevent later deformity. In the occasional case in which there is a transverse fracture through the shaft with displacement and there is instability, the fracture may be reduced and readily stabilized by an intramedullary Kirschner wire drilled through the distal end of the finger and down to the distal interphalangeal joint. Angular deformity of the distal phalanx should not be ignored since it may cause distressing disability (Fig. 197).

If the fracture is directly across the base of the finger and seems quite unstable, the wire may be passed across the joint and down into the middle phalanx. In this instance the finger should be immobilized in the position in which the fracture is most stable, preferably in a few degrees of flexion. The threaded wire should be removed as soon as healing has accomplished stabilization, which would be at two or at the most three weeks. If the fracture involves the articular surface in the nature of a "T" fracture or fracture across one angle of the base, this may be transfixed by drilling the wire laterally across the finger after reduction of the fracture. If reduction cannot be obtained otherwise, open reduction should be done using a transverse incision distal to the fracture. Great care should be taken not to involve the nail root lest deformity of the nail result.

Fractures of the base of the phalanx involving the dorsal or palmar surface are almost always *avulsion fractures* in which the flexor or extensor tendon pulls off a segment of bone as the distal phalanx is hyperflexed or extended. In fractures of the dorsal surface involving the tendon, so-called *baseball finger* (Figs. 198 and 199), it may be possible to immobilize the finger by flexion of the proximal and extension of the distal interphalangeal joint. I have been unable to hold this satisfactorily by simple splint fixation and have not been particularly pleased with the method of passing an intramedullary Kirschner wire down the distal phalanx and across the extended distal interphalangeal joint, out through the palmar cortex of the middle phalanx to transfix the proximal phalanx (Fig. 200). I have had better success in passing the Kirschner wire across the extended distal joint and down into the middle phalanx, stopping short of the proximal joint. One must supplement this by splinting, holding the middle phalanx flexed. I believe most of these fractures should be treated by open reduction and internal fixation. If the fragment is large enough, it may be reduced and held by a transfixion pin through the fragment and into the distal phalanx. If the fragment is too small for this, it may be held by wire suture passed through the fragment including the tendon attachment. The wire should be passed through the fragment from the fracture line back through the tendon and looped back to emerge into the fracture line again. It then passes through holes drilled in the distal phalanx to emerge on the palmar surface of the finger. It is then tied over a button. A pull-out wire will permit its easy removal after healing. Great care must be taken not to cause pressure necrosis on the skin of the palmar surface of the finger by the button.

Figure 198.   Baseball finger. Note (*A*) fragment is not reduced by extension of the phalanx, nor does it widely separate by flexion (*B*). However, the patient lacked complete extension. Treated by open fixation.

Figure 199.   Baseball finger showing (*A*) the deformity, (*B*) poor position by hyperextension of the finger, and (*C*) poor result with dislocation of the phalanx because of improper immobilization. It should be noted that this fracture involves over half of the articular surface.

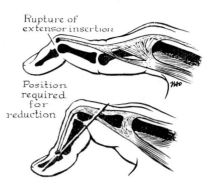

Figure 200.   Drawing illustrating the method of maintaining overextension of the distal phalanx and flexion of the proximal interphalangeal joint by immobilization with Kirschner wire. (Modified from Ochsner and DeBakey, "Christopher's Minor Surgery.")

Avulsion fracture of the flexor tendon attachment may be fixed in a similar manner with the finger in flexion. Again, my preference is open reduction, fixation either with a small pin through the fragment and distal phalanx or by wire fixation utilizing a pull-out wire. In this instance the wire may be passed directly through the nail bed over a button on the fingernail. In either instance, surgical repair should be supplemented by appropriate splinting, in the first instance with the distal phalanx extended and in the latter instance with the distal phalanx flexed.

OPEN FRACTURES

Open fractures are quite common in the finger due to the fact that the bone is so close to the skin, particularly on the dorsal surface. They should be treated as open fractures are elsewhere. If seen early enough, very careful and thorough lavage of the tissue may permit primary closure. If seen later, the wound should be left open and appropriate drainage used. This must be closed as soon as possible since longstanding chronic infection of the finger will result in stiffness of the interphalangeal joints. It is impossible to clean up a finger adequately without anesthesia, either local block or general. In the finger great care should be taken not to sacrifice any skin. Even if there is some question as to the vitality of the skin it should be saved, then a decision made later as the line of demarcation is formed.

Crushing injuries may present a considerable problem and this is particularly likely in the distal phalanx. If the crushing open injury includes avulsion of the nail and comminution of the distal fragment with tearing of the nail bed and root, the nail bed and root should be removed, the comminuted fragment should be removed and the palmar surface which is usually intact can be pulled back over the somewhat shortened distal phalanx to permit suture without tension. If it is possible to preserve the fingernail, this should be done.

One must be extremely penurious in sacrificing the length of the finger simply to effect closure. It will be far better to use a primary split graft and get the wounds to heal, then decide later on definitive treatment, including amputation. It is not proper to rush a patient with such an injury to the emergency room and clip away the distal tip of the finger until one has analyzed very thoroughly the situation in regard to blood supply. In many instances what may appear to be a hopelessly unsalvageable finger tip may actually be quite viable when properly replaced. I have witnessed many instances in which a seemingly lost finger tip was saved by replacement of the avulsed portion as a full thickness graft. Extreme conservatism must be practiced in sacrificing any tissue in the finger.

CHAPTER

13

Injuries of
the Chest

RIBS

ANATOMICAL CONSIDERATIONS

In discussing functional anatomy it is very difficult to separate the trunk from
the extremities and the various parts of the trunk from each other since, by the very
nature of their function, the extremities depend to a large extent upon the trunk
not only for stability but also for mobility (Figs. 201 and 202). So, in the chapters
on the upper extremities we have perforce included a good deal about the chest.
The discussion in this section will be largely confined to injuries of the chest proper,
excluding the spine but including the sternum.

The thorax is the most rigid part of the human trunk. Not only are the vertebrae much more firmly integrated in the dorsal spine than in other areas but the
formation of a rough oval by the spine, ribs and sternum serves to stabilize the
whole structure. Each rib articulates with its appropriate vertebra and is firmly
attached by strong ligaments not only to this vertebra but to the one above and to
its fellow ribs above and below. The end of the rib abuts directly against the articular
process on the body of the dorsal vertebra on the lateral surface of the pedicle, and
the articular tubercle of the rib articulates on the anterolateral tip of the transverse
process of the same vertebra. The capsular ligaments hold the rib firmly against the
body of the vertebra and against the transverse process. There also are dense ligaments extending vertically from the transverse process above to the upper surface

Figure 201.   Upper skeleton, viewed from the front. (From Anson, "Atlas of Human Anatomy.")

of the rib below so that the ribs are not only held firmly against the vertebrae but are bound to each other and to the adjacent transverse processes. These attachments are so firm that they are rarely damaged.

The oval of the chest is much smaller at the top. The first ribs together with the first thoracic vertebra and first piece of the sternum form a much smaller and more circular ring than those below. The ribs down to the 7th are progressively longer. The upper seven ribs are attached directly to the sternum by the costal cartilages. The costal cartilages are short in the upper three or four ribs, becoming progressively longer in the lower ribs. Whereas the costocartilage on the first rib may be no more than a fingerbreadth in length, the lower ones extend for several inches. The ribs are relatively horizontal at the top, running more and more obliquely downward until the 12th ribs may actually be more vertical than horizontal. The 8th, 9th and 10th ribs do not attach to the sternum but each of their costocartilages attaches to the costocartilage of the rib above. The distal tips of the

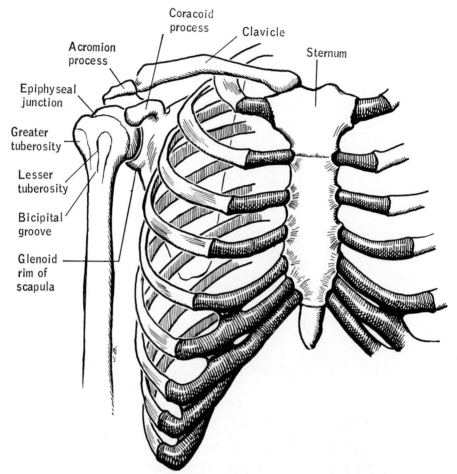

Figure 202.   Anatomical view of sternum, ribs and costocartilages, showing the relationships.

11th and 12th ribs are ordinarily free of any bony or cartilaginous attachment to the thoracic cage. The general alignment of the ribs is obliquely from above, downward and forward.

The muscles which elevate the ribs, consisting of the intercostals and many other accessory muscles, serve to pull the ribs upward and forward so that the anteroposterior diameter of the lower chest is increased by elevation of the ribs. Correspondingly, the anteroposterior diameter of the chest is diminished by depressing or compressing the rib cage. The ribs are quite elastic in a child and become increasingly brittle as age advances. In the young athlete there still remains an amazing degree of elasticity. Some of this results from the shape of the chest itself. Some of it is in the costocartilages but there is a good deal of "spring" in the structure of the rib proper.

The ribs are largely subcutaneous in the anterior one-half and are covered by the muscles of the back posteriorly. There is a shingling effect in the intercostal muscles since they attach posteriorly on the superior surface and anteriorly on the inferior surface of the rib. The intercostal vessels and nerves pass directly under the rib between the two layers of intercostal muscles and so are readily damaged by injury to the rib above. The nerves are also quite available for local injection. They are much more closely applied to the undersurface of the upper rib than to the rib below. The abdominal muscles are attached to the inferior more flexible ribs.

The ribs are further secured each to the other by the intercostal membrane. The anterior intercostal membrane is an extension of fascia over the external intercostal muscle. This muscle extends from the articular process of the vertebra around to cover about four-fifths of the rib, the remaining cover being the intercostal membrane which extends forward to attach to the sternum. Similarly, they are held together posteriorly by the posterior extension of this membrane, the posterior intercostal membrane. The internal intercostal muscle is in two layers, the more superficial layer extending from the sternum two-thirds of the way backward to be continued in the spine as the posterior intercostal membrane, so that the ribs are held together by this membrane both posteriorly and anteriorly.

The sternum is in three pieces (Fig. 202), the manubrium, the body and the xiphoid. The first rib articulates on the manubrium, the second on the junction of the manubrium and body, the third, fourth, fifth and sixth on the body, and the seventh on the junction of the xiphoid and body. These costocartilages are firmly adherent to the sternum and to each other by interdigitating ligaments, the so-called sternal intercostal ligaments.

CONTUSION

Contusion of the chest is frequent, its nature depending upon the location of the trauma. Contusion of the anterior one-half of the chest is likely to be either to the skin or to the bone itself, whereas posteriorly the muscles of the back cushion the blow and the injury will be to these muscles. The history is that of a direct blow with resultant pain. If the blow is severe enough, the "breath is knocked out" and subsequent muscle spasm may make breathing quite difficult for a short period. As soon as these preliminary symptoms are over, the patient becomes aware of a localized area of the chest that is tender to palpation. This does not interfere with breathing unless extremely deep breaths are taken. Examination at this time will reveal an area of localized tenderness, either directly over a rib or in the skin. If the periosteum is involved there will be considerable tenderness on the rib itself, whereas if the skin is involved the tenderness will be more superficial. This distinction can be made by sliding the skin upward or downward over the rib. If the tenderness remains constant in the skin, one can assume that the contusion is of the skin and subcutaneous tissues. If the tenderness remains on the bone, regardless of what area of skin is over the bone, one can assume the damage is to the bone.

Contusion of the chest wall does not often require extensive *treatment*. If there is a complicating hematoma, it may be aspirated. There is much more likely to be infiltration of blood and this may be injected with hyaluronidase early and a corticoid preparation later.

Another complication is fracture of the ribs. If several ribs have been fractured, the diagnosis can be made quite readily on the basis of severe pain on breathing, crepitation, ecchymosis and edema along the chest wall. If, as so frequently happens in athletes, a single rib is broken the adjacent ribs with the intercostal muscles splint it well and the major finding will be tenderness over the rib. However, if compression of the chest is carried out by placing one hand over the back of the chest and the other over the front of the chest, pressing from front to back, there will be pain along the point of contusion if the rib is broken or cracked. Rarely, lateral compression will cause pain. This sign is not significant, however, if pressure is made directly over the bruised area.

If there is no complication accompanying the contusion, no splinting is required. If the player is to continue in competition, particularly in a contact sport, an adequate protective pad should be placed over the contusion to prevent re-injury.

In the muscular areas of the chest, particularly on the posterior one-third, there may be painful contusion as the muscle is caught between the ribs and the striking force. This is treated as a muscular contusion anywhere, including the complication of hematoma. Myositis ossificans is not common in the muscles in the back of the chest. In the front of the chest, the lower portion is almost entirely subcutaneous. The superior anterolateral portion of the upper chest is covered with the pectoral muscle which fans out over all of the upper ribs as it extends out to its attachment on the humerus. This muscle is subject to all the injuries inherent in the muscular system and may receive a painful contusion with hematoma formation. Some of the fibers may be avulsed from the attachments to the ribs. This becomes essentially an injury to the shoulder rather than the chest, however, since the disability is primarily in use of the arm.

Overlying the pectoral muscle is the breast. The breast of most males is a recessive structure but it may receive a painful contusion. This may result in inflammation locally centered around the nipple and areola with redness, tenderness and local heat. The breast which has been quite inconspicuous may become quite prominent. On examination there is a palpable hard ring surrounding the nipple which is tender to touch. Serous fluid may exude from the nipple. This is really an inflammatory condition resulting from contusion and should be treated as such with local heat and protection. The acute symptoms may subside leaving a firm, palpable area around the nipple which may be moderately tender and should be protected by contact pads. Occasionally a painful fibrous nodule remains which may require excision.

With more participation in athletics by girls, a few words should be said about the female breast. The adolescent with immature breasts needs no particular protection but any injury to the breast should be treated promptly and adequately and athletic competition eliminated until inflammation has subsided. Early application of cold followed by heat and protection and support by a binder or brassiere should be maintained as long as there is swelling or inflammation. The more mature breast should be protected by an adequate brassiere during strenuous athletic competition. This not only will tend to protect the breast from direct blows but will prevent overexuberant motion of the breast during strenuous activity. Any contusion of the breast that does not respond promptly to local treatment will require consultation with a physician experienced in the management of breast conditions. The adolescent girl will tend to avoid any mention of a breast injury. The coaches and advisors should advise the girls to report promptly any discomfort in this area.

Be very wary of any persistent localized nodule in the female breast. Of equal importance are the symptoms of generalized chronic mastitis with aching pain, deep tenderness, and a tendency for "caking" of the gland.

STRAIN

Since a multitude of muscles attach to the chest, almost any manifestation of strain may occur. Strain may be caused by violent exertion or by overstretching of the muscles. The symptoms will depend entirely upon the area involved. In the long muscles of the back of the thorax, this condition may be indistinguishable from, or may be part of, a lumbar strain. In the front of the chest the strain may involve the muscles of the abdominal wall where they attach to the lower ribs. Strain may also involve the intercostal muscles although this is not frequent since they are well protected by other muscle structures and these muscles do not often act forcibly enough to rupture their fibers. A strain is much more likely to involve an area connecting to the chest than the chest itself. This is particularly true of the scapular muscles, i.e., strain of the rhomboids will occur either at the scapular attachment or along the spine much more frequently than at the costal attachment. Similarly, the serati may more likely be injured in their substance or at their attachments to the shoulder than in their costal origins. Careful analysis of the active motion that causes the pain will usually determine the proper muscle group although it may be quite difficult to relate it to a specific muscle.

Strain of a muscle at its attachment to the rib is likely to be more painful than it is disabling. There may, however, be considerable attendant muscle spasm which will tend to splint the chest and interfere with deep breathing. It actually may prevent certain types of activity. A strain of the abdominal recti attached to the lower ribs may interdict a sport such as rowing or wrestling where forcible use of the abdominal muscles is required. Similarly, spasm of the shoulder muscles may interdict throwing.

Treatment. Since most of the attachments to the chest are diffuse muscular ones, they do not lend themselves well to local injection. After one has determined what muscular activity causes pain, this activity should be restricted, either by appropriate splinting or simply by reducing the activity of the individual. If the muscles attaching to the scapula are involved, the arm should be put in a sling. If there is serious involvement of the abdominal muscle attachments, the patient should be put to bed with the head rest and knee support elevated in order to flex his spine and relax the abdomen.

Treatment will depend entirely on the muscles involved. Local treatment may be of some value. In the early stages application of ice will minimize the inflammation and blood infiltration. Later, local heat will give considerable comfort and promote improved circulation. Many of these injuries will be relieved by wearing a snugly fitting binder on the lower ribs. Any webbing band such as a rib belt (Fig. 203) or elastoplast strapping or, indeed, simply wrapping the lower chest with an elastic bandage may relieve the symptoms considerably. As with many muscular strains, complete recovery may be very tedious. Just about the time the player begins to get rid of his muscle spasm and have some expectation of recovery, he is likely to step up his activities to the point where he reactivates the process. The classic measures of rest, heat and gradual rehabilitation are quite pertinent here.

If after the first week or ten days there remains an area of persistent tenderness, local injection of this area with a long-acting local anesthetic plus one of the corticoid preparations may dramatically relieve the symptoms. Infiltration of several levels along the origin of the muscles to the ribs may be necessary. This may be

Figure 203.   Drawing of rib belt on a patient.

quite effective even in the early stage but is particularly so later if the symptoms have persisted. Our method usually has been to outline the areas of tenderness to palpation and check against active contraction and passive stretching of the involved muscle. If these measures cause pain in the area where there is palpable tenderness, one may assume there is local inflammation at this spot. These areas are carefully infiltrated with a local anesthetic. Proof of the effectiveness of the procedure will be complete elimination of pain on palpation, active contraction and passive stretching. If the pain is not relieved, at least while the anesthetic is effective, the involved area has not been adequately infiltrated. If the pain is relieved, this same area should be infiltrated with a corticoid and the patient should be encouraged to continue his activities but to avoid excess of either active or passive motion.

An example of the condition just described is found in the serratus posterior which rises from the lower ribs and passes over to the lumbar aponeurosis in the midline. There may be an area of tenderness extending from the inferior angle of the scapula directly down over the ribs which corresponds to the attachment of this muscle. Complete expansion of the chest or leaning toward the opposite side will cause discomfort here. Actively pulling toward the involved side will also cause discomfort in the same area. If these feelings of discomfort can be eliminated by injection of a local anesthetic, one may assume he has reached the area of the trouble. This local treatment should be supplemented by inductive heat. In many cases, support by appropriate strapping will be of value.

Muscle ruptures are unusual about the thorax. They are very difficult to diagnose unless they involve the small attachment of a single large muscle such as that of the latissimus dorsi to the upper extremity. This does not directly involve the chest since the chest component of this muscle is an extremely extensive attachment to many ribs and is not susceptible to strain.

FLOATING RIBS

Some mention should be made of the characteristics of the 11th and 12th ribs—the so-called floating ribs. The tip of the 12th and many times the 11th rib does not reach the sternal attachment and has no costocartilage as such. These ribs articulate with the spine with a single articular facet having no tubercle and no head so that there is much less stability and comparatively free motion at the spine. They are invested in the abdominal musculature and completely surrounded by muscle attachments. These ribs do not actually participate in respiration to any major extent and are more likely to be involved in injury of the spine than of the chest. They will be discussed in relationship to injury of the spine.

SPRAIN-SUBLUXATION-DISLOCATION

The areas subject to ligament injury in the chest are primarily at the vertebral and the sternal attachments of the ribs.

Vertebral Attachment

As has been mentioned above, the ribs are bound firmly at their vertebral attachments. The degree of motion in this area is necessarily quite restricted and the forces which cause tension against these ligaments are primarily compression forces against the chest or rotation forces. The excursion of movement is relatively small so that there is no forcible lateral bending at a costal vertebral joint, such as might occur at the knee. A direct blow on the rib itself is more likely to break the rib than to knock it loose at either end. A compression force applied to the whole thorax in the athlete is usually from front to back and the major strain of this force is applied at the angle of the ribs owing to flattening of the oval of the chest by the compressing force. The greatest strain is correspondingly felt at the widest extremes of the oval. There are instances of damage to the vertebral joint. In this case the symptoms will depend upon the degree of involvement. If the sprain is mild, there will be point tenderness over the injured ligament and but little discomfort on movement of the chest. In the athlete, this area is well covered by the lumbar muscles, making the diagnosis of a mild sprain virtually impossible.

If the sprain is more severe, there may be some pain on deep inspiration or on forced rotation motions of the chest. Here, also, the isolation of the injury is extremely difficult since other conditions may cause essentially the same symptoms. It is difficult to separate forceful motion against the ligament of the joint from overstretching of a neighboring muscle. Active contraction of a muscle may cause pain in the injured joint in the same manner as it would if the muscle itself was injured.

I have never seen a complete dislocation of the proximal end of a rib in an athlete. It is possible that subluxation or spontaneously reduced dislocation may occur and be unrecognizable. *Treatment* in any event will be symptomatic: early application of cold followed later by heat and protection against that motion which causes pain. If deep inspiration causes discomfort, a rib belt (Fig. 203) may be used to restrict inspiration. If rotation or flexion motions of the chest causes pain, these may be eliminated by adequate strapping of the back. Strapping in this instance should consist of strips extending from the shoulders to the pelvis and parallel to the spine. It is my practice to use 3 inch tape with three or four strips to each side, each overlapping about 50 per cent. These strips can be anchored by circumferential tape. They will to a considerable degree restrict forward or lateral bending and are equally applicable for ligament sprains and muscle strains. Physical therapy particularly with inductive heat will expedite the recovery. Active participation in sports may be impossible for several days while the condition is acute but after a lapse of a week or ten days, particularly with adequate strapping, participation may be resumed in the ordinary case.

Anterior Attachment

Ligament injuries at the anterior end of the rib are considerably more frequent than posteriorly, or possibly it should be said they are more often recognized. Although the ribs are firmly bound to the sternum, these ligaments are more subject to sprain than the posterior ones by virtue of the forward thrust which occurs with lateral compression or by direct force applied to the sternum, driving the sternum backward while the ribs swing forward (Fig. 202). A sprain of the costosternal joint should be distinguished from injury to the costochondral junction, which will be discussed under fractures.

The player will complain of tenderness in the chest localized over the area of injury. This area is readily palpable since it is subcutaneous. Often, these symptoms may be confined to a single costosternal articulation. Pressure directly over the joint or pressure over the adjacent sternum will usually cause discomfort. The symptoms will vary with the degree of injury. If the sprain is a mild one, there will be local tenderness and possibly a little local swelling—and that is all. If the injury is severe but still short of avulsion of the ligament, the local symptoms will be more intense. There will be no displacement. The tenderness will be more diffuse and will be accompanied by local swelling. There may be infiltration of blood or even formation of a hematoma directly over the joint. In case of a moderately severe injury, deep inspiration will be painful. The pain will be definitely localized to the involved joint. If there has been an actual subluxation of the joint or spontaneously reduced dislocation, the symptoms will be still more severe. The subluxation may tend to recur on deep inspiration or on lateral compression of the chest. Some degree of subluxation may remain, apparently caused by the dehiscence of the anterior ligament while the posterior ligament remains intact so that the rib will slide forward in relationship to the sternum and there may be palpable prominence. In the early stage this may be reduced by direct pressure. This movement may cause an audible snap and will certainly cause pain.

Treatment of these injuries to the costosternal area is quite unsatisfactory. The mild degree of injury may be handled without support but with local injection of an anesthetic plus hyaluronidase and application of heat locally. In the more severe injury where there is pain on motion of the chest, the chest should be strapped with adhesive or a suitable rib binder to prevent further stress on the ligament. The binder should not be put on tightly enough to increase the pain but should be used primarily to prevent wide expansion of the chest. If there is subluxation, it will be virtually impossible to hold the involved rib down in its normal position. One must be satisfied to immobilize the chest to eliminate pain and accept the minimal deformity caused by undue prominence at the tip of the rib. The injury may be extremely tedious to the player because of its chronicity and there will be many disheartening episodes of recurrence of pain following forceful activity.

The technique of injection of the costosternal area is quite simple. Repeated infiltrations should be used until all pain and tenderness are eliminated. Because of the interdigitation of the ligaments, the injury may be more widespread than first suspected. It may be advisable to infiltrate into one or more rib ends. I do not find it necessary to infiltrate the joint itself as frequently as I do the surrounding ligament. Once the pain and tenderness are eliminated, these same general areas should be carefully infiltrated in the early case with hyaluronidase and in the more chronic case with a corticoid—or a mixture of the two may be used.

In the chronic case, as has been mentioned above, player participation in sports is often not permissible. If the rib binder is applied snugly enough to prevent deep breathing, it may seriously interfere with the player's ability since it will be necessary for him to breathe deeply in the course of his participation. One must carefully evaluate the source of the discomfort. If it is from direct pressure or direct contact, the discomfort may be prevented by a suitably placed fiber board pad. If the pain is actually caused by compression of the chest, I know of no appliance that will completely eliminate it. However, a snugly fitted rib belt or corset will tend to hold the chest in a more circular position and so may well eliminate the stress at this particular point. If on the other hand the pain is caused by deep inspiration, it can be checked by a suitable binder. In most conditions I do not approve of local injection to permit participation but in this particular condition, and especially if it is restricted to one or two ribs, it is difficult to believe that injection to eliminate the pain would increase the hazard of further injury. One may give the player substantial relief by local infiltration. I do not believe this should ever be done, however, if the elimination of pain symptoms might increase the hazard of injury, as to the ligaments of the knee or ankle. The question of surgical treatment of these conditions does not often arise. If the pain seems to be from a chronic traumatic arthritis of the joint or from calcification in the anterior fissure of the joint, one may be persuaded to resect a portion of the costocartilage adjacent to the sternum. I have never had occasion to do this as a result of athletic injury or in order to permit participation.

A frank dislocation of the rib that persists should be reduced at the earliest possible moment. Dislocation of an isolated rib is rarely seen but it may be more frequent than is apparent because so often the dislocation reduces spontaneously. If seen, the deformity should be promptly reduced. For reduction, either local or general, anesthesia is usually required since, if the dislocation would readily reduce, it probably would have been reduced before it reached the doctor. After injection of a local anesthetic, the rib may be snapped back into the position by pressure over the chest and direct pressure with the thumb over the rib end. If it cannot be reduced by manipulation it may be reduced by making a small incision across the costosternal joint paralleling the rib. The rib can be gently levered into place with an elevator. Following open reduction an attempt should be made to repair the ligaments. If the rib tends to slip back out of joint it may be fixed by a suitable transfixion pin through the head of the rib and into the body of the sternum. Such treatment is rarely necessary. Following open reduction, a rib belt should be applied with a felt pad directly over the dislocated rib.

FRACTURE

Fractures of the ribs are relatively common in athletes. They usually are caused either by a direct blow from a blunt object, in which instance there is likely to be a fracture of a single or at the most two ribs, or by forceful compression of the chest in one of its diameters, in which case there may be single or multiple fractures. In the first instance, the player will give a history of a blow on the chest which may be forceful enough to "knock out his wind" and cause severe localized pain. As he gets his breath and tries to breathe deeply there is severe pain and the muscle spasm tends to splint the chest, preventing deep breathing. The result is rapid, shallow breathing, due to the combination of air hunger plus pain on inspiration. In the second instance the player may give a history of being crushed in a pile-up or of falling forcibly on his side with the ball or another player between him and the ground. Here again he will have difficult breathing accompanied by severe pain. Careful examination at the time of injury will elicit tenderness localized directly over the rib or ribs. There is pain in this same area on deep breathing. Compression of the chest, even though avoiding direct pressure on the involved rib, will neverthe-less cause pain. For example, if the 6th rib is broken at the anterior axillary line, pressure made directly backward on the sternum will cause pain in the area of the fracture and deep inspiration is painful. Any attempt at coughing or sneezing is disastrous. The player grabs his chest and attempts to restrict its motion manually. There may be a palpable defect in the rib if the fracture is complete, and it may be possible to elicit crepitation.

Fracture can be differentiated from a simple contusion by the fact that a con-tusion does not usually cause pain on motion of the rib. X-ray examination must be made (Fig. 15, page 39) but is often unsatisfactory in the early stages and a negative x-ray does not rule out a fractured rib. The obliquity of the rib, the depth of the thorax, the intervening soft tissues, together with the oblique nature of the fracture line and the frequent lack of displacement make the fracture very difficult to recognize. An exception is the unusual complete fracture in which the ends are separated.

Treatment.   COMPLICATED FRACTURE.   The vast majority of fractured ribs are uncomplicated by any more serious condition. In the occasional case, how-ever, the complications may be more critical than the injury itself. Fortunately, the bones of the young athlete are elastic enough that they do not usually splinter and present sharp-pointed fragments. When splintering does occur in the fractured rib, the sharp fragment may damage the internal mammary artery, or penetrate the lung and cause pneumothorax, or even penetrate the pericardium. A more frequent injury is damage to the intercostal vessels and nerves which will result in rather marked local swelling and formation of a hematoma.

Following an injury to the chest, if the patient does not promptly recover from the initial period of difficult breathing one should carefully investigate the possi-bility of internal injury. The patient may remain short of breath, may become some-what cyanotic, may complain of increased difficulty in getting enough air. All of these things suggest decreased lung capacity. If these conditions come on rapidly, a critical situation may arise in which immediate decompression of the chest is necessary. In such a case the patient should obviously be taken at once to the hos-pital where, after careful x-ray study to determine the degree of collapse of the lung or shift of the mediastinum, a decision is made on aspirating the air or blood (Fig. 204). If the hemothorax is small, it is probably better left alone. If the hemopneumothorax only partially collapses the lung, closed drainage of the pleural cavity will be the likely course. The vast majority of these cases fortunately are not emergent in character and ample time may be taken to complete the diagnosis. In cases of doubt, consultation should be obtained from one versed in the treatment of such conditions in the chest.

There will occasionally be subcutaneous emphysema from fracture of the ribs, with leakage of air into the soft tissues causing diffuse swelling which extends along under the skin and causes characteristic crepitation. This condition may reach alarming proportions, even to the extent of a swelling of the neck that extends to the level of the angle of the jaw, but rarely does it require any very radical or specific treatment. If there is any likelihood of internal injury, the patient should be hospitalized until all doubt concerning the presence of a serious complication has been resolved. Needless to say, x-ray study should be repeated since there may be quite rapid changes in the chest which may change the indications for treatment.

UNCOMPLICATED FRACTURE.   In the absence of any complication, local treatment may afford the player considerable relief. If there is a marked pain and muscle spasm, local anesthetic may be infiltrated into the intercostal nerve, at least a hand's breadth proximal to the fracture (that is, toward the spine). The needle is inserted directly under the margin of the rib, the plunger carefully withdrawn to be sure there is no blood, and 4 to 5 cc. of the agent is injected. The injection of a single rib may be quite effective, but it is usually necessary to inject two or three or even four ribs before relief is complete. If a long-acting anesthetic is used the relief may be quasi permanent since a good deal of the pain was caused by the

Figure 204.   X-ray (retouched) showing collapse of right lung following trauma. Note absence of lung markings in periphery of lung.

muscle spasm pulling at the fracture site. While the spasm will be relieved by injection, the recurrence of pain can be prevented only by support of the chest.

Once the pain is relieved, the chest should be properly immobilized to prevent motion of the rib. In any injury below the upper two or three ribs, the support should be circumferential and to the lower chest. It is not necessary to strap directly over the fractured 5th rib, for example. The purpose of the dressing is to splint the chest, prevent expansion of the thorax and elevation of the ribs. This can be done by pressure around the lower ribs and never needs to be any higher than the top of the xiphoid. I see little to be gained by strapping half of the chest since this certainly does not restrict expansion to any marked degree. I do not like adhesive tape because of the inevitable irritation of the skin due to the constant sliding of the skin on respiration. A commercial or homemade rib belt, which need not be more than 4 to 6 inches wide, can be pulled snugly around the chest and may be adjusted by the patient himself. His discomfort index is a very good criterion for the tightness of the dressing. He may loosen it at night when he is breathing easily and may want to tighten it during the day when his activities are more extensive.

Another advantage of the rib belt is its usefulness in strapping the female chest. Nothing is more futile than trying to strap adhesive over the breast. In the first place it cannot be placed tight enough to give any real restriction and in the second place there is such insecure foundation that it has little effect on the underlying structures. In addition, it is extremely uncomfortable. If the lower chest only is constricted, the problem of the pressure on the breasts is eliminated.

The strapping should be continued as long as the discomfort in the ribs is greater than that from wearing the restraint. This will vary considerably in different individuals. For at least six weeks a binder should be worn during any contact sport. Into the binder should be incorporated a local rigid pad to prevent a direct blow on the area. The rib may remain quite tender for many weeks. I do not believe one is justified in injecting the intercostal nerves in order to permit participation of the player with recently fractured ribs.

In the case of injury to the upper two or three ribs, the pain may be more closely related to motion of the shoulder and neck than it is to expansion of the chest. This can be readily checked by appropriate test movements. If chest expansion does not hurt, there is no advantage in using a rib binder. There may be some value in strapping directly over the shoulder, the straps beginning in the back and crossing behind the base of the neck, over the clavicle and down over the front of the chest. This strap tends to minimize elevation of the shoulder girdle when the arm is thrown up in the air. Considerable comfort may be obtained by carrying the arm in a sling. The support of the sling is not so important as the fact that the sling limits the use of the arm to routine movements with the arm at the side and, hence, forcible activity of the shoulder girdle is restricted.

Nonunion is not a complication of fractured ribs. Malunion is of little importance. If there is troublesome pain and discomfort from a malformed rib that rubs against its fellow, this segment of the rib may be removed without noticeable disability. Before this is undertaken, diagnostic check should be made by intercostal nerve block to make sure that the pain can be relieved.

Fracture of the Ribs Below the Diaphragm

As has been mentioned above, the lower ribs, particularly the 11th and 12th, have no firm fixation anteriorly and participate more in the abdominal muscle mechanism than in the chest. It should be emphasized here, however, that blows over the lower chest involving injury to the ribs below the diaphragm are potentially abdominal injuries and should be treated as such. The danger of complication is much more real than is the danger of the injury to the rib itself since the underlying structures of the spleen on the left and the liver on the right might well be injured. This will be discussed in detail under injuries of the abdomen.

COSTOCARTILAGE INJURY

The rather unusual anatomical situation in which the anterior end of the rib attaches directly to the corresponding end of the cartilage sets the stage for an annoying and sometimes quite disabling injury to the chest.

Acute Injury

Following trauma, instead of rib fracture there may be an actual dislocation at the junction of the cartilage and the rib. Occasionally the same general circumstances will arise in fracture through the costocartilage itself. The symptoms vary depending upon the level of involvement. If the injury occurs in any of the upper seven ribs where there is direct attachment to the sternum, it can usually be diagnosed quite readily (Fig. 202). The dislocation may be incomplete and without displacement and will be manifested only by tenderness at the costochondral junction with pain on forceful expansion of the chest or on direct pressure. Such a condition will usually subside without the necessity of treatment.

If the dislocation is complete there may be an actual offset and overriding so that the tip of the rib rests in front of the costal cartilage. In many cases I am sure that the dislocation is originally complete and is spontaneously reduced. The patient will present himself for examination complaining of pain in the anterior chest, which is particularly notable on coughing or sneezing. Since the area is readily palpable, he will have determined that he has a spot of localized tenderness and swelling one or two fingerbreadths lateral to the sternum. Careful examination will reveal the localized character of the lesion with pain on direct pressure, pain on pressure against the corresponding rib in the axillary line, and pain on pressure downward on the sternum. There may or may not be a palpable deformity and it may be possible to elicit a click as alternating pressure is applied on the sternum and on the involved rib. The subluxation may be minimal and be very difficult to determine, or the rib may completely dislocate. X-ray is of little value in this condition. The costal cartilages are not visualized by x-ray. The rib deformity is not sufficient to be revealed by even the stereoscopic film.

Treatment.   If there has been no demonstrable displacement or if there is no palpable click, one may assume that at least a major portion of the ligamentous investiture is intact and treatment can be directed toward preventing further injury and relieving the discomfort. The latter is accomplished by local injection of a long-acting anesthetic agent. The chest should then be firmly bound in the lower one-half either with a rib belt, elastoplast or similar strapping. The purpose of strapping is to prevent wide excursion of the ribs. If there is any possibility of recurrence of the subluxation, a direct pressure pad may be incorporated in the strapping with a piece of felt 1½ by 2¾ inches placed over the inner end of the rib but not overlapping onto the cartilage. In the male this can be strapped firmly in place with adhesive strips. This part of the dressing is quite uncomfortable. Straps over the shoulder should be used if the lesion is high and insecurity is apparent at this level, otherwise not. Adequately protected, this lesion may heal within six to eight weeks. Costal cartilage union is very slow.

Chronic Subluxation

Far too often the player does not present himself until the condition already has become chronic and one is then faced with a different problem. Here again, *treatment* will vary according to the amount of instability in the area. If there is no instability so that the major complaint is pain, the condition may respond well to injection of a local anesthetic and a steroid in the usual fashion; that is, the anesthetic agent is injected until the area is symptom-free, after which the same area is infiltrated with a corticoid preparation. The patient should be warned that he may have increased pain beginning after several hours and continuing for several hours. He may then expect improvement. If none is seen after three days the chances are that this treatment will fail. If there is improvement but after a week or ten days the symptoms recur the area should be reinjected. It may be necessary to repeat the injection four to six times, and one expects to obtain longer and longer periods of remission of symptoms after succeeding injections until finally but little residual remains. In the occasional case a single injection may be effective permanently. There is no necessity for repeating the injection if the symptoms do not recur.

In the case with or without displacement in which the symptoms persist and are severe enough to be disabling, one has to consider surgical intervention. The symptoms in such a circumstance are due to a pseudarthrosis with, in effect, a chronic traumatic arthritis in a false joint. This may be remedied by means similar to those used at the acromioclavicular joint, namely, resection of enough of the opposing surfaces so that they do not actually rub together. One must be careful, however, that in so separating the bone and cartilage he does not end up with instability and a snapping joint. After ½ to ¾ inch of the cartilage is resected the chest should be put in various positions and subjected to various pressures to make sure that the ribs and the cartilage do not interfere on chest movement. Fusion of the rib to the cartilage surgically is extremely difficult, and I can think of no justification for internal fixation in an effort to obtain union in an old case.

If the chronic case includes subluxation or dislocation, instability is already present and treatment must be based on different principles. Whereas in the case without subluxation the symptoms are presumably due to chronic irritation with minimal amount of motion, the case with subluxation contains a built-in aggravator since every time the rib slips over the cartilage the irritation is increased. It should be emphasized that the mere fact that it is slipping is not sufficient justification for surgical treatment. In the occasional case the slipping makes the patient so nervous that there may be sufficient justification but the justification is then the nervous tension and not the slipping itself. If the slipping is symptomatic so that it causes pain or spasm or local swelling, there is little hope of cure short of surgical intervention. Local measures such as injection and heat may be palliative but the chances are they will fail. There is no justification for strapping in the chronic case. The relief given will be purely temporary and indeed the strapping may be more of an aggravation than a relief. If the symptoms justify it, treatment is surgical removal of the costal cartilage or the end of the rib so that the two do not impinge. The fact that the end of the rib remains somewhat unstable will usually not be a problem since it is a single joint. This rib is firmly bound to the one above and below and does not have wide excursion. In fact, it may actually slip less after resection since there is no lever action to slide it up over the costal cartilage and catch it in this position.

Costocartilage injury is usually not severe enough to require elimination of athletics. In the acute case, however, the dislocation should be reduced and held by strapping. Following the reduction, contact sports should not be permitted during the six weeks required for union to become secure. Fortunately, this condition is not a common athletic injury.

STERNUM

ANATOMICAL CONSIDERATIONS

The most anterior portion of the chest is the sternum which in the newborn is in many segments corresponding to the ribs. These segments later fuse to form three distinct portions of the sternum. The upper one, the manubrium, carries the attachment of the first rib and the upper portion of the second; the middle portion, the body, contains the attachment to the 3rd, 4th, 5th, 6th and sometimes the 7th ribs; and the lower portion, the xiphoid, hangs from the distal end of the body, its upper portion giving attachment to the 7th costal cartilage. The 7th rib usually attaches along the junction of the body and the xiphoid. The bone is subcutaneous throughout anteriorly and is readily palpable. Posteriorly, it protects the vital structures of the upper mediastinum.

Since in athletic injury we are usually dealing with young individuals it is of some importance to recognize the considerable variations in the time of fusion of the four segments which make up the body. In the young child under 6, the sternum will usually present six different segments much as the sacrum does (Fig. 208). As growth progresses, the third and fourth segments of the body are fused around the 7th year. Hence, an x-ray of a 10 or 12 year old youngster will show definite segmental lines between the first, second and third pieces of the body. The second and third will fuse around the 14th year and the first and second are not fused until age 21. Any one of these segments may delay in fusion, particularly the first and second. Contrariwise, there may ultimately be a fusion between the body and manubrium and indeed between the body and xiphoid so that in an elderly person the sternum may appear as a single, solid bone. Hence developmental facts are important from the standpoint of injuries since one must be wary not to interpret a persistent fusion line as a fracture.

The superolateral angle of the manubrium carries the articular facet for the clavicle. Just below this is the facet for the first costal cartilage. The second costal cartilage, on the other hand, fits into the notch between the manubrium and the body. The manubrium is a heavy, thick bone. It is prominent and bulges forward at the lower end so that the most prominent portion of the sternum is the junction of the manubrium and the body. The body is somewhat thinner and elongated, roughly rectangular in shape and tends to slope slightly forward so that the lower ribs are more prominent at the costal cartilage junction than are the upper ones. The xiphoid process may actually be recessed behind the body and its proximal end may be somewhat posterior to the distal end of the body. The tip of the xiphoid hangs free in the infrasternal notch carrying the attachments for the lineae albae and abdominal muscle aponeuroses, particularly the recti. There is usually free motion at the xiphisternal junction. There is no demonstrable motion between the manubrium and the body.

There are many aberrations in rib attachments which are not particularly significant clinically as long as one keeps in mind that the ribs do not necessarily attach in a consistent pattern. For example, the 2nd rib may be horizontally attached to the manubrium and the 3rd may attach at the manubrial-body junction. Whereas usually the 7th rib is the last rib to attach directly to the sternum, it may carry attachments also to the 6th rib and the 6th rib may attach directly to the 5th.

CONTUSION

Since the sternum is directly subcutaneous it is readily subject to contusion. The periosteum or skin is damaged by a blow from a hard object. If the blow is a severe one, there may be considerable shock reaction so that the player breathes with difficulty and will believe he has had a serious injury. However, the shock is well cushioned by the bony thorax and the intrinsic organs are well protected so that the effect is transient. After this transient period the patient will note tenderness along the sternum, usually localized in a particular area. There may be local swelling, infiltration of blood and symptoms similar to those of contusion of any subcutaneous bone. If the condition is uncomplicated, deep breathing or compression of the chest will not increase the tenderness.

Treatment is usually not necessary. Local treatment, if used, is by local injection and cold followed by heat. There is no need to strap the chest but a protective pad should be worn unless the athletic equipment carries such protection. In football the shoulder pads protect the sternum very well, the injury frequently occurring when the players are without pads. One may expect uncomplicated and complete recovery.

SPRAIN-SUBLUXATION-DISLOCATION

The same forces causing contusion of the sternum may cause sprain. We have discussed elsewhere sprain of the costochondral junction (page 311). Sprain of the ligaments connecting the manubrium and body is possible but quite unusual since there is seldom enough motion at this joint to permit ligament damage. Sprain will frequently occur by actual subluxation; that is, the body will be displaced rather than angulated backward on the sternum. The same force that would break the

Figure 205.   Fracture through upper portion of body of sternum with distal fragment overriding proximal one. Similarly the body and manubrium may overlap. (Redrawn from DePalma, "Fractures and Dislocations.")

bone may separate the connection between the two causing a ligament injury, hence the lesion is really subluxation. The general contour of the chest causes the subluxation to be spontaneously reduced.

The patient presents himself with pain directly at the sternal angle and examination at the time will reveal tenderness here. Rarely, pain may be elicited by alternate pressure on the manubrium and body. Ordinary breathing does not cause discomfort but there is sharp recurrence of the pain on balottement with the heel of the hand against either the body or the manubrium.

Treatment.   If the condition is acute, contact sports should be eliminated for the first week or ten days. Subsequently a tailored fiber board pad may be placed over the sternum, hollowed out to protect the sternal angle and diffuse the force over the entire anterior thorax, particularly out over the adjacent ribs. This will usually be adequate to prevent recurrence of the trauma. If the condition is more chronic, injection of a local anesthetic plus a corticoid with the usual physical therapeutic measures will be effective.

If the dislocation is complete and persistent (Fig. 205), with the one bone caught over the other, it can readily be reduced under anesthesia by appropriate measures, first to separate the bone and then to slip one over the other (Fig. 206). Usually the bones will maintain themselves in a stable normal position unless the injury has been a major one—and this is not likely in athletes. It may be possible to reduce the dislocation without use of an anesthetic. The supine patient is positioned with a sandbag transversely under his shoulders slightly below the spine of the scapula. The arms are raised above the head and allowed to drop backward, thus overextending the dorsal spine. As the head drops backward the dislocation will frequently reduce. The dislocation is almost always of the manubrium over the body so that, if it does not go into position, manual pressure placed against the dislocated edge of the bone and directed toward the head will usually effect reduction.

If the dislocation will not reduce by manipulation even under anesthesia, open reduction is required. A transverse incision is made directly across the sternal angle.

This will permit one to lever the fragment gently back into position. Following open reduction the junction, if it seems unstable, should be fixed by three or four wire loops which extend only through the anterior cortex of the sternum.

Since only a major force will dislocate the sternum one should be alert to the possibility of a visceral injury. Even if the immediate shock reaction with difficulty in respiration and a tendency toward collapse is only brief, the patient should be placed in bed for careful observation. X-rays of the chest should be made to determine the possibility of an injury to the structures beneath the sternum, and a careful check is indicated for hemoptysis. One may expect difficulty in respiration from the dislocation itself if it is acute.

Sprain at the xiphisternal junction is not common since the anterior posterior motion at this junction is quite free in the young individual. A blow in the substernal notch may seem quite severe but usually the resultant disability is small. There is little likelihood of any dislocation at this joint.

FRACTURE

The same forces that cause dislocation of various pieces of the sternum may also cause fracture. The manubrium, a large bone almost cuboid in shape, will successfully resist almost any force tending to break it transversely. The fracture is usually through the upper portion of the body of the sternum and is caused by the identical forces applying in manubrial-body dislocation. The body is driven forcibly backward while the manubrium is held forward by the rigid first and second ribs so that the upper portion of the body tends to override the lower. This fracture may be complete or incomplete, with or without displacement (Figs. 205 and 206). The complete fracture has undoubtedly had displacement at one time. Since there is a strong tendency for the chest to resume its normal contour, the displacement corrects itself.

Figure 206.   Method of reduction of fractured sternum. If necessary an assistant may apply traction by grasping patient's arm at the axilla and pulling cephalad. Insert shows detail of the forces applied in reduction. (Redrawn from DePalma, "Fractures and Dislocations.")

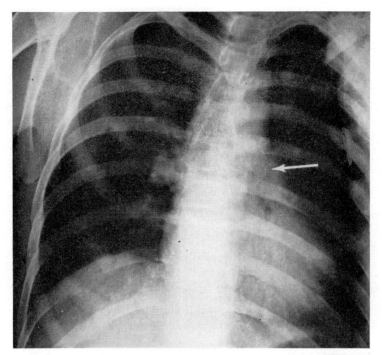

Figure 207.   Fracture across body of the sternum. Note fracture line across the body, not through the line of fusion.

The history will be of a severe blow with immediate loss of breath. There is a relatively prompt recovery from the general symptoms but pain persists in the sternum. If the fracture is complete there will be pain on even ordinary respiration so that respiration will be shallow. If the fracture is incomplete, normal respiration will not cause pain but deep inspiration will. Examination will reveal tenderness in the immediate area of the fracture site, with local swelling. Any deformity, if present, will be readily palpable in the early stages. Such a patient should be promptly x-rayed. Adequate x-ray visualization of the sternum is difficult but by positioning the patient in a few degrees of rotation with the sternum toward the cassette one can shift the sternum to the side of the spine and get a satisfactory anteroposterior view (Fig. 207). The lateral view may be instructive if there is displacement. X-rays may be quite deceptive, however, since the various symphyses of the body of the sternum may be interpreted as fracture lines (Fig. 208). A spontaneously reduced fracture is usually not unstable but alternate pressure above and below will often cause pain at the fracture site.

Treatment is local with application of cold, followed by heat and compression of the chest by a rib binder or by circumferential adhesive. The test of effectiveness of the dressing is relief of the discomfort on normal breathing or ordinary activity.

A displaced fracture in which the fragments are caught or locked on one another should be reduced. If the fracture line is oblique the displacement will tend to be minimal and is not important. The degree of disability will depend almost entirely on the stability with or without strapping. Contact sports should not be permitted the first few weeks unless the patient is completely pain-free on

Figure 208.   A, Lateral view of sternum in a child showing unfused separate segments. B, Note the closing spaces between the segments of 2-3-4 which will fuse to become the body and the much wider space between 1 and 2 which will persist. B is of an older child than A.

deep breathing and on direct compression of the chest. The sternum can be protected from direct blow with padding, as indicated above, the heavy fiber board pad resting on the anterior ribs and protecting the sternum from direct contact. However, this dressing will not eliminate chest expansion so it must be supplemented by adequate strapping.

Complications.   One must be constantly aware that acute fracture is a major injury and may be accompanied by damage to the underlying structures with hemorrhage into the pleura, pneumothorax or subcutaneous emphysema. These conditions may develop insidiously over several hours. For this reason the patient with a sternal fracture should be kept recumbent in a hospital and carefully observed for signs of intrathoracic injury such as increasing difficulty in breathing, impending shock or acceleration of the pulse, so that definitive treatment may be carried out if needed.

PENETRATING WOUNDS OF THE CHEST

A penetrating wound of the chest is not an athletic injury but may occur in the athlete. Any suspicion of penetration of the chest by a sharp instrument demands immediate hospitalization for careful clinical and x-ray study and prompt attention by a surgeon competent to handle conditions of the heart and lungs. There is no time for vacillation in penetrating chest injuries. One should assume that the worst has happened until he can prove that it has not.

Injuries in the
Area of the
Abdomen

ANATOMICAL CONSIDERATIONS

THE AREA under discussion is that from the diaphragm above to the pelvis below (Figs. 209 and 210). Like the chest, the abdominal area has two functions. One is as a cavity to support and protect the contents. The other is as a continuation of the trunk to support the body weight and to transmit musculoskeletal forces from the lower extremities to the body. Posteriorly, the lumbar spine gives the necessary skeletal support. In this area the massive bones completely surrounded by heavy muscle form a solid buttress which has some degree of mobility but provides a sturdy trunk with which to support the chest, upper extremities and head. It also serves to protect the abdominal contents from damage. Before the erect position was assumed, the great majority of insults to the abdominal area were posterior ones which the back is well constructed to withstand.

Extending from behind-forward are the abdominal muscles which traverse in several crisscrossing layers to converge into the fascia in front which in turn splits to include the vertical recti muscles and then converge at the linea alba in the midline. Superiorly, the lower ribs protect the upper part of the abdominal cavity and overlie the major portion of the liver, pancreas and spleen. Inferiorly, the abdominal cavity terminates in the pelvic cavity which has a strong, bony structure

319

Trapezius m.

Infraspinatus m.

Latissimus dorsi m.

Teres minor m.

Teres major m.

Pectoralis major m.

Serratus ant. m.

Sheath of rectus m.

Ext. oblique m.

Iliac crest

Figure 209. Lateral view of abdominal area showing the interdigitation between the muscles of the back, shoulder and chest at the top and attachment to the iliac crest below. Note the external oblique attachments along the many ribs. The front attaches to the fascia extending in front of the recti to converge at the linea alba in the midline in front.

Clavicle

Deltoid m.

Pectoralis major m.

Ext. oblique m.

Pectoralis minor m.

Serratus ant. mm.

Rectus abdominis m.

Transversus m.

Internal oblique m.
Post. rectus sheath

Rectus abdomini muscles (cut)

Pubic symphysis

Pyramidalis muscles cut

Figure 210. Note the intimate relationship between the muscles of the chest and abdomen. Also, the ingenious attachment at the pubis in the insert. Note the tendinae contained within the recti which may be subject to strain. Note the layers attaching to the iliac crest with the transversalis coming well forward on the crest while the obliques come only part way forward.

for protection of the urogenital tract. Anteriorly, the two recti muscles passing from the lower ribs to the pubis serve to help support the erect position by acting as guy wires. They also serve to assist the anterior spinal muscles in forward flexion of the spine. Thus, we have a massive group of muscles posteriorly, a relatively thin layer of muscle anteriorly and several overlapping layers extending peripherally from posterior to anterior. The whole makes an extremely synergistic muscle mass that permits motion in any direction—forward, backward, lateral, rotatory, or any combination of these—on the relatively flexible trunk of the lumbar spine.

Hence, it can be seen that injuries to athletes will fall into two very distinct categories although they may occur together: first, injury to the abdominal wall; second, injury to the abdominal content.

INJURY TO THE ABDOMINAL WALL

The abdominal walls are subject to those injuries peculiar to a musculoskeletal structure. We will later discuss injuries to the posterior portion of the abdomen, namely, the lumbar spine (page 370). We have also elaborated upon thoracic injuries (page 298) but some further word is warranted on the subject of injuries to the lower ribs.

Contusion

Contusion of the abdominal wall is frequent but with the exception of certain specific areas the damage to the wall itself is not usually a serious condition. The muscles of the anterior and lateral abdomen are resilient. They overlie the soft abdominal content and, hence, are not severely injured by a direct blow. Occasionally a contusion against the tightly contracted rectus, as when a pitcher is struck by a batted ball, may cause a painful injury that may even cause some bleeding into the recti muscles. Under these circumstances the treatment must be directed toward the muscular injury, namely, cold followed by heat and protection of the muscles until such time as the tenderness has disappeared. The physical condition of the athlete is such that he is not likely to have a severe contusion of the abdominal wall.

Contusion over the iliac crest at the attachment of the abdominal muscles may be extremely distressing. This will be discussed elsewhere (page 390).

Contusion of the upper abdomen may involve injury to the ribs. The twelfth, the eleventh and to a lesser extent the tenth ribs are much more mobile than the ribs above. Since the proximal end is relatively free and the distal end does not have a bony attachment, an isolated fracture of these ribs is not common. The rib simply moves away from the blow. The contusion may cause periosteal reaction with a subperiosteal hematoma which may require local injection and some protection. It is extremely unusual to see any displacement of the fragments of a fractured rib in this area since in this instance the rib is well enclosed by the muscle mass and the stresses are such that there is no overpull on one fragment as compared to the other such as may be found in a clavicle.

The one fact of overriding importance in contusion of the abdomen is not injury to the wall but to the abdominal contents.

Strain

Since under our definition strain involves the musculotendinous unit and since the abdominal wall is essentially muscular, strain is a frequent occurrence. The symptoms will vary according to the location of injury. Thus, a strain may involve the recti with pain at or near the upper attachments or at the pubic attachments below or at the horizontal fibrous bands within the muscle itself. The strain may be from a sudden, violent effort which may actually cause rupture of the muscle fibers or some of the tendon attachments or it may be from continued overuse. In the first instance the onset will be acute with pain, muscle spasm, some rigidity and dysfunction. This may be readily distinguished from injury to the abdominal contents since the rigidity is localized to the muscle involved or at least to the group involved. Pain is aggravated by active contraction or passive stretching of the muscle. There occasionally may be some concern as to whether the painful muscle is due to acute inflammation of an underlying organ (appendix, for example) but with diagnostic acumen there should be no real confusion between them. Painful muscle spasm on the right side suggests appendicitis. However, the clinical symptoms are quite different since the patient with a diseased appendix will have signs of inflammation, some degree of peritonitis, positive laboratory findings and fever, none of which will be present in the acute strain.

In the great majority of cases, strain does not actually tear the muscle fibers and recovery is relatively rapid. In those instances of musculotendinous injury at the ribs, pubis, or iliac crest, the symptoms may be quite prolonged and result in a distressing degree of disability since resumption of athletics inevitably causes recurrence of the symptoms. The pole vaulter or high jumper who has strained his abdominal wall by excessive stress may require many weeks before he can return to active competition. In fact, he may never be able to return as long as he keeps trying to compete. The best treatment for this condition is to rest the muscle until the symptoms have subsided. This is not incompatible with rehabilitation since activity may be allowed so long as it is kept within the limits of pain. The primary problem, then, in abdominal strain is that of diagnosis, and careful attention to the actual physical findings will usually rule out any intra-abdominal complication.

It is difficult to use any appliance to protect the abdominal wall against strain and still permit competition. A well fitted corset (see Fig. 248, page 374) will serve to give abdominal support and will restrict motion enough that passive tension on the injured area can be eliminated. The corset does little, however, in preventing the vigorous muscle contractions responsible for the symptoms.

Actual muscle or tendon rupture in the abdominal wall is an unusual injury, the exception being avulsion of the muscle from the iliac crest. As far as I know, this is the only indication for surgical repair in an acute injury.

Hernia.   There is no necessity here to discuss in detail the various hernias involving the abdominal wall. It seems quite unlikely that any of them are caused by athletic injuries. However, it is inescapable that many hernias will become symptomatic by increased abdominal tension such as the straining of weight lifting or the violent exercise of the oarsmen. I believe that if a player has a symptomatic hernia and that if the symptoms are made more severe by athletics, either the hernia should be repaired or athletics discontinued. This is not to say that because the patient has a suspected hernia he should lead a sedentary life. I would recommend that this patient see a capable surgeon and be guided by his judgment as to whether or not the hernia should be repaired. Following successful repair I see no reason for interdiction of sports.

INJURY TO THE ABDOMINAL CONTENT

In the abdominal area by far the most significant injury is the visceral one. When, following a blow or occasionally from violent exercise, abdominal symptoms arise, it is imperative to determine at the earliest possible moment the exact nature of the injury. *An intra-abdominal injury is an acute surgical emergency.* The team physician who is not a capable abdominal surgeon and who is not prepared to handle the extremely complicated situations which may arise from intra-abdominal injury will be unwise to carry out a policy of "watchful waiting" over any prolonged period. If there is *any* doubt in his mind as to whether or not there is injury to a viscus the patient should be transferred immediately to the care of the physician who will provide the definitive treatment should the need arise. These injuries are extremely infrequent in athletics but when they occur they may be disastrous, even fatal. This is another instance when timely diagnosis makes a simple problem out of what may otherwise develop into an extremely complicated one.

The injury may involve a solid viscus, such as the spleen, liver, kidney or pancreas. It may involve any portion of the gut. It may involve the peritoneum or mesentery, the bladder, or in the female the genitalia. While in the final analysis it is extremely important to determine just what the nature of the injury is, by far the most important consideration is to determine whether or not *any* intra-abdominal injury is present. It is the problem of the abdominal surgeon to determine the diagnosis and the definitive treatment and he must be given this opportunity at the earliest possible time.

Diagnosis

History.   History is of vital importance, not only as a guide to what injury to expect but also to ascertain the progress of events up to the time of the examination. A detailed description of the accident is important. Was this a direct blow by a blunt object and if so what was the object? Was it the helmet, was it the knee, was it the heel? What was the position of the body at the time of the blow? What was the location of the injury? Was it over the back which is well equipped to protect against trauma or was it in the flank or anterior abdomen? Were the muscles tense and the player alert or was he relaxed and unguarded? The period of time from the blow to the examination and what happened during that time is of vital importance. Did the patient think he had a serious injury? Was he brought immediately to the doctor or did he report late manifestations, having minimized the original injury? Information should be obtained as to whether or not he has recently eaten. Was his bladder full or empty? Has he had a recent stool?

Observation.   Observation of this patient is important. It may be that you were fortunate enough to be present at the time of injury and so were able to observe the actual development of the symptoms. The rapidity of their development is significant. The patient who has received a blow on the stomach or the so-called "solar plexus" may immediately present agonizing symptoms with air hunger, severe pain and cramping, which may lead to involuntary defecation and urination. If seen at once he may show symptoms of early shock. However, these symptoms subside rapidly, usually before medical attention can be obtained. Such a patient may be essentially well when he is examined by the doctor and is usually not cause for worry. However, the fact that he has survived the acute injury does not rule out the possibility of late manifestations from injury to a solid organ. The left lobe of the liver lying directly under the xiphoid is particularly vulnerable (Fig. 211). While such a patient ordinarily presents no real problem he should be warned to report any recurrence of his symptoms.

If the patient is in immediate collapse and does not respond rapidly with or without treatment, he has an extremely severe injury that demands emergency care and immediate transportation to a hospital. In the less emergent situation the patient should be observed for pallor and cold, clammy skin; his respiration should be noted; he should be watched particularly for signs of impending shock which together with other symptoms will suggest hemorrhage.

Palpation.   Careful palpation will be extremely informative in abdominal injury. Rupture of a hollow viscus or indeed bleeding into the abdomen will almost always cause peritoneal irritation and muscle rigidity. This ordinarily will be diffuse. Localized rigidity in a certain area of the abdomen suggests a walled-off lesion with local bleeding or leaking from a viscus. If the abdomen is not tense and not rigid, one may proceed with a more detailed examination, palpating for tenderness around the spleen, liver and kidneys. Loss of peristaltic sounds may be quite significant since this is a frequent sign of early hemorrhage or other intra-abdominal injury.

Lung

Spleen

Hilus of kidney

Descending colon

Diaphragm

Liver

Kidney

Psoas m.

Posterior view

Figure 211.   Indicating the position of the spleen on the left side to demonstrate why a blow on the lower rib on the right might damage the liver and on the left the spleen.

Laboratory.   The laboratory may be of considerable value. In case of doubt, one should not wait for laboratory reports. Bloody emesis, bloody urine, bloody stool, all have significance. Change in the blood count usually will be only confirmatory since by the time hemorrhage is manifested by reduced hematocrit or hemoglobin, the decision should long since have been made that there was injury within the abdominal cavity.

X-ray.   X-ray examination is important but only in a positive way. A negative x-ray by no means rules out abdominal injury. Fracture of the lower ribs on the left may suggest damage to the spleen; on the right to the liver (Fig. 211). Fractured lateral processes may suggest kidney damage. Free air in the abdomen demands immediate attention (Fig. 212). Other findings such as obliteration or enlargement of the splenic shadow (Fig. 213), blurring of the psoas margin, change in the level of the diaphragm, generalized dilatation of the bowel (Fig. 214) and dilatation of isolated loops of the bowel all have significance.

Specific Diagnosis

Although we are not at this stage primarily concerned with an exact diagnosis, a few words might be said about this problem. As a rule, injury to a solid viscus will be suggested by the history of the blow which makes one suspect the injury, by the location of the abdominal pain over liver, kidney or spleen, or by localization of tenderness and rigidity. The other significant findings are usually due to bleeding and as such are not particularly diagnostic as to the organ involved. They consist of the signs of blood loss, such as rapid pulse with low pulse pressure, dizziness, fainting, finally syncope, and the signs of impending shock. Examination may reveal shifting dullness in the abdomen due to free fluid. It should be recalled that nausea

Figure 212. Ruptured diaphragm. Note air under left diaphragm and scattered throughout abdomen. Severe crushing injury to the chest.

Figure 213.   Flat plate of abdomen. Note the enlarged spleen in the upper left quadrant. Following injury this would suggest intracapsular hemorrhage.

Figure 214.   Ileus. Note tremendous dilatation of bowel.

and vomiting frequently accompany any type of abdominal injury and do not necessarily mean injury to the gastrointestinal tract.

Splenic injuries are particularly likely to be insidious since the symptoms here
are due entirely to bleeding. This bleeding may be walled off and may actually
stop only to be re-initiated by some other activity at a later time. The physician may
be faced with the situation in which his patient is doing very well and then goes
into a relatively sudden collapse. Splenic injury should have an extremely low
mortality since the spleen can be removed without apparent handicap to the individual if done before dangerous collapse has occurred.

Liver injuries on the other hand are much more likely to be rapidly dangerous
and carry a high mortality. As might be expected, the patients who die do so quickly
before they have had a chance to receive supportive treatment. There may be secondary abdominal symptoms from bile leakage as a late sequela to a relatively minor
liver injury from which the patient has apparently recovered.

Pancreatic injuries are very uncommon in athletes.

Gastrointestinal tract injuries are extremely uncommon in athletes or at least
they are not commonly diagnosed. Contusion of the abdominal wall may well cause
some contusion to the underlying stomach or intestines but these organs are pliable
and usually "give" with the blow enough that they are not caught between the
abdominal wall and the spine. This also is made much less likely since the player's
stomach and intestine are usually empty.

The stomach is the organ most frequently injured. Following such an injury
there may be tarry stools or possibly coffee-ground vomitus which would make
one suspect intrinsic damage to the stomach or bowel. Either of these should put
one on the alert but neither is necessarily serious. The injury of sufficient caliber
to rupture the bowel will give immediate, serious symptoms with abdominal pain,
tenderness and spasm, nausea, vomiting, ileus and other signs of peritonitis. Since
such symptoms could occur without actual viscus rupture, some confusion may
arise as to whether or not these symptoms are from the immediate shock of the
blow or from the resultant complications. Here the rapidity of development of the
symptoms is extremely important. If the vomiting is simply a process of emptying
the stomach and if the symptoms of shock rapidly diminish, one may be permitted
more latitude. Persistence of such symptoms and, more particularly, accentuation
of these symptoms constitute an emergency which demands immediate hospitalization with appropriate examination and treatment.

Treatment of Injuries to the Abdominal Contents

It is not our intention here to give the detailed care of the patient with intra-
abdominal injury. As indicated above, there is a diagnostic problem in determining
whether or not the patient should be placed under the care of a competent surgeon.
Some generalities about treatment are pertinent, however, since they serve to emphasize the necessity for diagnosis.

Treatment of any intra-abdominal injury is basically surgical. That is not to
say that every patient must be operated upon but in the presence of a real or suspected intra-abdominal injury, surgery must be immediately available. It follows

that the responsible surgeon must be in close touch with this patient and ready to carry out whatever procedure is indicated or may become indicated.

In the period prior to a definitive diagnosis, the cardinal points for treatment are bed rest under constant observation and repeated examinations by the physician who notes the local condition of the abdomen and the general condition of the patient. The patient should be covered but heat should not be applied to either abdomen or extremities. The patient's head should be lower than his feet. If he has abdominal distention, a gastric suction tube should be passed. If he is unable to void, an indwelling catheter should be used. His apprehension should be quieted but he should not be heavily sedated. Morphine or any of its modifications or derivatives should be avoided since they serve to lower the blood pressure still further. Of even greater importance is that opiates may screen vital symptoms. Barbiturates may be used. If the patient is obviously seriously injured and awaiting transportation to the hospital or arrival of the surgeon, certain other measures should be taken. An intravenous infusion should be started which not only gives the patient some support but also has the advantage of a patent vein which may be hard to obtain if the patient should go into collapse. Blood should be matched for transfusion if possible. Oxygen and suction should be available.

None of these measures is ordinarily necessary in abdominal injury received by direct blow in the athlete. If they are necessary, a very serious injury is indicated.

INJURY TO THE KIDNEY

It is probable that a mild degree of kidney injury is relatively common in any contact sport. In fact, it has been shown that red blood cells are frequently present in the urine from violent exertion alone. This has nothing to do with trauma to the kidney proper so that the mere finding of red blood cells in the urine does not necessarily indicate a kidney injury. Certainly everyone who has pain in the flank does not have an injury to the kidney. On the other hand, anyone who has this type of injury does deserve examination to rule out the possibility of kidney damage.

Contusion

The most common injury to the kidney is contusion. This may be the result of a blow from a knee or helmet with the shock penetrating the muscles and transmitted to the kidney. The result of a minor contusion is slight kidney damage (Fig. 215) with local extravasation of blood under the capsule. This causes only

Figure 215.   Anatomical view of kidney showing various types of injury.

mild pain persisting a few days. Red blood cells may be recovered from the urine. Such an injury is of no serious consequence and need not make the athlete over-cautious once complete recovery has occurred.

Late manifestations are possible, principally localized infection in the hematoma area. This will be indicated by the general symptoms of infection plus local signs of urinary tract infection. In any kidney injury it is advisable to examine the patient and make a urinalysis some two weeks after the injury to determine whether any complication is developing.

A more violent blow may cause serious damage to the kidney (Fig. 215). The capsule may rupture with development of perirenal hematoma. There may be sub-capsular hemorrhage which goes on to kidney necrosis. The rupture of the kidney may actually extend into its substance even to the extent of penetrating the kidney pelvis. The symptoms and signs will be related to the type of injury. In extrinsic hemorrhage, unless this is quite severe, the signs will remain quite localized with pain and muscle spasm in the flank and lumbar muscles together with painful function of these muscles. It may be difficult to distinguish this from muscular hematoma or contusion and the two may well co-exist. It may be impossible to de-termine the underlying kidney injury unless there are renal symptoms, particularly blood in the urine.

If the kidney substance itself is damaged, urine extravasation may occur. This must be extremely unusual in an athletic injury. In case of doubt, careful study by a competent urologist is in order. There may occasionally be serious hemorrhage from an injured kidney. Not only is it important to determine the severity of injury but also the location since a major vessel may be damaged. The most outstanding signs here are those of hemorrhage. First these are local: signs of hematoma forma-tion, extravasation of blood along the flank with tenderness, swelling, possibly posi-tive x-ray findings. If these are accompanied by systemic signs of bleeding one is dealing with a surgical emergency.

INJURY TO THE BLADDER

Bladder injuries are extremely uncommon in athletics. The nervous tension of the athlete prior to competition is axiomatic. It is almost always manifested in re-peated trips to empty the bladder. Since the collapsed bladder is practically never injured, the scene is not set for bladder rupture.

Contusion of the bladder may cause blood cells in the urine but otherwise no symptoms except some indefinite tenderness above the pubis.

Rupture of the bladder (see Figs. 216 and 217) is an extremely serious but quite unlikely complication. The patient should be asked to void. If he is unable to void a catheter should be inserted and left in place. An intravenous cystogram is easily made but may be quite unsatisfactory. Most urologists frown on injection of a measured amount of fluid into the bladder, followed by an attempt to recover the same amount. This is not only inaccurate but may lead to further extravasation if the bladder is damaged. Signs of shock with lower abdominal pelvic pain are danger signals.

Figure 216.   The intact bladder.

Figure 217.   Severe fracture of pelvis with extravasation of urine from ruptured bladder.

Injuries of
the Spine

THE SPINE is readily subdivided into the cervical, dorsal (thoracic) and lumbar sections (Fig. 218). We shall consider these areas separately since the management of their injuries varies in many particulars.

CERVICAL SPINE

ANATOMICAL CONSIDERATIONS

From the standpoint of the athlete, the cervical spine is by far the most important part of the spinal column. It has two major functions. The first is the musculoskeletal function that provides support to the head in such a fashion as to permit the person to utilize the various sense organs, such as the eyes, ears and nose, to the best advantage. This requires enough stability to support the weight of the head, yet sufficient flexibility to permit the extreme ranges of motion which are necessary. From the evolutionary standpoint the neck has been one of the most adaptive areas. In various mammals there are wide differences, from the extreme length and flexibility of the neck of the giraffe whose small head perches an amazing distance from the trunk, to the apparent absence of neck in the pig whose snout seems to extend right back into his body.

The other major function of the neck is to transmit the major nerves from the head to the rest of the body and to give them adequate protection. The requirements for these two functions are to a great extent contradictory. The best protec-

331

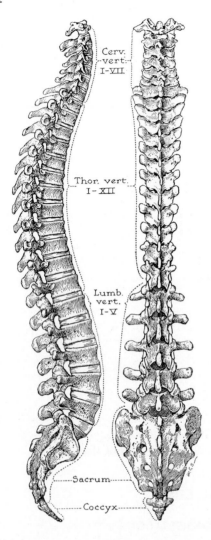

Figure 218.   The vertebral column as seen in lateral and posterior view. (From Jones and Shepard, "Manual of Surgical Anatomy.")

tion would be a rigid tube with the spinal roots and cord inside. The musculo-skeletal function, which demands extreme flexibility, is ill designed to protect the nerves. The amazing ingenuity by which this is accomplished merits comprehensive study which cannot be given here.

Free flexibility of the head demands much more cervical motion than is available anywhere else in the spine. The degree of rotation that can be obtained from the oval vertebrae rotating each on the other is strictly limited. While this is very much greater in the cervical spine than in other areas by virtue of the relatively flat articular processes, still any major degree of rotation will simply subluxate or dislocate one facet on the other. Similarly, a much more localized range of flexion and extension is necessary to nod the head than can be obtained in any one ordinary vertebral joint or series of joints. Hence, the two top cervical vertebrae are entirely different in structure and function from the remaining ones. The first cervical vertebra (atlas) is a large ring bearing on its anterolateral half the articular facets, those above articulating with the skull, those below with C-2. The area elsewhere occupied by the body of the vertebra is an extension forward of the neurocanal which is separated from the canal by a strong fibrous band. This space forms a socket to receive the odontoid process of C-2. Developmentally the odontoid is the body of the first cervical vertebra which has detached itself from the first vertebra to become a portion of the second. The superior articular facets of C-1 are long and shallow and on these facets the head can nod with a hinge motion. There is no rotatory or lateral motion between the cranium and the first cervical vertebra. This wafer of vertebra would readily dislocate were it not for its firm fixation to C-2 by the odontoid.

So much for the flexion and extension of the head. The rotatory motion of the head which in the human is equally, if not more, important is provided at the atlanto-axial junction. The head and first cervical vertebra rotate as a unit around the pivot of the odontoid process of the second. The comparatively elongated articular processes permit this sliding motion between the atlas and axis.

The remaining cervical vertebrae are very similar to the dorsal vertebrae in general structure. There are certain variations characteristic of the function required. The massive cervical spinal cord with its extreme vulnerability to injury requires a large ring so that the cord can be suspended in the middle of the ring without direct contact with the surrounding walls. The other and opposing requirement, namely mobility, is obtained by the articular processes which in the cervical spine are relatively horizontal. The rather flat convex upper surface fits into the shallow concavity of the inferior articular surface of the vertebra above in a much more horizontal plane than in the dorsal area. The angle of these facets is about 45 degrees from the horizontal. This is much less secure than the hooks on any of the vertebrae below the cervical spine since in the dorsal and lumbar spine these articular facets are vertical. The bodies are relatively light since the weight to be carried is only that of the head. The spinous processes are long and extend horizontally backward in the upper portion of the neck but obliquely downward in the lower portion. They are bifid to add further to the area available for the attachment of the multitude of ligaments and muscles that provide good stability and yet free mobility. The seventh cervical spinous process is longer and more prominent and, hence, the most vulnerable to injury. The transverse processes of all are short and light because the massive muscles that attach lower in the spine are not present in the neck. Mobility is more important than strength. The foramina through which the rather large cervical nerve roots pass are relatively shallow. The nerves pass almost horizontally through the nerve root canals and so are quite subject to traction injury. The discs between the vertebrae are relatively shallow and much less strong than those below since there is less weight involved.

The vertebrae are bound together by the annular ligament with its dorsal and ventral thickenings that hold the bodies snugly but not rigidly together. The ligamentum nuchae extends from the external occipital protuberance to attach along the tips of the cervical vertebrae as far as C-7 and then extends downward as the supraspinous ligament. This ligament is a thin septum, wide from behind-forward, which serves to separate the muscles of the posterior portion of the neck at the midline. The interspinous ligaments lie between the spinous processes. The ligamentum flavum secures the laminae. The capsular ligaments bind the vertebrae at the articulations. Together, these ligaments stabilize the vertebrae in their relative position, each to the one above and the one below. In the neck they are much less stable than anywhere else in the column. This combination of extreme mobility plus the necessity for protection requires an amazingly intricate interdigitation of muscles as well as the support of many ligaments.

The muscles of the vertebral column are extremely massive in the lower back, becoming less massive but with wider excursion as the cervical spine is reached. Since the neck is an isolated column it requires support in the nature of guy wires in each direction. The fact that these musculotendinous guy wires can be varied in length permits the neck and head to be moved in any direction while maintaining a constant degree of support. Nowhere is the synergistic use of muscles better demonstrated than in the neck where the function of each muscle depends altogether upon the position of the head at the time the contraction takes place. It is not advisable here to discuss in detail the individual muscles of the neck since their number is legion. It suffices to say that the muscles are so arranged as to permit traction to be applied in any position of the head or the spine so that with appropriate contraction of one group and relaxation of others, synchronous motions occur. As might be expected, the heaviest groups of muscles are posterior. Many of the muscles of the neck pass distally to attach to the muscles in the shoulder girdle as well as to the trunk itself.

In front of the neck lie many vital structures that are poorly protected in the upright position. The veins and arteries on either side, the esophagus behind, the larynx and trachea in front are all quite vulnerable unless the head is held down to permit the chin and thorax to protect the front of the neck.

EMERGENCY MANAGEMENT

Injury to the neck has extremely serious connotations for major disability. If there is any question at all as to the severity of a cervical injury, it should be assumed that the most severe injury is present. Under no circumstances should the patient be asked to sit or stand. If he is lying on the ground with a possible serious injury to his neck he should not be moved until an evaluation of the situation has been made. This may require some time but delay of the game is of no consequence under such circumstances and the physician must not be hurried in his evaluation and permit what may be fatal movement. If the player is conscious, a few words will determine his own feelings in regard to his neck. One should determine whether he has normal function of his hands and feet. This does not require a detailed physical examination but does entail sensible evaluation. The patient should then be moved to a stretcher and for this adequate help must be present so that it can be done without any motion between his head and trunk. Under ordinary circumstances the athlete will be conscious and he is better placed on his back with his head carefully supported. On occasion this may serve to dramatize and overemphasize what turns out to be a relatively minor injury. On the other hand, it may save a life or prevent lifetime paralysis.

Once the player has been moved to a place for better examination, detailed study should be made at the end of which the physician should have a definite impression as to the severity of the injury. He should observe such deformity as may be indicative of unilateral or bilateral dislocation. He should attempt to localize the pain. If it is decided that the injury is only relatively severe and the patient can be moved to the hospital for evaluation, great care must be taken in his handling. The head may be stabilized by a sandbag on either side or by someone sitting at his side holding his head. It may be stabilized quite well by a simple head halter which may be made by a muslin strip under the occiput and another under the chin with a weight hanging over the end of the carrier or bed. If it is decided that x-rays should be made, they must be made under the same precautions. Under no circumstances should the x-ray be made with the patient sitting up until one can be sure there is no instability of the neck. Once a diagnosis is made of a serious injury to the neck, consultation should be sought immediately with whatever person is going to carry out the definitive care. This may be the orthopedic surgeon or neurosurgeon, or both. I cannot emphasize too strongly that the patient must not be asked to sit up. He must not have forceful manipulation of the head to see how well it will move. He must not be allowed to walk from the field. If he already is sitting or standing, this position may be maintained, again with greatest precautions.

In spite of utmost care, symptoms may develop insidiously. The patient receives his injury but may seem quite well, only to succumb to some inadvertent motion later. Any complaint of the neck by any player demands that he be removed from the contest and a definitive examination made. This will tend to minimize the tragedies that occur in the locker room or at home following the initial injury.

CONTUSION

Contusion in the vicinity of the neck has many serious connotations, not in relation to the integument since the skin is rarely damaged but because of the vital underlying structures. In the back of the neck, the blow may be received on the spinous processes, particularly in the lower cervical area, and since these are long the leverage exerted at their bases may be quite powerful. If the blow is received with the neck in forward flexion, the combination of tension on the ligament and muscle plus the striking force may break off a spinous process anywhere from its tip to its junction to the body. Such an injury will be painful. There will be local tenderness, particularly on dropping the head forward. Palpation will usually be unrewarding in fracture but careful x-ray study will reveal the lesion. A word of warning. X-ray of the lower cervical area is difficult and one must be sure he is visualizing the area of involvement. It is worthwhile to insert a hypodermic needle into the tender area at the time the picture is made in order to localize the tender spot in the x-ray.

If a fracture is found it should be treated appropriately as indicated below. Contusion of the bone without fracture is treated according to its severity. Ordinarily no treatment is necessary. Painful bruising of the cervical muscles may cause the usual complications of muscle contusion with hematoma formation (Fig. 219), muscle spasm, stiffness, pain, etc. In such an instance local treatment is of value with application of heat, pain-free massage and local analgesic balm. Some degree of protection with a cotton collar may speed up the recovery. Muscle spasm can be relieved by antispasmodics and participation in athletics should be minimized.

Occasionally a blow on the back of the neck will have a direct effect on the spinal cord and the resultant *shock* may cause transitory paralysis. Much more

Figure 219.   Calcification superficial to ligamentum nuchae following neck injury with hematoma. This mass does not move with the spinous process.

often there simply is a generalized feeling of numbness which is extremely transitory and of little significance. In case of persistent neurologic symptoms such as numbness and paresthesia a more thorough search for interspinal injury should be carried out. Certainly the patient should be protected by observation and no contact permitted so long as there is any doubt. Concussion of the cord may be quite alarming but complete recovery is the rule.

At the side of the neck contusion is less frequent but may cause distressing symptoms by a direct effect on the brachial plexus with the feeling of shock to the neck and numbness in the arm. This is usually quite transitory and the player is able to shake it off. Occasionally there may be permanent damage to some of the components of the brachial plexus. Frequently the contusion may occur with the neck flexed in the opposite direction so that there may be strain as well as contusion.

In the front of the neck contusion may be quite severe. The athlete usually learns to protect the neck by carrying his chin low and forward so that the interval between the chin and sternum is relatively narrow. Given an opportunity, he will protect himself further by dropping his head forward when the blow is impending. The structures most likely to be damaged by a direct blow are the *larynx* and *trachea*. A blow to the throat may cause extreme distress, even to the extent of systemic shock. The player is speechless with severe dyspnea. He struggles for breath, is completely unable to phonate and for a period has the feeling of impending doom. Under ordinary circumstances he recovers quickly, the spasm of the vocal cords subsides and he is able to breathe more easily although the hoarseness may persist. Immediate treatment should be complete bed rest with a cold pack on the neck. Body activity should be discouraged in order to cut down on the oxygen requirement. Reassurance is vital but sedation should be given cautiously, particularly if there are signs of systemic shock. Recovery may be complete within a very few minutes with no damage done and the patient may be able to resume play

In the more severe case, there may be a hematoma, either intrinsic in the larynx or extrinsic from the muscles in the neck. If severe, this can be a dangerous complication. It usually is not. There may actually be *fracture of the thyroid cartilage*, of the hyoid or of the trachea but this is not common in young athletes since these structures are quite resilient. If there is persistence of symptoms beyond the day of injury, careful laryngeal examination should be carried out, particularly if dyspnea persists. In case of doubt the patient should be hospitalized where oxygen, suction and intravenous therapy are available. Laryngoscopy is indicated if there is any question as to intrinsic injury. If signs of increasing intrinsic bleeding appear the patient should be carefully observed since the neck will not tolerate much pressure either from the bleeding or from the attempt to arrest this by a pressure pack. It is axiomatic that if there is any persistence of these symptoms, the patient should be kept at rest and under careful observation.

It probably is not advisable to attempt to aspirate a hematoma in the neck unless all the facilities of the hospital are available together with a trained laryngologist. If the bleeding appears to be increasing and pressure more severe and ice packs do not control the situation, consultation is mandatory.

STRAIN

Muscular strain in the cervical area may be extremely complex. The large number of small muscles with multiple attachments are capable of different functions in different positions of the head. It is an area quite subject to strain. It may be very difficult to distinguish between strain and sprain or between sprain and muscle spasm caused by secondary nerve root involvement. While the athlete is quite subject to strain of the cervical muscles by violent movement of the head, he is also the subject of sprain of the joints with its attendant complications. Indeed, the strain and sprain may well coexist.

Diagnostically, there is some value in the history although it may be quite misleading. While strain may follow overuse of the muscles of the neck, it is even more likely to be the product of an avulsion force against a muscle resisting a violent motion. Since this same violent motion may cause sprain, subluxation, dislocation or fracture, a muscular strain may well be a secondary consideration. When strain occurs as a separate entity active function as well as passive stretching of the involved muscle will be painful. The exact diagnosis becomes somewhat academic if the injury is a serious one. In the more minor injuries, diagnosis is not so difficult. The muscle spasm that follows this injury is a universal accompaniment of any injury to the neck and is of little diagnostic significance. Tenderness within the muscle itself or at its attachment may give a clue.

If the strain seems to be relatively mild, the *treatment* may also be mild. Local heat, rest and reduction of activity are important. All too often, what begins as a minor strain ends up as a rather severe spastic type wryneck which may be completely disabling while it lasts. The actual injury seems at the time to be minimal. It is not until 24 to 48 hours later that the constant irritation of the injured muscle causes spasm of all its fellows. This case requires more definitive treatment. Bed rest with light cervical traction, 4 to 6 pounds, is preferable to massive traction in the upright position (Fig. 220). It also has the undoubted value of being good

Figure 220.   Patient in cervical traction. The traction apparatus is placed at the foot of the bed instead of at the head, with the type of halter as shown. Note that the bed is positioned so that the neck is held in extension.

treatment for any injury to the neck so that if one's diagnostic acumen has been somewhat at fault, at least the treatment is suited to whatever lesion may be present. Bed rest, cervical traction, local heat, muscle relaxants and mild sedation will result in prompt relief of symptoms. The danger is recurrence. If the strain is indeed quite mild and recovery is complete within 24 to 36 hours, no protection need be applied to the neck. The patient should be advised against forceful activities, told to move his neck as freely as he can but strictly within the limits of pain and not against resistance. If the case seems to be more severe and traction has been needed for several days, a cervical support such as a cotton collar (Fig. 221) may be necessary for two to three weeks. As in any strain, careful rehabilitation is needed to prevent prompt recurrence of symptoms. The protective factor here is not against motion of the neck as in sprain but against overuse of the muscle involved. This requires a cooperative patient who understands his problem. The posterior spinal muscles are the ones most commonly strained—the result of forcible extension of the spine against resistance as in the wrestler. However, any of the muscles may be involved in strain.

Figure 221.   Cotton collar. The collar illustrated is a single wrap of tapered quilted outing flannel, small end 3 inches enlarging to 6 inches and 6 feet long. Same can be made of alternating wraps of sheet wadding and gauze. This should extend far enough to support the occiput and chin.

SPRAIN-SUBLUXATION-FRACTURE-DISLOCATION

Injuries to the spine are difficult to subdivide into specific categories of sprain, subluxation, dislocation and fracture since one extends indistinguishably into the other and there is often a combination of all four. A much more serviceable classification can be made on the basis of the mechanism causing the injury. While there is a great deal of overlap and the motion may be much more complex than simple motion in one direction, nevertheless there is a predominant motion in one direction which is almost always the major cause of the damage. I suppose it is virtually impossible to have pure flexion of the neck without some degree of rotation or vice versa. Nevertheless, the injury characterizes itself by the prime mover.

Whereas the strain discussed above is caused by overuse of the muscle, sprain is caused by forcing a joint through an abnormal range of motion and the ligament designed to prevent this motion is damaged. Sprain of the neck is a very common injury and may be mild, moderate or severe. The mild injury is of little significance and will require but little treatment. The moderate injury in which there has been some loss of ligament strength will require primarily protection from the forces that caused the injury. Much more complicated is the severe injury in which there is complete loss of integrity of the ligament. As this ligament loses its function, the motion that it is designed to prevent is unrestricted. The forces that ordinarily are controlled by this ligament are then transferred to other areas of the lever. This ligament injury may progress into subluxation in which the joint partially dislocates; or indeed the capsular ligament may tear completely and the joint completely dislocate. Other ligaments in the spine that are not related directly to the articulations may be involved. The interspinous ligament posteriorly restricts flexion of the neck. The anterior longitudinal ligament anteriorly prevents anterior separation of the bodies of the vertebrae. There is usually some combination of ligament damage so that, when the one ligament tears, the force being shifted to another ligament damages this one also. This may continue until there is complete disruption of all the supporting ligaments and complete dislocation of one vertebra on another. So also a fracture may supervene. That is, as the ligament gives way one place, a fracture may occur elsewhere or, as the ligament holds, the edge of the bone comprising the fulcrum or counter-lever may give way. Some attempt will be made to describe these injuries under the categories of the forces applied.

Flexion Injury

Interspinous-Supraspinous Ligament Injury (Sprain). The supraspinous and interspinous ligaments which attach along the spinous processes from the occiput to the dorsal spine serve as a checkrein to prevent overflexion of the head. Although they are somewhat elastic, their fibers are not tight when the neck is in extension. They become increasingly tight as the neck flexes forward. The mechanism causing sprain is a forcible hyperflexion of the neck. As this force is applied, the cervical bodies are forced together. The vertebrae rotating on the sagittal axis of the articulations force the spinous processes to separate (Fig. 222). This force is arrested by the combination of the pressing of the intact bodies together and the checking action of the dorsal muscles and the ligamentum nuchae. If the force con-

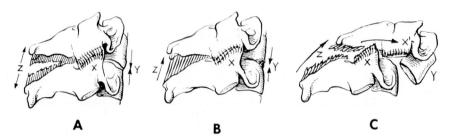

Figure 222.   Flexion force. *A,* Forcible hyperflexion. The cervical vertebra rotates on the axis of the apophyseal joints (x). The cervical bodies (y) maintain their integrity. The interspinous ligament (z) ruptures.

B, Same force. The ligament (z) holds. The rotation is around (x) and the adjacent edges of the bodies of the cervical vertebrae buckle.

C, Same force. The interspinous ligament (z) gives way. The bodies (y) maintain their integrity. The center of rotation (x) advances to (x') as the interarticular ligaments rupture to slide the inferior articular process of the upper vetebra in front of that of the lower with subluxation or dislocation.

tinues and the bodies maintain their integrity, the ligaments may tear (Fig. 222, *A*). This sprain may be mild, moderate or severe.

The MILD sprain is of little consequence. There will be no particular weakness in the ligament. All the symptoms will be local with tenderness and pain at the site of injury. Ordinary cervical flexion within normal range will be pain-free. Forcing the neck beyond this range may cause some distress. This injury is not likely to arouse muscle spasm since the symptoms are mild.

In a MODERATE sprain which involves some loss of function of the ligament, a portion of the ligament has actually been torn away. This may be within the ligament itself or may be at its attachment to one of the cervical processes. In this instance the symptoms will be more severe. The patient holds his head in extension and resists any attempt to flex it forward because of pain at the site of injury. There is localized tenderness. After the passage of several hours, there is likely to be muscle spasm of the posterior spinal muscles (Fig. 223); and the neck, instead of being pulled to one side or the other, is held in extension. The direction of force applied may indicate the expected location of injury. If the patient can rotate his atlanto-occipital joint, that is, nod his head without pain, one may assume the injury is below C-2. A further guide is the location of tenderness.

If there is sharply localized tenderness in the spinous processes or ligament, injection of this area by a long-acting local anesthetic plus hyaluronidase if the patient is seen very early and a corticoid preparation if he is seen later may give substantial relief. This injection may need to be repeated several times. In this case, traction is ordinarily not indicated since holding the head up will relieve the tension. However, this becomes quite tiresome and tension headache is common with spasm of the posterior cervical muscles. This patient will be relieved by a cervical collar that holds the chin up (Fig. 224). He may be more comfortable at night in light cervical traction although usually this is not necessary. Physical therapy is of value here. Great care should be taken that any manipulative treatment is pain-free. This injury may be quite disabling to the athlete since six to eight weeks will be needed for the ligament to heal, which is enough to seriously disrupt his season. A well fitted cotton collar may permit him to participate much sooner.

Figure 223.   X-ray, lateral view, made with the neck in forward flexion. Note reversal of the curve, caused by muscle spasm of the lower cervical segment so that this is held in extension while the upper part of the neck flexes forward. This is indicative of muscle spasm such as accompanies strain or sprain.

The collar must be carefully fitted so that the ligament will not be reinjured by forward flexion of the neck.

If the ligament injury is a SEVERE one, there is complete separation of the ligament. The ligament may be torn off a single spinous process and the main body of the ligament may remain intact. This is a much less serious injury than that occurring when the ligament itself is pulled in two. If the ligament is ruptured either in its substance or off one of the processes, the symptoms will be quite severe with sharply localized pain. If palpated early, a defect may be felt in the ligament, particularly if the head is forced into some degree of flexion. Further flexion will be bitterly resisted. The patient will feel that his head is insecure and will tend to hold

Figure 224.   A, An adjustable cervical brace. B, A plastic cervical collar.

Figure 225.   Avulsion fracture of the tip of the spinous process of C-7 following acute
flexion injury.

his neck quite rigid. Painful spasm soon supervenes and the head is pulled into
hyperextension. At this time it may be quite difficult to determine the exact nature
of the injury. Careful x-ray study may reveal an avulsion of a portion of the bone
with the ligament (Fig. 225). X-ray made with the head and neck in flexion may
reveal unusually wide separation of the spinous processes at some level. This is
quite suggestive of ligament injury, particularly if this coincides with the level of
local symptoms. There is normally a wide variation in the amount of separation of
the spinous processes in the normal neck at different levels.

Treatment for avulsion of the tip of one of the spinous processes is surgical
removal of the fragment and repair of the ligament. This treatment seems to be
well accepted, especially since the diagnosis can be confirmed by x-ray. The same
treatment would be ideal for complete ligament avulsion. Usually, however, this
condition is not diagnosed in the early stage and is treated nonsurgically as a sprain.
Indeed, if the head is kept in hyperextension, thereby bringing into contact the tips
of the spinous processes and with them the ligament ends, the ligament may grow
together at near normal length. If this same force breaks the spinous process at the
lamina or if it fractures the spinous process without displacement, uneventful healing will occur by simple immobilization of the neck in extension. Avulsion of the
tip is very prone to nonunion since the separation is usually wide. The treatment
of a painful nonunion is excision of the fragment. Athletic competition should not
be permitted until union is complete—either union of ligament to bone if the
fragment is removed or bony union of the fragment to the vertebra.

Other Flexion Injury (Subluxation-Dislocation).   In the more severe flexion
injuries of the neck, the damage is usually not confined to the interspinous liga-

ment. As the neck is flexed, the cervical discs compress. The bodies are forced together in front and apart posteriorly and excess of motion occurs at the apophyseal articulations. If the interspinous ligament gives way while the body remains intact, the force is received on the laminal and articular ligaments as well as the posterior longitudinal ligament, which is relatively weak. As long as the front of the body remains intact, the dislocating force will separate the articulations, rupture the capsular ligaments and a subluxation of the cervical vertebrae will occur. (Fig. 222,C). Indeed, this may happen without actual rupture of the posterior longitudinal ligament. As the flexion is continued there is a shearing force of the head forward on the trunk that causes the superior articulations to displace forward over the ones below. If some of the ligaments are left intact—either the interspinous or the laminal or possibly the articular ligaments plus the anterior and posterior longitudinal ligaments—a great deal of stability is still present in the spine and the articular process of the vertebra above slips in front of the superior articular process of the vertebra below. This dislocation locks in the unreduced position. Subluxation followed by spontaneous reduction probably occurs quite frequently in flexion injuries of the neck. This is one of the reasons, already mentioned, why the neck should be carefully protected against a repetition of the flexion shearing force in order that complete dislocation does not occur with a subsequent injury.

In bilateral dislocation (Fig. 226) the head is characteristically held thrust forward in hypertension. The spinous process of the vertebra below is prominent with a corresponding defect above, while the proximal portion of the neck will appear to be flexed. The patient is usually extremely apprehensive and will resist any attempt to move his head in any direction. Indeed, he will often hold his head with his hands. I well recall being called to the hospital one Saturday afternoon to see a man who had ridden in his car to the hospital holding his head in his hands following an episode with a bull. He absolutely refused to take his hands away from his head, making the statement that "if he did his head would fall off," nor would he relinquish his grasp to permit examination until he was supine in bed and even then only reluctantly.

This injury has serious potential for cord and root damage and a careful examination should be made for the presence of a neurological deficit. This absolutely must be done before any attempt at reduction is made. The injury is obviously a serious one but fortunately it is extremely infrequent in the athlete. It demands the prompt care of the orthopedist. In the interim, the patient should be placed supine and the head should be protected by sandbags on either side. Since the exact nature of the injury will not be evident until x-ray study has been made, precautionary traction of a few pounds with head halter is imperative as soon as it can be applied. Needless to say, transportation must be made with extreme caution. Definitive care demands reduction at the earliest possible moment, hence the necessity for early diagnosis.

The same flexion, forward shearing force that causes the dislocation mentioned above may continue with the destruction of the remaining ligamentous support at this level so that one body may slide forward on the other until the back of the neurocanal of one vertebra is at the level of the front of the neurocanal of the one

Figure 226.   Fracture-dislocation of C-6 on 7 from tackling. *A*, Anteroposterior view. Notice lateral displacement of mass of C-7 with rotation of C-6 forward. *B*, 24 hours in traction reduced the dislocation. *C*, Lateral view in traction shows no displacement, no obvious fracture. *D*, Recent lateral films in flexion and extension showing subluxation, with persistent collapse of disc between C-6 and C-7. This boy developed latent neurological deficit in the long thoracic nerve which has persisted.

below (Fig. 228). This applies a shearing trauma to the cord and may cause complete quadriplegia. With this injury there is such instability that the neck will frequently fall back into correct apposition and local physical and x-ray examination may be entirely negative. One must not be misled as to the severity of the injury by the negative x-ray. The same dislocation may have been complete and reduced and without cord damage only to have cord damage occur because the injury was not recognized and subsequent activity caused a dislocation.

Figure 227.   Fracture-subluxation of C-5 on 6 with fracture of the articular process of C-5. The deformity was corrected under traction, recurred in the brace and has persisted. Neurological deficit was persistent with hypesthesia in the right thumb.

Figure 228.   A, Complete dislocation of C-5 on 6 without fracture. The intact arch caused transection of the cord and complete quadriplegia. B, Postoperative picture showing complete reduction with internal fixation from C-4 to 6 plus bone graft. Partial laminectomy at C-5.

As this dislocation occurs, the posterior portion of the neural arch may break and remain posterior (Fig. 229). This break may take place at the pars interarticularis or further back on the lamina. In any event, this protects the cord to a considerable degree since the shearing action of the posterior portion of the ring is prevented as the ring itself expands. This accounts for the case of complete dislocation of the vertebra forward with no neurological symptoms. Careful x-ray examination will often reveal that the arch has remained posterior. Such cases serve to emphasize

Figure 229.   Fracture-dislocation of C-2 on C-3. Note that the fracture separated the arcs and lamina from the body which relieved the tension on the cord and there was no neurological deficit. This picture shows the reduction and plaster fixation. Complete healing. Asymptomatic.

the importance of intelligent handling of the cervical injury. The same force that causes bilateral dislocation with forward flexion and shearing may well cause fracture of the articular processes which may complicate the recovery and result in painful joints.

A unique type of injury that may occur from forward stress is dislocation between the first and second cervical vertebrae (Fig. 230). It will be recalled that the odontoid is held firmly to the anterior portion of the body of C-1 by the transverse ligament, which keeps the body of C-1 from displacing forward. On a sharp forward

Figure 230.   Fractured odontoid with forward subluxation of C-1 on 2. Only transient neurological deficit. Treated in traction, cast, brace with complete clinical recovery but some persistent subluxation.

thrust of the head, particularly combined with some forward shearing, the odontoid is forced sharply against this ligament. If the ligament tears, the articular ligaments also give way and dislocation occurs leaving the odontoid within the neurocanal of the first cervical. The large vulnerable cord of this area is very likely to be damaged and death ensue. Occasionally there is a congenital shortness of the odontoid so that it can slip forward under the transverse ligament without actually tearing it. This is the so-called somersault dislocation caused by sharp hyperflexion of the neck. Many of these cases will not have serious nerve involvement. They may actually be in the nature of recurrent dislocation and slip forward and spontaneously reduce. If they do not reduce spontaneously, they can usually be reduced. Owing to the very large brain stem at this level, reduction is better done by mechanical traction with weights than by manipulation. The traction should first be with the neck well flexed, then gradually moved toward extension. This dislocation may be very difficult to distinguish from fracture of the odontoid since the latter, when it accompanies dislocation of the first cervical vertebra, is not readily seen in the antero-posterior x-ray. Careful study after the deformity is reduced will reveal the character of the lesion.

A much more frequent injury appears to be the fracture of the odontoid from the body of C-2. In this instance there is much more leeway for the cord and it is much less likely to be impinged. This fracture may be complete or incomplete. The patient usually realizes that he is seriously hurt. The usual careful management should be carried out. Definitive diagnosis is made by x-ray. The severity of this major injury demands early, adequate treatment, which may well be surgical. Of some consequence is the incomplete tear with damage to the transverse ligament. The initial relatively minor injury may be followed by a fatal accident at a later time.

Fracture.   Aside from the laminal fractures mentioned above, which are essentially a component of dislocation, there may be fractures of other portions of

Figure 231.   Fracture of the ring of the first cervical vertebra without displacement. No neurological deficit. Treated by plaster immobilization.

Figure 232.   *A*, Compression fracture of C-7. This does not require reduction but requires protection so that the body does not collapse laterally. A period of traction until the spasm subsides and then a Minerva cast would be adequate treatment.

B, Inadequately treated cervical fracture-dislocation. This is a flexion film made some months after the injury, showing posterior dislocation of C-6 and compression of C-7. The upright view shows no dislocation.

the vertebrae. It has been mentioned that the spinous process may break rather than the ligamentum nuchae tear. As the flexion force is applied and the spinous processes separate, the bodies are forced together and a fracture of the body may occur (Fig. 232, *A*). In fact, a fracture of the cervical body is more frequent than a complete tear of the posterior longitudinal ligament. If the fracture is not accompanied by a dislocation, the body may compress as much as 75 per cent. The front part of the body will be down to 25 per cent of its normal height and the posterior part will maintain its normal height. Since the axis of rotation is at the articulations which are adjacent to the posterior portion of the body, the force is primarily applied at the extreme front. These cases are not often accompanied by cord damage since the neural canal is not impinged upon. The patient will have extreme forward flexion of the neck, severe pain, with the feeling of insecurity that accompanies severe ligament injury or dislocation. The same careful study described above will reveal the fracture.

The fracture will require definitive treatment by traction to restore the body contours and prolonged immobilization to permit union.

Roentgenographic study of the neck presents many difficulties and the team physician would be wise to consult a competent radiologist or orthopedist before concluding that the x-ray of the neck is negative. The potentialities of permanent disability are so great that one can ill afford to "wait and see" in these injuries (Fig. 232, *B*).

Figure 233.   *A,* Fracture of anterior inferior quadrant of C-2 with anterior rotation of the fragment. No neurological symptoms. *B,* Five months later solid union. All manipulative efforts to replace the fragment failed. This was undoubtedly an extension injury.

Extension Injury (Dorsiflexion)

Anterior Longitudinal Ligament Injury (Sprain).   The anterior longitudinal ligament extends throughout the cervical spine and serves to prevent separation of the anterior margins of the cervical vertebrae by hyperextension of the neck. As the neck moves into extension, the spinous process tends to impinge and, as the force continues, the lever changes from the first degree with the fulcrum at the cervical articulations to the second degree with the fulcrum at the tip of the spinous processes. Distraction force is applied to the anterior longitudinal ligament and to a lesser extent to the articular ligaments. This results in some degree of damage to the anterior longitudinal ligament. The anterior ligament may tear or avulse a fragment of the body (Fig. 233). If the ligament maintains its integrity there may be a fracture of the spinous processes. If the spinous processes hold, the ligament may tear. The tear may be of any degree and if it is severe enough may permit actual dislocation of the cervical spine. If the force is arrested the neck returns to its normal position and there are relatively few symptoms since the normal position of the neck puts no strain on the anterior longitudinal ligament. Usually the player knows that he has had a neck injury and examination will reveal that the pain and tenderness are anterior and that his symptoms are aggravated by extension of the neck.

If the injury is a MILD one, no particular treatment is indicated except that as a hedge a cotton cast should be applied. If the injury is MODERATE, the same treatment may be used as for the posterior sprain except that the neck should be placed in some degree of flexion rather than extension, whether it be in traction or a collar. The motion to be prevented by the brace is extension rather than flexion.

If the injury is SEVERE and there has been actual tearing of the anterior longitudinal ligament (Fig. 234), the symptoms will be more extreme and protection must be prolonged. This is the reason for mentioning that in the mild injury it is well to protect the neck until it is pain-free. The ever present danger is repetition of the force that caused the original injury. Riding in a car, participation in scrimmage, etc., should be ruled out without protection of the neck to prevent this motion. If muscle spasm supervenes, the head will be pulled forward by the bi-

Figure 234.   Extension injury of the cervical spine.
    A, Hyperextension forces the spinous processes together at (z), dislocates the front of the vertebra at (y). The center of rotation changes from (x) to (x") as the spinous processes impinge and the vertebrae are torn apart.
    B, Continuation of the same force dislocates the articulations, rupturing the discs, anterior and posterior longitudinal ligaments and a frank dislocation may occur.
    C, With application of the same forces, the spinous processes break which relieves the tension and the vertebrae fall back together without major damage to the cord.

laterally tight sternomastoid muscles. This may be extremely painful and to a considerable extent disabling since the patient has difficulty in raising his head to the erect position. It must be determined by examination that the difficulty is not actually from weakness of the dorsiflexors but from tightness of the forward flexors.

    The severe case will require the same careful handling as any potentially serious injury of the neck. The patient should be put at bed rest with the neck in a position of slight flexion and light traction applied. Muscle relaxants, sedation and local heat are all important. Attention should be called to the fact that the symptoms are very similar to those resulting from bilateral dislocation of the articular facets and careful x-ray study is needed to rule out possible bone or joint damage. Physical examination will help since in this instance forward flexion very carefully, even gingerly, applied will be pain-free whereas an attempt to extend the neck will cause increased spasm in the sternomastoids. On the other hand, with a dislocation of the neck the patient is quite willing to dorsiflex his head. A few hours of traction with local heat and sedation will serve to relax the spasm and a more definitive diagnosis can be made. The patient must be protected for several weeks against dorsiflexion of the neck. This would seem to be quite incompatible with active athletics.

    Subluxation-Dislocation.   If this same extension force continues, the anterior edges of the bodies are separated, the disc is disrupted (Fig. 234, B), the posterior longitudinal ligament tears, the articular ligaments tear and the vertebra may actually displace backward over its fellow below. This hyperextension type of injury is extremely serious and accounts for many of the cases accompanied by complete paralysis below this level, yet with entirely negative x-rays. The cord will tolerate posterior displacement even more poorly than it will anterior. This injury is not a frequent one in athletics. There is a limiting factor in that the lever of the spinous process is potentially a weak one and it may well give way (Fig. 234, C) at any time during the application of this posterior flexion. This buckling of the process may save the cord since it permits the vertebrae to rotate near the spinal canal rather than to open up on an axis of the posterior tip of the spinous process. The patient with paralysis will present no great problem to the examining physician since it is obvious he has a major injury. More puzzling is the injury that does not cause primary paralysis. Examination may be relatively negative. X-ray findings are negative. An incautious or unrestricted motion may lead to disaster. One should try to determine whether or not the direction of the force that caused the injury was extension or flexion. The initial traction in bed followed by a cervical brace should be designed to prevent extension of the neck. Permission to resume active athletic participation, if ever, will depend upon the individual case.

A present concern in the causation of extension injuries is the modern HEAD-GEAR. There can be no reasonable doubt that today's headgear is a great improvement over the types previously used, particularly in the area of preventing blows to the head and face. There has been an unwelcome dividend from this improvement that is particularly related to cervical injuries. The plastic headgear is extremely solid and unyielding. Its posterior edge is no exception. In many of the headgears, the posterior edge strikes the upper cervical area so that, with the head in complete extension, the edge of the headgear drives toward the spinous processes. A major improvement in the headgear has been utilization of the face bar which has markedly diminished facial injuries. However, the long bar projecting well forward, as preferred by many, presents a convenient handle that the opponent may consciously or inadvertently grasp in his contact with the player. Indeed, he does not need to grasp it. The blocker coming up with the shoulder or elbow may catch the bar and forcibly extend his opponent's neck. The hazard is greatly increased if the bar extends well forward. A severe force is applied to the back of the neck by the combination of the leverage action on the front of the helmet and impingement of the unyielding back of the helmet against the spinous process. This may actually break off a spinous process, which is not of transcending importance. Much more vital is the fact that the back of the helmet may tend to support the tip of the spinous process so that it maintains its fulcrum as the front of the bodies of the vertebrae are separated. The force is concentrated at a single point, further encouraging extension injury. This can be alleviated by better designing of the helmet.

Until lately the designers of helmets have concentrated on protecting the head of the wearer. Little thought has been given to the effect of the helmet on other portions of the player's or his opponent's anatomy. A recent modification of the helmet is designed to improve these conditions. A comparison of the helmet previously used by the University of Oklahoma and the one used now is seen in Figure 235. In Figure 235, A, the headgear is of solid, unyielding plastic with a small leather roll over the back edge of the helmet, with no padding over the top of it. The new helmet (Fig. 235, B) has had the plastic back of the neck cut away and replaced with an apron so that it is impossible for the edge of the plastic to impinge against the neck proper. This same helmet has a strip of plastic foam beginning at the forehead and extending up over the crown of the helmet, about 6 inches wide, to serve as protection for the opposing player. The helmet also has plastic pads inside. While the players complain of it being somewhat hotter, it certainly seems to be more protective. The addition of the external and internal padding accounts for an increase of but 1 ounce in weight. Incidentally, the single face bar for protection has been supplanted in many places by double ones. These do not need to extend as far forward since they cover more of the facial area and so reduce the leverage somewhat. They are harder to grasp because of the spread between the bars. The blocker is also less likely to get his elbow, shoulder or knee under the bars since the lower one is considerably further toward the chest. The second bar adds about 10 ounces

Figure 235.   A, The older style helmet. Note the hard posterior edge of the helmet is directed at about C-6 and 7. However, it is at least 2 inches away from the spinous process with the head forcibly extended by pressure on the face bar.

B, The new style helmet. Note the soft leather roll against the skin with the hard plastic edge 1½ inches away so that the hard plastic edge is 4 inches from the bone. This is the same player.

to the weight of the helmet but this probably can be reduced in newer models by using lighter weight material. These efforts to improve the protective helmet and face bar are certainly much more valid than condemning them and recommending their abandonment.

Rotatory Injury

Sprain.   This sprain is usually the result of rotation of the neck so that the head is forcibly turned beyond the tolerance of the vertebra involved. The chin is pulled toward the opposite shoulder and excess strain is placed upon the ligaments as the neck is not only flexed to the side but rotated the same direction. These capsular ligaments tear to some degree. The force is released. The result is some damage to the ligament fibers with hemorrhage into the capsule and, indeed, into the joint. In the vast majority of cases, no actual subluxation occurs. As soon as the head resumes its normal position, the spasm subsides but soreness will persist. In many cases, if the examination is made early, the level of involvement can be determined by palpation directly over the joint. Active function of the cervical muscles will not cause pain, even against resistance. If the sprain is on the left side of the neck, forcibly pulling the head to the left or right against resistance will not be painful. On the other hand, passive flexion and rotation to the opposite side to reproduce the force that caused the injury will cause pain.

If the sprain is a MILD one the symptoms will be few. The player will shrug it off. On the following day he will have soreness and stiffness in the neck but will usually recover completely without either treatment or protection.

If the sprain is MODERATE and some portion of the ligament is actually torn, the symptoms will be much more pronounced. Although the injury may not have appeared to be serious at the time of its occurrence, on the following day muscle spasm will intervene. Spasm of the muscles will have pulled the head toward the involved side and will resist any effort toward reproducing the motion that caused the sprain. The pain may become quite severe, not primarily from the ligament injury but from the resulting muscle spasm. The patient may present himself several days later with the ear pulled toward the shoulder on the same side and the chin rotated toward the same side with pain and spasm along the same side (Fig. 236, A). The treatment of this condition at whatever stage seen will depend upon the severity. If there is painful spasm, the best way to relax the spasm is by bed rest and light cervical traction, accompanied by local heat. Muscle relaxants will give relief. Indeed, the treatment is the same as that indicated for strain above. Here, too, the extent of the treatment will depend upon the symptoms. It may be that the spasm will subside in a few hours or a day or so but be assured that this spasm will return if the patient is allowed unprotected activity. This patient must wear a cotton collar or metal or plastic brace to protect the ligament against reproduction of the motion that caused the injury. Athletic competition cannot be permitted for several weeks if the injury was serious. If it appears to be less severe, the player should be protected with a cotton collar during the time of his participation.

Subluxation. If this force continues, subluxation or unilateral dislocation may occur. The spontaneously reduced subluxation gives the symptoms of the sprain mentioned above. In the cervical spine, the articular process may slide partially off and become locked in this position rather than dislocate entirely forward. This patient will have the same history of injury and the same complaints of pain as one with sprain, but the pain is usually more severe. He will have sharply restricted motion of the neck immediately so that he is unable to rotate his neck at all to the affected side. The chin will have turned toward the opposite side and the head will be tilted to the opposite side. The sternomastoid muscle on the involved side will be tight. The essential problem here will be muscle spasm due to tightness of the muscles that prevents replacement of the dislocation. Subluxation

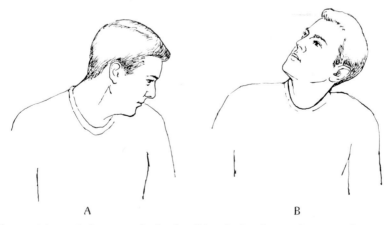

A B

Figure 236. A, In sprain the head will be tilted and rotated in same direction. B, In wryneck the chin will be rotated toward the opposite side and the head tilted toward the affected side.

may occur without actual ligament damage if the ligaments of the neck are somewhat relaxed. In the athlete it ordinarily occurs as an acute injury and with some damage to the ligaments. The reason for separating the two is that in the subluxation without actual ligament damage the joint is not affected and once the subluxation is reduced the patient is essentially asymptomatic, usually with no residual. This may be compared to the recurrent dislocation of the shoulder which has become so loose that it slips out without further damage to the ligament and, once the dislocation is reduced, it is pain-free. These recurrent subluxations may well be the result of an untreated sprain in which the ligament was allowed to heal with redundancy.

The case that is seen as an acute injury without previous history of subluxation should be treated as a severe sprain. It is important first to reduce the subluxation. This is accomplished not by massive overhead traction but by bed rest with 4-pound cervical traction, accompanied by local heat, muscle relaxants and sedation. I have yet to see one of these cases of subluxation persist overnight if the patient slept. This is not a complete dislocation and the articular processes are not locked. Reduction of a subluxation does not heal the ligament injury. As soon as the reduction is accomplished, the condition should be treated as a sprain and the neck protected against recurrence of the injury until the ligament healing is complete. This will take six or eight weeks.

Dislocation-Fracture. If this same force continues, a complete dislocation of the articular process occurs on one side. In this instance the articular process slips forward and lodges in front of the superior articulation of the vertebra below, where it is held securely in position. The patient will have had severe pain located at the side of the neck. Muscle spasm will be immediate. At examination the chin is turned away and the head is tilted away from the dislocation. The patient obviously has a serious injury and should be handled as such. True enough, if the injury was due to a rotatory force and the major ligaments are intact, the patient is in little danger. One cannot be sure, however, that the injury is not major and the same care should be assumed in management as in the case of complete bilateral dislocation.

Ill advised attempts at manipulation should be discouraged. In the first place, manipulation is almost uniformly unsuccessful and in the second place it may cause irreparable damage. Definitive treatment should be carried out by the surgeon skilled in this type of injury. If manual manipulation is to be attempted under anesthesia or without, the earlier it is done the more successful it will be. For manipulation without anesthesia the patient is sedated heavily and the head is tilted forward and rotated in the direction to increase the deformity until the vertebra is unlocked. The cervical spine is slightly flexed, traction is increased and the head is carefully turned and tilted back toward the injured side and into hyperextension. Repeated efforts to do this without anesthesia are unjustified. Under anesthesia the same manipulation may be carried out but must be done with utmost precautions, bearing in mind that the safety factor of the patient's muscles has been eliminated.

Many of these dislocations may be reduced by cervical traction although one is inclined to fear that, if reduction is too easy, one or both of the articular processes may be fractured. Following reduction of the deformity, light traction may be continued with the neck in extension or the patient may be promptly put in a Minerva

Figure 237.   The Minerva jacket for high cervical fracture-dislocation. The forehead and parietal regions are included to limit rotation and nodding of the head which take place chiefly in the occipito-atlas and atlanto-axis articulations.

type jacket (Fig. 237). The head should be placed in some hyperextension. The chin should be supported and the cast should extend over the forehead and rest on the iliac crest. Anything short of this cannot immobilize the neck. It should be borne in mind that the dislocation entails a ligament injury that will require the usual period for healing.

Many of the rotatory injuries are accompanied by lateral stress so that, as the head is twisted to the opposite side, the articular process slides forward on the involved side. A great deal of force is applied to the lateral mass of vertebra of the opposite side from the inflicting force—that is, on the side toward which the head is turned and flexed. This may cause a fracture of the articular processes on the opposite side (Fig. 227) or any portion of the lateral mass. If this patient is treated as indicated above, the fracture will not particularly complicate the picture since it will have healed by the time the ligament injury has. Casual treatment of the ligament injury combined with overlooking of the fracture may court disaster.

Unilateral subluxation and dislocation are extremely difficult to visualize by x-ray, particularly if they occur around C-6 and 7 where the intervening shoulders, particularly in a muscular individual, interfere with good visualization. Oblique views, repeated anteroposterior and lateral views and stereoscopic views may be necessary to determine the nature of the damage.

Many of these rotatory injuries are relieved by simple repositioning of the spine. It may be extremely difficult to persuade the eager athlete that he has an injury that demands prolonged treatment. One must exert every effort to prevent him from injudicious exercise in his effort to hasten his rehabilitation since this only results in prolongation of his recovery and even may result in permanent disability.

Torsion Injuries to Nerve Elements

Brachial Plexus and Nerve Root Injuries.   While flexion and extension of the neck account for the major dislocations, in twisting injuries there may be serious involvement of the nerve roots. As the neck is forcibly rotated in one direction and flexed the same way, undue tension is placed upon the cords of the brachial plexus, particularly if traction is applied at the same time to the outstretched arm. For example, when the player is being tackled by his right arm and someone else is pulling his head to the left, considerable tension is placed upon the nerve structures. This may result in transitory paralysis of the arm with the familiar numbing or shocklike feeling which within a few seconds or minutes completely disappears. It may, however, result in more serious neurological pathology, even to the extent of tearing the nerve roots from the cord. This is an irreparable injury. Damage to the cords of the brachial plexus also may occur. This latter may well be remediable.

Following such an injury, any evidence of nerve involvement of the extremities that persists more than a few hours demands very careful study with an attempt to delineate the exact root or trunk involved. Frequently there will be a generalized involvement of the arm with diffuse numbness and a feeling of heaviness of the arm which gradually recovers. Certain specific neurological defects may be persistent, however, and may easily be overlooked. Damage to the posterior cord affecting the use of the triceps, for example, may be easily overlooked since the arm will readily fall into extension by the effect of gravity and several days may pass before the physician realizes that a loss of function of this muscle is actually present. It behooves him to make a careful neurological examination of the extremity after such an injury. The earlier this is done the better, since it provides a base for measuring the progress of the condition by successive examinations. In case of increasing involvement, surgical neurolysis may be indicated. The neurosurgeon should have the opportunity to determine the necessity and decide on the best time for the procedure.

Major tears of the roots are extremely rare. When they occur they are manifested by complete loss of function of the components involved. Unfortunately, they are not amenable to surgical repair. Fortunately, one is usually able to distinguish between damage to the more peripheral portions of the brachial plexus and damage to the nerve root. This is of vital importance since the plexus injury may be reparable.

ASSOCIATED CERVICAL INJURIES

Nerve Root Injury

Any of the above described forces may cause damage to the nerve roots ranging from brief irritation with a transient numbing, shocklike feeling in the arm, to complete severance of the root. As a rule, the important consideration is to determine if possible the exact nature of injury, so as to know what should be done with the patient. Once he gets well developed nerve root symptoms he is a problem for the neurosurgeon or the orthopedist. There is nothing specifically diagnostic about nerve root pain. It may be caused with equal facility by the pressure of a cervical disc, by fracture of a portion of the nerve root foramen, or by pressure on the nerve root from hematoma or hemorrhage within the nerve. Certainly a diagnosis of nerve root syndrome is no more specific than one of bellyache or headache.

The nerve root symptoms caused by a sudden twist of the head that are transient and disappear rapidly are usually of little significance. Exceptionally they indicate a subluxation, particularly if the symptoms were the first of their kind to occur in this patient. Some players have repeated episodes of pain in the neck with nerve root symptoms into the arm which seem to be accompanied by no particular pathology in the neck. These must be interpreted as resulting from an impingement on the nerve, either due to hypermobility of a joint or to narrowing of the nerve root canal so that the nerve is pinched by a motion that ordinarily would leave it amply free. So also may adhesions about the nerve root cause traction on the nerve on an unguarded motion which ordinarily is prevented by protective muscle tension. While careful study may be rewarding in eliminating some remediable lesion, one is often in a quandary as to whether or not athletic participation should be permitted. The decision will depend partly on the patient's desire, mostly on the physician's own judgment of the situation.

Scalenus Anticus Syndrome

The scalenus anticus syndrome, like many other syndromes, has become much less frequently diagnosed as more specific diagnoses such as cervical rib, cervical disc and various vascular conditions are made. The symptomatology arises because of occlusion of the artery or vein and/or pressure of the brachial plexus caused by spasm of the anterior scalene muscle. Certain anatomic characteristics make this more frequent, particularly the presence of a cervical rib. The symptoms are usually of the lower roots of the plexus, with pain along the ulnar distribution, particularly whenever the arm is over the head. This is combined with a tendency toward vascular occlusion so that one is unable to work with his arms higher than his shoulders because of pain and the feeling that the arm "goes to sleep." This is not an athletic injury. It is mentioned here since it may at times be confused with cervical injury. A little attention to the history will help. A classical test is obliteration of the radial pulse as the arm is pulled over the head and the neck is pulled to the opposite side. A well established syndrome will require extensive treatment.

Cervical Rib Syndrome

This is mentioned along with the scalenus anticus syndrome since the two are quite similar. The presence of a cervical rib makes injury to this area of the plexus at the base of the neck somewhat more likely. A blow at the base of the neck over a cervical rib may well cause a sharp accentuation or may, indeed, initiate the neurological and vascular symptoms of cervical rib. Recognition of the possibility of a cervical rib will usually permit adequate diagnosis and treatment (Fig. 238).

Injury to the Long Thoracic Nerve

Frequently occurring in conjunction with sprain or other injury at the base of the neck is injury to the long thoracic nerve. This nerve comes directly off the nerve root and does not participate in the brachial plexus. It passes down and supplies the various serrations of the serratus anterior. Bruising or damage to this nerve may occur and pass unrecognized until distressing winging of the scapula is noted (Fig. 239). The cause may be a sharp blow at the base of the neck laterally that

Figure 238.   Bilateral cervical rib C-7. This is congenital and not necessarily disabling.

Figure 239.   Photograph illustrating winging of scapula.

impinges the nerve against the lower cervical vertebrae. Since this is primarily a motor nerve, there is usually little pain or discomfort to guide the physician. There may be weakness or complete paralysis of the nerve, resulting in loss of fixation of the scapula to the chest wall so that, as the arm is pulled forward, the vertebral border of the scapula swings outward.

The ideal treatment for this condition has not been found. If it is recognized early recovery would probably be expedited by immobilization of the arm in abduction and external rotation in order to hold the scapula against the chest wall and protect the muscles from undue strain. Since it is usually recognized quite late, there is some question of the value of immobilization. Surgical treatment is not acceptable since recovery will usually take place without it. The injury is usually a contusion rather than separation. Since the involved area is extremely inaccessible, making any sort of repair virtually impossible, neurolyses should probably not be attempted, even in late involvement. After a period of a few weeks there is no reason to forbid active use; in fact, athletic competition within the patient's capacity should be encouraged.

Injury to the Spinal Accessory Nerve

The spinal accessory nerve, located as it is somewhat superficially near the surface in the trapezius muscle, may be injured by a direct blow across the trapezius muscle. This injury may be confused with contusion of the muscle. The player may have difficulty elevating the shoulder toward the ear and will have severe aching pain. The injury requires no specific treatment other than physical therapy. Heat and superficial massage will usually relieve the symptoms and restoration of the motor function of the trapezius muscle is rapid. For a few days there may seem to be serious paralysis.

Snapping Neck

Another and more common condition in the cervical area may give the player and the physician a good deal of uneasiness. This is the presence of an audible and palpable click or snap of the neck on certain rotations. The cause of this popping or snapping is varied. It may be due to irregularity at the articulations. Much more commonly it is due to forcible snapping of a tendon over a bony prominence. As with most conditions of the neck, there is a very considerable apprehension factor which does not seem to be present in joints more distal from the head. The player who can pop his neck on certain rotatory movements is quite certain that he has gross pathology. He usually holds the neck stiff. He may become amazingly adept at this snapping since, if he learns to hold certain muscles tight, the audibility of the snapping becomes much more notable. There is undoubtedly a functional component in this condition and the player has a well nigh uncontrollable impulse to pop his neck whereupon he proclaims that he gets great relief.

The treatment for this condition is to prevent the snapping and with an understanding patient it can usually be stopped simply by having him stop demonstrating it. A word of warning should be sounded, however. One must make sure that no underlying pathological condition is present that needs to be treated, such as irregularity of the articular facet, tenosynovitis of a tendon, or muscle spasm that tends to bow the tendon across the bony prominence. For this reason, a fairly extensive regimen of physical therapy should be instituted. In the true "snapping neck," pain is not an important symptom while apprehension is. A very careful physical examination together with x-ray study may be followed by a frank conference with the player in which the situation is thoroughly explained. He is assured that he has no serious condition and that many joints are prone to snap. He should then be urged to avoid, if possible, getting in the position where the phenomenon occurs. Frequently after a suitable period either the snapping disappears or the player learns to ignore it.

DORSAL SPINE

ANATOMICAL CONSIDERATIONS

The dorsal (thoracic) spine (Fig. 218) is the most stable section of the vertebral column. No detailed description of the anatomy need be given here other than to mention a few pertinent points. The 12 dorsal vertebrae together with the ribs and sternum combine to form the bony thorax. The whole structure of the thorax is such that it tends to limit motion of the spine. The general contour of the spine is one of dorsal convexity, and extension from this position is resisted by the thoracic cage. The spine itself has a good deal of intrinsic stability, the vertebrae being very firmly bound together by the various ligaments. The articular processes are vertical and face in such a manner that the inferior processes of the vertebrae above lock behind the superior processes of the vertebrae below to completely prevent any forward displacement of the upper vertebrae on the lower unless there is a fracture of the arch. Sufficient displacement to permit the articular processes to displace upward the full length of the articulation is necessary before the joint becomes dislocated. The angle of these processes is such that the inferior processes on the superior vertebrae above fit within the arc of the superior processes of the lower vertebrae, the articular face of the lower vertebrae facing inward almost 45 degrees. The bodies themselves are slightly higher behind than in front, which causes the convexity and again adds to stability. The ribs, articulating as they do between the two vertebrae, tend to reinforce the column at the level of the back of the bodies. The column is also supported by the very immobile articular processes.

The disc spaces are narrow and the disc itself has much less elasticity than either the cervical or lumbar discs. The spinous processes, rather than extending backward as in the cervical and lumbar spine, extend downward, overlapping each other as shingles on a roof. In many instances one actually rests upon its fellow below so that the leverage on the interspinous ligaments is greatly increased because these spinous processes actually have to separate as the spine flexes forward. These processes immediately impinge as the spine is flexed backward. They are subcutaneous at their tips.

The stable dorsal spine serves for attachment of many of the muscles (Fig. 240) of the trunk, shoulder and arm. The trapezius muscle attaches to the spinous processes from the upper cervical well down to lower dorsal. In the lower part of the dorsal spine, it overlaps the long attachment of the latissimus dorsi, which attaches to the spinous process beginning mid-dorsal and extending to the pelvis. These are the most superficial layers of the muscles in the back and serve to enclose

Figure 240. Anatomical drawing of muscles of back.

the deeper layers. These latter are broad, flat muscles and are not frequently subject to injury. The scapular muscles including the levator scapulae and rhomboideus major and minor underlie the trapezius in the upper portion of the dorsal spine and extend down toward the level of the upper limit of the latissimus dorsae. Still deeper are the muscles running from the spine to the ribs—until we reach the sacrospinalis group which is a combination of many muscles whose course essentially parallels the spinal column. The sacrospinalis group fills the sulcus between the spinous processes and the body of the vertebrae and arc of the ribs. They interdigitate in such a manner that each tends to support the other. These muscles make up the so-called lumbar mass of muscle that extends from the occiput to the sacrum just lateral to the spinous processes. They all have multiple actions depending upon the inter-relationship between them. In one instance they may serve to stabilize the spine in a certain position while another portion moves; in another they may serve to move the spine; in yet another they may serve to anchor the spine while other muscles move some other portion of the body. The nerve supply is direct from the spinal roots and so is well protected and seldom damaged.

CONTUSION

Contusion of the spine is relatively common but is not often severe. The subcutaneous spinous process may receive a blow that crushes the skin against the protruding bone beneath or may damage the underlying bone. However, the most common contusion of the spine is of the muscles lateral to the spinous processes. These muscular contusions are similar to contusions elsewhere. One should make an effort to determine whether or not there is some underlying pathologic condition. The contusion may cause a hematoma within the muscle that will require the usual treatment with cold pack, local injection and pressure, followed by heat.

The most common complication of contusion of the muscle is residual stiffness, which causes aching pain and restriction of motion for a few days subsequent to the injury. This should be treated by heat, pain-free massage and careful exercise. If the contusion is over the spinous process there may be some periosteal reaction or reaction in the supraspinous ligament which will leave a painful, tender area very sharply localized to the involved area. It may be painful enough to suggest the possibility of a fracture. Indeed, there may be an infraction or crack in the spinous process which cannot be demonstrated by x-ray but which may be diagnosed clinically. The resultant painful area can usually be relieved by physical therapy. Local injection of a long-acting anesthetic and a corticoid is of considerable value here and should give rather prompt relief, although more than one injection may be necessary. If athletic participation is to be continued following contusion, a localized protective pad should be placed over the area.

STRAIN

The spine is particularly susceptible to muscular strain because of the multiplicity of muscles involved in holding the body erect. Strain of these muscles may be extremely distressing. In the early stages it may be rather difficult to distinguish strain from contusion since the contusion may cause some hemorrhage within the muscle and may well cause pain on function of the muscle. However, the early history may be a valuable guide in diagnosis. The patient will mention some unusual occurrence. In athletics it is usually a major effort while he is somewhat off balance, such as the shot putter throwing a 16 foot shot from an imperfect stance. Strain in the athlete does not as a rule result from simple repetition of a motion, as it does in the industrial worker, since the athlete is usually in good enough shape that his muscles will tolerate the degree of strain he puts upon them in athletic use. Basically, the strain is caused by violent contraction beyond the strength of a muscle against a fixed resistance or by overstretching as the muscle attempts to resist this stretch.

On examining the patient with such an injury it is quite difficult to identify the exact muscle involved. In the shoulder girdle, where one may be able to check a certain specific function, as for example the rhomboid or levator scapulae, and find painful function limited to one motion, such identification may be quite simple, but in the spine one will consider himself fortunate if he can determine which group of muscles is involved and in some instances even which side of the back is involved since there is a great deal of generalized muscle spasm. There will be tenderness over the involved muscle and pain caused by passive stretching or active contraction. If, for example, the spinalis group is involved on the right side, one will find tenderness just to the right of the spinous process. Pain is elicited by passive forward flexion whereas active forward flexion within limits even against forceful resistance is pain-free. Passive backward bending will be pain-free since the involved muscle relaxes in this motion whereas active backward bending against resistance (as for example with the patient lying prone and raising his chest from the table) will cause pain. Passive flexion to the right is pain-free. Active flexion to the right against resistance will cause pain. To the left side passive flexion is painful and limited active motion even against resistance is not. If the condition is fairly severe and well established there will be tenderness and spasm in the whole group of spinal muscles as they endeavor to restrict the motion of the spine and to reduce the pain. In this instance the spastic muscles themselves may become painful, even though not originally involved. Diffuse pain in the back is the result. The patient presents himself with a poker spine that will resist motion in any direction.

Treatment is general and local. If there is muscle spasm, muscle relaxants are of considerable value. Preparations are available today that have minimal sedative effect and these may suffice. The tranquilizers such as meprobomate may be used if there is an element of apprehension or nervous tension in the individual. Local treatment is directed at the local lesion and to relieve muscular tension. If there is an isolated tender area, a so-called "trigger point," local injection of an anesthetic agent into this area will tend to break the reflex arc and relax the tension. Similarly, if there is evidence of rupture of the muscle fibers with hematoma formation, local injection of hyaluronidase is of value. Physical therapeutic measures are important and should consist of local heat, massage and careful active motion limited to that which is pain-free. The patient may be placed in the prone position and hot packs used in a manner similar to the blanket packs in acute anterior poliomyelitis. Body whirlpool, if available, may be used although I think that heat is more effective when the patient is lying down. For this reason I prefer diathermy, infra-red, electric pad, or electric baker.

As soon as the muscle spasm is subsiding, rehabilitative measures may be commenced but should be carried out strictly within the limits of pain. Far too often in the athlete, the urgency of his participation persuades the doctor or trainer to rehabilitate him too rapidly, with recurrence a discouraging aftermath. It is difficult to protect the upper dorsal spine by a corset. The lower dorsal spine may be fairly well protected by a full length corset which the participant should wear whenever he is in active competition. Adhesive strapping of the back to limit the motion involved is quite valuable. Since the strain is usually of the posterior muscles, the strapping should be applied so as to prevent forward flexion and lateral flexion. I believe that parallel strips are very much more effective for this than crisscross strips on the back. The back should be carefully prepared and shaved and the skin cleansed with ether before the strips are applied. One may use tincture of benzoin on the skin if he so desires. The most effective way of the strapping is shown in Figure 241. Strapping so applied is much more effective in limiting motion of the back than is a corset and is of course much less expensive if it is to be worn a relatively short time. Elastic adhesive with a sideway stretch may be substituted for regular tape and is considerably stronger. Elastic adhesive with long way stretch is not adequate in this instance since its longitudinal stretch does not give enough support. Heat can be given right through adhesive tape. The tape is changed only when it becomes ineffective. Any adhesive that is dependent upon adherence to the skin for fixation will become ineffective if the patient perspires unduly. As the condition improves and less support is needed, one may shift to elastoplast or to a cor-

Figure 241. Six to eight strips of heavy 3 inch tape are cut long enough to extend from the base of the neck to the pelvis. The first strip is placed parallel with the spinous processes and just adjacent to them. A strip is placed on either side of the spine. This is anchored below by a circular strip placed just at the level of the trochanters and extending entirely around the trunk. The pubic hair is protected by a cotton pad. Transverse strips should be overlapped. It is important to get the first strip low enough to protect the inguinal canal. The second pair of vertical strips is then applied overlapping the first by one-half. The second horizontal strip is applied overlapping about one-third. This is continued until the strapping extends 4 to 6 inches on either side of the spine. This will require three or four pairs of vertical strips. It is not necessary to use cross lap strips above. Cross-stretch elastic tape is good here. Long stretch is useless!

set, but some protection of the muscles should be continued for several weeks to prevent re-injury.

The *chronic back strain* represents a major problem. It is frequently the result of an acute strain that was not adequately treated. Every recurrence of the condition makes the final cure more difficult. It is frequently cured only after the season's athletic competition is over. The best treatment is physical therapy and protection. One is quite prone to accuse a player of being "chicken" or "dogging" it since in these back strains there are few, if any, positive findings. Little is to be gained, however, by insisting on strenuous activity in the presence of a painful back unless this seems desirable to establish the diagnosis. In the chronic condition there is usually not enough localization of pain to justify local injection. Frequently, the so-called fibrositis, which can be described as irritation of the fascial planes of the back, may be relieved by general therapy. We frequently use a combination of a muscle relaxant, salicylates and a cortisone derivative. Cortisone is well tolerated by the young athlete if the dose is small and is not continued too long. One should avoid long-continued use of any cortisone preparation.

SPRAIN

Many of the statements we have made about strain may also be applied to sprain. It may be difficult in the spine to distinguish between the two. The same force that causes muscular strain may tear some of the many ligaments of the spine. Many of these ligaments are deeply placed such as those around the articular processes and between the lateral processes and those extending between the lamina and the vertebrae. About the only ligament that can be palpated easily in the dorsal spine is the supraspinatus, which extends along the tips of the spinous processes. Injury to this ligament can be determined by localized palpable tenderness either along the course of the ligament itself or at its attachment to the bone. Extension of the spine should be pain-free but forward flexion will cause pain at the involved area if the supra- or interspinous or interlaminal ligaments are involved.

The direction of the motion that causes pain is the key for diagnosis of spinal ligament injuries. Given right side involvement with damage to the capsular ligament, one would expect the local tenderness and spasm to be on the right side in an effort to prevent stretching of this involved ligament. Forward flexion, either active or passive, is painful. Backward flexion, either active or passive, is not. Homolateral flexion to the right should relieve the symptoms and, indeed, the patient will stand pulled toward the right side. Contralateral flexion to the left will increase the pain unless it is prevented by the spastic muscle. X-ray is of little importance in the diagnosis of sprain although x-ray should be made in a serious injury in order if possible to rule out bone damage. The one condition in which x-ray may be valuable is rupture of the supra- and interspinous ligaments. In this instance, as noted above, the tenderness will be right on the ligament. Sometimes a palpable defect may be felt. If the tear is complete, forward flexion may reveal greater separation of the spinous process than at the one above and below. This is an extremely unusual injury in the dorsal spine.

Treatment of a ligament injury of the dorsal spine is the same as that of ligament injury elsewhere, that is, protection of the ligament against stretch until it is healed. A period of bed rest may be necessary if the injury is severe. The back should then be strapped in a way to prevent the motion that causes the pain (Fig. 241). This is a good test of the effectiveness of the strapping. One should be extremely careful not to discard the protection too soon since recurrence is as likely in the spine as at the ankle or knee when the injury occurs in the latter.

DISLOCATION

The ultimate of sprain is dislocation (Fig. 242). This is extremely unusual in the dorsal spine. Even in the mayhem caused by the modern automobile, the dorsal spine is infrequently dislocated. As mentioned in the discussion of the anatomy, the vertebrae are very securely bound together and have a good deal of bony as well as ligamentous stability. If there is dislocation, the injury will obviously be a major one. I do not comprehend the so-called "dislocation" of the "manipulators," who will make an x-ray film and glibly describe a dislocation in a normal appearing spine. Following manipulation, this "dislocation" is reduced. Anatomically and physiologically such a thing is virtually impossible in the dorsal spine.

FRACTURE

Fracture of the dorsal spine is more common than dislocation but is extremely unusual in ordinary athletic competition such as football, basketball, baseball and track. Some of the more violent sports such as automobile racing, polo playing and the like do cause spinal fractures. The fracture may be of the body or of the arches or of the spinous processes.

Figure 242. *A,* Fraction-dislocation of D-12 on L-1. Note backward displacement of L-1 and complete dislocation of the articular facet. *B,* Reduced and held with wire around transverse processes and spinal fusion. Neurological symptoms in lower extremities completely disappeared. *C,* Fracture-dislocation of D-11 on D-12. Paraplegia. *D,* Postoperative film showing internal fixation and graft. *E,* Complete dislocation of D-11 on D-12 without apparent fracture which resulted in complete paraplegia.

Compression Fracture of the Body

Fracture of the body is usually caused by sharp forward flexion, the so-called "compression" fracture (Fig. 243). The patient will give a history of sharp forward flexion such as falling violently on the buttocks or of having his head forcibly pushed between his knees. This tends to flex the very rigid dorsal spine, the posterior ligaments hold, and the force is taken by the anterior portion of the body of the vertebra. This cancellous bone gives way to a greater or lesser degree. The anterior corner of the vertebra may be broken off or more commonly there is compression of the vertebra so that the cancellous bone may be impacted into itself.

There is nothing about the ordinary compression fracture of the dorsal spine that will prevent ambulation so that the patient may actually be up and around in spite of his back complaint. On examination, although it may be difficult to determine the exact degree of injury, forward flexion will ordinarily cause considerable complaint. This may be elicited by having the patient lie supine. When the operator flexes his neck with the chin against the chest, there will usually be localized pain at the fracture area. This test will also be positive for ligament injury. Motion in any direction will probably cause pain, even in an impacted fracture.

Careful x-ray study will usually reveal this lesion although it may be easily overlooked if the deformity is mild and the x-ray film inadequate or inadequately studied. In the x-ray the vertebrae should be carefully measured anteriorly to determine whether a single vertebrae is narrower than its fellows. This may be extremely misleading, however, since frequently one or more dorsal vertebrae will be of smaller size than the others. Of more importance is the appearance of the bone itself. A fracture line may be visible. The bone may be compacted so that this particular vertebra not only appears smaller but seems more dense than its neighbor.

Treatment. If the compression is definite and amounts to as much as 25 per cent of the height of the body, I think an attempt should be made to reduce it in the young athlete. In the older person this amount of compression may be accepted in order to speed up healing but I do not believe this is acceptable in the

Figure 243. A spinal injury with compression of D-9. The patient suffered persistent localized pain. *B*, Careful study of D-9 reveals unilateral compression on the right. This can be seen in the lateral view (*A*). Note that the superior surface of D-9 presents two cortical shadows whereas the inferior surface shows a single shadow.

Figure 244.   *A,* Severe compression fracture of L-1, preoperative view. *B,* Correction by the jack method. The "X" marks the head of the jack which actually is one vertebra above L-1. These x-rays were made with a surgical portable machine without a Bucky diaphragm, which accounts for their fogginess.

youngster. The exact area involved is determined and an effort is made to correct the vertebra by manipulation. This will not correct in a simple convex bed if the bone is impacted. The usual methods of hyperextension in which the entire back is extended are needlessly handicapping to the patient since to be effective the extension must proceed to the point where all of the anterior ligaments are taut before there is any effect at all upon the broken vertebra. Local hyperextension is much more effective.

For local hyperextension I think the various modifications of the "jack method" are by far the best. In this method, with the patient supine on a suitable fracture table, the jack with suitable protective cap is placed directly under the spinous process of the vertebra involved. By elevating the jack the corrective pressure is applied to this vertebra alone and the back is locally extended (Fig. 244). This causes some local hyperextension of the adjacent vertebrae but it is not necessary to hyperextend the entire spine. Once the vertebra has come up to its normal height, a suitable plaster jacket can be applied, again without generalized hyperextension but with local extension, the pressure points being the pubis and sternum in front, the fracture site behind.

The patient, assuming that he is an athletic individual who can well tolerate bed rest, should be kept recumbent for four to six weeks since it is very difficult to apply a plaster jacket that will completely eliminate recurrent compression of the vertebra if weight bearing is allowed. In any event there may be some loss of correction—a fact that prompts some surgeons to believe that no attempt should be made to correct a compression fracture. The cast should be worn for six to eight weeks to be followed by an adequate brace. Indeed, a brace of the three point hyperextension type with pressure on the pubis and sternum and over the involved vertebra posteriorly may be substituted for the cast. X-ray examination will determine when union is complete but athletic competition should not be permitted for at least four months and probably six would be better. There is some danger of late aseptic necrosis of this vertebra if weight bearing is permitted too soon.

In minimal compression fractures of the vertebral body, rehabilitation can be much more rapidly carried out if the compression deformity is accepted. In these cases a protective brace need be worn only a few weeks until the fracture is well consolidated. In fracture of the anterior corner of the vertebra a differentiation should if possible be made between a snubbing fracture caused by flexion and an avulsion fracture caused by hyperextension, since in the latter protection should be in flexion rather than in extension. Often the history of the injury will provide a valuable guide. The increased pain on backward bending as compared to forward will also be significant. Sometimes the picture made on backward bending will show actual separation of this fragment.

Arch Fracture

Fracture of the lateral processes of the dorsal spine is extremely infrequent since they are well protected by the ribs. If it does occur, a corset, brace or body jacket may be worn until union has taken place. Fractures of the laminae or interarticular portions of the bone or of the articular processes themselves require very careful examination by x-ray for diagnosis. Adequate support by brace or cast should be worn for six to eight weeks to prevent painful excessive formation of callus or nonunion. In fracture of the spinous process, protection should be against forward flexion. If there is separation of the fragment, a good deal of time will be saved by its early removal (Fig. 245) as a primary measure rather than to wait for nonunion and then remove the fragment if there is resultant pain. Separation is much more frequent in the upper dorsal spine and may be the result of avulsion of the tip by

Figure 245. "Sprain" of the upper dorsal spine with persistent complaint. Early x-ray studies had not adequately visualized this area. More careful x-ray technique revealed the ununited fragments of D-1 and 2. Uneventful recovery followed removal of the fragments but months of disability might have been prevented by more careful early treatment.

sharp forward flexion of the neck and upper spine or by a direct blow. It is occasonally caused by muscle jerk as described under the so-called "clay shoveler's fracture" in the cervical spine.

LUMBAR SPINE

ANATOMICAL CONSIDERATIONS

Whereas the dorsal vertebrae have a good deal of inherent stability as indicated above, the lumbar spine (Fig. 246) lying between the rigid pelvis and thorax is so designed as to permit greater mobility and yet provide this quality of inherent stability. The vertebrae in this area are massive. The convexity of the spine forward of this area is caused by very heavy bodies which are taller and slightly wider apart in front than behind. The entire arch is massive with heavy lateral processes extending well away from the midline to add additional leverage for the muscle attachments. The laminae are heavy. The articular processes, which in the dorsal spine angulate to form a diagonal line with the body, in the lumbar spine are much more in the sagittal plane. While the processes on the vertebrae above do lock behind the one below they are at a good deal flatter angle. Hence, the mobility in the spine is largely in flexion and in extension in which the intervertebral joints serve more or less as an axis with motion permitted by compression and expansion of the disc and by separation and apposition of the spinous processes. There is but little rotatory motion in the lumbar spine.

The muscles of this area of the back (Fig. 247) are very massive. The sacrospinalis group interdigitating up into the dorsal spine consists of heavy muscles arising from the pelvis to attach to the spinous process and to the vertebral bodies and act as firm stabilizers of the trunk over the pelvis. The muscles of the abdomen complete the stabilizing effect in front. These muscles extending from the pubis to the ribs serve as anterior guy wires to provide active forward flexion and to prevent overextension. The heavy mass of spinal muscle also serves to protect the posterior portion of the abdominal cavity and prevent injury to the kidneys, spleen and liver.

CONTUSION

This area of the spine is frequently contused but fortunately the injury is usually not particularly severe. The only subcutaneous bones in this region are the tips of the spinous processes. These lie in a sulcus between the two erector spinae muscles so that the muscle ordinarily will absorb the blow unless it is by a relatively small object. Contusion of the muscle suffers the same complications as contusion of muscle anywhere. The history is of a blow with localized tenderness at the area of the blow and moderate pain on function. After a few hours muscle spasm supervenes which tightens up the whole group of muscles on that side, apparently in an attempt to prevent painful motion. At this time the differentiation from strain may be very difficult. In a simple contusion, active muscle contraction is not especially painful.

Figure 246.   Skeletal view from the front and from behind. In both figures certain of the ligaments of the trunk and extremities are shown. (From Anson, "Atlas of Human Anatomy.")

Rectus capitis posterior minor

Rectus capitis posterior major

Obliquus capitis superior

Obliquus capitis inferior

Semispinalis capitis

Longissimus capitis

Longissimus cervicis

Iliocostalis cervicis and thoracis

T 6

Semispinalis thoracis

Multifidus

Erector spinae

Splenius capitis

Semispinalis cervicis

Splenius cervicis

C 7

Iliocostalis cervicis

Longissimus cervicis

Iliocostalis thoracis

Spinalis thoracis

Longissimus thoracis

Iliocostalis lumborum

L 1

Figure 247.　　The chief muscles of the back. (From Hollinshead, "Functional Anatomy of the Limbs and Back.")

If any *treatment* is necessary, application of ice followed by heat is indicated. If a massive hematoma appears to be present, an attempt can be made to aspirate it and inject it with hyaluronidase although the indication is difficult to determine in these heavy muscles. If the contusion seems to be severe, attention should be paid to the underlying structures to determine the possibility of a fracture of the lateral or spinous processes.

STRAIN

Muscular strain results either from overstretching or from overuse of the muscle. It may be difficult to distinguish from sprain. Fundamentally, any active motion of the involved muscle against resistance will cause pain even though the ligament is not put on tension by actual movement. For example, if you have the patient stand erect and ask him to bend sideways and you resist this motion so that he does not actually bend, he should have a complaint of pain if the involvement is in the muscle but no complaint if the involvement is in the ligament. The muscle involved is palpably tender and passive stretching of the muscle will cause pain. If the strain is on the right side of the spine, active flexion to the right against resistance will be painful whereas in ligament injury it should not be. Passive flexion to the opposite side will be painful as soon as the injured muscle is put under tension. Backward bending against resistance will be painful and forward flexion will become painful only when the excursion is sufficient to stretch the muscle.

The *treatment* of the acute strain is quite similar to that of sprain; that is, rest, protection and local heat. Protection is necessary, however, against active use of the muscle rather than against excessive range of motion. This is a good deal more difficult to accomplish. The patient should be instructed not to make any movement causing pain. If the area can be treated promptly and adequately, recovery will be prompt.

Unfortunately this condition is often inadequately treated and chronic strain supervenes with all its implications. The only cure for the chronic strain is prolonged rest until recovery is complete, after which gradual rehabilitation of muscle can be carried out. If the rehabilitation is too rapid the pain will recur. If athletic participation is begun during the recovery period a single over-movement may start the whole cycle over again. Localized trigger areas in the muscle may be present and, if so, injection of a long-acting anesthetic followed by injection of a corticoid preparation into this area will be of benefit. This treatment is of little value in the case of diffuse muscle involvement, however. Muscle relaxants are useful, particularly in conjunction with physical therapy. Rehabilitation must be gradual, persistent, and kept within the limits of pain.

The actual protection of the back can be accomplished first by bed rest, later by a cast or brace, lastly by taping (Fig. 241). It is important to bear in mind, however, that taping is not as effective in strain as it is in sprain because, while the taping protects against overstretching of the muscle, it will not protect against muscle contraction.

A chronic strain tends to recur and can be extremely troublesome to the athlete. In many cases we advise a lumbosacral corset to help support the back and protect against overstretching—the same measure that is used in a case of chronic

Figure 248.   The lumbosacral corset.

sprain. This is more effective than adhesive since with the latter the skin becomes quite irritated, particularly after repeated applications. The corset should go well up over the lower ribs, particularly posteriorly, and well down on the sacrum if it is to provide much protection (Fig. 248).

SPRAIN

Sprain is frequent in the mobile lumbar spine with its many ligaments giving support of the various joints. The supraspinous ligament, which extends along the tips of the spinous processes, is particularly susceptible. This sprain can be diagnosed by the presence of tenderness over the ligament or over the tip of the spinous process where the ligament attaches. Active contraction of the muscles to pull the spine into hyperextension is pain-free, as is passive extension. Active flexion of the back, as in attempting to sit up from the supine position, is pain-free until tension is put on the process by forcing the head toward the knees. Passive hyperflexion of the spine will cause pain. This condition is treated by protection against overflexion by strapping. Activity can be permitted so long as the ligament is protected. Occasionally the ligament will be pulled in two or will be avulsed from the bone and more extensive treatment will be indicated. In this instance immobilization in extension in a brace or with a plaster jacket is in order. If the fragment of the spinous process does not unite, it may be removed. Primary early repair of the ligament would be advisable but so infrequently is the condition diagnosed in the early stage that this is seldom practical.

Injury to the other ligaments of the back is much more difficult to determine with exactitude. The interspinous ligament is not frequently damaged because it has elastic fibers and is not readily overstretched. However, the articular ligaments around the apophyseal joints are frequently damaged, as is the anterior spinal ligament or the lateral spinal ligaments. Whether or not the ligamentum flavum is damaged by hyperflexion is problematical since it, too, is an elastic structure and probably will allow as much motion without damage as the range of flexion of the back will permit. Diagnosis of these sprains is on the basis of tests bringing stress upon certain areas. In the diagnosis of sprain it should be remembered that passive movements which put stress on the involved ligament will cause pain so that sprain of the capsule on the left would cause pain on flexion to the right or on flexion forward, etc.

Treatment of the acute sprain is to place the ligament at complete rest. Unfortunately this is not often done and a chronic sprain ensues. In the acute sprain, muscle spasm is a characteristic symptom. Ideally the patient should be put at bed rest, given muscle relaxants, inductive heat or electric pad until the acute symptoms subside at which time he should be treated by elastic strapping or corset to protect the area until the ligament is healed. During this time athletics should not be permitted. A sprain is easier to protect than a strain since, if the range of motion is limited, there is no stress on the ligament. For this reason, competition can be allowed much earlier in a sprain of the back than in a strain.

DISLOCATION-SUBLUXATION

Sprain of the lumbar spine rarely goes on to actual dislocation. There may be subluxation, which occurs when the interspinous ligament tears and the articular processes tend to disengage. If this is spontaneously relieved, it should be treated as a sprain. Unilateral dislocation in the lumbar spine is extremely rare and is not usually to be considered an athletic injury. A frank dislocation of the lumbar spine occurs only after severe violence, such as a fall from a height or motor accident. This is a serious injury. X-ray will reveal the deformity (Fig. 249) and in most cases open reduction will be required. This type of dislocation may cause severe neurological deficit. However, it is not as damaging in the lumbar spine as it is higher because the cord proper does not extend into the lumbar area and so is not

Figure 249.   *A,* Complete dislocation of L-2 on L-3. This was treated by open reduction and graft. There were no permanent neurological sequelae. This is possible in spite of the intact lamina because the medullary portion of the cord stops just above this level and the cauda will tolerate much more trauma than will the spinal cord. *B,* Results six months later. The distortion of the body of L-3 may well be due to damage of the epiphysis since the original film does not show any compression here.

primarily involved. The peripheral nerves in the cauda will stand a great deal more trauma than will the substance of the cord.

FRACTURE

Fracture may occur in the body of a lumbar vertebra, a lateral or spinous process, or in some portion of the arch.

Figure 250.   A, Severe compression fracture of L-4 following violent jack-knifing. B, Eight months later note complete restoration of vertebral height by "jack" decompression.

Figure 251.   A, Relatively mild compression fracture of the superior portion of the body of L-1 at eight weeks post injury. B, Note persistent deformity following failure to correct compression. This relatively mild fracture has comparatively severe residual whereas the very severe fracture in Figure 250 is pain-free.

Fracture of the Body of the Vertebra

Fracture of the body of the vertebra (Fig. 250) is extremely rare as an athletic injury. It is a major injury and is readily recognized as such. X-ray examination will reveal the deformity and anything beyond minimal deformity should be reduced as indicated above under dorsal spine. Failure to correct the compression may be disabling (Fig. 251). Athletic competition will be limited for many months.

Fracture of the Lateral Process

Fracture of the lateral processes is quite common in athletes. It should be noted that the lumbar vertebrae have spikelike lateral processes, some of which are quite thin or have a narrow neck. These processes are ruptured by two different mechanisms—a direct blow as a complication of contusion, and violent exertion of the muscle; or by a combination of the two. There is a difference of opinion as to the relative frequency of the two causes since the combination of a blow and exertion often prevails. However, I think it is quite possible that a direct blow will account for the breaking off of a single lateral process. Fractures of multiple processes are almost always of the avulsion type (Fig. 252). In any event the significance of the fracture is not the broken bone but the muscle injury. The distal fragment frequently separates quite widely and nonunion is often the result. The patient reports a history of a blow on the back by the knee or foot, usually at the time of pretty violent exercise during play. This causes immediate pain in the back which may be quite severe or may be relatively minor. As participation continues, the pain increases and muscles become more spastic. The player's body will be pulled toward the same side. This is more noticeable after a period of rest and then re-initiation of activity. There is localized tenderness over the area of injury. Stretching of the involved side by contralateral bending causes pain. Homolateral bending

Figure 252.   Fracture of transverse processes of the left second and third lumbar vertebrae.

against resistance also is painful and passive forward flexion will cause pain. Active backward flexion will be painful.

Treatment depends almost entirely upon the symptoms present. If the patient is having severe pain and is seriously disabled he should be placed at bed rest with application of cold, followed by heat. In two or three days when the most acute symptoms have subsided (immediately if the primary symptoms are not too severe), some support should be applied to the back. Here again there is a great difference of opinion as to just what the nature of this support should be. I think this depends entirely upon the symptoms. If the patient is having severe pain and marked muscle spasm, a light weight body jacket will give him good protection. He can wear this ten days or two weeks and then substitute a corset. If the symptoms are not too severe, the back may be strapped or a corset applied which limits the activity somewhat and gives some degree of support although not as adequately as the cast. Ordinarily the symptoms will subside within three to six weeks. Infrequently in cases of nonunion there will be persistent pain to the point that removal of the fragment becomes necessary.

The player may be allowed to participate in sports just as soon as the back does not hurt him. The pain level is a good indication for continuing or discontinuing the treatment. After recovery there is no need for any restriction of activity even if nonunion of one or more processes is persistent.

Fracture of the Spinous Process

Fracture of the spinous process in the lumbar spine occurs from three different causes. One cause is sharp hyperflexion that pulls off the tip of the process; another is sharp hyperextension that impinges one process against the other and breaks one or the other. The third cause is a direct blow that mechanically knocks off one of the projecting processes. The condition may ordinarily be diagnosed clinically

Figure 253. Avulsion fracture of the inferior border of the spinous process of the third lumbar vertebra.

Figure 254. Vertical fracture through the lamina and articular process of L-5 visualized only on this right oblique view.

by the sharp localization of pain, occasionally by the unstable spinous process. It can be confirmed by x-ray made with a technique to visualize the spinous processes (Fig. 253). If there is actual separation of the fragment in the distal 1 inch of the process, a great deal of time and trouble will be saved by removing this fragment since it will be very slow to heal and the case will likely terminate with pain on violent exertion. If the fracture is near the base of the process or in the arch, it will heal much more rapidly and completely, provided the spine is immobilized in extension, preferably by a plaster cast. Athletic competition is interdicted until healing is complete.

Arch Fracture

Any fracture involving the arch of the vertebra is potentially serious because of the danger of neurological involvement. The fracture may be between the articular processes (Fig. 254). It may be through the arch at the base of the process. It may actually be of the articular process. In any event, once the fracture is recognized the patient must be immobilized to permit it to heal since painful function may result if union is imperfect. This is a serious injury which should be treated as such. Athletic competition is forbidden until healing is complete.

NONTRAUMATIC DEFORMITIES OF THE SPINE

KYPHOSIS DORSALIS JUVENILIS (SCHEUERMANN'S DISEASE)

This condition is essentially a disturbance of the growth of the vertebra. It is often generalized as evidenced by wedging of many dorsal vertebrae with osteochrondrosis of the bodies ofttimes going on to fragmentation (Figs. 255 and 256). Occasionally only a single vertebra or adjacent ones may be involved and this may

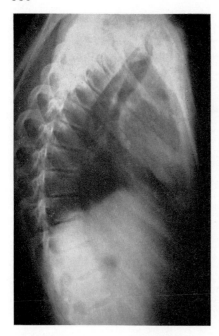

Figure 255.   Generalized dorsalis juvenilis epiphysitis. Note wedging of all the dorsal and lumbar vertebrae.

cause some confusion in the early stages. There is usually no particular problem in diagnosis. There is no evidence that this condition is actually caused by a single injury. However, it seems quite apparent that malformation of the vertebrae is definitely increased by active or passive forward flexion and by exercise.

The patient should be protected by a hyperextension brace to place the weight back on the arches and articular processes and to take it off the defective portion of the anterior body. The problem here will be with that person who wants to con-

Figure 256.   Localized vertebral epiphysitis involving D-12, L-1 and 2. Note characteristic deformity with interference of growth. A, The extreme involvement between L-1 and 2 may lead to erroneous diagnosis. B, Healing six months later. C, Final result six years later shows amazing restoration of architecture with only minimal kyphosis due almost entirely to wedging of L-3. This boy had prolonged protection against anterior weight bearing which I think was the factor in his good recovery.

tinue athletic competition. Certainly in the active stage of this condition, athletics should be banned. As the replacement phase of the condition develops, as evidenced by improved density of the vertebrae and coalescence of the fragmented areas and by the absence of pain, the patient may be allowed to participate although he should wear protection against flexion until the bodies are completely reconstituted. I recall one young man who was an ardent baseball player. Toward the end of the course of the involvement, we permitted him to play baseball in a body jacket. He was a catcher and used the cast for a chest protector much to the detriment of the cast but apparently with no bad results to his back (Fig. 256). These cases resemble Perthes' disease in that they cause very little discomfort and yet may give rise to marked deformity (Fig. 257). They occur in a slightly older age group (12 to 15 years) than Perthes' disease and *limiting* activity at this age may be extremely difficult when the patient is not actually having many symptoms. Nevertheless it should be done.

Of more difficulty diagnostically is the localized manifestation of the same condition in which one or two or three of the vertebrae may be involved with quite major changes and yet be essentially pain-free, until an injury calls attention to this area or until the area becomes spontaneously painful. It may be that the injury is entirely coincidental. Here again it is necessary to reduce the patient's activity and by serial x-rays determine when the bone is repaired sufficiently to permit the stresses of athletic competition.

One does not add to his popularity by refusing permission to these young men to participate. Nevertheless a firm stand is vital, particularly if there is any major involvement, since increasing deformity may result in a persistent gibbus.

Figure 257. Untreated dorsal epiphysitis of only moderate severity but note extreme deformity.

Figure 258.   Spina bifida occulta in first sacral vertebra. This is asymptomatic and of no significance.

CONGENITAL DEFORMITIES

Congenital deformities are much more common in the lower back than in the upper, specifically about the fourth and fifth lumbar and the first sacral vertebrae. These deformities are not caused by athletic injuries. However, they often become a problem to the athlete since when recognized following an injury a decision must immediately be made on the advisability of his continuing in athletics and, indeed, on the treatment of the acute condition. The great majority of these conditions do not affect the function of the spine enough to require restriction of activity.

Spina Bifida Occulta

The most common of these deformities is spina bifida occulta in which there is failure of fusion of the arch of one or more of the vertebrae posteriorly (Fig. 258). This is a common finding and is ordinarily of no significance. The player should not be alarmed or be told that he has a dangerous condition of the lower back or that he should be careful the rest of his life. Exceptionally, a wide open spina bifida involving several vertebrae may be of sufficient concern to require the use of additional support or even the recommendation that some less strenuous activity be followed.

Spondylolysis or Spondylolisthesis

Spondylolysis (Fig. 259) is the failure of fusion of the arch of the vertebra, usually between the articular processes. Spondylolisthesis (Fig. 260) is spondylolysis in which there is displacement of the superior vertebra forward on the one below. This laminal defect does, indeed, cause weakness of the spine but of an

Figure 259. Spondylolysis. No slipping of the body forward although there is some narrowing of the disc space posteriorly. The arch defect was confirmed by the oblique view (not shown).

Figure 260. A, Grade 3 spondylolisthesis. Note the narrow disc space, the juxta-chondral sclerosis, the spurring, all indicating a chronic process.

B, Grade 1 spondylolisthesis. Note arch defect even in the lateral view. Note failure of fusion of S-1 to S-2.

extremely variable degree. Many persons have spondylolysis or spondylolisthesis all their lives and never know it. However, if the athlete is having trouble in the lower back and spondylolysis is discovered, I think one is justified in restricting him to some of the less active sports. Athletics basically should not cause serious damage to the spine but he probably will have discomfort to the point that he will not be very effective. After the pain is relieved he should be advised to wear a lumbosacral support or sacroiliac belt during periods of active competition.

In actual spondylolisthesis there is separation at the line of defect, and here again it may be difficult to decide on the proper procedure. If there is sufficient pain, one should seriously consider treatment of the condition rather than interdiction of athletics. However, if the pain occurs only on violent exercise such as football, I think one is justified in discontinuing the football to see how the patient gets along with his condition. If he continues to have pain, treatment should be recommended. The boy of 14 or 15 years of age with spondylolisthesis who is already having pain in the back almost inevitably will come to treatment at a later time in spite of any recommendation that he decrease his activities, since degenerative changes will certainly occur as the years pass. It is quite unlikely that he will become pain-free as he gets older. In such a case one cannot assume that simple banning of athletic competition will mean that the boy is inactive. If he is an active, energetic type he will occupy himself with an equally strenous occupation. If he is the indolent type, one questions the advisability of encouraging further indolence to protect a condition that might be remedied surgically.

Variations in Sacral Fusion

As has been noted above, the sacrum originally is made up of five bones which during adolescence fuse into a solid mass. Various anomalous conditions may arise as a part of this process. The lower lumbar vertebra may participate to some extent in the sacral fusion and, indeed, may completely fuse so that there is *sacralization of the fifth lumbar vertebra* (Figs. 261 and 262). This is of no significance activity-wise. If the fusion is incomplete, with one side fusing and the other not, some imbalance may arise in the lower back and occasionally pain will be present. The same can be said here as was said of spondylolisthesis, namely, that a boy having pain in his early teens will inevitably have pain when he becomes older. One should therefore proceed to complete the fusion, after which unlimited activity can be permitted. A symptom-free unilateral sacralization is of no significance— and most of the cases are symptom-free. The same is true of *lumbarization of the first sacral vertebra*. If a portion of the sacrum fails to fuse this is of no significance (Fig. 260, B). Certainly the fibrous fusion is extremely firm and highly unlikely to be damaged by any type of athletic competition. I would not recommend the wearing of a belt or brace or other support. On the other hand, a sprain of the back in which there is a congenital anomaly may be somewhat more resistant to treatment than uncomplicated sprain and protection should be given, not for the congenital anomaly but for the accompanying sprain.

Other Anomalies

Other conditions such as hemivertebrae (Fig. 263), scoliosis (Fig. 264), kyphosis (Fig. 265) and increased lordosis (Fig. 266) must be managed on an individ-

Figure 261.   Unilateral sacralization of the fifth lumbar vertebra. *A,* Note the massive formation of sacral ala on the left side with relatively normal transverse process on the right. *B,* Lateral view showing the very narrow disc space and the massive arches.

Figure 262.   Complete sacralization of L-5.

ual basis. In many instances, such as extreme lordosis, athletic competition may be valuable from the standpoint of posture. It must be accompanied by instruction in the treatment of the primary condition. The patients must be judged symptomatically. The deformity itself is not necessarily disabling if it is not accompanied

Figure   263.   Hemivertebra   of   the
lumbar spine.

Figure 264.   A, Moderate scoliosis, asymptomatic. B, This asymptomatic scoliosis was
found incidentally in a college athlete who had ruptured his knee cartilage while playing
varsity football.

Figure 265.   Moderate dorsal kyphosis, probably from asymptomatic mild dorsal epiphysitis although it may be postural.

Figure 266.   Typical   adolescent lordosis in nine year old boy. The vertebral epiphyses have not yet ossified but these vertebrae are normal for this age. Note that the separate pieces of the sacrum have not yet fused. This condition presents no contra-indication to athletics. On the contrary, physical fitness should be encouraged.

by signs of secondary involvement such as nerve root pressure and muscle contracture. There is no justification for making a chronic invalid out of a patient because of an x-ray diagnosis of a spinal anomaly.

SPINAL DISC LESIONS

In recent years the diagnosis of disc rupture with attendant nerve root injury has been a major development and consequently must be considered in the treatment of athletes. In my experience this condition has rarely resulted from athletic participation. However, once a ruptured disc is present it tends to be recurrent, and strenuous athletics should be banned until the condition is corrected. The disc is the pad lying between the two vertebrae. The periphery of the pad, the so-called annulus fibrosus, is the firm ligamentous and cartilaginous structure that forms a ring within which is enclosed the softer nucleus pulposus. This arrangement acts as a hydraulic shock absorber between the bodies of the vertebrae. Infrequently the annulus may be subject to damage by excessive motion. Compression of the two vertebrae forcing the bones together puts pressure on the inner mass and causes it to bulge so, theoretically, the disc could rupture. However, the normal annulus is so strong that excessive pressure in a single violent effort usually will break the disc into the body of the vertebra or compress the vertebra rather than rupture the annulus.

Classical ruptured disc has its origin in a degenerative annulus. The disc commonly ruptures posteriorly owing to the lordosis of the lumbar spine, which causes eccentric weight bearing with an inordinate amount of weight on the back margin of the disc. It is probable that pressure on the disc causes it to rupture or herniate through an area of the annulus already defective. This pressure may be caused by anything that raises the pressure within the disc, such as leaning forward to tie the shoe, but is more likely to be caused by lifting—and particularly lifting in a rather strained position, the same sort of effort that would cause muscular strain. The athlete is not in the common age bracket for ruptured disc; additionally, his splendid muscular condition takes a good deal of strain off the disc itself.

The classical symptoms will not be reiterated here. One should suspect disc involvement in an injury in which the pain follows the sciatic distribution in the leg and is increased by coughing or sneezing or by raising interspinal pressure by pressure on the jugular veins. The difficult case will be the mild one in which there are few nerve root signs. There is some stiffness in the back but not at a disabling level. Shall this patient be allowed to participate in sports? I think the case must be individualized and some balance struck between the urgency for his participation and the danger of it. If athletic competition will accentuate his discomfort he probably will require definitive treatment anyway, so he likely is doing himself no major harm by participating. Whether or not he is effective is a wholly different thing. Thus, while a ruptured disc must be considered in many conditions of the back, it is not really a major problem in the treatment of athletes.

16

Injuries of the
Pelvis and Hip

IT IS CONVENIENT to include both the pelvis and hip under a single heading, since these areas are closely related anatomically.

ANATOMICAL CONSIDERATIONS

The pelvis is a uniquely devised mechanism designed to transfer the body weight from the single weight-bearing axis of the trunk to the bipolar weight-bearing of the lower extremities (Fig. 246). It is designed to have a whippletree effect. Thus, the spine attaches to the pelvis by a single connection to the sacrum and for stability is anchored in all four directions by various combinations of ligaments and muscles. Through the bony ring of the pelvis the weight is transferred from the spinal column to the two lower extremities so that of necessity the pelvic ring must be intact in order to give stability. The primary function of the pelvis including the bones, joints, ligaments and muscles is this mechanical transfer of weight. A secondary function of the bony pelvis is protection of the pelvic viscera. Enclosed within the pelvis are the bladder, the female genitalia, the rectum and the great vessels and nerves extending to the lower extremities.

At the lumbosacral level the spinal muscles descend to attach to the sacrum and the wings of the ilia. The hip joint is an extremely stable ball-and-socket joint—stable, that is, from the standpoint of dislocation. However, by virtue of the fact that it is a ball and socket there is no bony restriction of motion in the hip as in other joints. The functional stability of the hip depends entirely upon the muscu-

389

lature about the hip. The strong capsule and capsular ligaments maintain the ball within the socket but the stability of the thigh in relation to the pelvis and hence to the trunk is entirely controlled by muscle. There is no stable position in the flail hip as there is, for example, in the flail knee. The knee can be locked in extension by the stabilizing effect of the posterior capsule and collateral ligaments with no muscle action involved. Not so the hip. To effect stability the hip is surrounded by a great mass of muscle which must be adequate to support the trunk in the erect position, and indeed in many other positions. The muscles must also serve to propel the trunk by action of the lower extremities and to give powerful impetus to the lower extremities in relation to the trunk, as in kicking.

The various muscles have wholly different effects as the relative position of the trunk and lower extremities is altered. Careful analysis of the types of force involved will often give a valuable lead as to the injury to be expected.

CONTUSION

Contusions about the pelvis may be of almost any kind or degree since in some areas the pelvic bone is subcutaneous and other areas it is surrounded by masses of muscle, Contusions in general should be managed as is contusion anywhere, depending upon the degree of injury. The local area may be injected with a long-acting anesthetic agent plus hyaluronidase. A compression bandage and cold compresses in the early stage, followed by heat, are useful. Protection against re-injury is by contact pads rather than by strapping.

Muscular contusion frequently involves the buttock and if severe enough may be quite disabling for a period. In a severe contusion with major local symptoms, careful investigation should be made for a possible fracture of the underlying bone. The contusion may result in a deep-seated hematoma which is virtually impossible to diagnose in the early stages. It is not common for a hematoma in the pelvic muscles to progress to myositis ossificans. Occasionally a contusion of the tuberosity of the ischium will cause an ischial bursitis or an ischial periostitis progressing to actual spur formation. Of major importance in contusion is the ruling out of a more serious injury. Subcutaneous hematoma along the crest of the ilium may be extremely tender and require protective padding all season. It can be distinguished from deeper injury in that functional movement of the muscles attached to the iliac crest does not cause increased pain.

Because the types of injury to the pelvis vary greatly depending upon the anatomical structure of the area involved, they will be discussed on a regional basis.

INJURIES IN THE VICINITY OF THE ILIAC CREST

Contusion and Strain

A pelvic area that is particularly susceptible to injury is the iliac crest. This area extends from the anterosuperior spine in front over the crest of the pelvic bone (ilium) to the posterosuperior spine in back. Along its outer margin attach the large muscles going to the lower extremities and on its inner margin the group of muscles going to the abdomen and spine (Fig. 267). The area between is largely subcutaneous.

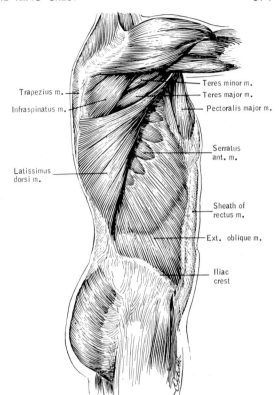

Trapezius m.

Infraspinatus m.

Latissimus
dorsi m.

Teres minor m.

Teres major m.

Pectoralis major m.

Serratus
ant. m.

Sheath of
rectus m.

Ext. oblique m.

Iliac
crest

Figure 267. Drawing of iliac crest, subcutaneous but with the hip muscles below and the trunk muscles above. (From Anson, "Atlas of Human Anatomy.")

The vast majority of injuries about the pelvic crest are contusions that will respond promptly and well to the simple measures outlined below. A definitive diagnosis should be made at the time of injury to rule out a more serious injury. Too often a more serious injury is detected only after ordinary measures fail to give relief. This results in a delay in definitive treatment for the serious condition that may well prolong morbidity and cause greater permanent disability.

Injury along the pelvic rim—the so-called *"hip pointer"*—may consist of a contusion of the bone of the iliac crest, a periostitis of the iliac crest, a strain, an avulsion of the muscles attaching to the crest, or other pathology. It is of considerable importance to determine the exact nature of the injury since the treatment, particularly the protective treatment, and also to a considerable extent the immediate prognosis may depend a great deal upon the muscles involved. The injury frequently damages the attachment of the abdominal muscles along the anterior and inner portion of the iliac crest. This is caused by forceful contraction of the abdominal muscles while the trunk is being forced to the contralateral side. This results in some degree of detachment along the iliac crest, the separation varying from a few fibers to complete detachment of the entire muscle from the bone (Fig. 268).

I recall one case of a high school boy who threw himself in front of an opponent in making a block. He had immediate severe pain along the iliac crest with severe disability. When examined a few hours later he was able to walk with the hand on the involved side dangling below the knee with the rib cage drawn down into the pelvis. Any effort to straighten him up from this position was strenuously

Figure 268.   Drawings showing degrees of detachment of the aponeurosis at the iliac crest. *A,*
    A small tear. *B,* An appreciable tear with bare bone exposed. *C,* Avulsion of the caput.

resisted because of severe pain. Examination revealed extreme tenderness along
the entire iliac crest. When we were able to get him to relax a little, a palpable
defect was found above the iliac crest. At operation an incision was made completely encircling the iliac crest. There had been complete avulsion of the aponeurotic attachment to the crest of the ilium, so that the attachments of the iliacus and
the abdominal muscles remained together but were completely pulled away from the
iliac bone. The whole medial crest and interior surface of the ilium were denuded.
The damage was easily repaired by placing drill holes along the iliac crest and pulling
the detached cap snugly back into position on the crest. The boy had a good recovery
and went on to play varsity collegiate football without disability. This is admittedly
an unusual case but I think it explains the variation in degree of "hip pointer" and
shows why treatment is so often disappointing.

    At examination to determine the type of injury, certain findings are of extreme
importance. The location of the tenderness is not particularly diagnostic since tenderness will be noted in both contusion of bone and avulsion of muscle. In contusion, however, contraction of the involved muscle will not cause pain. On the
other hand, if the athlete has pain on contracting his abdominal muscles or on
flexing to the opposite side, one must assume some degree of damage to the muscle
attachment. Similarly, if pain is caused by active abduction or extension of the
thigh with the patient lying on his side, one must assume some damage to the
gluteal attachments or possibly to the tensor fascia femoris or to the lateral abdominals. Careful check must be made of the muscles that attach in the involved area.
Once it has been determined that muscular involvement is present, the next step
is to determine its degree. This may be extremely difficult. If there is complete
avulsion, surgical repair should be carried out promptly. Fortunately complete
avulsion of the iliac crest seldom occurs and I have diagnosed only this one case
in many years of observation of this type of injury. I am sure that more do occur
than are diagnosed. A great many of these injuries never actually reach the doctor

and are treated by the athlete himself or by the trainer, often without true recognition of the nature of the injury.

If the avulsion is less than complete, treatment should be that of any muscle strain. The muscle should be put at rest. In the early stage one should use cold and compression; after 24 hours heat and protection. Since we are assuming some degree of avulsion of the attachment, local treatment may be of considerable value. Any hematoma should be aspirated first, then a long-acting anesthetic agent is injected and followed by hyaluronidase. Protection must be given to the muscles at the attachment to the iliac crest. Even though the trunk is strapped to hold it toward the involved side, which in itself is difficult, this does not prevent active forceful contraction of the muscle but simply prevents overstretch. So if there is pain on active use of the abdominal or thigh muscles, a period of inactivity is necessary in order to restore normal function. Rehabilitation should be within the limits of pain and this can be determined readily by the patient himself. When activity is resumed, strapping of the flank as described in Figure 269 may be undertaken although its accomplishment is quite difficult. Properly applied, this strapping gives considerable restriction of motion. Indeed, it may be so restricting as to be a considerable handicap to the player but it will give good protection against overstretching. A good plan is to begin the strapping with cross-stretch and progress to long-stretch elastic tape as healing progresses and more activity is permissible.

Figure 269. Strapping of flank. The strapping is done with adhesive applied with the patient in the erect position with the trunk flexed toward the involved side. Broad strips of long-stretch or cross-stretch elastic tape are used. The former stretches on its long axis and allows considerable motion, while the latter stretches on its cross axis and gives more restriction of motion; so that the one which should be used depends upon the degree of fixation desired. Various methods can be used for application. A good method is by crosshatching of the strapping, one strip beginning in the region of the substernal notch extending diagonally downward and backward across the anterosuperior spine and over the trochanter to terminate on the back of the thigh, and another beginning in the back, starting at the lateral margin of the opposite lumbar muscle mass and crosses downward over the trochanter to end on the anteromedial thigh. These strips should cross at about the level of the trochanter. Successive parallel strips extending backward and forward forms crosshatching of the adhesive. The crossed strips begin at the trochanter and extend up to the lower ribs. For additional support this dressing can be given an underlying foundation of vertical strips as illustrated on the left. At the completion of the strapping, the tape should be secured by circumferential straps.

Contact sports of any kind should not be permitted without very effective protective padding over the iliac crest since the crest will remain extremely sensitive. This protection should be used for the remainder of the season.

A tendency toward recurrence of these lesions is a disheartening factor. I am sure that the majority of them are undertreated rather than overtreated since they are considered to be simple contusions when they are actually muscular avulsions.

Fracture

Fracture of the *wing of the ilium* (Fig. 270) is not frequent as an athletic injury. It is usually caused by a direct blow against the wing of the ilium. In most sports in which such a force is likely, the iliac crest is protected by padding to prevent injury to the bone. The most frequent sport in which this occurs is horseback riding, often in the manner described in the illustration. This, as may be imagined, is an extremely painful injury, not only at the time of the blow but in the immediate period after the injury. It will ordinarily be recognized as a serious injury. Examination reveals extreme tenderness along the iliac crest and down onto the wing of the ilium, the area depending upon the extent of the fracture. The patient will usually not permit deep enough palpation that one can actually feel a defect along the rim, although this is occasionally possible. Any attempt at function of the involved muscles is extremely painful and even involuntary spasm of the abdominal or hip muscles may cause acute distress. It is necessary to have the patient completely relaxed mentally and physically before a definitive examination

Figure 270.   Linear fracture of ilium. This young lady was riding a horse which headed for the stable and turned through the gate so abruptly that she bumped the ilium on the center post.

can be done. If a lesion of this severity is suspected, an x-ray examination is in order. The fracture can be completely overlooked in the ordinary anteroposterior view of the pelvis. If the trunk is rotated 45 degrees to the involved side, however, an antero-posterior view of the wing of the ilium will reveal the lesion.

This fracture may be treated by complete bed rest, and with a tranquil patient this is usually adequate. Even with some degree of displacement of the fragment, reduction is not necessary. Reposition would of necessity have to be by open reduc-tion with internal fixation. This is a more formidable procedure than is usually justified. If simple bed rest does not give adequate relief of pain, a pair of plaster pants extending from above the knees to above the rib margin may give substantial relief of discomfort and permit mobility of the patient in bed. A simple corset may suffice or adhesive strapping may relieve the patient. It should be borne in mind that if there is real, measurable displacement of the fragment, a compression dress-ing with a corset or strapping may increase the pain and in fact increase the dis-placement. The patient should be kept in bed about four weeks and then allowed to be up in a corset.

Another injury in the region of the iliac crest is fracture of the *anterosuperior spine of the ilium* (Fig. 271). This fracture is almost always an avulsion fracture, the fragment being pulled off by the sartorious and tensor fasciae femoris attach-ments. The history is usually of unusual muscular violence in running or jumping—occasionally jumping down from a height. Examination reveals local pain and ten-derness at the anterior spine. This can be distinguished from a contusion in this area by the fact that function of the involved muscle attachments is painful and active flexion of the thigh or passive overextension of the thigh will cause pain

Figure 271. Avulsion of the ante-rior spine of the left ilium with flexion contracture and pain on active flexion or passive extension. The x-ray shows avul-sion of the rectus femoris attachment, which was treated nonsurgically with good recovery.

directly at the area. If one examines the patient early he may be able to palpate a separate fragment of bone which may be 1 inch or more below the location of the attachment at the anterosuperior spine. X-rays should be taken. An anteroposterior view of the ilium rather than of the pelvis may be necessary if the fragment is not to be missed. An avulsion of the tendon may occur without a fragment of bone being displaced.

Treatment of this condition is primarily surgical. If it is diagnosed promptly, surgical correction is relative atraumatic and easy. The fragment can be drawn back into position and fastened by whatever type of internal fixation seems most effective in the individual case. It may vary from a single screw fastening the fragment of bone to the pelvis to direct suture through drill holes. If the avulsion is incomplete or if for some reason surgery is inadvisable, treatment should be by immobilization with the thigh flexed. This can be accomplished by bed rest with the knees elevated or by plaster fixation in the appropriate position. I believe it is more simple and less traumatic to carry out prompt open reduction with definitive fixation than it is to immobilize the patient for the period necessary to permit healing to become complete. If nonsurgical treatment is selected, local measures consist of aspiration of the hematoma, injection with hyaluronidase, compression bandage, cold early, heat after 24 hours.

Following surgical repair, the degree of activity to be permitted will depend upon the security of the internal fixation. If firm fixation is obtained, I prefer to use a short single spica running from the knee on the affected side around the pelvis with the thigh flexed slightly. The patient should be allowed up on crutches within a day or two and rehabilitation promptly commenced. This includes isometric contraction of the involved muscles. At the end of two weeks, the spica is removed. The wound is dressed and if it has properly healed, a spica of elastic adhesive bandage is applied with the patient standing and the thigh and knee slightly flexed by putting the foot on the involved side on a 4 inch block. This permits rehabilitation of the hip joint to proceed. Ordinarily active running should not be permitted short of six weeks and in the case with less secure surgical fixation a longer period may be required.

If at operation the fragment is found to be small or comminuted it should be removed, rather than repaired, and the muscle sutured to the bone. Indeed, there is some argument in favor of routinely removing the fragment and obtaining muscle-to-bone healing rather than waiting for bone-to-bone union. The latter requires considerably longer and will prolong the rehabilitation. Unless I can get anatomical reposition and very positive screw fixation, I generally remove the fragment and repair the attachment to the ilium through drill holes.

INJURIES IN THE VICINITY OF THE POSTERIOR SPINE OF THE ILIUM

Injuries to the posterior spine of the ilium are not frequent since the attachments here are such that there is no acute avulsive force applied. The most frequent injury in this vicinity is simple contusion of the posterior superior or inferior spine. While this may be somewhat distressing it is not particularly disabling and responds well to local treatment by heat and other means of physical therapy.

INJURIES IN THE VICINITY OF THE SACRUM AND SACROILIAC JOINTS, INCLUDING THE COCCYX

The sacrum is the keystone of the arch of the pelvis. The two innominate bones are attached to the sacrum at the sacroiliac joints. The sacroiliac joint is one of extremely irregular contour. the bones fitting together with interdigitations much like the rachets in the ordinary desk lamp bracket. There is no true articular motion between these two bones but there is articular cartilage and often a synovial lined capsule so it must be classified as a diarthrodial joint (Fig. 272).

Contusion

Contusion in the vicinity of the sacrum and sacroiliac joints is a common injury, so frequent that sacral pads are a required part of the equipment for contact sports. The sacrum itself is largely subcutaneous on its posterior surface, as is the postero-inferior spine of the ilium. A direct blow to the unprotected sacrum may cause an extremely painful injury. Examination reveals tenderness over the sacrum which may be diffuse or may be sharply localized on the sacrum or on one of the iliac spines. If the injury appears to be acute, an x-ray should be made since it is not unusual to crack the sacrum or to fracture one of the spines by direct trauma. If fracture can be ruled out, treatment should be by early application of cold and compression followed by heat and support. Actually this injury, while it is quite painful, is not particularly disabling. As long as the sacrum is tender it should be protected against direct contusion.

Fracture

A fracture of the sacrum is usually transverse or stellate in type and will respond quite well to conservative treatment (Fig. 273). This will require a period of bed rest followed by support. Ordinarily a corset will be adequate. Healing will usually be complete within four weeks but residual tenderness and pain may last another month.

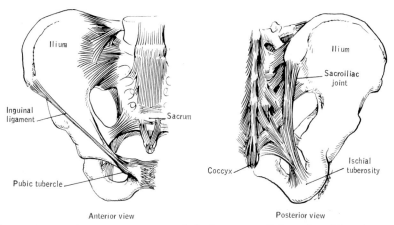

Ilium

Inguinal ligament

Sacrum

Pubic tubercle

Anterior view

Ilium

Sacroiliac joint

Ischial tuberosity

Coccyx

Posterior view

Figure 272.   Anteroposterior view of the ligaments of the pelvis. Note the complete investiture of the sacroiliac joints by a continuous band of very heavy ligament. This includes also the ligament attaching the third lumbar vertebra to the ilium. Note that the entire pelvis is firmly bound down with strong ligaments. (From Anson, "Atlas of Human Anatomy.")

Figure 273.   Transverse fracture of sacrum just below the sacroiliac joint, caused by force-ful blow against the lower portion of the sacrum. *A,* Anterior view. *B,* Lateral view.

Sprain

A sprain of the iliosacral ligaments is possible. It may be of the ligament extending from the posterior projection of the wing of the ilium to the posterior sacrum, or of the ligaments within the pelvis. It should be borne in mind that many of the conditions that used to be called sacroiliac sprain were actually other entities. It was a "wastebasket" term. The sacroiliac ligaments are so strong, particularly in the young athlete, that ordinary stresses will cause damage to the lumbosacral ligaments more readily than to the sacroiliac ligaments. One should, therefore, be very wary of the diagnosis of sacroiliac sprain.

Following injury in the vicinity of the sacroiliac joint there will be pain localized about the joint. There also may be pain referred to the groin, hamstrings, or back of the thigh. It will not ordinarily be along the sciatic distribution. If this condition is suspected, great care must be taken to localize the lesion to the sacroiliac joint. Many of the tests that will elicit pain in the sacroiliac joint will also be positive in such conditions as ruptured disc, sciatic neuritis and lumbosacral sprain, so that the mere fact that the tests cause pain is of little significance. The greatest significance is in the location of the pain. In an acute injury this may be extremely difficult to determine accurately. The common tests such as straight leg raising (Fig. 274, *A, B*) which put torsion force on the sacroiliac joint or the similar test of forward flexion of the trunk with the knees straight will cause pain in sacroiliac joint involvement but will also be positive in many other conditions. Some tests are designed to stress the sacroiliac area particularly. The popular Gaenslen test (Fig. 274, *C*), in which the opposite thigh is flexed on the abdomen in order to

Figure 274.   A, Straight leg raising. Note the extended right thigh. The left lower extremity is flexed with the knee extended.

B, Straight leg raising test with dorsiflexion of the foot (Lasègue).

C, Thigh flexion test (Gaenslen). Note the right thigh held in extension. It may be dropped off the table in hyperextension while the left thigh is flexed.

D, The heel to knee test. The left pelvis is fixed by the examiners left hand. With the right heel on the left knee, the right knee is pushed down toward the table.

E, F, G, H, Iliac compression or separation. E, Lateral decubitus. With the opposite thigh flexed for stability, the right iliac crest is compressed toward the table. F, With the patient supine, the examiner's hands force the iliac crests apart. G, With the patient supine, the legs are widely abducted. H, Examiner forces crests together.

immobilize the pelvis in forward flexion and then the involved leg is pushed into hyperextension, causes rotatory stress on the sacroiliac joint. Obviously it would also strain other areas so again the mere positive test is not diagnostic.

Of rather more significance are tests designed to compress or separate the iliac crests (Fig. 274, E-H). With the patient lying on his back, simple compression force across the crests will put some stress across the sacroiliac joint. The opposite maneuver of forcing the crests apart can be applied in a thin individual by locking the heels of the hands against the inner portion of each anterior spine and attempting to separate the spines. A similar test is to have the patient lie on his side with the inferior thigh flexed to 90 degrees to fix the lumbosacral area. Compression downward against the upward iliac crest will throw stress on the sacroiliac joint.

If the sprain is acute, the pain will be relieved by bed rest. Local treatment consists of injection of the tender area with an anesthetic and a corticoid preparation followed by compression made by a constricting elastic adhesive dressing wrapped around the pelvis or by a sacroiliac belt or by a simple corset. Heat will relieve the attendant muscle spasm. As in back injuries, muscle spasm may be relieved by enteric antispasmodics. The duration of immobilization in bed depends upon the severity of the injury. The patient may be permitted up as soon as he can get up without pain. If the injury is actually an acute sprain of the ligament three to four weeks will be needed for the ligament to repair and the area should be carefully protected during this time.

Dislocation

Actual sacroiliac dislocation occurs only as the result of a massive injury that is ordinarily not athletic in origin, although it could occur by being thrown from a horse or similar severe trauma. The treatment will be that of a fractured pelvis which is not within the scope of this work.

Subluxation

Our "manipulative brethren" frequently make a diagnosis of sacroiliac dislocation and often obtain dramatic relief by manipulation of the pelvis. It is probable that in certain circumstances of relaxation of the iliosacral ligaments some of the interdigitations of the joint become caught with a minimal degree of displacement undetectable by x-ray. In these cases simple manipulation may cause them to "snap back into place" and give relief. This happens too frequently to be ignored but I am sure that many times the relief by manipulation is either relief of the muscle tension or is psychic. The exact manipulation may vary. One of the most effective maneuvers is the forceful application of the Gaenslen test (Fig. 275, A) in which one thigh is sharply flexed and the other hyperextended. Another manipulation (Fig. 275, B) is carried out with the patient lying supine on the table. Instruct him to reach over and catch the left edge of the table with the right hand over his left shoulder. The left thigh is then grasped and with the knee in extension the thigh

Figure 275.   Sacroiliac manipulation. A, Forceful flexion of thigh with opposite thigh fixed. B, The patient fixes the upper trunk by grasping the edge of the table with the right hand while the left lower extremity is forced up into flexion and adduction, thus rotating the pelvis on the hip.

is flexed to 135 degrees and then adducted and internally rotated. This rotates the pelvis toward the left. This maneuver can be carried out in either direction. Sometimes it is rewarded by an alarming snap and dramatic relief, but alas, most often with no result at all! Manipulation should not be attempted casually by the uninitiated and by no means under anesthesia. With the patient awake his muscular resistance will usually prevent any actual damage. However, with him relaxed under anesthesia, the leverage applied may cause serious damage to the hip or spine.

As is frequent with ligament injuries there is a tendency toward recurrence, so once the injury has been treated and the patient rehabilitated a well fitting sacroiliac belt should be worn in contact sports for the remainder of the season. It should be emphasized again that before diagnosis of sacroiliac sprain can be made the burden of proof remains with the examiner to show that the condition actually is a sacroiliac sprain and not something else.

Coccyx

There will occasionally be injury to the coccyx although this too is not a common injury in sports. It usually occurs by falling in a sitting position or by a blow (inadvertent) from a shoe. While this is an extremely painful injury, it is not especially disabling and usually requires no specific treatment other than local application of heat. The pain may be severe enough to prevent competition for two to three weeks. Local protection is advisable in the nature of a fiber pad, and some degree of constriction helps. Something like a panty girdle will be valuable for this purpose. A suitable pad can be inserted at the appropriate area in the girdle to give local protection. Ordinarily a moderate amount of displacement is of little importance, particularly in the male. The fracture will heal promptly.

There will occasionally be involvement of the sacrococcygeal joint by subluxation or traumatic arthritis. If pain is persistent and disabling, coccygectomy may be justified. Great care must be exercised to be sure that the coccyx is actually the seat of the trouble and that the condition is truly local. I cannot recall having removed a coccyx damaged as a result of athletic injury.

INJURIES IN THE VICINITY OF THE BUTTOCK AND PERINEUM

Contusion

The most common injury to the buttock is from a direct blow. This does not usually cause injury to the skin because of the ample underlying padding. Contusion of the muscle is a common occurrence and usually is of little consequence. In most of the areas of the buttock there is a thick muscle mass with relatively little danger of catching a muscle between two unyielding objects. As a result the condition is usually diffuse without gross hematoma formation in the muscle. A tender, painful muscle mass results which may be uncomfortable but is not actually disabling. The buttock is usually not protected in athletic competition by any padding other than that inherent in the anatomy and so superficial contusion is relatively common here. One should be wary of the condition that appears to be unduly severe or that causes other than local symptoms.

A *contusion of the sciatic nerve* may result in pain in the buttock extending down the back of the thigh into the calf and foot similar to sciatic pain from other causes. This is nonradicular in character and follows the whole distribution of the sciatic nerve rather than that of any single root. Straight leg raising causes pain in the area of the contusion. During the acute period, hyperesthesia of the skin may be evident in the lower portion of the extremity. This contusion is not frequent. The ordinary contusion of the sciatic nerve will require no particular treatment other than protection against stretch. Physical therapy may give considerable relief. A word of caution should be said about inductive heat. If deep therapy such as short wave diathermy causes increase in the pain it should be promptly discontinued. Sometimes local tension in the nerve will be increased by congestion due to the heat. This does not ordinarily occur with the whirlpool bath or infrared radiation.

Another area of the buttock in which a complication of contusion may arise is over the ischial tuberosity. Here the bone is essentially subcutaneous although it may be protected by an overlying layer of muscle of greater or lesser thickness. A contusion here may cause a *fracture of the tuberosity* in which case there will be severe localized pain. The pain is increased by straight leg raising or by any local pressure. More commonly the result of the blow will be periostitis or fibrositis over the roughened surface of the bone. In other cases there will be involvement of the ischial bursa. It may be impossible in the early stages to distinguish between these conditions. Treatment should be local heat and rest. Usually the symptoms will subside promptly. In the case of periostitis or bursitis there will be persistent pain and extreme local tenderness. In these cases local injection into the area with attempt to aspirate fluid from the bursa is advisable. If the bursa can be entered, injection of a steroid will often give substantial relief. If not, the area should be infiltrated with a long-acting anesthetic. Indeed, the proper corticoid may be diffused throughout the area, a soluble preparation being preferable to the suspension.

If the symptoms persist, x-ray examination should be made. The injury may occasionally result in spur formation or in calcification within the bursa (Fig. 276).

Figure 276.   Calcification within ischial bursa.

Figure 277. This 14 year old girl fell astraddle the gymnasium rail, receiving a severe perineal contusion, immediate, severe pain and disability with terrific adductor and hamstring spasm. The x-ray was negative. Three weeks post injury it shows osteomyelitis of the ischium, the result of stagnation of blood from contusion of bones. A high febrile course began one week post injury, subsided under antibiotics. The abscess later required drainage.

If there is calcification of the bursa and if this does not respond well to aspiration and local injection, surgical excision of the bursa is justified. Usually relief is prompt and complete following surgical excision. If the irritation results in ossification and spur formation which does not respond to treatment and which is constantly disabling, the spurring should be removed surgically. Completely atraumatic technique must be used. Access is readily obtained to this location by placing the patient in the lithotomy position with a folded sheet beneath the sacrum. This presents the tuberosity of the ischium in its subcutaneous position. One is able to expose the tuberosity and the ascending ramus of the ischium or whatever area is primarily involved without extensive dissection. If careful attention is paid to hemostasis by proper coagulation, an extremely dry field may be obtained and the exact pathology determined. If there is bursitis, the bursa may be readily removed and the underlying periosteum examined. If on the other hand there is irregularity of the bone or spur formation, the muscle attachments may be stripped away subperiosteally, the bone carefully smoothed off and hemostasis secured with bone wax. The incision need only be as extensive as is required for the lesion encountered.

Occasionally the ascending ramus of the ischium or descending ramus of the pubis will be injured by a direct blow such as a fall astraddle a bar. This may be an extremely painful injury but ordinarily recovery is complete without specific therapy other than local measures. This treatment should depend upon the severity of the condition. Usually cold applications followed by heat and a period at rest will suffice. In the case of serious injury, x-ray study should be made to determine possible fracture. At the time of injury the patient will feel that a major disaster has befallen him since the injury is painful and distressing—and often humiliating. He may try to avoid embarrassment over his ineptitude by appearing to be badly injured.

Injuries to the deeper structures of the perineum hardly fall into the scope of this work since they are very infrequent in athletic pursuits. Probably the most common of them is contusion from falling forcibly on a hard object, with resulting painful hematomata (Fig. 277). In injury of any consequence, careful examination should be made to be sure there is no serious damage to the underlying structures. In the male the cavernous muscles and urethra may be damaged. In the female the genitalia. Suitable consultation should be obtained from a competent urologist or gynecologist particularly if there appears to be subcutaneous bleeding or open laceration. So too there may occur damage to the anus and rectum and if any question is present, a rectal examination should be carried out immediately to observe local tenderness, presence of bleeding or even the presence of a palpable defect in the sphincter or wall.

Strain

This same ischial area is quite subject to muscle strain, a common one being strain at the origin of the long head of the biceps on the tuberosity of the ischium. This may result in avulsion of the ischial tuberosity, particularly if the epiphysis in this region is not yet closed. It usually occurs as result of forcible flexion of the hip with the knee extended, as in the leading leg of the hurdler (Fig. 278). Extremely forceful straight leg raising is the same mechanism and throws a heavy pull on the origin of the long head of the biceps. The result may be irritation at the attachment of the muscle or complete avulsion from the bone (Fig. 279). Symptoms are localized pain on pressure over the ischial tuberosity, pain on flexion of the thigh with the knee extended, and pain on active forceful contraction of the biceps muscle. X-ray examination may or may not reveal the nature of the injury.

Treatment is that of avulsion anywhere except that replacement of the avulsed fragment may not be necessary. It should be replaced if the separation is wide and complete. Immobilization of the leg with the knee flexed and avoidance of thigh

Figure 278.   Avulsion of a portion of the ischium by the attachment of the biceps muscle. Following a relatively acute period of two or three weeks, he had recurrence of pain on running or jumping. The fragment was removed and the muscle sutured to the bed with a good recovery.

A, Preoperative. B, Postoperative.

Figure 279.   High school baseball pitcher who injured his leg throwing. He threw left-handed. This is his kick-off leg. He had pain and soreness but was able to complete the game, pitching a one hitter. Subsequently was unable to play. Now (eight weeks later) he is getting a good recovery. The injury represents an avulsion of the attachment of the semi-tendinosus.

flexion will usually suffice for protection. In fact, in many instances, simple elimination of forceful activity is enough. If the symptoms are persistent, local injection and physical therapy are of value. A painful nonunion of the fragment may be relieved by removal of the fragment although this is seldom necessary. As is true of many avulsions, this one is not compatible with athletic competition. A period of rest from strenuous activity is imperative but under ordinary circumstances there will be no permanent disability. The same surgical technique may be used here as indicated above for ischial bursitis. In some instances, however, the lithotomy position may be inadvisable because it may overstretch the hamstrings. This can usually be minimized by extending the thigh somewhat from the acutely flexed position. The same approach can be utilized with the patient lying prone with a large pillow under the pelvis of the involved side and with the knee flexed.

A straddling injury caused by forceful abduction of the thighs may cause damage to the adductor muscles. They are particularly vulnerable at their attachments to the ischiopubic rami. Following this type of injury the symptoms are readily recognizable since there will be localized tenderness along the subcutaneous edge of the ramus and to the lateral side. The diagnostic test is pain on passive abduction of the thigh and on forced active adduction, each of which causes pain localized at the origin of these muscles along the puboischium. This same force will occasionally cause avulsion of one of the adductors, usually the adductor longus (Fig. 280), in which case the symptoms are more pronounced and there may be a palpable defect between the bone and the muscle belly. I have seen instances in the athlete in which the longus muscle has been ruptured at a distance from the

Figure 280.   Partial avulsion of the attachment of the adductor longus and gracilis from the pubic ramus. This gave chronic recurrent pain and terminated a player's basketball season. Local injection and physical therapy relieved the symptoms.

insertion, usually about 2 inches from the attachment at the pelvis. This may simulate a contusion and is often difficult to distinguish from it. If the condition can be recognized, prompt surgical repair of the rupture of the attachment or muscle is indicated. Detachment or rupture may be recognized by the bunching up of the adductor longus muscle a short distance away from the pelvis and by a tender, firm mass which is more noticeable on active adduction of the thigh against resistance. If several weeks have passed, any attempt at repair is doomed to failure because of the inability to get secure enough suture within the muscle substance to overcome the shortening of the muscle. In this instance the condition should be carefully explained to the patient, pointing out that the mass is of no consequence in itself. In most instances the athlete will accept this without insistence on further treatment. Should the pain be persistent and to some extent disabling, late surgery may be justified. At this time the fibromuscular mass should be removed and the remaining muscle belly sutured to the adjoining adductor magnus. An injury of this severity is rather unusual but prompt relief may be obtained by definitive treatment. It is important to point out to the athlete that this treatment will not add to his muscular strength or ability or agility but is simply designed to relieve his pain.

As indicated above, by far the most common injury is a strain at the muscle attachment. In this instance the symptoms are similar to this condition anywhere and are relieved by the same measures. If the patient is seen immediately after the injury there may be some virtue in application of cold. Ordinarily the symptoms are not called to the doctor's attention for several days when the patient is seen because of persistent pain and discomfort. At this time local measures should consist of local injection with long-acting anesthetic and a corticoid preparation, application of heat by sitz baths, whirlpool, diathermy and rest. Injudicious exercise in an attempt

Figure 281. This 14 year old girl was learning a new dance step when she did an anteroposterior split with immediate, severe pain in the buttock with disability. X-ray revealed complete avulsion of the semitendinosus origin. Treatment by surgical replacement of the fragment resulted in complete recovery.

to improve the range of abduction will only prolong the symptoms. Constant effort should be made to avoid forcible abduction of the involved thigh.

Pubic Symphysis

Damage to the pubic symphysis is not frequent except in major accidents involving the pelvis. However, one may get a painful contusion over the subcutaneous anterior surface of the symphysis. This may result in considerable local swelling and even hematoma formation but it is not a dangerous or crippling injury. We have recently seen a girl who fell heavily forward on her mons pubis while ice skating (Fig. 282). The result was the prompt development of a hematoma the size of a small orange which was alarming and distressing to the patient. The actual disability, however, was minimal, the pain being present only on direct pressure. Because of the unsightly swelling, an attempt was made to aspirate it. This was unsuccessful because of infiltration of blood through the fibrofatty pad and ultimately it was necessary for the gynecologist to evacuate the hematoma. This case

Figure 282. Injury of the mons pubis by a fall on the ice, with resulting hematoma.

is mentioned particularly since the condition may seem quite alarming and drastic remedies may appear in order whereas it is a relatively superficial hematoma and ordinarily will respond to the local measures used for hematoma.

In the adolescent the pubic symphysis is not nearly as firmly fixed as it is in the adult and sprain of the ligaments connecting the two pubic bones can occur by forceful abduction of both thighs. This must be distinguished from a contusion which is considerably more common since, in a strain of the pubic ligaments, the force applied is one that separates the pubic bones rather than a direct blow to the local area. The treatment is quite different in the two instances since the treatment in sprain of the pubic ligaments must be designed to hold the pelvic ring together and to prevent wide abduction of the thighs. Early treatment should consist of local injection, application of heat and rest. This can be accomplished by circumferential adhesive strapping or by a well fitted lumbosacral corset. As with any sprain, several weeks are required for healing, and protection should be continued for many weeks, particularly if any sport is indulged in that causes tension on these ligaments, such as horseback riding or water skiing. The prognosis is quite favorable if the condition is recognized and treated adequately.

INJURIES IN THE VICINITY OF THE GROIN

Contusion

In this area we find the tunnel formed by the bridging of the anterior pelvis by Poupart's ligament, which runs from the pubis across to the anterior superior spine on either side (Fig. 283). Under this ligament pass the vascular sheath, the femoral nerve, the inguinal canal, the cord and some muscle groups, particularly the iliopsoas. A direct blow over this area may cause damage to any of these structures. This is ordinarily not severe but may be relatively painful. It may cause a few minutes or hours of disability, then go on to a good and complete recovery.

Permanent vascular damage after a blow to the groin is infrequent. Traumatic phlebitis and even phlebothrombosis from a direct blow over the femoral vein are remote possibilities. Trauma to the femoral nerve may cause paresthesia along the front of the thigh which is worrisome to the patient but of little significance

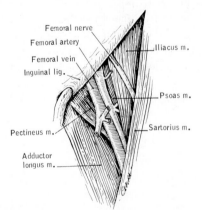

Femoral nerve
Femoral artery
Femoral vein
Inguinal lig.
Iliacus m.
Psoas m.
Pectineus m.
Sartorius m.
Adductor longus m.

Figure 283.   Note compartment formed by the inguinal ligament above, the iliopsoas laterally, adductors medially, the compartment housing the femoral artery, vein and nerve. The sartorius and rectus attach to the anterosuperior spine while the adductor muscles attach along the pubic ramus. Note also how the psoas and iliacus blend to form the iliopsoas tendon which attaches to the lesser trochanter of the femur. (From Anson, "Atlas of Human Anatomy.")

from the standpoint of disability. The well trained athlete has been taught to protect his abdomen and groin by flexion of the thigh so injury in this area is not as frequent as might be expected from its relatively exposed position.

Strain

Muscular strain in this area is relatively frequent, the most frequent being *strain of the iliopsoas tendon.* This may occur at its attachment to the lesser trochanter of the femur or in the musculotendinous junction. It is not caused by a direct blow to the groin but by overactive contraction of the iliopsoas with the thigh fixed or forced into extension. The patient complains of severe pain in the groin and holds the thigh in a flexed adducted position. Any attempt of the examiner to extend or to rotate the thigh causes severe pain. So does active contraction of the iliopsoas muscle. Tenderness will be found at the area of the injury. If it is at the lesser trochanteric attachment the tenderness will be below the groin, along the upper anteromedial aspect of the thigh. Careful x-ray study should be made of the lesser trochanter to determine whether there has been an avulsion of the bone (Fig. 284). This is particularly true in the adolescent in whom the epiphysis of the lesser trochanter has not united with the shaft. If the avulsion is complete it should be treated by surgical repair, either removing a small fragment of bone and suturing the tendon to the femur or, if the fragment is large, by firm internal fixation of the fragment to the femoral shaft. If the lesion is incomplete, as it most frequently is, treatment should be by bed rest with the thigh flexed and externally rotated with application of cold compresses in the early stage followed by local heat. After a few days, better determination can be made as to the severity of the injury. Duration of treatment will depend upon the symptoms. This is an extremely disabling condition since any effort to run or jump causes excessive strain on this tendon, with resultant pain. The patient's athletic endeavors must be terminated for whatever period is required for the symptoms to subside, usually several weeks.

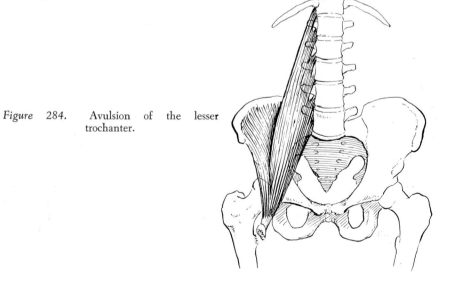

Figure 284.   Avulsion of the lesser trochanter.

Because of the complexity of the various flexors of the hip, it is sometimes difficult to determine whether or not complete avulsion of the tendon has occurred. In case of persistent pain with chronic irritation, treatment by local injection into the tender area may be tried. This area is relatively inaccessible and skillful manipulation of the needle is needed to reach the involved area. The iliopsoas is an important flexor of the thigh and complete recovery is necessary before unrestricted function can be permitted. Strapping that holds the thigh in slight flexion will prevent overstretching of the muscle but does not prevent overactivity and so is relatively ineffectual. Plaster fixation is ordinarily not necessary since the thigh readily assumes the position of flexion which puts the muscle at rest. This position is all too often held even after the lesion has healed so that troublesome flexion contracture of the thigh may be the result. In order to minimize this danger the patient should be encouraged to extend the thigh actively within the limits of pain several times each day. After the acute symptoms subside a daily period spent lying prone in bed is desirable.

Also susceptible to damage in this area is the abdominal muscle group which attaches along Poupart's ligament. Strain of these muscles must be treated by rest, heat and protection—the same type of treatment necessary for similar injury along the iliac crest. Occasionally there will be a painful strain of the conjoined tendon of the abdominals at the attachment to the pubis at the inner end of the Poupart's ligament.

INJURIES IN THE VICINITY OF THE TROCHANTER

Contusion

The significant area of contusion in the vicinity of the hip is over the trochanter. In this area the bony trochanter is covered only by the iliotibial tract and the skin. The tract is separated from the trochanter by the trochanteric bursa, which is a constant structure of considerable size lying beneath the muscle and tendon of the tensor fasciae femoris. Contusion may result in damage to the muscle or to the bursa. The symptoms are the same as in contusion elsewhere and the treatment presents no unusual elements.

A trochanteric *bursitis* may be caused here by a direct blow, by infection or by friction between the adjacent bursal walls. In many instances contusion of the trochanter may result in bursitis and the symptoms will gradually change from those of a contusion to those of involvement of the bursa. In this instance there will be tenderness over the trochanteric area with pain on forcible activity of the thigh. In the course of flexion and extension of the hip or of rotation of the extended thigh, the tensor fasciae femoris slides backward and forward over the trochanter and in the presence of an inflammatory reaction this will cause pain.

On examination there is local tenderness over the bursa often with crepitation on motion. Pain is elicited by adducting the thigh with the knee extended to put the tensor under strain as it passes over the trochanter. In this position, internal and external rotation of the extremity will cause the trochanter to slide back and forth under the tight tensor and pain will be caused on this maneuver which would not be present with a simple contusion.

The so-called "snapping hip" should be mentioned in this connection. This is due to chronic bursitis with thickening of the bursal walls and spasm of the tensor so that on each step, as the tensor slides back and forth over the trochanter, an audible and palpable snap will occur. This is quite distressing. The condition is much more common in girls since, with their wide pelves and prominent trochanters the tensor bows over the trochanter at a more acute angle than in the narrower pelvis of the male. X-ray examination is ordinarily of little value although it may occasionally show calcification within the bursa.

Treatment of the acute bursitis is by rest and local heat. Early injection into the bursa of a local anesthetic may give prompt relief. There is a decided tendency toward recurrence and, in the occasional case with chronic recurring bursitis resistant to treatment, excision of the bursa may be necessary. If the chronic bursitis is accompanied by a snapping tensor tendon or by undue tension between the tensor and the trochanter at the time of operation, it will be advisable either to divide the tensor and make suitable repair or to shift it anteriorly or posteriorly. The indication for this operation is extremely uncommon in the male but is relatively frequent in the female although not ordinarily as the result of athletic injury.

Strain

There may be strain of the muscles attaching to the trochanter, particularly the gluteus medius (Fig. 285). This is ordinarily caused by overactivity of the gluteus medius and is usually chronic rather than acute. Symptoms in such a case will be pain on active contraction of the gluteus medius against resistance. Such contraction will not cause pain if the involvement is of the bursa alone. Similarly, a tendinitis of the rotators of the hip joint attaching along the posterior margin of the trochanter will cause local tenderness at the area of their attachment, with pain on active external rotation or passive forceful internal rotation of the hip. These

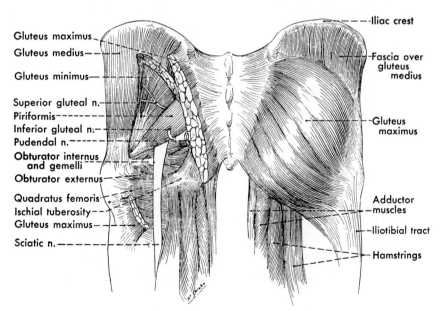

Figure 285. The musculature of the buttocks. On the left side, the space between the inferior gemellus and quadratus femoris is exaggerated so that the insertion of the obturator externus can be shown. (From Anson, "Atlas of Human Anatomy.")

Figure 286.   Avulsion of the anterior portion of the trochanter six months post injury with
nonunion.

Figure 287.   Avulsion of the trochanter by violent, active abduction against resistance.
This minimally displaced fragment held without surgery. This is borderline for internal
fixation.

conditions are treated by local heat, some sort of inductive heat being necessary to reach the area of involvement (diathermy or microtherm). Local injection is relatively simple here and the use of a long-acting local anesthetic plus a suitable corticoid frequently will give very good results.

In the adolescent in whom the trochanteric epiphysis is not united with the shaft an *avulsion* (Figs. 286 and 287), complete or partial, of the trochanteric epiphysis is not infrequent. This is a relatively serious injury and analogous to complete avulsion of the tendon attachment. If the avulsion is incomplete and the epiphyseal plate appears to be only a little bit wide it should be treated by immobilization with the thigh in abduction and slight external rotation. This position is maintained at least six weeks and activity is resumed gradually. If the avulsion is complete it should be treated by surgical replacement and fixation by long wood screw or similar appliance. Similar treatment is advisable if the trochanter is broken and displaced. Following firm internal fixation, support is needed only during the period of wound healing but athletic activity should be eliminated for at least six weeks.

INJURIES TO THE HIP JOINT PROPER

From an orthopedic standpoint and indeed from the standpoint of the traumatic surgeon, the hip is extremely liable to injury. Fortunately athletic injury to the hip joint is almost a rarity, in contrast to the knee, which is highly vulnerable. Owing to the extremely free motion of the hip joint, sprain of the ligaments of the hip is very uncommon. Strain of the muscles and tendons about the hip has been discussed previously and nothing needs to be added here.

Fracture and Dislocation

Fracture about the hip is unusual in the adolescent and young adult. The bone is exceptionally resilient and the hip is much more likely to dislocate than it is to break. For this reason we may see a *dislocation* of the hip in an athlete although fortunately it is of great rarity. If it occurs, it is obviously a major injury and represents a medical emergency. The patient is completely disabled at once. He has severe pain in the hip and resists any attempt to manipulate the limb. The extremity is usually held with the thigh internally rotated and adducted with the knee resting above and against its fellow on the opposite side (Fig. 288). The trochanter appears quite prominent. Any attempt to move the thigh from this position of flexion adduction and internal rotation causes severe pain. Diagnosis is confirmed by x-ray and the film should be carefully studied to be sure there is not an accompanying fracture. This is quite infrequent in youth. The posterior acetabular margin, which is vulnerable in the adult, is seldom damaged in the adolescent or young adult.

No attempt should be made to reduce the hip on the field. The patient should be taken immediately for x-ray examination, after which the dislocation must be reduced *under anesthesia* and *at the earliest possible moment*. While these two requirements may seem incompatible they are vital and there is good reason for both. The most important complication of dislocation of the hip is aseptic necrosis of the head of the femur. It has been shown definitely that the frequency and degree of aseptic necrosis of the head varies in direct proportion to the length of

Figure 288.   Drawing showing patient with dislocated hip. Note that the leg is shortened, internally rotated, adducted, with tendency to rest the affected foot on top of the opposite foot, with prominence of the greater trochanter laterally. (From DePalma, "Fractures and Dislocations.")

time the hip has remained displaced. Even minutes are of vital importance prior to complete reduction. On the other hand, experience has shown that it is virtually impossible to reduce a complete dislocation of the hip without profound relaxation and any effort to do so may cause considerable damage to the vulnerable cartilage of the femoral head.

A third consideration is that it seems unwise to attempt reduction of the dislocated hip until one can be reasonably sure there is no other injury such as would be demonstrated by x-ray examination. Clinical examination will determine whether the sciatic nerve has been damaged after reduction. It is very distressing to discover a nerve deficit that may or may not have preceded the manipulation. In spite of the patient's discomfort, a few simple movements of the foot will demonstrate an intact nerve. If active motions in plantar flexion, toe flexion and inversion are present, the tibial portion of the nerve is not severed. If the patient can actively dorsiflex and evert the foot, the peroneal division is intact. A rudimentary sensory check may also be made. If the nerve seems completely afunctional and remains so after reduction, an early exploration is advisable since the traumatized area of the nerve may be readily exposed by the posterior approach. On the other hand, if the lesion is incomplete or if the deficit develops gradually, one may safely assume that the injury is a contusion and compression rather than severance. In that case watchful waiting is the best treatment. The deficit may recover in a few days, or a few weeks. If there has not been definite improvement within three months the sciatic nerve should be explored. During the waiting period it is important to protect against drop foot or knee flexion by a suitable brace (Fig. 289).

Following dislocation of the hip it is imperative that the hip be immobilized for sufficient time to permit the capsule to heal. There seems little justification for overly prolonged denial of weight bearing, however. It has been recommended in the past that weight bearing should not be permitted for at least six months in the

Figure 289. Short leg brace for drop foot.

hope that aseptic necrosis would not develop. Recent studies have shown that the die is cast by the time the hip is reduced, that weight bearing itself is not a factor in the development of aseptic necrosis. Immobilization should be continued for four to six weeks and then active rehabilitation encouraged. Active participation in sports should not be permitted for at least three months following a complete dislocation of the hip.

It must be obvious that there are cases in which the hip dislocation is incomplete and goes unrecognized. The head either does not entirely leave the socket or is spontaneously reduced. The true pathology can be very easily overlooked. The patient usually complains of immediate severe pain at the time of the injury which promptly subsides and at the time of the examination there may be essentially no positive findings. Explanation for the lack of symptoms rests in the fact that by examination of the hip joint it is very difficult to put the ligaments of the hip on strain. In the normal hip, subluxation or dislocation cannot occur without laceration of the capsule. This usually occurs posterosuperiorly. This capsular tear is not put under stress by ordinary manipulation of the hip. The significance of this condition is that if one can be reasonably sure subluxation has occurred, the hip should be put at rest for a period of about four weeks in order to permit the capsular tear to repair (Fig. 290). If it does not repair or if it repairs with redundancy, this may well be the cause of repeated episodes of incomplete dislocation of the hip. A diagnosis of incomplete dislocation of the hip is extremely uncommon, especially in the athlete, but it is probable that many such diagnoses are missed.

In the adolescent with an unfused capital femoral epiphysis there is occasionally a fracture through the epiphyseal plate (Fig. 291). This is a serious injury and requires adequate treatment. The symptoms of this injury, if the displacement is complete, are those of a fracture of the femoral neck. There will be severe pain in the hip, shortening of the extremity, external rotation, and abduction of the thigh. However, the dislocation is frequently not complete and this characteristic position will not be assumed. It possibly may even resemble that of dislocation of the hip, another reason for careful x-ray study before any manipulative measure is carried out. If this is an acute traumatic dislocation of the epiphysis, it should be treated as a fracture of the femoral neck with reduction and internal fixation.

Figure 290.   Calcification of hip capsule following "sprain." This was probably an
unrecognized subluxation or spontaneously reduced dislocation.

Special Conditions

A related condition for which one must be on guard is a *slipped femoral
epiphysis* (Fig. 292). An apparently minor injury may be the precipitating cause
of the slipping and careful study should be made in any case of injury about the
hip to determine whether there is damage involving the epiphysis or epiphyseal
plate. The treatment of slipped femoral epiphysis may be quite different from that

Figure 291.   *A,* An acute epiphyseal dislocation analogous to fracture of the neck of
the femur. Note that this patient has none of the stigmata of slipped femoral epiphysis.

B, Uneventful healing followed reduction and fixation with Lorenzo screw. The screw
was used to avoid undue trauma to the head. This picture was at one year but the epiphysis
had closed by four months after the fixation.

Figure 292. Slipped femoral epiphysis. *A,* In the anteroposterior view the lesion is readily overlooked. *B,* In the lateral view the degree of slipping on the left side is revealed. (Note the osteochondritis dissecans of the acetabular roof on the same side.) *C,* One year after reduction and internal fixation with premature closure of the epiphysis. The osteochondritis dissecans has healed.

of acute epiphyseal fracture. In any of these conditions about the hip, time is of the essence. If the diagnosis is uncertain, consultation should be sought at the earliest possible moment since disaster with loss of function of the hip frequently results from delayed diagnosis.

Involvement of the acetabulum is not frequent in the athlete. Although chondral fractures can occur along the margin of the acetabulum, it is much more likely that the fragments seen in the x-ray are developmental. Careful study should be made of both hips before diagnosis is made of fracture of the rim of the acetabulum.

Osteochondritis dissecans (Figs. 292, B, and 293) infrequently develops in the acetabulum or in the femoral head, or at least it is infrequently diagnosed. Even in a joint permitting ready x-ray visualization, such as the knee or ankle, osteochondritis dissecans may be extremely difficult to recognize. In the hip it is doubly difficult, not only because of the depth of the joint surrounded by soft tissue but because of the fact that the head is enclosed within the acetabulum and there is superimposition of bone. Special x-ray studies may be required such as stereoscopic pictures or scanograms.

The hip joint is not frequently subject to *traumatic synovitis*. However, it may be that effusion of the hip is more common than is recognized since it is rather difficult to determine whether there is actual distention of the hip capsule by fluid. One infrequently makes the diagnosis of synovitis of the hip. This again is probably due to the fact that the hip itself has such freedom of motion that it is not subject to the same forces that damage the knee and ankle.

Figure 293.   Typical osteochondritis dissecans of superior portion of the acetabulum. The osteocartilaginous fragment is surrounded by a translucent area.

17

Injuries of
the Thigh

THIS CHAPTER covers the thigh proper. Injuries in the vicinity of the knee and hip are discussed under these headings elsewhere. Anatomically the thigh consists of a single bone completely surrounded by very heavy muscle. One would expect the common injuries to be concerned with the muscle and such is the case. Injuries to the skin are not frequent in the thigh since the skin is well protected by the resilient muscle pad beneath.

CONTUSION

Contusion of the thigh is a frequent injury in contact sports such as football since the thigh often receives the brunt of the collision between participants. The thigh is extremely well suited for this, however, since its thick muscle surrounding smooth bone can absorb a tremendous amount of impact without apparent damage. Ironically, contusion of the muscle is often caused by the edge of the mis-placed thigh pad which is designed to protect the anterior part of the thigh from a direct blow.

The *symptoms* of contusion of the thigh are much less localized than in the more subcutaneous areas. The patient is usually not disabled at the time of the blow. He is able to continue playing but at the end of the contest complains of aching and soreness within the muscle. There is disability and pain on passive stretching of the muscle involved. By far the most frequent area of involvement

419

is in some portion of the quadriceps, usually the lateralis or intermedius. The rectus is less frequently involved in a contusion since it is protected by the muscles beneath it.

Upon *examination,* diffuse tenderness along the anterior and lateral portion of the thigh, may be sometimes accompanied by muscle spasm, elicited by deep palpation. A point of sharply localized tenderness is not commonly present. Partial flexion and extension of the knee are not particularly painful but forced flexion beyond a right angle will cause tension in the swollen muscle fibers and some distress. Active extension of the knee against firm resistance may cause rather minor and undramatic discomfort. Some degree of hematoma is probably present in any contusion of the muscle although the bleeding may be more in the nature of an infiltration in the muscle than of pooled blood. An actual hematoma of the thigh, unless it is quite extensive, can be diagnosed only with extreme difficulty, because it is so deep-seated.

Treatment will depend upon the severity of the lesion, and the same principles apply here as in other areas. If there seems to be infiltration of blood or hematoma formation, an attempt at aspiration under aseptic precautions is justifiable. The area is then infiltrated with several ampules of hyaluronidase and a firm pressure bandage is applied. The bandage may be very snug and firm on the thigh of the athlete. If there is some concern about the swelling distal to the pressure bandage, the bandage may be started at the toe, run to the knee and then applied with increased pressure above the knee. After the application of the compression bandage the thigh should be carefully packed in ice and the extremity elevated and immobilized by bed rest. Since infiltration of the thigh may be quite extensive, I consider it important to encourage absorption of the blood and this we do by local injection of hyaluronidase into the immediate area. Intramuscular injection of an enzyme, 1 cc. for two or three days, is of value. Following this an oral enzyme is used. There is a wide divergence of opinion as to the value of these enzymes since a controlled series is hard to come by and each of us is inclined to judge by his own experience. I believe they help materially and use them freely where blood infiltration is a factor.

Examination the following morning will give good insight into the extent of involvement. If the thigh is tense, swollen and quite painful, immobilization should be continued along with the pressure bandage. After 24 hours, heat should be substituted for cold on the assumption that any active bleeding has stopped and increased circulation is desirable. The degree of immobilization will depend entirely upon the location and extent of the area involved. A good rule of thumb is that no motion should be permitted which is painful. While the patient is in bed, simple elastic compression is adequate. When he is allowed to get up one should immobilize the knee by cotton cast or other similar type dressing until the acute stage of the contusion and hematoma has passed.

Rehabilitation is extremely important and should progress as rapidly as possible but within the limits of pain. There is no excuse for forcible stretching of a contused muscle unless muscle healing is complete. On the other hand, the quadriceps muscle normally extends functionally from its resting position so that gentle flexion of the knee up to the limit of pain does not necessarily put any stress on the injured area and will aid immeasurably in rehabilitation. *There is no place for massage in the early treatment of contusion of a muscle.* The so-called "working it out" or "rubbing it out" simply increases the damage. On the other hand, after healing has progressed for 10 to 14 days massage may be used as a rehabilitative measure, again within the limits of discomfort. A major problem in management is the contusion of lesser extent. The player is anxious to continue his competition and practice and one is hesitant to hold him out when he contends he can use the muscle quite well. Critical judgment is important since a short period of complete inactivity will usually pay dividends in the long run.

MYOSITIS OSSIFICANS

The thigh is particularly prone to myositis ossificans. In my opinion this is due to the fact that the symptoms of muscle injury are often so mild that the player is allowed use of the muscle much beyond the limit set by his injury. This results in chronic irritation in the injured muscle with the reparative response of calcification and ossification. Some degree of ossification is extremely frequent and I am sure this is increased by unwise early treatment.

Treatment. Overenthusiastic massage to "knead out the knotted muscle," forceful passive flexion of the knee, too early active use of the quadriceps, intensive exercise—all are important aggravating factors. Myositis ossificans in the thigh is not necessarily disabling when only a small plaque of bone is present in the muscle. However, it can be and frequently is extremely disabling, and the mass may reach an amazing size (Figs. 294 and 295). Once ossification occurs in contusion, the management requires even more patience than before.

Rehabilitation may progress within the limits of pain but manipulation under anesthesia and similar measures are to be condemned. *It can be stated unequivocably that early surgical removal of the mass of bone simply invites recurrence and magni-*

Figure 294.   Calcification in the quadriceps lateralis which spontaneously regressed and disappeared.

fies the extent of the lesion itself and also the extent of disability. This has been demonstrated too often to require further substantiation (Fig. 296). If the plaque requires removal because of disability it should be excised only after the lesion is completely mature as demonstrated by clinical findings and x-ray examination. Six months is a minimum and frequently a longer time is needed, particularly if over-treatment has been carried out in the interim. At the proper time, with the proper care, operative excision is extremely gratifying.

At operation, an adequate incision that will expose the entire mass to view must be made so that it can be removed without the necessity of scraping, curetting, etc. The mass is not ordinarily covered with periosteum so I do not believe it necessary to carry out sharp dissection leaving the capsule attached to the bone. This does not apply when the parent bone is reached and great care should be taken not to strip the periosteum away from the femur as the mass is detached from the femoral shaft. The location of the lesion will determine the approach and one should fit the approach to the lesion, not the lesion to the approach. We recently removed a mass from the anteromedial aspect of the femur (Fig. 297). This was readily removed by an anterior approach whereas it would have been extremely difficult, if not impossible, to handle adequately by the more stereotyped antero-lateral approaches. Atraumatic surgery in these conditions is extremely important.

After the incision is made through the skin, meticulous hemostasis is obtained by electrocautery. A very careful atraumatic approach through the intervening muscle mass is important. If it is at all possible, the penetration should be muscle-

Figure 295.   Typical extensive myositis ossificans illustrating plaques in the muscle separated from bone. This case was treated by complete excision of the plaque with some recurrence of the mass. This is quite likely to happen in an area which is this extensive. It may to the urgings of the player, coach and parents with the result (B) that the recurrence was more extensive than the original lesion. These masses must not be disturbed until they are completely mature.

Figure 296.   Myositis ossificans. *A,* Preoperative. This mass was obviously immature at the time of the operation which was only a few months after injury. The surgeon succumbed to the urgings of the player, coach and parents with the result (*B*) that the recurrence was more extensive than the original lesion. These masses must not be disturbed until they are completely mature.

splitting rather than muscle-dividing. The division of a muscle, if it must be done, should be by sharp dissection, obtaining careful hemostasis as the operation proceeds. Care is taken to coagulate only the vessels and not a great deal of the muscle mass. The method of making a small buttonhole through the muscle and then proceeding to tear it open by so-called "blunt dissection" is to be condemned. In this method an index finger is placed at each extremity of the wound and the muscle is forcibly pulled apart. This is much more disrupting and traumatic to muscle fibers than is sectioning them with a sharp instrument. It results in many torn blood vessels and muscle fibers, a condition very similar to that occurring at the time of the original contusion to the muscle.

As the bony mass is approached by careful division of the overlying structures there is a temptation, when reaching the mass at one point, to strip the tissues away from it. This temptation must be resisted. The whole purpose of the procedure is to remove the mass of bone in its entirety and leave as little dead space, as little necrotic tissue, and as little infiltrated blood as possible. After the mass is thoroughly exposed it is divided from the femur by a sharp, curved osteotome, care being taken

Figure 297.   A, Calcification of front of upper femur (myositis ossificans), in this instance the result of partial avulsion of the iliopsoas tendon with resulting hematoma and calcification. B, Six months postoperative, asymptomatic.

to leave the femoral surface smooth. In the ordinary case one can readily distinguish the line of division between the recent ossification and the femoral cortex. In the occasional case the ossification may surround the shaft and blend so intimately with the femoral cortex that no line of cleavage can be found. These cases are not ordinarily symptomatic. The femur is simply larger than normal and surgical removal if necessary is very difficult. It may only increase the pathology.

After the mass is removed, complete hemostasis should be secured, including the vessels on the femoral surface. As a rule this surface does not bleed but if it does the bleeding can be controlled by judicious application of bone wax. Any shreds of muscle should be carefully clipped away. At the end of the procedure the wound should be dry, clean looking, with well defined margins. Closure is then carried out in layers. The periosteum of the femur is sutured first, if possible. The muscle should then be carefully closed in layers, great care being taken not to leave dead space. In placing the sutures it is important that they not constrict large masses of muscle. After closure of the vaginal fascia and the skin, a firm pressure bandage is applied from the toes to the groin. It is my practice to utilize a heavy posterior plaster splint from the toes to the gluteal fold supported by a lateral stirrup running from high on the inner aspect of the thigh under the foot and up to the trochanter laterally (see Fig. 315, page 455). This is bound snugly to the thigh and gives uniform pressure throughout the lower extremity. The patient is placed in bed with the foot elevated. One cubic centimeter of a suitable enzyme is given intramuscularly for three days. An oral enzyme, one tablet every four hours, is used post nauseam and continued for five to eight days, depending upon the degree of local reaction.

Active *rehabilitation* is not initiated in the thigh for at least three weeks. This does not interdict isotonic contraction of the quadriceps and hamstrings. We urge frequent periods of contraction of the calf and of the other muscles of the leg and foot. Unless the rectus femoris is primarily involved we initiate active physical therapy to the hip on the involved side on the first or second day. It goes without saying that the rest of the muscles of the body are rehabilitated from the first. The wound is inspected at appropriate intervals. At the end of 12 to 14 days the stitches are removed but the stirrup splints are continued for three weeks—longer if there is any undue reaction in the muscles of the thigh. After removal of the splints at three to four weeks, graduated active exercises are carefully begun and may need to be continued for three or four months before complete flexion of the knee is obtained. By this time the quadriceps should be of normal size.

Surgery for myositis ossificans of the thigh is not justified unless one is prepared to take the time and the pains required to make the necessarily rigorous regimen a success. This fact must be fully accepted by the surgeon and carefully explained to the player, his parents and the coach so that there can be no misunderstanding as to the time and effort required. Active participation in contact sports cannot be permitted until rehabilitation is complete.

It bears repeating that in its early stages myositis ossificans may resemble a tumor and precautions must be taken to avoid uncalled-for surgery, as indicated in Chapter 4.

MUSCLE RUPTURE

The muscles of the thigh are sometimes ruptured, a particularly susceptible one being the rectus femoris which extends from above the hip to below the knee. This often occurs as the result of a forcible blow on the muscle while it is in firm contraction so that the two ends of the muscle are firmly fixed. The muscle mechanism will tolerate a certain degree of stress without rupture. If while the muscle is under maximum stress additional tension is caused by sharp flexion of the knee, the muscle gives way somewhere along its length. This is illustrated by the running athlete as he suddenly reverses the direction of the knee motion from extension to flexion by falling or by having his knee forcibly flexed.

Figure 298.   Silhouette view of the front of the thigh while the patient is holding the quadriceps contracted. Note bulging mass of the lower end of the rectus resulting from partial avulsion of the rectus attachment to the quadriceps tendon.

The additional massive force causes the muscle to give way. The most frequent sites for rupture are at the attachment of the rectus at the hip and to the conjoined tendon above the patella.

If the tear is complete and recognized early, surgical repair will be quite gratifying. Ordinarily the condition is diagnosed as a contusion or hematoma and it is not until the local swelling and local reaction subside that the true nature of the condition becomes apparent. By this time repair is probably not possible if the rupture is within the muscle fibers. If there is actual avulsion of the attachment at the hip, it can be repaired even though rather late. Frequently the muscle is torn off the tendon at the junction of the lower middle third of the thigh or it may be separated at about the level of the trochanter. In either instance the muscle bunches up on contraction and presents a definite tumor mass (Fig. 298). This swelling subsides when the muscle is relaxed. Attempts at repair after several weeks may be extremely disappointing since we have found it impossible to suture the muscle down firmly enough to obtain any additional length.

The typical patient will present himself with a painful swollen thigh with rather localized tenderness in the muscle. Following treatment for contusion the soreness will persist and the muscle mass will appear. There may be substantial disability for many weeks. After the local reaction appears and the nature of the condition is recognized, the surgeon should carefully explain the situation to the patient, assuring him that the rupture will probably cause no actual disability, that the pain and tenderness will completely disappear, but that the bunched-up mass of muscle will remain. He will notice that the muscle of this thigh is different from that of the other thigh. Usually careful explanation of the nature of the condition is satisfactory and he will condition himself to the asymmetry and is little the worse for his lesion. Occasionally persistent pain will remain, apparently from chronic myositis or constricting fibrosis of the detached muscle ends. In this case careful surgical removal of the detached portion of the muscle eliminates the mass and will relieve the symptoms of pain (Fig. 299). One can only justify this procedure after very thorough trial of physical therapy and rehabilitation. This type of surgery probably adds no strength to the thigh but serves only to reduce the muscle mass and to relieve the pain.

This same situation occasionally arises in the adductor muscles, particularly the adductor longus (Fig. 300). The signs will be present at some point between pubis and the medial condyle of the femur. In this situation, however, if it is the attachment that is avulsed repair is quite satisfactory. If the tear is within the muscle itself, repair must be carried out within the first two weeks to have much hope for success. This same condition also occurs in the hamstring muscles but avulsion of either origin or attachment is more frequent than tear in the muscle.

A good deal of acumen is needed to recognize an isolated muscle rupture. This is particularly true when the ruptured muscle is one of several muscles carrying out the same function: for example, the rectus femoris muscle, one of the adductor muscles, or one of the hamstrings. The telltale sign of bunching up of the muscle because it has lost its attachment is usually well screened by the associated local swelling during the early stages of the condition.

The extremely heavy muscles of the thigh receive tremendous strain in almost any athletic competition. The very fact that the muscle ruptured in a given athlete would suggest excessive strain in the area involved. For this reason athletic competition must be sharply curtailed following such an injury. Certainly during the acute period no active use of the extremity should be permitted. As in so many instances of muscle damage, premature attempts toward strenuous activity can result only in disappointment and prolongation of disability. A minimum of four weeks is needed for the healed tissue to even approach maturity and even at this time the scar is very susceptible to injury. Actually, the best criterion for active use lies in the patient himself, since pain-free activity does not do any harm. The difficulty is that he may go along with ordinary pain-free activity and a sudden burst of exertion may cause re-injury. It would seem advisable to restrict activity sharply for at least six weeks. This is not to say that rehabilitation cannot be proceeding within the limits of pain. Protection of the muscle by padding or strapping is extremely difficult since active contraction may cause the damage.

Figure 299. This athlete gave a history of running hard, received "pulled muscle" in the thigh. No treatment was given other than advice to "work it out." He was examined six months after the injury. He had been sent in for Baker's cyst and the notation was that it was a little high. On examination a firm mass was palpable in the posteromedial thigh just above the knee. This mass was nonpulsating and on flexion of the knee against resistance it moved downward and became more prominent. This was accompanied by aching pain. The patient's complaint was that on running hard he had pain of increasing severity in the back of the thigh. At surgery six months post injury, this mass was found to be muscle belly with a long tendon below and a spindle-shaped upper end which was attached only by loose areolar tissue (*A*). Further dissection revealed the neurovascular bundle entering the mass in the posterosuperior aspect (*B*). The upper end detached (*C*). Note nerve entering muscle at superior end. The symptoms were caused by traction on the nerve in the neurovascular bundle as the muscle contracted. Muscle was entirely removed, relieving the symptoms.

Figure 300.   An 18 year old boy was injured at water skiing when his ski turned outward throwing his thigh into forced external rotation-abduction. Severe knifelike pain occurred on the inner side of the thigh with immediate disability. He was treated expectantly with heat and rest after a diagnosis of ruptured vessel. He was seen four months post injury because of a firm mass in the upper inner thigh. The mass itself was not painful but varied in size and was disabling because, when the youth would run, the mass would tighten up and contuse the testicle. Running was interdicted thereby. On examination there was a soft but firm mass along the adductor muscle just below the pubis extending about 5 inches distally. On contraction of the adductor, this mass would travel upward and become more prominent and more firm. Diagnosis was made of ruptured adductor, either adductor longus or gracilis. Surgery was recommended because of the disability.

A, The muscle at rest. *B,* With the adductor contracted showing impingement against the scrotum. *C,* The muscle dissected out showing complete detachment of the lower end from its femoral attachment and rounding off of the end. Note the tendinous attachment of the adductor longus with the intact gracilis lying inferior to the longus.

D, Pinching the branch of the obturator nerve to the longus. Note contraction of the muscle into the spherical shape suggested in *B.* Uneventful recovery. Early diagnosis and surgical repair might have saved this muscle.

FASCIAL HERNIA

The muscles of the thigh are completely invested in one continuous sheath of fascia—the so-called vaginal fascia of the thigh. This contains the voluminous muscles in a well defined envelope. The fascia itself is inelastic but may change shape as the enclosed muscle mass shifts about. Therefore, it is not easily torn and a traumatic defect in the fascia of the thigh is not common. It may occur, however, and present itself as a fascial hernia usually along the anterolateral aspect of the thigh where the fascia becomes thinner anterior to the iliotibial band. The ordinary symptoms of fascial hernia may be present. There is a palpable tumor mass, particularly notable when the muscle is relaxed. In some instances if there is not too much subcutaneous tissue a linear defect in the fascia may be detected. When the quadriceps muscle is contracted to extend the knee, the tumor mass will disappear and the defect be less noticeable. If this rent is large enough it probably will be asymptomatic. A small tear may cause some discomfort by bunching of the areolar tissue or fat between the tight edges of the split.

Treatment is usually not necessary. If the symptoms are too severe the condition may be treated surgically by repair of the rent provided the edges are well defined and reparable. If repair of the defect is impossible, relief may be obtained by simply enlarging the slit to a length of 3 or 4 inches. This condition is ordinarily not disabling and treatment can usually be postponed until a convenient time. Usually the patient becomes accustomed to the condition and it becomes asymptomatic.

FRACTURE OF FEMORAL SHAFT

Fracture of the shaft of the femur is a very serious injury but fortunately is not frequent in athletes. The fracture occurs as result of excessive force, usually rotatory in nature, applied to the lower extremities, and as a rule the ankle, leg or knee will give way before the thigh. If the fracture is complete the disability is immediate and usually there is little difficulty in recognizing the lesion. Incomplete fracture requires an x-ray examination. In the presence of a serious injury to the thigh, the patient should be taken on a stretcher to the hospital and a definitive diagnosis made by x-ray if the fracture is not obvious. For transportation a traction splint is applied, the most useful being a Thomas splint with half ring that rests against the ischial tuberosity, with the traction applied to the foot. For short periods this can be applied by a Jones' hitch (Fig. 301) tied around the ankle and foot and twisted to tighten the rope. Great care should be taken not to constrict circulation of the foot for a long time by this apparatus. Treatment of fracture should be instituted at once.

It is not necessary here to define the various methods of *treatment* of fracture of the femur. It will be borne in mind that the athlete is usually a young healthy male, that his healing potential is good and that he is very anxious to be rehabilitated promptly. He will of course lose the current season of competition.

Rehabilitation is extremely important in this type of fracture. The patient should be carefully instructed in exercise of the other extremities and in the use of whatever muscles of the involved extremity are available. If he is treated by traction he can keep the knee mobilized to a considerable degree. If he is placed in a plaster cast, isotonic contractions will help and he should be instructed to contract all the

Figure 301. Traction splint for fractured femoral shaft, a half-ring splint with Jones hitch. This type of traction should not be used for a long period and care should be taken to preserve the circulation to the foot.

muscles within the cast as by "shrugging" the patella and "setting" the calf. If he is treated by intramedullary fixation and this is successful enough to obviate the necessity for external fixation, rehabilitation can proceed much more rapidly. The rod will probably need to be removed before athletic participation can be resumed.

One should emphasize again that, although rehabilitation may proceed rapidly, active competition must not be permitted until the fractured femur is solidly united and the muscles of the thigh and calf are as large and strong as those on the other side. The range of the motion in all the joints must be normal. The strain on the fractured femur is magnified tremendously if there is any restriction of flexion of the knee and re-fracture is certainly a distinct possibility due to the increased leverage. Knee flexion must be essentially complete in range before any activity is permitted that could cause forcible flexion of the knee.

CHAPTER

18

Injuries of
the Knee

ANATOMICAL CONSIDERATIONS

THE KNEE is probably the most vulnerable joint of the body from the standpoint of athletic injury. The articular cartilage of the femoral condyle at the lower end of the femur is divided into two areas in its posterior and distal aspect, one covering the medial condyle and the other the lateral whereas in front the two become confluent to form the patellar groove. While functionally the knee joint is a hinge joint, physiologically it is a gliding joint, the femoral condyle rolling over the saucers of the tibial plateau which are slightly deepened by the semilunar cartilages. The patellofemoral joint particularly is a gliding joint, the patella sliding up and down in the femoral groove as the knee is flexed and extended. The posterior ligament serves to prevent overextension of the joint (Fig. 310). The lateral ligaments (Fig. 309) prevent lateral motion. Anteriorly, support is given by the quadriceps mechanism, the tone of which permits constant tension on the ligamentum patellae, no matter what position the knee is in so long as the quadriceps is in tone.

The knee is enclosed in a capsule that is very closely applied to the ligaments posteriorly and laterally (Fig. 310). In front it becomes more redundant to permit flexion of the knee. It is tight anteriorly only with the knee in complete flexion. The superior fold of the knee capsule continues into the suprapatellar pouch, the two being divided to a greater or lesser extent by the plica semilunaris. This anterior structure is quite taut with the knee in flexion but becomes quite redundant with

431

the knee in extension. There is a cone-shaped fat pad which fills the gap between the patellar tendon and the joint. This is fastened back to the intercondylar notch by the ligamentum mucosum to give it some degree of fixation. The only intra-synovial structures in the knee are the semilunar cartilages and the popliteus tendon. The cruciate ligaments, the fat pad and all of the other ligaments are extrasynovial.

This anatomically unstable joint is reinforced mainly by muscular structures. The quadriceps muscles covering the entire front of the thigh converge to attach into the patella, with some of the fibers of the aponeurosis extending medially and laterally as the patellar retinaculum to become continuous with the fascia of the leg. This gives extremely powerful extension to the knee. The anatomical position of the quadriceps is with the knee in extension. The muscle has to be extended from its resting position in order to function as an active knee extensor. The hamstring muscles running from the back of the femur and pelvis to below the knee and attaching on either side of the joint are powerful flexors of the knee. These muscles contract within their resting length in order to flex the knee. The fact that the internal hamstring tendons sweep around the medial side of the upper tibia to attach in front gives a lateral stabilizing component to the hamstrings. They also aid in preventing anterior displacement of the tibia on the femur.

The medial collateral ligament has many divisions but from the standpoint of function there are essentially two layers. The short fibers run from the femoral condyle to the upper tibial margin and extend forward only to the midlateral line. Posteriorly this blends into the posterior ligament of the knee. The more superficial portion of the medial collateral ligament passes down to attach to the tibia 2 to 3 inches below the upper tibial margin. Anteriorly this becomes continuous with the patellar retinaculum. It blends with the deep fibers usually at about the line of the joint. A superficial portion is continuous with the vaginal fascia of the thigh. The fact that this attaches below the tibial margin and anteriorly allows an arc of motion that permits the knee to bend while the ligament remains constantly tense.

On the lateral side is a strong band running from the fibula to the femoral condyle—the fibular collateral ligament—which is supported by the iliotibial tract. The iliotibial tract helps to stabilize the knee laterally. A portion of it running from the femoral condyle to the upper tibial plateau is ligamentous and forms the lateral tibial collateral ligament.

With the knee in flexion the femoral condyles are somewhat protected against a direct blow by the patella. The margins are quite vulnerable on either side of the patella, however.

The medial and lateral menisci are intrasynovial and serve to deepen somewhat the fossa of the upper plateau of the tibia. They are not essentially weight bearing but tend to fill the crevice left by the lack of congruity of the arcs of the condyles of the femur and plateau of the tibia. The actual weight bearing is on a relatively small area of the femoral condyle and a similarly small area of the tibial plateau. It should be noted that the menisci have a bony attachment anteriorly and posteriorly, the medial meniscus being "C" shaped and attached well toward the front and well toward the back of the upper surface of the tibia, whereas the lateral meniscus is more "O" shaped and attaches within the two attachments of the medial meniscus.

The anterior cruciate ligament arises from the nonarticular area on top of the tibia in front and extends upward, backward and outward to attach to the medial side of the lateral condyle of the femur well posteriorly in the intercondylar notch. The posterior cruciate ligament, on the other hand, arises anteriorly in the inter-condylar notch on the lateral side of the medial condyle right at the cartilage margin and extends backward, downward and outward, passing over the back edge of the tibia through a well defined groove to attach to the posterior surface of the tibia near the midline.

The popliteus hiatus is a defect in the coronary ligament that attaches the lateral meniscus to the upper tibia through which passes the popliteus tendon as it comes forward from its origin on the back of the tibia to attach to the lateral surface of the lower femur just superior to the chondral margin.

The entire knee is subcutaneous. In many instances bursae lie between the skin and underlying bone. Posteriorly the gastrocnemius muscle and the hamstring tendons lie between the skin and the underlying bone. The vessels and nerves crossing the popliteal space are well protected by their deep position between the two femoral condyles which project much further posteriorly than anteriorly.

CONTUSION

Basically, a contusion about the knee should be treated in the same manner as a contusion in any other location. There are certain characteristics of contusion of the knee joint, however, that deserve more detailed consideration. The knee is a highly vulnerable joint and is particularly liable to contusion either by a fall directly on the front of the knee or by a blow from the side, and one of the major considerations must be the differential diagnosis.

Diagnostically, we identify a contusion by local swelling, local tenderness, ecchymosis and overlying abrasion. Of greater importance, however, are the negative findings since it is most important to distinguish major injuries from the simple contusions. Thus, an injury along the front of the upper tibia may be called a contusion when actually it represents a tear of the tibial attachment of the medial collateral ligament. An injury over the patella may be interpreted as a contusion although there actually has been damage to the quadriceps mechanism in the nature of sprain or strain or even fracture. It is most important, therefore, in any given injury to check carefully the function of the underlying structures. Tenderness over the internal condyle of the femur may be simply the result of an opponent's boot. On the other hand, it may represent a serious injury to the femoral attachment of the medial collateral ligament. Careful attention to detail in examination will largely eliminate this diagnostic hazard. In case of doubt the knee should be treated as if it had received the more serious injury.

If it is concluded that the injury is a contusion, *treatment* is basically the same whatever area is involved; aspiration for hematoma, local injection with hyaluronidase, cold packs and compression are indicated. In the ordinary contusion splinting of the part to prevent motion is not necessary. Usually motion itself is not an aggravating element. Athletic participation need not be interdicted since under ordinary circumstances the part can be protected adequately. Protection should be designed to prevent repetition of the direct blow to the injured part. An additional knee pad, a doughnut made of sponge rubber or a plastic guard is ordinarily all that is necessary.

The conditions most likely to be confused with simple contusion are partial tears of the ligament attachments, either to the tibia or femur, strain of the attachment of the quadriceps tendon or patellar tendon to the patella, strain of the patellar tendon at its attachment to the patellar tubercle of the tibia, and early Osgood-Schlatter's disease. It bears repeating that the injury should be treated as the more serious of the two should the diagnosis be in doubt. One should become quite suspicious of a contusion that does not promptly heal. The contusion may be the precursor of a bursitis or tenosynovitis or very frequently of hematoma formation with later calcification or ossification.

STRAIN

The vicinity of the knee is quite subject to muscular and tendinous strain since violent muscular activity is involved in the normal function of this vulnerable joint.

Extensor Mechanism

Strains involving the extensor mechanism are most likely to occur in certain definite areas. In the patellar tendon the strain is usually at the lower attachment of the tendon to the patellar tubercle of the tibia or to the upper attachment at the lower pole of the patella. In both instances, the symptoms will be essentially the same except for the different areas of local manifestation. On examination, observation will be negative. Palpation will indicate a definite area of tenderness which may be directly over the patellar tubercle in one case, around the periosteum at the lower one-third of the patella in the other. Forced extension of the knee against resistance is painful, as will be forced passive flexion if the strain is acute. There is ordinarily no local swelling, local heat or any other sign of superficial inflammation. The symptoms may be quite insidious, becoming evident only after explosive activity. The player may notice them only when he runs forcibly or when he kicks the soccer ball or when he suddenly squats. This condition can be most annoying since it frequently is not severe enough to actually disable the person, yet it cuts down his effectiveness so that he cannot operate at his maximum level.

In a similar manner, strain may occur anywhere in the attachment of the quadriceps mechanism to the top of the patella. This may be in the rectus femoris or in one of the vasti. It is not frequent in this location but is often accompanied by a contusion which may complicate the diagnosis. Tenderness directly over the margin of the patella rather than over the bone itself and pain on active contraction of the quadriceps are diagnostic points.

Hamstring Mechanism

In the hamstring mechanism the strain may be in any location in the various tendons. Thus, it may be about the head of the fibula near the attachment of the biceps. It may be at the musculotendinous junction of the biceps. It may be anywhere along the internal hamstrings. The most common location is at the biceps attachment to the fibula where it may be easily confused with bursitis of this area. It can be distinguished from bursitis by the fact that active function of the biceps tendon will ordinarily cause pain whereas in a bursitis it should not. Frequently in the hamstring tendons the strain may be accompanied by tenosynovitis in which case treatment should be directed toward the tenosynovitis as well as the strain. The treatment is quite similar for the two conditions. Another frequent location for strain is the attachment of the internal hamstrings through the pes anserinus where it may be readily confused with damage to the attachment of the medial collateral ligament to the tibia. Here again, diagnostic points are pain on function of the tendon and absence of pain on stress of the ligament. A distressing strain of the knee occurs at the musculotendinous junction of either the biceps or the semitendinosus which causes pain in the back of the thigh and may become completely disabling as a result of spasm of the involved hamstring muscle. A more obscure type of strain is that of the popliteus tendon where it attaches to the femur just above the articular margin of the lateral condyle. This may be very difficult to distinguish from sprain of the lateral collateral ligament or damage to the lateral meniscus.

Treatment of strain of the knee is complete rest to eliminate active function of the muscle involved. In some cases this will require the use of a splint and in others merely the avoidance of strenuous activity. Either measure is incompatible with continued athletic participation. Direct therapeutic measures consist of the injection into the area of a long-acting local anesthetic followed by a corticoid preparation. Use of local heat such as diathermy is in order. Whirlpool baths, hot packs, analgesic balm, all may be useful. In the final analysis, in a relatively severe strain of the tendons about the knee complete nonparticipation for an interval long enough to permit definitive treatment may well return the player to active sports whereas continued participation in sports may render him quite ineffectual. The danger is in recurrence since it is difficult to eliminate the cause of the strain and not ground the athlete. Once recovery is complete, recurrence need not be anticipated. Straps, wraps and pads will have little effect in preventing reinjury.

It is worth emphasizing again that one should spare no effort to make a specific diagnosis in these conditions about the knee. Proper diagnosis is the antecedent to proper treatment.

BURSITIS

It was noted in the general discussion of bursae that while many of them are relatively constant many others are adventitious. As a basic concept, a bursa develops in order to permit friction-free motion between contiguous moving parts. There is a wealth of bursae about the knee (Fig. 302) and a detailed anatomical description of them all is not pertinent here. With a few exceptions only those which are consistent in their formation and are particularly prone to involvement in the athlete will be discussed.

BURSITIS ON THE ANTERIOR ASPECT OF THE KNEE

Prepatellar Bursa

Anteriorly the bursa most commonly involved is the prepatellar (Fig. 302). This bursal sac lies between the skin and the anterior surface of the patella and serves to permit free sliding of the relatively thin skin over the underlying subcu-

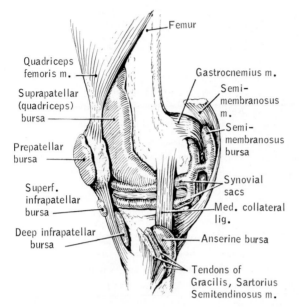

Figure 302.   The bursae about the knee. Medial aspect.

taneous bone. This bursa is particularly susceptible to damage by direct trauma, as by falling on the flexed knee. Whereas in its normal state this bursa is somewhat smaller than the underlying patella, it may reach amazing size when its sac is distended. Involvement of this bursa may be acute or chronic.

Acute Prepatellar Bursitis.   Acute involvement will usually begin as an area of tenderness, reddening and inflammation directly over the kneecap. The skin becomes extremely red and warm and sensitive to touch. If the knee is examined very early, snowball crepitation can often be elicited between the walls of the bursa as the skin is moved over the patella. This inflammation progresses rapidly to the formation of effusion so that there is tense, hot swelling localized directly over the patella (Fig. 303). Ordinary motion of the knee is pain-free but flexion to the point of skin tension will cause pain. This condition can be readily distinguished from involvement of the knee joint by its definite localization in front of the patella.

TREATMENT in the acute stage is that of any acute inflammatory reaction. Immobilization of the knee in a posterior splint (Fig. 315, *A*) and a warm saline dressing will usually suffice. If there is definite fluid in the sac, aspiration will distinguish between gross pus and bursal fluid. A culture of the fluid, if any is obtained, should be made. Ordinarily the inflammation will subside quickly with only a slight residual thickening of the lining, the period of disability being only a few days. It is unusual for acute bursitis to go on to acute suppuration, but if this occurs drainage is carried out through a short (1½ inch) vertical incision through the skin ½ inch lateral to the patella on either side. Great care is taken to restrict the incision to the skin and bursa to avoid any possibility of opening into the knee joint. Through-and-through rubber tissue drainage together with moderate pressure and continuation of the hot pack will suffice in most local situations. A broad-spectrum antibiotic is given until definite sensitivity of the organism to a specific antibiotic can be determined.

Following acute bursitis, adequate protective padding over the knee should be used since recurrence is a strong possibility owing to the extremely vulnerable location of the bursa.

Chronic Prepatellar Bursitis.   A much more frequent involvement of the prepatellar bursa is chronic bursitis. This may develop as a sequel to repeated attacks of acute bursitis but is more likely to be the result of repeated mild traumata which cause thickening of the bursal wall, oversecretion of fluid and gradual filling of the bursal sac. Examined early the knee will be asymptomatic, the only finding being the well outlined discrete sac of fluid very obviously subcutaneous and not involving the knee joint (Fig. 303).

TREATMENT at this stage should consist of aspiration of the fluid, injection of a corticoid and a firm pressure dressing. Since the condition is relatively asymptomatic, however, and since a pressure dressing is not consistent with active sports participation, it is unusual for the player to seek or accept this particular plan of treatment. Usually the condition is allowed to continue and, as he repeatedly falls or kneels on the distended bursa, pressure on its wall causes it to stretch and the sac to expand. A bursa which actually is much smaller in diameter than the patella may distend to cover the whole anterior surface of the knee, not infrequently reaching 6 to 8 inches in diameter. It presents itself as a loose, floppy, fluctuant tumor mass causing symptoms largely by its very bulk. Once a bursa has reached this stage no treatment short of surgical excision is adequate. Surgical excision is relatively simple, a transverse incision being made slightly above the midline of the patella and extending from 3 to 6 inches depending upon the size of the bursa. The bursa is carefully dissected out. This is particularly difficult directly over the patella where the skin is very thin. Care should be taken not to buttonhole the skin. It is important to remove the whole lining of the sac and this is facilitated by opening into the sac

Figure 303.   Prepatellar bursitis of the patella in its normal position with swelling between patella and skin.

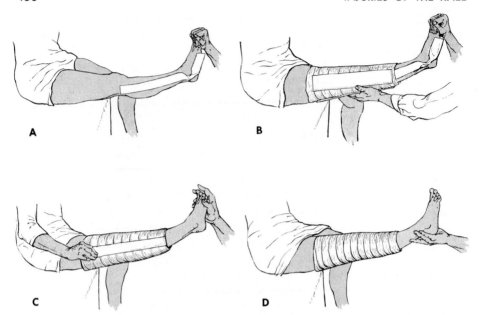

Figure 304.   Cotton cast. *A,* The leg is shaved from the knee to the ankle and 3 inch adhesive strip is applied to either side. *B,* The knee is wrapped in regular sheet wadding, usually five or six rolls, slightly longer than the length of the yucca board. A moistened yucca board splint is applied on either side and posteriorly, centering at the knee. *C,* Yucca board splints have been wrapped snugly in place with 3 inch gauze. The two adhesive strips are pulled back firmly over the ends of the two lateral boards. *D,* The finished cotton cast, the adhesive strips having been wrapped down snugly with gauze and the whole protected by spiral 1 inch adhesive tape.

and using the finger within the bursa to determine its limits. Following excision it is advisable to tack the skin to the underlying fascia over the patellar retinaculum and the quadriceps in order to prevent development of dead spaces. If the bursa was quite large the two angles of the wound should be drained for 48 hours by strips of rubber tissue. Recurrence of the fluid postoperatively is to be avoided if possible since an adventitious bursa may develop that may have all of the characteristics of the original one.

Following excision of the bursa the knee should be supported in a dressing such as the cotton cast (Fig. 304) in order to prevent excess motion between the skin and patella until such time as the space is completely obliterated. This usually requires about three weeks. It is important that the area be inspected at frequent intervals during the early postoperative period since any fluid that accumulates must be promptly aspirated. It is discouraging to the surgeon, and I dare say even more to the patient, to have the bursa recur. Those most likely to recur are the large ones. For this reason it is recommended that the bursa should be removed as soon as it can be definitely determined that irreversible chronic bursitis is present. The removal of a small, sharply localized bursa is relatively simple and very effectual whereas some of the larger ones may present a major problem.

I recall a case of a football player who insisted on playing without knee pads. He carried his prepatellar bursitis through an entire season, being treated only by repeated aspirations and some feeble attempt at pressure. At one time over a quart of fluid was removed from the bursa. At operation it was found to be of tremendous size, extending as high as midthigh and down to about 4 inches above the ankle. The player was cured by surgical excision of the sac (which could hardly be called a bursa) and suture of the skin to the underlying fascia. In spite of care at the original operation there was a small area of recurrence which required a second excision. The player had remarkably little disability even during the period of extreme distention of the sac. One of the complaints was a sloshing up and down of the contained fluid as he ran.

Characteristically the wall of an extremely expanded bursae will upon examination present the picture of a very chronic synovitis, usually without villous thickening. It has a shiny, almost plastic appearance interspersed with areas of petechiae the size of the end of the finger. The superficial appearance of these areas is similar to that of psoriasis on the skin. The pathological report has uniformly been "chronic synovial inflammation." During the chronic stage of this noninflammatory type of bursitis it may be necessary to aspirate the sac repeatedly, continue pressure bandages and allow participation until a more convenient time for surgical removal. However, if the sac is widely distended it is not desirable to permit competitive athletics for the reasons noted above. In carrying out aspiration it must be remembered that the sac is just beneath the skin and great care should be taken that the aspirating needle does not inadvertently penetrate into the knee joint. This is particularly important if there is an acute inflammation, in which case also the accident is much more likely to happen since there will be edema, tension and considerable inelasticity of the tissue. Prepatellar bursitis treated nonsurgically is prone to recur hence adequate padding of the knee is mandatory in order to prevent direct trauma over the patella. After surgical excision also, even though there appears to be complete cure, it is wise to insist that a player wear knee pads whenever he is engaged in competitive or contact sports.

Infrapatellar Bursa (Deep Infrapatellar Bursa)

The infrapatellar bursa lies behind the patellar tendon and in front of the infrapatellar fat pad (Fig. 302). It does not ordinarily communicate with the knee joint, being separated from the knee by the fat pad. The etiology of infrapatellar bursitis is quite different from that of prepatellar bursitis. The prepatellar bursa is frequently traumatized by a direct blow upon the hard patella which makes up its floor, whereas the infrapatellar bursa is not particularly subject to direct trauma since it lies behind the thick patellar tendon and in front of the soft fat pad. Occasionally the lower part of the bursa, which extends down over the front of the upper end of the tibia, may be traumatized but inflammation of this bursa is ordinarily due to friction between the patellar tendon and structures behind it (upper tibia and fat pad), the result of overactivity.

The *symptoms* are usually pain on complete passive flexion and on active complete extension of the knee. Tenderness surrounds the patellar tendon and is particularly notable under its edges. If the tendon is picked up between the thumb and forefinger and the thumb and forefinger are permitted to slip behind it, direct pressure will cause pain.

Diagnosis.   Infrapatellar bursitis must, if possible, be distinguished from involvement of the infrapatellar fat pad which lies directly behind it. In inflammation of the bursa which has proceeded to the point of fluid formation it may be possible to demonstrate fluid in the sac lying directly behind the patellar tendon, which bulges out on either side. Pressure on one side will cause it to bulge out on the other. Similarly, flexion of the knee will cause the patellar tendon to compress the sac and make it balloon out on either side. Inflammation of the infrapatellar fat pad, on the other hand, will seem to be deeper, more posterior. Passive extension of the knee should be pain-free in infrapatellar tendon bursitis whereas, if the fat pad is inflamed and swollen, complete passive extension may be impossible or will cause pain. Complete flexion of the knee will cause pain in either instance. One distressing symptom of both conditions is the sharp twinge of pain on pendulum extension of the knee which is particularly distressing to the place kicker since in completing this kick there is snap extension of the knee whereas in the punt or ordinary running there is much less of this particular motion. If the involvement in infrapatellar bursitis is severe enough it will seriously interfere with active motion of the knee, particularly in extremes in either flexion or extension. The condition must also be distinguished from so-called Osgood-Schlatter disease (page 520). In Osgood-Schlatter disease the pain and tenderness are more specifically in the tendon or in the patellar tubercle. However, the same clinical tests will cause discomfort, namely, extension of the knee against resistance, overflexion of the knee, and direct pressure over the area.

The *treatment* of infrapatellar bursitis is that of bursitis anywhere. In the early stages local heat and splinting of the knee in extension will reduce the inflammation. Aspiration of the bursa with removal of any fluid encountered, followed by injection of a corticoid, is particularly effective if done early. If effusion is recurrent and resistant to local treatment the bursa may readily be excised, incision being made usually on the inner side of the patellar tendon. The bursa can usually be removed entirely through the single incision. If the bursal mass should appear to be more extensive laterally, incision may be made on the outer side of the patellar tendon. Following careful removal of the entire bursal sac, the fat pad is sutured to the back of the patellar tendon to obliterate the dead space. The knee is splinted in extension with a type of dressing that gives both immobilization and compression (cotton cast). The dressing must be maintained for at least three weeks.

Suprapatellar Tubercle Bursa (Superficial Infrapatellar Bursa)

Another bursa on the anterior aspect of the knee that may become symptomatic lies between the skin and patellar tubercle of the tibia (Figs. 302 and 305). This is not a consistent bursa nor is it frequently involved. In a young individual there may be some difficulty in distinguishing inflammation of this bursa from early Osgood-Schlatter disease; indeed, many of the cases of Osgood-Schlatter disease which have apparently been relieved by local injection may well have been involvement of this pretibial bursa.

Symptoms of involvement of this bursa are sharply localized pain and tenderness directly over the patellar tubercle. They vary from those of infrapatellar bursitis in that active function of the knee does not cause pain since the attachment of the patellar tendon is not involved. In the acute type local inflammation will be the characteristic finding. I have yet to see an extensive collection of the fluid in this bursa.

Figure 305.   Calcification of the suprapatellar bursa. *A,* Silhouette view of patella, apparently showing an osteochondritic fragment in the joint. *B,* Lateral view showing the calcification in the patellar tendon attachment. Although in the silhouette view this appeared to be under the patella, it was actually some 4 inches away. This illustrates the value of very careful interpretation of the film. The fact that this fragment did not show under the patella in the lateral view was suggestive. (Note the normal fabella, a sesamoid bone lying within the gastrocnemius and articulating with the femoralcondyle.)

Since active function of the knee is not affected, protection against direct trauma is the most pertinent point in prevention of recurrence. Following local treatment there is no particular indication for immobilization of the knee, hence the importance of distinguishing this condition from Osgood-Schlatter's disease, strain of the patellar tendon attachment, infrapatellar bursitis and other neighboring conditions which do require immobilization and do cause disability.

BURSITIS ON THE MEDIAL ASPECT OF THE KNEE

Anserine Bursa

Another bursa consistently present but not so frequently involved is the anserine bursa (Fig. 302). While this bursa may have the usual variants and may be single or multiple, it ordinarily lies between the aponeurosis of the attachment of the internal hamstrings and of the long fibers of the medial collateral ligament and the underlying anteromedial face of the upper end of the tibia (Fig. 302). Under normal circumstances the pes anserinus and the long fibers of the collateral ligament attach to the tibia some 3 inches below the superior articular surface. The bursa serves to separate these freely sliding portions of the tendon and ligament from the periosteum of the tibia. Bursitis in this area is typically of the friction type although it may be initiated by an external blow impinging the bursa against the hard tibia beneath. The resulting congestion and inflammation cause the same reaction that occurs in tenosynovitis or any friction bursitis.

Original *symptoms* are pain from the contusion, which is persistent and rather sharply localized. Symptoms are aggravated by flexion and extension of the knee. Since the symptoms will be located on the upper anteromedial face of the tibia they may be confused with those of injury to the medial collateral ligament. However, they are quite distinguishable under careful examination, the tenderness being located not at the attachment of the tendon and ligament but under their unattached portion. Crepitation if elicitable is diagnostic.

Treatment is application of local heat and immobilization of the knee. Recovery can be expedited by injection of a corticoid into the bursa. While this condition may be quite acute it seldom causes suppuration. In fact, I have never seen a case of acute suppuration in this bursa. The involvement does tend to be chronic, particularly if full activity is allowed too early. Protective pads against contusion are of little value since real protection requires elimination of motion of the knee joint and so will demand nonparticipation in athletics. I have never been able successfully to aspirate fluid from this bursa nor have I seen fluid develop to the point that it could be demonstrated as fluctuation. I think one explanation for this is the tension that exists between the tendon and ligament structures and the tibia, allowing for no redundant fold of bursa that can be filled with fluid. Similarly, I have noted in complete rupture of the collateral ligament that it is very unusual for blood to accumulate under the pes anserinus.

Semimembranosus Bursa

More posteriorly on the medial side is the semimembranosus bursa (Fig. 302) lying between the attachment of the semimembranosus muscle to the upper tibia and medial capsule of the joint. This position is slightly posterior to the midline of the tibia and extends about 1 inch below its upper end. Further posteriorly is the gastrocnemius bursa lying between the tendon of origin of the medial head of the gastrocnemius and semimembranosus tendon. There may also be bursae between the tendons of the semimembranosus and semitendinosus and gracilis. All of these are subject to involvement, the symptoms depending upon the location and the degree of involvement. Inflammation of the semimembranosus bursa may be confused with damage to the medial collateral ligament but is distinguished by the fact that tension on the medial collateral ligament does not cause increase in pain. The tenderness is distinctly over the semimembranosus tendon just short of its attachment.

BURSITIS ON THE POSTERIOR ASPECT OF THE KNEE

Baker's Cyst

Posteriorly, the most common involvement in athletes is the so-called Baker's cyst. The confusion which so frequently accompanies the use of eponyms is certainly evident here since the term "Baker's cyst" has been extended to include almost any synovial hernia or bursitis involving the posterior aspect of the knee.

One type of "Baker's cyst" is bursitis of the semimembranosus or of the medial gastrocnemius bursa (Figs. 302 and 306), a bursa which lies between the medial head of the gastrocnemius and semimembranosus tendon. Involvement of the bursa causes expansion of its wall, usually posteriorly since there is no particular obstruction to its expansion in this direction. It presents itself as a large soft tumor mass in the popliteal space. The appearance of the mass is usually preceded by a varying period of chronic, aching type pain in the back of the knee. Since the bursa frequently communicates with the knee, often by a valvelike arrangement,

Gracilis m.

Semitendinosus m.

Semimembranosus m.

Bursa

Gastrocnemius m.

Biceps femoris m.

Semimembranosus muscle

Semimembranosus bursa

Gastrocnemius m.

Synovial sac

A   B

Figure 306.   Baker's cyst showing the semimembranosus bursa lying between the semimembranosus and medial head of the gastrocnemius. The actual enlargement of the sac may be palpable at any level. If it protrudes proximally, it will appear in the midline. If it protrudes in its distal portion, it will appear medial to the midline. The medial gastrocnemius bursa (not labeled) lies under the tendon.

the swelling may come and go and present great difficulty diagnostically. As a consequence of the valvelike connection with the knee joint, sufficient fluid may collect to make a sizable tumor. This fluid then concentrates to the characteristic jell contained in a synovial hernia. Later as a result of trauma or other cause it may be discharged into the knee, where the concentrated fluid becomes an irritative factor and causes synovitis. We frequently have found a to-and-fro connection between the knee and bursa so that increased fluid in the knee will distend the bursa and, as the knee recovers, the bursal fluid may remain only to be discharged back into the knee and cause recurrence of the joint effusion. It has been my observation that this bursal involvement is frequently the result of chronic trauma and is too often related to posterior damage to the medial meniscus to be entirely coincidental. Whether the trauma actually opens up the space between the bursa and knee or causes exudation of fluid that discharges into the bursa rather than into the suprapatellar pouch varies with the individual case. The patient with Baker's cyst, therefore, may present himself with a perfectly benign, asymptomatic swelling back of the knee or he may have swelling incidental to internal derangement or to chronic synovitis of the knee. So it can be seen that in this one entity, namely, the involvement of the medial gastrocnemius bursa and semimembranosus bursa, there may be several different conditions that can be called Baker's cyst.

So also may Baker's cyst be the result of a synovial hernia off one of the tendon sheaths, specifically, the semitendinosus. Add to this the fact that the cyst may also result from a true synovial hernia from the back of the joint due to a defect or degeneration in the posterior capsule similar to the formation of a ganglion anywhere and we have several different etiological conditions giving the same terminal diagnosis. One should if at all possible avoid the eponym "Baker's cyst" and be more specific in the diagnosis, since specificity of diagnosis will aid in treatment.

Diagnosis.   This condition must be distinguished from other tumor masses, such as aneurysm of the popliteal artery, arterial venous aneurysm or soft tissue tumor. Occasionally wholly benign conditions may present a confusing picture. I well recall my humiliation at confidently exposing the mass of a "Baker's cyst" only to find that in this singularly well muscled individual the "cyst" was an unusually low lying belly of the semimembranosus muscle. The only pathologic finding in this instance was a preoperatively diagnosed posterior tear of the medial meniscus. As a rule, these conditions present no emergency and time and patience will permit diagnosis. If it is necessary to operate upon the knee for some other cause, as in the case mentioned above, exploration of this area cannot be condemned since a second operation must thus be avoided. On the other hand, one would be quite chagrined to operate under a primary diagnosis of Baker's cyst and find only over-redundant fat or overdeveloped muscle.

Treatment.   If the pathology is that of a synovial hernia off the joint then dissecting out the mass and carefully closing the defect into the knee joint will ordinarily institute a cure. If it is an involvement of the bursa with an open connection into the knee joint, removal of the bursa must include careful suture of the defect in the joint capsule. If it is a result of involvement of the medial meniscus, removal of the Baker's cyst or of the medial meniscus alone will be disappointing. On many occasions we have been able to demonstrate the opening extending into the bursa back of the knee in the course of exposing the posterior compartment for complete removal of the medial meniscus.

If the Baker's cyst is primarily an irritative bursitis of the bursa lying between the semimembranosus and gastrocnemius, removal of the bursa should be followed by careful suture of the semimembranosus to the gastrocnemius, thus eliminating the irritative friction point between these two muscles. I have done this on many occasions and have yet to see any untoward symptoms as the result of suturing these structures together.

If this discussion of treatment for Baker's cyst seems somewhat confusing it is because of the heterogenous group of conditions that are lumped together under this name. Carefully analyzed it will be seen that the treatment recommended is the treatment for the basic underlying condition. If bursitis, excision of the bursa. If hernia of the joint or tendon, repair of the hernia. If a defect in the posterior capsule or medial meniscus, appropriate treatment for the underlying lesion. In this situation, as in many others, the proper treatment will depend upon accurate diagnosis. In many instances this diagnosis may not be made preoperatively and one must be alert at operation to determine if at all possible the basic underlying pathology so that he can remove the disease as well as the symptoms.

Following surgical correction it is advisable to hold the knee in compression immobilization (Fig. 304) for a period of at least three weeks. As in synovial hernia or ganglion elsewhere, recurrence may be prevented by adequate repair. If the condition was a true bursitis, recurrence may be prevented by permitting complete healing of the structures involved. In my hands nonsurgical management of these swellings in the back of the knee has not been satisfactory. I have occasionally aspirated the mass for diagnostic purposes and at other times have seen the tumor disappear spontaneously but have been dissatisfied with treatment by aspiration, local injection and immobilization.

BURSITIS ON THE LATERAL ASPECT OF THE KNEE

Bursae About the Head of the Fibula

On the lateral aspect of the knee are several bursae, any one of which may cause symptoms. The most common are bursae about the upper end of the fibula. A rather consistent bursa, the bicipital, lies between the fibular collateral ligament and the biceps just adjacent to the fibular attachment. Since each of these strong, fibrous structures splits to encompass the other, there may be several bursae in this area to permit active motion between them.

Diagnostically, inflammation of these bursae may present a considerable problem since they are consistent neither in size nor location. Characteristically the pain is proximal to the head of the fibula with tenderness around the fibular collateral ligament and the biceps. However, the same findings may be present in a strain of the biceps tendon or a sprain of the fibular collateral ligament. In many instances it is impossible to distinguish between these conditions and in other instances they co-exist. Only in the unusual case does synovial effusion develop in sufficient amount to permit palpation of a fluctuant mass. However, local swelling in this area, even though it may be diffuse, is much more common in bursitis than it is in the other conditions commonly found here. Thickening of the bursal wall plus effusion with local irritation may become severe enough to cause pressure on the peroneal nerve as it winds around the back of the fibular head. Symptoms are of pain along the distribution of the nerve; on occasion an actual peroneal palsy develops. Bursitis in this location is not commonly prone to calcification. The presence of a hard, calcified mass contained within the constricting walls of the bursa may be exceedingly painful and may indeed cause pressure on the nerve. In case of unexplained peroneal neuritis one should suspect bursitis about the head of the fibula.

Treatment of bursitis in this area is local heat, rest and local injection. It should be noted that this treatment is similar to that of strain or sprain and in many cases one may not have distinguished between these conditions. This is particularly likely since active motion of the knee will cause pain in all of them. Strictly speaking, active flexion against resistance should hurt more in a strain or tenosynovitis of the biceps tendon than it should in a true bursitis, whereas direct pressure or passive extension of the knee might be expected to be more painful in bursitis. Bursal pain may also be elicited by activity within a range of motion that does not cause strain on the tendon. It should be realized that these are more impressions than diagnostic certainties. Involvement in this area may be particularly disheartening since it is exceedingly prone to recur because of the previously mentioned anatomical relationships with two bifid attachments interdigitating with each other to make multiple friction points.

If pyogenic bursitis develops it should be treated appropriately for the infection. If the response to antibiotic therapy is not reasonably prompt, the best definitive treatment for pyogenic bursitis is early drainage with identification of the organism and institution of specific antibiotic therapy. If one succumbs to the

Figure 307.   Calcification of bursa about the fibular head with nerve involvement. This patient developed soreness around the outer side of the knee which was attributable to increased activity. The pain gradually became more intense and lancinating in character down the peroneal nerve distribution. Physical examination revealed inability to straighten the knee with peroneal nerve pain on attempting to straighten it, and palpable tumor in the vicinity of the head and biceps tendon. X-ray revealed calcification in the bicipital bursa. Excision of the mass resulted in dramatic relief with uneventful recovery.

temptation to treat the condition by antibiotics alone it is very apt to terminate in excessive thickening of the bursal walls and painful scar formation even if the acute infection subsides. It is much more likely to go on to chronic suppurative involvement with a long period of disability. If calcification develops in the early stages it may respond to aspiration and injection with a corticoid whereas in the later stages it must be surgically removed. I recall one instance in which exceedingly distressing peroneal pain had been attributed to many other things including psychoneurosis. The patient, a woman, had a very large calcifying bursitis and at operation the peroneal nerve was found to be tightly stretched over the firm, solid mass of the bursa full of calcium. Excision of the bursa and saline neurolysis of the nerve gave prompt and complete relief (Fig. 307).

Popliteal Bursa

A little higher up on the fibular collateral ligament a bursa will be found lying between the popliteus tendon and the fibular collateral ligament slightly above the line of the knee joint. Another relatively consistent bursa lies upon the lateral head of the gastrocnemius located slightly behind the biceps tendon. Any of these lateral bursae may connect with the knee joint, particularly the one between the lateral condyle of the femur and tendon of the popliteus and the one between the popliteus and fibular collateral ligament. In this area, too, a specific diagnosis may present great difficulty because of the variety of structures which present a similarity of symptoms. It has been said that the popliteus muscle is the overlooked structure of the knee since its lesions are so infrequently diagnosed. Differentiation between popliteal bursitis, popliteal tenosynovitis, strain of the popliteus muscle or tendon, and involvement of the adjacent bursae is difficult. It is sufficient to state that treatment of the lateral aspect of the knee is local treatment of the tender area: injection, local heat, and protection against any motion that causes pain. This whole lateral complex of lateral meniscus, fibular collateral ligament, popliteus muscle and biceps tendon may present well-nigh insuperable obstacles to diagnosis. Fortunately, as has been mentioned, the basic treatment is essentially the same in the incipient case and the more advanced cases will present more specific diagnostic points.

Other Bursae

As one proceeds posteriorly he encounters the *lateral gastrocnemius bursa* lying between the condyle of the femur and the lateral head of the gastrocnemius. Involvement of this bursa is infrequently diagnosed. As to its frequency or whether it occurs as part of another pathological symptom complex I have no information. I have never been able to diagnose inflammation of the *bursa lying beneath the popliteus muscle* since in acute conditions it is indistinguishable from other conditions in the back of the popliteal space and in chronic conditions I have never seen it sufficiently distended with fluid to provide a clue.

SPRAIN

It must be remembered that a ligament is a fibrous structure designed to prevent abnormal motion of a joint. Any injury to a ligament caused by abnormal motion may be defined as a sprain. It should be obvious, then, that a sprain can vary from a complete dislocation of a joint with total loss of integrity of the ligament at one extreme to a slight tearing of a few isolated fibers with no loss of function at the other. Properly it should include avulsion of the ligament from bone with or without a small fragment of bone (sprain-fracture) (Fig. 308), partial avulsion of the

Figure 308.   Acute avulsion of fibular collateral ligament from the femur with a flake of bone.

ligament from the bone, or tearing of the ligament within its substance either transversely, obliquely or longitudinally. In the last instance the ligament will be elongated although it may appear to be intact. The function of the ligament depends not only upon its strength but upon its length, and a ligament that is elongated does not carry out its function of preventing abnormal motion of the joint. Since we are primarily concerned clinically with the function of the ligament, it matters little in what way but a great deal to what extent this function is disturbed. It is apparent that the severity of the injury is of much more significance than the exact location or type of the tear. It follows that the determination of the degree of loss of function of the involved ligament at the earliest possible moment is of prime importance.

Ligamentous Anatomy of the Knee

The anatomical drawings (Figs. 309 and 310) will serve as a review of the ligamentous structures of the knee. The knee consists essentially of two long bones meeting end to end without benefit of either the deep ball and socket of the hip or the mortise and tendon of the ankle. The bony stability of the knee derives solely from the fact that the femur is a bipod with two separate distal condyles, and lateral instability will be present only when one or the other foot of the femur has been lifted from the tibia. This bipod provides lateral stability with much less

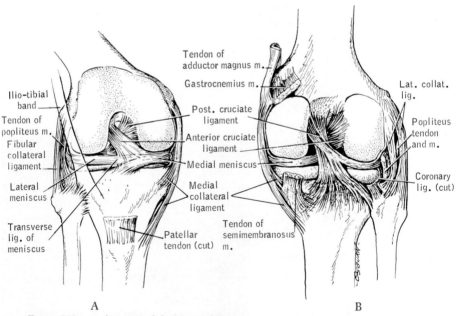

A   B

Figure 309.   Anatomical drawings of knee.
A, Anterior view. Patellar tendon is sectioned and the patella reflected upward. Knee flexed. Note that the cruciate ligament rises in front of anterior tibial spine, not from it. Note also that the medial meniscus is firmly attached to the medial collateral ligament.
B, Posterior view, knee extended. Note that the posterior ligament has been removed. The two layers of the medial collateral ligament are shown diagrammatically, also the tibial portion of the lateral collateral ligament. The posterior cruciate ligament rises behind the tibia, not on its upper surface. Observe the femoral attachment of the anterior cruciate ligament at the back of the notch.

Figure 310.   Anatomic sketch illustrating posterior capsule of the knee joint. This is
an extremely dense fibrous structure attaching above the condyles clear across the back of the
femur extra-articularly. It attaches below the knee all the way across the tibia and onto the
fibula. This structure is tight in extension (left), at which time it adds materially to the
stability of the knee in all directions except flexion. It is an extremely positive check ligament
to prevent overextension. With the knee flexed (right), the ligament becomes redundant, so
that it no longer has any stabilizing effect in any direction.

demand upon ligament strength than would be necessary if there were but a single
condyle. Nonetheless, real stability of the joint depends in major degree upon the
intricately designed and ingeniously arranged ligaments of the knee.

The LATERAL LIGAMENTS (Fig. 309) and the POSTERIOR LIGAMENT (or capsule) (Fig. 310) actually are a part of the great investiture of the joint by ligamentous structures which are massive and very strong laterally and posteriorly but
which become thinned in front to form the patellar retinaculum and so permit
motion of the joint. These ligaments are supported and their strength greatly aug-
mented by the CRUCIATE LIGAMENTS (Fig. 309) which are very strong, fan-shaped
structures, each twisted on itself to permit motion but to provide maximum stability. The anterior cruciate ligament arising anteromedially from the tibial plateau
in front of the anterior tibial spine extends backward, upward and outward to attach
to the femur posterolaterally in the intercondylar notch. While it has other functions, its primary function is to prevent forward displacement of the tibia on the
femur. The posterior cruciate ligament, on the other hand, arises from the back of
the tibia, actually posterior to the articular surface. It extends forward, upward and
inward to attach to the anterior edge of the intercondylar notch on the medial side
just adjacent to the articular margin. The primary function of this ligament is to
prevent backward displacement of the tibia on the femur.

All the ligaments of the knee—both collaterals, the cruciates and the posterior
capsule—are taut in complete extension of the knee and in this position the knee is
the most stable. Varying degrees of relaxation occur in the different ligaments as the
knee is flexed. This is particularly exemplified by the posterior capsule which loses

its stabilizing function completely with only a few degrees of flexion. The knee ligaments act synergistically to support each other in preventing abnormal mobility of the knee while at the same time permitting normal motion. Functionally the knee joint is a hinge joint although anatomically the motion is much more complicated than this. The ligaments of the joint are designed to prevent abnormal lateral motion, abnormal rotatory motion and abnormal forward and backward displacement of tibia on femur. The heavy posterior ligament serves to prevent overextension of the joint. The anatomy of the menisci will be described later in this chapter.

Etiology

Sprain of the knee is caused by an abnormal motion of the joint that throws stress on the ligament or ligaments designed to prevent this motion. Forced motion beyond this normal limit will result in some degree of injury to the ligament primarily involved. This motion may be in any direction—adduction or abduction, overextension, internal or external rotation, forward or backward displacement—or almost any combination of these. Certain particular combinations are more frequent than others.

Although frequently it is not obtainable, detailed knowledge of the manner of injury can be of great importance since it may indicate the type of ligament damage and so permit early, definitive treatment. In the classical athletic injury of the knee, the foot is fixed to the ground, the thigh rotates inward and the leg outward, the knee is forced inward toward the opposite leg and the stress is primarily received on the ligaments on the inner side of the knee. It is generally caused by the familiar lateral blocking or by the "cut-back" motion of the running athlete, when the foot is forced into external rotation and stress is exerted against the medial collateral

Figure 311.   Photograph illustrating the forces causing "The Unhappy Triad," namely, sprain of the medial collateral and anterior cruciate ligaments and damage to the medial meniscus. (Permission to print granted by The Miami Herald, Miami, Florida.)

Figure 312. Classic injury resulting from forces shown in Figure 311. Note superficial layer and deep layer of medial collateral ligament torn near tibial attachment. Medial meniscus is ruptured and anterior cruciate ligament has torn completely.

ligament of the knee, the superficial layer of which takes the strain first. As this stretches, tears or gives way, the force reaches the deep layer, to which is attached the medial meniscus. If the force continues, the anterior cruciate receives the stress and it, too, may fail. In severe injuries, the posterior cruciate may also give way. We would expect in injuries of this causation to find sprain of the medial collateral and anterior cruciate ligaments and damage to the medial meniscus ("The Unhappy Triad") (Figs. 311, 312 and 313). Obviously, the injury may stop at any point in

Figure 313. "Unhappy triad." Classical injury with the medial collateral off the tibia, the anterior cruciate pulled off the femur with a fragment of bone. This is very favorable for cruciate repair.

this progression of events. In a similar manner the adduction and internal rotation type of injury places the stress against the lateral ligaments of the knee, the lateral cartilage, and the anterior and posterior cruciate (Fig. 314). Hyperextension of the knee throws initial tension on the posterior ligament of the joint, followed by stress against the posterior cruciate ligament and the posterior part of the two collaterals if the hyperextension continues. Direct forward motion of the tibia on the femur will injure the anterior cruciate while the opposite motion will damage the posterior cruciate.

Diagnosis

Diagnosis begins with a general evaluation of the situation. Did it seem to be a serious injury? Was the player immediately disabled, or was he able to keep going? Did he himself feel that he had received a serious injury? Was he able to leave the field under his own power, or was he carried? Was he suffering extreme pain, or was it relatively mild? This general evaluation is subject to further modification following examination but is often of considerable importance in determining the severity of the injury. Following this an early, careful and complete physical examination of the joint is of great importance. The earlier this can be done the better, since factors can often be determined then which become obscure after pain and swelling screen the symptoms. Note whether tenderness is at the joint line, above the joint, or below. Check the knee carefully for abnormal mobility in any direction, including rotation, lateral motion, anterior and posterior motion of the tibia on the femur. Observe the degree and the rapidity of swelling. Investigate whether the knee was actually locked at the time of the injury, and whether it is actually

Fibular collateral ligament
Lateral collateral ligament
Lateral meniscus
Anterior cruciate ligament

Figure 314.   Left, Lateral side injury, the succession being fibular collateral, iliotibial band, lateral meniscus, anterior cruciate. The biceps tendon may or may not be avulsed, depending on the level of the injury. Right, Note the iliotibial band repaired to the tibia through drill holes, the fibular collateral ligament to the fibula through drill hoes. The anterior cruciate is shown held by drill holes from the anteromedial face of the tibia. (O'Donoghue, D. H.: J. Bone & Joint Surg. 32-A:735.)

TABLE 1.   THE DIAGNOSIS OF KNEE LIGAMENT INJURY

Demands early, careful, meticulous examination
Note particularly:
1. Apparent severity of injury
2. Degree of disability
3. Restriction or pain on normal motion
4. Presence of abnormal motion
5. Location and extent of tenderness
6. Amount and rapidity of the swelling
7. Location of swelling—intra or extrasynovial
8. Deformity, either present or reported
9. Locking?

locked at the time of the examination. All of these findings are of extreme importance if they are obtained in the early stage before swelling, apprehension and pain obscure the true pathology. Often, in this initial examination, a definitive diagnosis can be made, not only as to the location but as to the extent of a ligament injury.

A summary of diagnosis appears in Table 1.

For purposes of diagnosis and treatment, the various ligament injuries may be classified according to their severity into three general groups—mild, moderate and severe (Table 2).

Mild Ligament Sprain

In a mild ligament injury (Table 3), there has been some tear in the ligament fibers but its strength has not been particularly impaired. There has been some degree of damage, either within the ligament itself or at one of its attachments. The *symptoms* of such a tear are tenderness at the site of the tear, pain on active use of the knee, local swelling at the site of the injury and pain on forced motion or on attempt to duplicate the motion which caused the tear. Negative findings of significance are no instability, no blood in the joint or infiltrated through the tissues, no effusion, no locking and no pain on normal motion.

If the injury is indubitably mild—and fortunately the great majority of ligament injuries fall into this classification—*treatment* can be based on the premise that the strength of the ligament is actually unimpaired. Prolonged and extensive treatment is not necessary; in fact, the injured person seldom reaches the doctor and practically never the specialist. The basis of treatment is, first, protection against further injury and, second, reduction of local reaction. Immediate application of a pressure bandage with an ice pack will minimize local swelling. These are

TABLE 2.   CLASSIFICATION OF KNEE LIGAMENT INJURY ACCORDING
TO SEVERITY

A. Mild—A few fibers of the ligament damaged
        No actual loss of strength of the ligament
        Little treatment necessary
B. Moderate—A definite tear in some component of the ligament
        Definite loss of strength of the ligament
        No wide separation of the fibers
        Treatment is primarily protective
C. Severe—Ligament torn clear across
        Complete loss of ligament function
        Potentially wide separation of the fragments
        Treatment: Restoration of ligament continuity

TABLE 3.   SYMPTOMS AND TREATMENT OF MILD KNEE SPRAIN

1. Symptoms
    a. Positive
        (1) Tender at site of tear
        (2) Pain on abnormal stress
        (3) Local swelling
        (4) Pain on forced motion
    b. Negative
        (1) No instability
        (2) No blood in joint
        (3) No effusion
        (4) No locking
        (5) No pain on normal motion
2. Treatment (Designed to relieve discomfort)
    a. Rest
    b. Local injection
    c. Compression
    d. Cold early
    e. Heat later
    f. Early, active use
    g. No immobilization
    h. Early activity permissbile

the cases in which apparently dramatic results may be obtained by local treatment. Even ethyl chloride spray may seem valuable. Local anesthesia inserted into the injured area will reduce pain and vessel spasm. Injection of hyaluronidase into the hematoma will speed absorption and reduce swelling and ecchymosis. Protective wrapping will permit prompt resumption of activity. Complete immobilization is neither necessary nor desirable. The patient may be rapidly rehabilitated without danger. *Warning!* Since the diagnosis may not be entirely certain at the time of injury the player should not be permitted to participate in sports immediately if a local anesthetic has been injected. The injection may screen his symptoms and permit re-injury.

Moderate Ligament Sprain

In moderate ligament injury (Table 4), it is postulated that the ligament has

TABLE 4.   SYMPTOMS AND TREATMENT OF MODERATE KNEE SPRAIN

1. Symptoms
    a. Positive
        (1) Immediate disability to some extent
        (2) Swelling at first localized, later within the joint
        (3) Pain in and about the knee
        (4) Pain on lateral or rotatory motion of the knee
        (5) Local tenderness at the point of injury
        (6) Locking may or may not be present
    b. Negative
        No abnormal mobility in any direction
2. Treatment
    a. Complete bed rest with elevation of the leg
    b. Aspiration
    c. Injection, local anesthetic plus hyaluronidase
    d. Compression—Cotton cast or elastic bandage
    e. Cold—Ice pack applied directly over compression bandage for 12 to 36 hours
    f. Later, heat (after 36 hours)
    g. Protection by long leg stirrup splints, to long leg cast, to cotton cast, to taping
    h. Rehabilitation

been partially torn. This group actually includes most of the sprains that require extensive treatment, ranging from a slight tear to tears with only a few intact fibers remaining. The strength of the ligament is impaired to a greater or less degree. The *symptoms* here are very similar in pattern to those of mild injury but are greater in degree, the groups shading imperceptibly into the other. The positive findings are: pain in the knee; tenderness at the site of the injury; disability of a greater degree than in the mild type; swelling at first localized at the area of damage, later spreading to a diffuse swelling of the joint; fluid or blood in the joint; pain on reproduction of the force and direction of the injury. There may or may not be locking due to meniscus damage. The findings not present in a moderate injury are excess lateral motion and increased anteroposterior slipping of tibia on femur with the knee flexed (positive drawer sign). These latter two tests each indicate complete loss of function of a ligament permitting abnormal motion and are not positive if the ligament is only partially severed.

Treatment is based upon the premise that there has actually been a significant damage to the ligament with weakening of its structure and considerable loss, or at least potential loss, of function. Therefore, treatment must be more comprehensive than in the mild group and the emphasis is on protection from further injury. A firm compression bandage should be used and ice pack applied. Aspiration of the

Figure 315. Stirrup splints. Note that the extremity is supported constantly by the foot and the thigh, permitting the tibia to drop backward and relax the anterior cruciate. *A,* A heavy posterior splint is applied first, wrapped with gauze and allowed to harden a little. *B,* The lateral splint is then applied and wrapped with gauze. After this has set, a single layer of sheet wadding is wrapped 6 inches above to 6 inches below the knee, and this is covered with a single roll of 6 inch plaster (*C*). *D,* The completed splint. The circular plaster roll *C* is applied only during the postanesthesia stage in the operative case. It is not used routinely.

Figure 316.   A method for strapping the knee to support the lateral collateral ligaments. The criss-cross straps should cross in the midline. Maximum support for this dressing is directly medially and laterally.

local hematoma or of the knee joint following injection of a local anesthetic is carried out. Hyaluronidase is valuable if hemorrhage is recent. Since the exact degree of injury may not be readily apparent, one must protect the joint against further insult as long as symptoms persist. Bleeding is reduced by immediate compression with elastic bandage and application of ice. Later, plaster splints (Fig. 315), graduating to cotton cast (Fig. 304) and finally to elastic wrap, as symptoms permit, will serve to promote healing and prevent further injury. If fluid in the joint persists, aspiration should be repeated as often as is necessary. Aspiration of bloody fluid should again be followed by injection of hyaluronidase, while aspiration of cloudy fluid is usually followed by a corticoid preparation. Protection must be maintained and insisted upon as long as symptoms persist. Contact participation should not be permitted without firm adhesive strapping (Fig. 316) which serves to protect the ligaments of the knee better than any available type of compression knee bandage.

It is difficult to state positively just how comprehensive treatment should be in a given case but it is quite apparent that the sprain which causes only moderate damage will not require as extensive or as prolonged treatment as one that is more severe. As a general rule, compression and ice pack should be continued for several hours or even longer if the swelling is severe. Use of one of the enzyme preparations systemically may be of value—for the first 24 hours intramuscularly, then orally for a few days. With discontinuance of the compression bandage and ice pack, decision should be made as to whether the injury was severe enough to require plaster splints from groin to toes or some type of coaptation splint (such as the cotton cast) from midthigh to midcalf. If the ligament is actually torn at least three weeks will be required for healing and there should be an additional period of protection. Here again the degree of the damage will be the governing factor, since, if the greater part of the ligament is intact, the ligament itself may serve to protect the injured portion while if the defect is a major one a longer period of external protection will be indicated to prevent reinjury. The posterior and stirrup long leg splints may be worn for seven to ten days and then be replaced by a long leg walking cast (Fig. 317) for another ten days. This may be followed by short splints and later by an elastic bandage, particularly if swelling or effusion persists. It merits repeating that the knee capsule should not be permitted to remain distended over a long period of time and that aspiration should be repeated as frequently and for as long as necessary. Worth emphasizing again is the caution that the procedure should be carried out with the same aseptic technique that one would use if the knee joint were to be opened surgically. I prefer a thorough soap (hexachlorophene) and water scrub, protective draping, use of sterile gloves. One need not fear infection if he anticipates its possibility and takes the proper preventive measures.

Opinions differ on the length of time the ice pack is beneficial. Since it diminishes bleeding and slows down metabolism, it should be continued as long as these two ends are desirable. In the ordinary case bleeding will stop after a few hours, at which time it is desirable to increase metabolism by the application of local heat by means of an electric pad, diathermy or hot bath. If a well equipped and well

Figure 317.   Long leg cast. Note that the extremity is supported by the thigh and the foot to permit the tibia to drop backward to relax the anterior cruciate. *A,* Posterior plaster slab. *B,* The completed cast with the foot in slight eversion, the ankle neutral, the knee at 20 degrees. *C,* The heel. *D,* Standing position. Note that the patient should have a shoe with heel of equal height on the good leg to balance the pelvis.

controlled training room is available, the dressing may be removed daily for the application of heat and controlled physical measures such as whirlpool, massage and careful motion. This must be under the protective eye of a qualified trainer. A typical set of rehabilitative exercises follows. There are obviously many that can be used.

REHABILITATIVE EXERCISES TO THE LOWER EXTREMITY
O'Donoghue Orthopedic Clinic

Each of the following exercises should be done deliberately and to a particular count. In each instance, raise the leg slowly to the count of 3, hold to the count of 3, lower to the count of 3 and rest. Repeat this series ten times. Rest. Repeat this through three series of ten times each, 30 times total. The exercises should be repeated two or three times a day, depending upon your tolerance. Whenever you are able to complete this series of 30, add weight and start a new series, gradually adding weight as your strength improves. Build this weight up to 25 pounds if possible. Chart your daily progress and record it. Continue this until the involved thigh is (*a*) as large as the normal side, (*b*) as strong as the normal side and (*c*) normal motion is reached.

The following exercises should be done as indicated above:

1. Lying on the back, raise the leg up with the knee straight and not flexing.
2. Lie on the opposite side. Raise the leg up with the knee straight.
3. Lie face down. Raise the leg up with the knee straight.
(N.B. In each instance, increase weight as indicated above.)
4. Sitting with the leg hanging and the knee at a right angle, go through the series of exercises with spring resistance or weight. If there is ligament damage, a spring or system of pulleys and weight is preferred to hanging the weight on the foot.
5. Lie face down with weight on the foot, flex the leg to vertical through the same series.

Active physical therapy, increasingly active use, protective strapping and re-education are all of importance. Injudicious overuse or too early return to physical activity will interfere with prompt and complete recovery. Reduction of pain and swelling by local injection must not be permitted to cover up the true nature of the injury since active stress must not be allowed until healing is complete. Ordinarily complete recovery should be expected, with no residual disability in the joint if treatment is adequate. After complete healing there is no justification for limiting the activity of the patient. It is the unusual or the untreated case that has permanent disability from a moderate sprain. "Once a sprain always a sprain" is an excuse to screen inadequate treatment.

Severe Ligament Sprain

In severe ligament injuries (Table 5), the *diagnosis* is based on the premise that one or more of the major ligaments of the knee are completely torn loose from their attachment, or torn through their substance. The mechanism of this injury is that previously mentioned, namely, forcing the knee through a wide range of abnormal motion beyond the tolerance of the ligament. Symptoms in this type of injury are much more severe. There is immediate disability, usually severe. There is the feeling that the knee has given way or dislocated. There is often extreme pain at the time of injury. Examination and evaluation reveal early disability, giving way of the knee joint, severe pain in the knee or leg, blood in the joint, blood infiltrating through the tissues (Fig. 318), and local swelling first at the site of injury and very rapidly into the knee itself. Confirmatory x-rays (Fig. 319) show abnormal lateral motion at the knee joint. Locking may or may not be present. While the above symptoms and signs strongly suggest a complete ligament avulsion, *the*

TABLE 5.   SYMPTOMS AND TREATMENT OF SEVERE KNEE SPRAIN

1. Symptoms
    a. Immediate disability, usually severe; patient apprehensive
    b. Knee "gives way" on attempt at weight bearing, particularly with flexion
    c. Severe pain
    d. Blood infiltrated in tissues but may collect in joint
    e. Marked swelling, first local, later diffuse about the knee
    f. Pain on stress (lateral, rotatory, anteroposterior)
    g. Abnormal mobility.
    h. Positive stress x-ray
2. Treatment (Designed to restore continuity of the ligament)
    a. Surgical treatment should be given if at all possible
        (1) Make prompt diagnosis and decision as to surgery
        (2) Operate as soon as feasible
        (3) Repair each torn ligament
    b. Nonsurgical (not desirable)
        Same as for moderate sprain, but longer protection

one single confirmatory finding is instability. One should be able to demonstrate by his examination loss of function of one or more ligaments of the knee. It should be noted also that a torn ligament, particularly a cruciate, may be present without the signs of major injury indicated above.

Increased abduction of the tibia with the knee in complete extension means loss of the medial collateral, anterior cruciate, and at least part of the posterior ligament (Fig. 319, *A*). A knee that is stable in extension but not at 30 degrees indicates that the medial or lateral collateral is gone but the posterior ligament is intact. Increased anterior-posterior mobility of the flexed tibia (90 degrees) on the femur indicates anterior or posterior cruciate ligament damage (drawer sign, Fig. 320). The importance of these findings cannot be overemphasized. If surgery is indicated for some other reason, such as a locked knee or a knee with positive lateral instability and questionable anterior-posterior instability, the cruciate ligament can be checked at the time of the operation. Appropriate measures can be taken for repair at that time without the necessity of a preliminary diagnostic anesthetic. In doubtful cases it is justifiable to induce anesthesia for diagnosis. Stress x-rays are illustrative and

Figure 318.   Appearance of leg 48 hours after injury with avulsion of posterior cruciate and posterior capsule from the tibia. Note extreme swelling, ecchymosis and hematoma formation

Figure 319.   *A,* X-ray of injury to medial collateral ligament of knee. *Left,* Neutral anteroposterior view; *right,* position of abduction of leg on thigh; arrow indicates increased tibiofemoral joint space.

B, X-ray illustrating damage to lateral collateral ligament. *Left,* Neutral anteroposterior view of knee; *right,* stress film showing rupture of fibular collateral and iliotibial band. Arrow indicates avulsion of tip of fibula.

confirmatory but usually are unneeded since if the x-ray is positive physical examination alone will reveal abnormal lateral motion in the knee.

Diagnosis must be early and be definitive in order to permit the proper decision as to treatment. If one waits three or four weeks until swelling and pain subside, instability becomes quite obvious. In the meantime the optimum time for treatment has passed.

Treatment. Treatment poses the question: Why is it essential that diagnosis should be made definitively and at once? The answer is basic in our approach to the problem of treatment. If all ligament injuries are to be treated by modifications of the same basic method, it may indeed be of academic interest only to define the exact pathology. It is agreed that certain basic measures are of value in the treatment of an injured knee ligament. We have seen that aspiration, local injection, compression, ice packs, immobilization, protection and rehabilitation are utilized to a greater or lesser degree, depending upon the severity of the injury. Under such a concept, whether the sprain be moderate or severe, treatment will require only some variation of the extent to which these measures are utilized.

Obviously, if there is no effusion, aspiration will not be necessary. If effusion is recurrent, aspiration will need to be repeated. If the injury is mild, compression may well be the only protection applied, to soon be discarded. If swelling persists, so must compression bandaging whether it be elastic wrap or cotton cast. If symptoms subside promptly, no protection by splint or cast is necessary. On the other hand, if symptoms remain severe, a cylinder for eight weeks may be required. The same concept applies to rehabilitation which can be perfunctory in the injury requiring only brief treatment but must be extensive if prolonged protection has been required.

Why, then, do we demand "careful, tender but meticulously complete examination" of every sprain of the knee? If the treatment is to be the same whatever

Figure 320. The drawer sign. The patient sits with her leg dangling from the table. The examiner is seated in front of her with the foot clasped between his knees, hands as shown. Forward pressure will demonstrate anterior cruciate instability; backward pressure, posterior cruciate instability. This motion should be made by slow, steady pull rather than by a succession of jerks, which will be painful to the injured knee. The inset shows a positive anterior drawer sign, the tibia sliding forward and downward in relation to the normal position.

the injury, why not initiate this treatment first and then decide as we go along just how extensively the injury must be treated? Severity could be judged by the manner in which the condition responds to therapy.

Such specious reasoning, by appearing reasonable on the surface, insidiously undermines one's actual understanding of the condition which he is treating. It is easy to see how the habit of treating these injuries "by feel" rather than by diagnosis becomes fixed. If one is called upon to examine a knee injury and responds by directing that it be "packed in ice" until morning, the next time the trainer or team physician encounters this injury, he will "pack it in ice" himself. Indeed, if the treatment is to be standardized into a certain pattern, he is perfectly correct in doing so.

Many of us have found through years of observation that nonsurgical treatment is not always the best treatment. We may differ substantially on how frequently surgery is indicated and how complete it must be but most would agree that at least some cases will require surgical treatment.

We have been able to show that early operation (within two weeks is distinctly more favorable than late operation (Fig. 321 and Table 6). In a series of 80 cases of knee ligament operations the vital factor governing the degree of recovery was not the severity of the injury, the location of the tear or the age of the patient. It was the time of the operation. Almost without exception the patient who was operated upon within two weeks obtained a better end result than the patient with a comparable injury operated upon later. Indeed, a more satisfactory

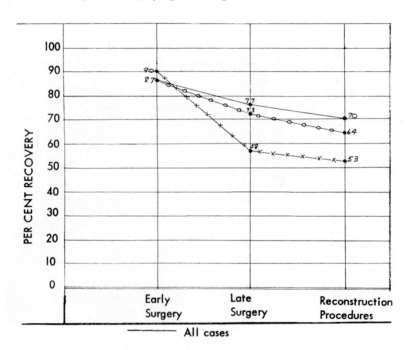

Figure 321.   Showing end results of operations on ligaments of the knee. (From The Journal of Bone and Joint Surgery, Vol. 37A.)

TABLE 6.   FOLLOW-UP CHART OF 80 KNEE LIGAMENT OPERATIONS
(Comparison by Age Groups)

	EARLY SURGERY	LATE SURGERY	RECONSTRUCTION PROCEDURES	TOTAL
Under 20 years				
No. of Cases	21	12	12	45
Grade	89 (average)	75 (average)	66 (average)	79 (average)
Over 20 years				
No. of Cases	23	8	4	35
Grade	84 (average)	78 (average)	60 (average)	80 (average)

Note that the result was essentially the same whether they were under 20 or over 20. There were consistently poor results from surgery delayed over two weeks. In this table "early" is under two weeks, "late" is two to six weeks.

(From The Journal of Bone and Joint Surgery, Vol. 37A.)

result was obtained in the severe case treated by early operation than in the milder case in which operation was late.

So if we grant these two premises, namely, that some cases need surgery and that early surgery is better than late, it follows that the decision whether to operate or not must be based on early, thorough, careful examination, under anesthesia if necessary. We must not treat all knee injuries alike if we are to treat them the best way. Attention to the exact diagnosis must be an integral part of the management of any knee ligament injury.

These injuries provide a classical example of the importance of the precepts mentioned in the Introduction, which must be constantly kept in mind. The goal of treatment must be 100 per cent recovery. The best treatment must be selected rather than the most convenient treatment. The decision must be entirely objective without consideration of extraneous influences. Above all, treatment must be prompt. A definitive decision as to the proper treatment must be made at the earliest possible moment.

Once the diagnosis of a complete ligament tear has been made, the method of treatment must be elected. It will not suffice to try so-called conservative treatment first and then proceed to surgery. Early surgical repair yields so much better and surer results than late repair or reconstruction that surgery must not be reserved for only those cases in which conservative treatment has failed. Modern anesthesia, operating room asepsis, highly skilled personnel and antibiotics have minimized the hazards to the degree that in the well run hospital with a competent surgical team, open surgery can confidently take its place alongside nonsurgical measures. In the absence of complicating factors the management chosen must be that which will give the best chance of complete recovery in the shortest time.

I believe that, when one can demonstrate complete severance of any single ligament or of any combination or ligaments of the knee, surgical repair is mandatory. The repair should include not only one ligament but all ligaments involved. It makes little sense to repair the collateral ligament and ignore the cruciate because it "adds to the severity of the operation" or is "too difficult" or "may not be essential." The cruciates are not vestigial. One has only to examine the splendid mechanism of the anterior cruciate, to note its size, to check its strength, to recognize its vital structure, in order to realize that it is not an evolutionary misfit ready for the discard. The cruciates play a living, vibrant part in that ingenious mechanism

Figure 322.   Both cruciates off tibia. Tibial end of medial collateral under medial meniscus. Tendon widely separated. (From The Journal of Bone and Joint Surgery, Vol. 32A.)

that is the knee. We may argue about their exact function but be assured they have a major one.

Even though we agree that the many interlocking ligaments of the knee act as a physiological unit and that a portion of this unit may be spared without great disaster, we must acknowledge that the knee without the cruciate is actually or potentially less than normal. The cruciate should be repaired since in no other way may a normal knee joint be attained.

Figure 323.   Tendon and medial ligament widely separated from the lower attachment. (From The Journal of Bone and Joint Surgery, Vol. 32A.)

Figure 324.   Anterior cruciate torn from tibia. Posterior cruciate from femur. Medial collateral torn from femur and lying on top of medial meniscus. (From The Journal of Bone and Joint Surgery, Vol. 32A.)

I examine many knees in which the only detectable complaint is cruciate instability. These patients seek surgical reconstruction because to them the condition is materially disabling. This in itself is evidence that the cruciate in a given case may be vital for adequate function.

Late cruciate reconstruction is highly speculative and should be done only when the stakes are high, as for example in a professional baseball player who is unable to play because of anterior-posterior instability or when the degree of anterior-posterior instability is actually disabling. Early cruciate repair is highly suc-

Figure 325.   Anterior cruciate avulsed from femur and lying on top of lateral meniscus. (From The Journal of Bone and Joint Surgery, Vol. 32A.)

cessful and should be done as a matter of course. The operation, which is not unduly technical, is within the capabilities of any competent orthopedist who properly prepares himself in the necessary technique.

In certain cases the ligament may heal spontaneously. This is particularly true of tears of the collateral ligaments. The real danger is in our inability to determine short of surgery which case will heal with normal length and which will not. At operation I have actually found the tibial end of the medial collateral lying in the joint underneath the medial meniscus (Fig. 322). I have seen the ligament torn with the ends disengaged and retracted an inch or more (Fig. 323). I have located the femoral attachment of the medial collateral ligament lying in the joint on top of the meniscus (Fig. 324); also the femoral end of the anterior cruciate lying over the lateral meniscus (Fig. 325). There are many other such situations which are unredeemable except by surgery. Anyone who has actually seen these or similar lesions at operation becomes very skeptical of the uniformly good results reported from nonsurgical treatment.

The results of surgical treatment recommend it. In 80 consecutive cases of ligament injuries,* early repair gave good results in approximately 90 per cent of cases (over 90 per cent in athletes), regardless of the severity of the injury. It was demonstrated that the promptness of the operation and the completeness of the repair were much more important than the nature or severity of the injury; failure of cruciate repair was the most common single cause of permanent disability in knee ligament injuries; and repair of the cruciates was highly successful early but very unpredictable late.

OPERATIVE TECHNIQUE

I will attempt in this section to indicate some of the more common surgical procedures for ligament repair, and to describe in detail those which I personally prefer. The exact pathology encountered may have many variants but the diagnoses nevertheless fall into more or less definite categories. The procedures may be grouped as follows on the basis of the diagnosis:

1. Technique for repair of the medial collateral, the medial portion of the posterior ligament, the anterior and/or posterior cruciate ligament, medial meniscus, medial hamstring tendons.
2. Technique for repair of the lateral components, namely, the iliotibial band (which in effect is analogous to the superficial layer of the medial collateral ligament), the fibular collateral ligament, the lateral portion of the posterior capsule and the cruciate ligaments; the lateral meniscus; the peroneal nerve; the biceps tendon.
3. Technique for repair of the posterior components—the posterior approach for either the posterior capsule or posterior cruciate.

The *preoperative preparation* for all these procedures is the same, namely, meticulous preparation of the skin. In the presence of a specific skin contamination this begins 48 hours before the operation, otherwise 12 to 24 hours before. If the operation must be delayed because of inability to obtain a hospital bed or for some other reason (such as irritative abrasions, cuts, etc.) we provide the patient with a hexachlorophene soap and instruct him to scrub his knee vigorously with very heavy

* O'Donoghue, Don H.: An Analysis of End Results of Surgical Treatment of Major Injuries to the Ligaments of the Knee. J. Bone & Joint Surg. 37A:1-13 (Jan.), 1955.

lather at least ten minutes twice a day. If there is a lesion on the skin, it must have healed as completely as possible. However, we sometimes plan our incision to avoid an abrasion on the skin rather than postpone an operation unduly. Infected skin is a definite contraindication to operative treatment.

Upon the patient's admission to the hospital on the evening before operation the leg is carefully shaved from the toes to the groin. (We frequently have the patient shave his own leg. He cuts it less.) The leg is then thoroughly scrubbed with hexachlorophene soap, first freely for five minutes, then with sterile gloves and sterile towels for five minutes more. Over this extremity is rolled sterile doubled stockinette, covering the leg from the toes to the groin. This is strapped in place at the top with adhesive.

On the day of operation the patient is taken to the operating room and anesthetized, after which the leg is suspended by a foot-holding apparatus (Fig. 326, A) which relieves the nurse or other individual from holding the heavy extremity throughout the period of the preparation. This apparatus is modified from that used to suspend fluids from a carrier and consists of a rather broad base with a vertical telescoping upright surmounted by a strong hook. The apparatus is placed on the operating table with the base beneath the mattress. A suitable loop is thrown around the foot and the leg is suspended as high as it will conveniently go (preferably at least 45 degrees from horizontal). Use of the suspension frame is more difficult in the prone position than in the supine but still is easier than holding the leg manually. The tourniquet is applied as high on the thigh as possible, because one is never sure of the extent of incision required. The tourniquet is fastened with adhesive so that it will not roll down the cone-shaped thigh. Employment of the leg holder permits the nurse to use both hands in the preparation and encourages a full length scrub time.

With the leg suspended in the apparatus, the stockinette wrapping is detached at the thigh and carefully rolled down the leg to just above the ankle so as not to contaminate the clean skin beneath. Surgical preparation is carried out with liquid hexachlorophene soap, the preparer wearing sterile gloves and using both hands with compresses to work up a very generous lather. This scrub is continued ten minutes by the clock. It does not include the foot. It is my belief that when the foot is included in the preparation, an inordinate amount of time is spent in cleaning the toenails and foot whereas, if the foot is draped out, the entire preparation may be concentrated about the knee. At the conclusion of the preparation the foot is grasped by the preparer and removed from the suspension apparatus (Fig. 326, B). The stockinette is removed from the foot. The leg is held elevated at all times to help drain the blood from the extremity. One of the gowned and gloved surgeons then lays a sterile towel over the foot. Over this is rolled the stockinette which from the toes to the calf is double. Immediately after passing the heel the stockinette wrapping is halted while a sterile towel is folded around the leg (Fig. 326, C), including the ends of the towel originally draped over the foot. This adequately protects the area where the scrubbed sterile leg and the dry unsterile foot meet since the soap would readily come through the doubled stockinette and theoretically these suds are contaminated. The stockinette is rolled over the towels and up the leg and thigh. A sterile towel is folded around the tourniquet (Fig. 326, D) and held with a clip. The stockinette wrapping is continued over this

Figure 326.   *A,* The leg suspended for preparation. Suspension apparatus permits the preparer to use both hands, avoiding an additional helper. Note that the tourniquet is high on the thigh. The double layer of stockinette wrapping placed on the leg following preparation the night before has been rolled down to permit access to the extremity from just above the ankle to the tourniquet. Care is taken not to touch the tourniquet or the stockinette with the gloved hand.

B, A towel has been placed over the foot by a scrubbed surgical assistant and the sterile double stockinette is pushed over the foot.

C, At this point a towel is folded around the leg to cover the junction between the sterile and the unsterile portions. The double stockinette now is rolled over this towel, the double part ending just below the knee, the single part continuing on up the thigh.

D, A sterile towel is folded around the tourniquet. Note the sterile drape under the leg. After this towel is applied, the stockinette is rolled up over the towel and a second towel is folded around the end of the stockinette.

E, As the foot is held elevated, a 4 inch Ace bandage is wrapped from toes to tourniquet and the tourniquet is inflated. After the tourniquet is inflated, a double fan sheet is fanned up over the anesthetic screen. An additional double fan sheet is placed under the leg; the top edge of it is clipped to the edge of the upper fan, but the bottom edge is not fanned downward. This permits considerable manipulation of the leg without exposing the unsterile area beneath the thigh. Note that the foot has been held elevated ever since preparation began.

towel and another towel is wrapped around the proximal end of the stockinette, thus effectively covering the tourniquet, the stockinette and the second towel. These steps accomplished, the leg is held elevated during the application of the drape and until the tourniquet is inflated. Appropriate table drapes are then placed and, with the leg still elevated, an Esmarch or ace bandage is wrapped firmly from the toes to the upper thigh (Fig. 326, E). The pneumatic tourniquet is then inflated and the time noted. From the moment of application of the tourniquet no unnecessary delays can be tolerated since the tourniquet time becomes all-important.

1. Technique for Repair of the Medial Collateral, the Medial Portion of the Posterior Ligament, the Anterior and/or Posterior Cruciate Ligament

Exposure for Definition of the Pathology.   A sweeping anteromedial incision is made beginning above the level of the superior pole of the patella and halfway between the medial epicondylar line and the patella (Fig. 327). It extends downward and forward toward the middle of the medial border of the patella, then is continued downward along the anteromedial aspect of the joint paralleling, and ¾ inch medial to, the patella and the patellar tendon. At the level of the patellar tubercle of the tibia it curves backward to end at the posterior border of the tibia about 3 inches distal to its articular margin. The medial skin flap is reflected backward in the superficial fascial plane to expose the entire anteromedial surface of the tibia, the joint and the femoral condylar area. (Fig. 328, A). The superficial layer of the ligament is thus revealed and may be inspected. The site of damage will be indicated by ecchymosis and hematoma within the fibers of the ligament, usually at or near its tibial attachment. This may be demonstrated also by rocking the tibia on the femur.

The incision is now carried through the patellar retinaculum along the line of the skin incision beginning at the superior pole of the patella and extending

Figure 327.   Medial incision for repair of the medial collateral ligament. Any part of this incision may be used. *a, b,* The portion of incision utilized for medial meniscectomy. It may be extended to *d* to further explore the knee joint or shave the patella, and extended down to *c* for repair of the medial collateral ligament.

Figure 328

A, The medial utility incision as drawn in Figure 327.

B, Incision has been made through the patellar retinaculum and the superficial layer of the medial collateral ligament reflected upward in the tenaculum revealing the joint line with irregular laceration of the deep layer of the medial collateral ligament which in this instance is torn off the femoral attachment.

directly distal along the anterior margin of the superficial layer of the medial collateral ligament. An instrument then can be passed beneath the superficial portion
of the ligament in order to better demonstrate the area of the damage. The tear is
defined usually either at the tibial attachment or just above this but below the
line of the joint, and the superficial layer is reflected proximally to expose the deep
layer. In many instances the superficial layer may be reflected as a separate layer
to a point above the line of the joint. At other times the superficial and deep layers
will blend just below the joint. As this layer has been detached and folded backward, the deep layer is exposed (Fig. 328, B). This layer must be inspected entirely
across the line of the joint from front to back. Again rocking the tibia may give a
clue as to the site of the tear. This tear is readily seen if the operation is done before
healing occurs.

Frequently, the ligament will be torn in an irregular fashion. A commonly
found tear begins at the midlateral line on the tibial attachment of the deep layer
and extends backward an inch or two and then vertically upward across the joint
and posterior medially across the femoral attachment. Another lesion frequently
seen is a tear of the deep layer from its tibial attachment all the way posteriorly
to include the medial one-third of the posterior ligament. In other instances the
ligament may tear at the joint line and the meniscus may be split, the upper part
going with the femur, the lower with the tibia. Frequently the ligament will not
give way from the midline forward since the medial ligament becomes very thin
here to permit flexion of the knee and so has enough redundancy to permit the
knee to "open up."

It is advisable at this stage to enter the knee by an incision through the
synovium along the medial parapatellar line. In some instances this incision may
be required to open the joint in order to specifically define the area of the tear,
which sometimes can be better demonstrated from within out than from without in.
At this point the deep layer of the medial ligament is reflected away from the
tear. In other words, if the tear is along the tibial margin it is reflected upward. If
the tear is along the femoral margin it is reflected downward. This gives ready
access to the medial meniscus, which should be routinely removed to permit shortening of the medial collateral ligament. This is particularly necessary if the detachment is from the tibia below the meniscus. An effort is made to leave about 1/16
inch of the cartilage intact to the medial ligament since it provides a very firm area
through which to place the plicating sutures.

After this exposure is made the knee can readily be examined (Fig. 328, C).
If the anterior cruciate ligament is torn the knee will open up more widely and
the pathology of the cruciate ligament may readily be determined. The posterior
cruciate ligament should also be carefully examined.

C, The medial incision, the superficial layer of the ligament reflected upward, the deep
layer reflected downward, the Russian forceps holding the anterior cruciate ligament which is
torn off the femur.

D, The medial incision. A ⅛ inch drill protected with a short sleeve is drilled through the
back of the intercondylar notch to emerge on the lateral epicondylar ridge. Two parallel holes
are made. If the knee will not open up sufficiently to approach from within-out, the drill holes
can be made from without-in. It is important to get the holes as far back in the notch as possible.

E, Heavy silk suture engaging the torn femoral attachment of the anterior cruciate ligament.

F, The lateral incision along the epicondylar ridge showing the two silk sutures as they
exit on the lateral side of the femur. (See page 472 for continuation.)

Figure 328 (*Continued*)

G, The medial incision. Drill holes are placed in the denuded medial femoral condyle through which mattress sutures are placed to hold the proximal end of the deep layer of the medial collateral ligament.

H, The deep layer is ligated to the lower femur by mattress sutures.

Repair of the Anterior Cruciate Ligament.   If the anterior cruciate ligament is torn from the femur an incision is made laterally to expose the epicondylar
ridge of the femur and two drill holes are placed extrasynovially. They extend diagonally downward and inward to emerge in the notch at the site of the femoral
attachment of the anterior cruciate ligament. These holes are about ½ inch apart
at the point of their entrance to the lateral femur and their exit in the intercondylar
notch should be as far back as possible. These holes will be in the posteromedial
aspect of the lateral condyle in the notch. In many cases, if the knee will open up
widely, the drill holes may be more easily made from within out (Fig. 328, D),
care being taken to encase the 8/64 inch drill in a short sleeve so that it will not
damage the cruciate ligaments or the articular cartilage in the course of the drilling.
At present I ordinarily use a drill with a twist of only about 1 inch on the end and
the rest of the shaft smooth, which attains the same objective.

A heavy suture (my own preference is No. 3 braided silk) is passed through
one drill hole, carefully plicated through the torn end of the cruciate ligament
(Fig. 328, E) and then passed out through the other drill hole (Fig. 328, F). We
use a ligature carrier made of a fine Kirschner wire, the end of which has been
folded over to make an eye, and for easy handling a small, knurled handle is applied.
Any other suitable ligature carrier may be used but an ordinary silver probe is a
little large for this hole. At other times we use an eye in the tip of the drill as a
ligature carrier. Occasionally, however, this will cut the thread as one pushes it
through the small hole. It should be emphasized that these sutures should be placed
while the knee is still wide open. This greatly facilitates the passing of suture
through the cruciate ligament. I prefer to use a so-called tonsil needle which is a
small, heavy, full curved round needle (we call them "knee needles").

If the cruciate is torn off the tibial attachment, drill holes are made from the
anteromedial face of the tibia up into the tibial origin of the cruciate ligament on
the superior surface of the tibia. This is considerably easier than the other repair.
Similar plication is done within the stump of the cruciate. If it is torn in the middle I frequently will make drill holes in both bones, pick up the tibial stump
through femoral drill holes and the femoral stump through tibial drill holes. I
believe this as a rule is more successful than direct suture although we sometimes
utilize the latter, too. The important consideration is to get good contact of the
torn ends. These sutures are placed but not tied. Similarly, if the ligament is redundant but not torn it can be plicated and shortened by passing heavy suture through
the drill hole and up into the substance of the ligament and out the other hole.
Sutures on the epicondylar ridge should be extrasynovial. None of these procedures
is formidable; and with proper tools should add no more than 15 to 20 minutes to
the operative time. After the placing of these sutures, they are not tied until the
medial ligament repair is completed, the leg position at 30 degree flexion and the
wounds are ready to close.

Repair of the Medial Collateral Ligament.   The immediate repair of the

---

I, A heavy stay suture is placed at the anterior edge of the reflected medial collateral ligament and is pulled snugly forward. This is about the level of the patellar tubercle.

J, Mattress suture placed through the periosteum of the tibia beneath the pes anserinus.

K, The superficial ligament is sutured into position.

L, Wound closed with subcuticular wire.

deep layer of the collateral ligament may be by one of several methods. If there is a direct tear in the ligament with two well defined margins, simple suture will suffice, with imbrication if feasible. If the ligament is avulsed from the bone, the best method of repair consists of a series of three or four superficial drill holes about ¾ inch apart at the site of the attachment to the tibial margin or femoral condyle (Fig. 328, G), as the case may be. Suitable suture is passed through the ligament into one drill hole out of an adjacent drill hole, and back through the ligament. When all of these have been placed the knee is positioned at about 20 to 30 degrees of flexion with the leg internally rotated, and all ligatures are tied (Fig. 328, H). As a rule, the superficial layer can be repaired by simple suture to its bed, overlapping the edges (Fig. 328, J) if possible. If this is not possible, a similar procedure may be carried out by drill holes at the level desired.

In the collateral repair every effort should be made to obtain maximum shortening of the ligament, and its tibial attachment should be pulled forward as far as is possible (Fig. 328, I). All loose tags are carefully sutured down (Fig. 328, K).

From this point onward the procedure is similar for the different types of incision and has already been described. I will discuss the postoperative handling of the extremity at the end of this section. All apparent bleeding points are coagulated and the wound is closed, sutures being cotton 4-0 for the synovium and cotton 2-0 for the retinaculum, cotton No. 1 for the collateral ligament, twisted silk No. 3 for the cruciates, 4-0 chromic for the subcutaneous tissues and No. 32 wire subcuticular for the skin (Fig. 328, L).

Repair of the Posterior Cruciate Ligament Through an Anteromedial Incision. If the posterior cruciate ligament has been avulsed from the tibia and additionally the medial collateral ligament has ruptured, repair will frequently be possible from in front. A drill hole starts in front of the tibia about ¾ inch distal to the articular margin and proceeds directly backward, paralleling the articular surface to emerge posteriorly at the midline near the attachment of the posterior cruciate ligament. A similar drill hole is passed parallel to and about ½ inch medial to the first. A suture can be passed with a suitable ligature carrier from front to back to emerge posteriorly. This suture is then placed in the knee needle and, since the knee will open up well, it is possible with some patience to plicate the ligature through the detached portion of the posterior cruciate ligament. The needle is then removed and a suture is again threaded in the ligature carrier and pulled out through the second hole to be tied in front of the tibia after the other portion of the repair has been completed (Fig. 322). We prefer to use a heavy suture for this since breakage on tightening is very distressing, necessitating taking down the entire repair in order to replace the suture.

Repair of the posterior cruciate that has been torn off the femur is very easy through the anteromedial incision (Fig. 327). The medial femoral condyle is already exposed. We simply denude an area extrasynovially along the epicondylar ridge and direct the drill holes from this area almost directly lateralward to emerge at the chondral margin in the front of the knee on the lateral side of the medial condyle of the femur. To put it another way, the drill hole emerges on the medial side of the intercondylar notch as far forward as possible. A similar drill hole is made ½ inch away, paralleling the first one. A ligature can be readily passed through this hole, plicated through the stump of the posterior cruciate and back out on the medial condylar margin where it is tied.

2. Technique for Repair of the Lateral Components

With the patient lying on his back with a sandbag under the buttock on the involved side to hold the leg in internal rotation, the same meticulous preparation and draping are carried out as indicated above. The incision begins at the level of the superior pole of the patella and about ¾ inch lateral to its lateral margin (Fig. 329). It proceeds distally at this distance from the patella and patellar tendon to the level of the patellar tubercle of the tibia, then swings downward and backward to terminate at the level of the fibular shaft about 1½ inches from its proximal end. The skin margins are reflected and stockinette is fastened to the skin edges with skin clips. The posterior flap is reflected backward to expose the lateral aspect of the knee, care being taken to take all the subcutaneous tissue with the skin flap.

Careful investigation is now made to determine the nature and degree of the injury. The upper end of the fibula should be carefully examined to see if there has been avulsion of the combined attachment of the biceps tendon and fibular collateral ligament. If the lesion is in this vicinity or if the fibular collateral ligament is avulsed from its femoral attachment, the flap should be resected far enough so that the peroneal nerve may be examined and suitably protected either by leaving it under observation in its normal course or by dissecting it free and protecting it with a rubber drain retractor. My personal preference is not to strip out the nerve unless this is necessary because of nerve injury. The attachment of the iliotibial band to the tibia should be carefully inspected. Frequently it will be found to be avulsed. The iliotibial band actually is analogous to the superficial layer of the medial collateral ligament. It becomes a ligament of the knee because of its firm attachment to the femoral condyle through the intermuscular septum so that the section of the band from the femur to the tibia is a lateral tibial collateral ligament.

After the nature of the lesion is defined the knee should then be opened along the line of the skin incision (lateral parapatellar) and the lateral meniscus carefully explored. If the knee will open up readily on the lateral side, this exploration

Figure 329. Lateral incision for approach to the knee joint. This incision parallels the fibular ilio-tibial band to within a fingerbreadth of the patella and parallels then the patellar tendon. This permits the ilio-tibial band to be split and reflected backward giving good access to the lateral compartment. It must be extended downward and backward below the fibular head for lateral ligament repair or for treatment of peroneal nerve injury.

is relatively easy. At the same time the popliteus tendon should be inspected. If there is serious ligament injury on the lateral side, it is advisable to remove the lateral cartilage for the same reason we remove the medial one on the opposite side, namely, to permit more positive plication of the ligament. The cruciate ligaments may be inspected from this incision and suitable repair carried out as noted on page 473.

From this incision it is easy to make the drill holes to repair the anterior cruciate to the femur without a separate incision. If the anterior cruciate is avulsed from the tibia there is no necessity for making a medial incision. Drill holes can be made from the lateral plateau forward, inward and upward to emerge on the medial side of the extra-articular portion of the superior tibial surface and a suitable suture passed through these two holes as indicated above. If it is necessary to repair the posterior cruciate to the femur a separate incision on the medial side will be necessary to permit drill holes to be passed through the medial femoral condyle and into the medial side of the intercondylar notch just at its anterior edge. If the posterior cruciate is detached from the tibia, a similar procedure can be carried out as indicated above for the medial repair.

After the sutures for repair of the cruciate ligaments have been passed, one then proceeds to the lateral repair. It should be emphasized that replacement of the fibular collateral ligament is in itself not adequate in lateral ligament rupture, since usually far greater damage is present. The same technique is used to repair the posterior capsule as on the medial side, the posterior capsule being pulled downward to the soft tissues at the back of the tibia with every effort made to get it as tight as possible with the knee flexed about 30 degrees. Similar repair of the fibular collateral ligament is made, either of the femoral attachment to the femur or the fibular attachment to the fibula. The latter frequently includes the biceps tendon attachment which must also be replaced. The tibial attachment of the iliotibial band should be carefully replaced even if this requires drill holes along the tibial margin. After all the sutures are placed the knee is positioned at about 30 degrees of flexion (150 degrees) and all sutures tied. The leg is permitted to externally rotate to beyond neutral while the thigh is kept in internal rotation by the sandbag under the buttock as the ligatures are tied. Closure is then carried out by usual methods.

3. Technique for Repair of the Posterior Components

The patient is positioned face downward with entire leg exposed, protected by sterile stockinette as previously illustrated. During a portion of the operation a folded sheet may be placed under the knee to hold it in complete extension. When desired, the sheet may be moved beneath the foot to flex the knee when this is necessary to facilitate the operation. The incision begins about 3 inches above the popliteal fold over the semitendinosus tendon, extends distally along the semitendinosus tendon to the level of the popliteal fold and then swings sharply laterally across the fold to the bicipital tendon and down the calf for about 3 inches along the posterolateral surface (Fig. 330). This curvilinear incision has no sharp angles and as it proceeds transversely across the back of the knee is slightly oblique.

The posterior approach is utilized for repair of the posterior cruciate ligament when avulsed from the tibia and for repair of the posterior ligament of the joint

Figure 330. Posterior incision. Note general line of incision. This can be extended proximally or distally or a shorter segment of it may be used. Two important points are that the vertical portion above the knee should be medial and parallel the semitendinosus tendon; the transverse portion should cross in the skin folds behind the knee with rounded rather than right angle corners. The vertical portion parallels the biceps tendon just slightly medial to it.

which occurs as a result of hyperextension of the knee. The posterior ligament may be avulsed from the femoral attachment above the femoral condyles but more frequently it is torn from the tibia. In this instance the whole attachment is peeled off the tibia as a cuff, leaving the upper end of the tibia denuded. It usually includes the posterior cruciate ligament. While the posterior portion of the meniscus can be exposed by this incision the approach is not a proper one for entering the posterior compartment to remove a foreign body or to complete removal of the posterior horn of either meniscus.

The popliteal fascia is exposed by reflecting both skin flaps. The classical landmark in this area is the posterior cutaneous nerve of the calf which uniformly lies beneath the fascia centering between the two heads of the gastrocnemius. The fascia may be split along the line of this nerve proximally as far as the fascial termination above the knee joint, where the nerve will be found to join with the tibial nerve. Following the tibial nerve proximally one may locate the peroneal as it comes off to the lateral side and extends down the lateral side of the popliteal space. This exposure is facilitated by the use of a tourniquet but care should be taken to clamp and coagulate or ligate any vessel which may be damaged in the area. The tibial nerve is located posterior (and so superficial) to the artery and vein so that it may be followed down across the posterior space to the bifurcation of the two heads of the gastrocnemius. It is ordinarily not necessary to dissect out the peroneal nerve so long as it is located and adequately protected. Since the peroneal nerve has a firm attachment, it is relatively immobile and will not tolerate forceful retraction, particularly toward the medial side. After these structures are located, careful dissection deeper into the space will reveal the popliteal artery and vein. These can be retracted toward the lateral side, which will expose the medial head of the gastrocnemius. The geniculate vessels crossing behind the knee in the popliteal space may be sacrificed as necessary depending upon the pathologic findings.

Having defined the medial head of the gastrocnemius by retracting the vessels and nerves laterally, the tendinous attachment of the medial head of the gastrocnemius to the femur is divided, leaving ½ inch attached to the femur for re-suture. It is extremely important that the approach be made from the medial side for, by sectioning the medial head of the gastrocnemius, the whole neurovascular bundle may be retracted laterally. The tibial nerve has much more retractability than the peroneal and it is not as satisfactory to remove the lateral head of the gastrocnemius in an attempt to enter the area between the peroneal and tibial nerves.

By this division and retraction of the medial head of the gastrocnemius and the vessels and nerves laterally, the posterior capsule of the joint is exposed. The posterior ligament of the joint is revealed and the pathology here may be defined. If the posterior ligament has been avulsed from the tibia by hyperextension of the knee, a very heavy, firm rim of ligament will be found with a free distal margin extending transversely across the lower portion of the popliteal space. This can be lifted up by a suitable instrument and the posterior surface of the tibia will be found to be denuded. In most cases the posterior cruciate ligament is included with this avulsed posterior capsule. If not, it may be readily examined by reflecting the capsule or cuff proximally to inspect the posterior part of the knee. If the posterior capsule itself seems to be intact or possibly only stretched, access to the posterior cruciate may be obtained by a vertical incision in the midline extending from the level of the femoral condyles to a point below the upper end of the tibia. By retracting the margins of the capsular incision the posterior cruciate is exposed as it arises behind the tibia on its posterior surface and courses upward, forward and inward to attach to the lateral margin of the medial femoral condyle anteriorly.

The posterior ligament of the joint actually is made up of many structures but usually it is torn en masse so that separate repair of each of these structures is not necessary. If it is necessary to carry out isolated repair of the posterior cruciate ligament, the exact procedure will depend upon the nature of the tear. If the avulsion is from the tibia, suitable drill holes are made in the back of the tibia and heavy suture is passed through the drill holes and mattressed into the end of the ligament. This is a favorable type of repair. At this point the knee should be flexed to facilitate relaxation of the tissues in the popliteal space. If the tear in the posterior cruciate is anterior, it will be necessary to make a second incision on the medial aspect of the lower thigh in order to expose the subcutaneous border of the medial femoral condyle and permit drill holes to be made into the intercondylar notch as indicated above. Although this seems quite formidable, it can readily be accomplished from the two incisions. Suture is passed through the drill hole in the femur with a suitable ligature carrier and recovered in the posterior incision as it emerges in the notch. It is then plicated through the posterior cruciate and passed back out through the second drill hole. As tension is put on this suture it replaces the posterior cruciate ligament against its attachment to the femur. If the posterior capsule is torn directly across, it may be repaired by direct suture. If torn away from the femur it also may be repaired by suture to the attachment of the gastrocnemius. A certain amount of ingenuity may be necessary depending upon the pathologic findings.

I would like to emphasize that one cannot count on simple flexion of the knee to approximate the separate edges of the torn capsule. A recent case illustrates this very well. When the knee was hyperextended the denuded part of the tibia was exposed, the whole posterior ligament and posterior cruciate ligament being torn away like a cuff. As the knee was flexed, this cuff did not slide down over the end of the tibia. Rather, it buckled into the back of the joint so that even if union had occurred it would have been with considerable redundancy of the ligaments. It is possible that with an intact posterior cruciate the torn posterior capsule might well heal spontaneously by simple flexion of the knee. As in the case of other complete ligament tears about the knee, however, there is no means of ascertaining short of operation the exact nature of the lesion. Hence, surgical repair offers a much better overall prognosis. Granted, there are instances in which a good result is obtained by nonsurgical measures following complete rupture, yet the percentage of these good results is substantially less than with surgical repair because of those cases which obviously cannot return to normal without the latter.

After all the ligatures are placed, the knee should be positioned at about 30 degrees of flexion (150 degrees) and all the sutures tied. Closure is remarkably easy in this posterior approach. The gastrocnemius head is sutured back to its tendinous attachment. No other deep sutures are necessary since, as the popliteal fascia is closed, the whole area is snugly pulled together.

Postoperative Care

After closure of the skin the management of the extremity varies according to the type of repair which has been made. Up to this time the leg has been positioned on the table at about 30 degrees flexion with the foot in internal rotation for medial repair, external for lateral repair, or neutral for posterior repair. If there has been damage to the anterior cruciate ligament the extremity must be supported from the thigh and the upper end of the leg be permitted to drop backward. The attendant holds the leg by the thigh and by the foot (Fig. 315). This position is maintained until the dressing is completed. If in addition to the cruciate the medial collateral ligament is torn, the lower leg should be internally rotated in relationship to the femur and held in this position until the external fixation is secure. If on the other hand the posterior cruciate ligament is involved, the support should be behind the calf rather than the thigh in order to hold the leg forward and relax the tension on the posterior cruciate ligament. If both cruciate ligaments have been torn a neutral position will be held by maintaining support under both calf and thigh. These measures are extremely important since the simple weight of the leg may be enough to pull out the rather insecure suturing through the cruciate ligament. If the combination is anterior cruciate and lateral collateral, the leg should be supported by the thigh and foot and with the leg externally rotated. If it is posterior cruciate and posterior capsule and the incision is posterior, a heavy posterior plaster slab may be applied to the leg in the prone position extending from the gluteal fold to the toes and the lateral stirrup applied after this has set.

After this careful positioning of the extremity by the attendants, the knee is wrapped in sterile sheet wadding. We prefer to use Webril at the top of the thigh since it does not fray out so badly. Do not use Webril over the knee. A posterior slab is placed from the gluteal fold to the toes (Fig. 315, A). Whether or not the leg is held in external rotation, the foot must be placed in the weight-bearing position, namely, slight eversion and neutral dorsal flexion. The plaster slab is wrapped in place with 3 inch gauze bandage and then supported by a lateral stirrup running from the perineum to the trochanter (Fig. 315, B). This is firmly wrapped in place with gauze.

At this point we have completed the stirrup splint (Fig. 315, C). However, the patient is usually an active athlete and in order to obviate the possibility of his flexing his knee abruptly through the opening in front of the splint as he awakens following the procedure, a single roll of sheet wadding is wrapped around the knee from 6 inches above the knee to 6 inches below. Directly over this is wrapped a single roll of 6 inch plaster of Paris bandage (Fig. 315, D). If the repair has been posterior and by a posterior approach the splint may be applied with the patient lying on his face. Preferably the very heavy posterior splint is applied and permitted to set. Then the patient is turned on his back for completion of the dressing. The advantage of this type of stirrup splint is that, as swelling occurs, it may be readily opened. As swelling regresses it may be kept snug.

By the time the patient is well awake that evening the plaster circular bandage is removed. If there is any doubt concerning the swelling, the entire dressing is split from the toes to the groin and the splint rewrapped. The dressing must not be split over the knee only. If swelling is severe enough to suggest an effusion, the dressing is removed under surgical precautions with the surgeon wearing cap, mask and sterile gloves and the knee aspirated. Injection of a corticoid preparation may be done if desired. This dressing is left for about two weeks at which time under ordinary circumstances the size of the leg will be static. The dressing is then removed, the stitches removed and a light weight, long leg plaster cast applied with the knee flexed 20 degrees (Fig. 317). The leg should be supported in exactly the same manner for application of this cast as for application of the original dressing since union of the ligament is quite insecure at the end of two weeks. This plaster cast is worn for three to four weeks. Frequently a walking heel is used if the repair seems stable and if the patient is reasonably agile. He may use the heel for weight bearing but is advised to continue his crutches. At the end of three to four weeks in the solid cast (five to six weeks postoperatively) it is removed and a cotton cast (Fig. 304) (Yucca boards over sheet wadding) applied. Aspiration and injection are repeated if indicated. This splint is removed in two weeks (seven to eight weeks postoperatively) and an elastic bandage utilized as indicated. If effusion persists, repeated aspiration and injection may be done. Most cases do not require even one aspiration.

For *rehabilitation*, quadriceps and straight leg raising of both legs are encouraged from the first day. The patient is in a wheel chair at 24 to 48 hours after the operation. He should be able to actively raise the leg, splint and all, at 72 hours and to walk on crutches in 3 to 5 days. Weight bearing is not permitted, however. After the solid cast is applied (two weeks postoperatively) he may walk with crutches on a walking heel if progress is good. In the meantime, exercise of all other available muscles is encouraged.

After the cotton cast is applied (five to six weeks postoperatively) the patient is urged to walk, gradually discarding his crutches. He is to continue his exercises. Two weeks later (seven to eight weeks postoperatively) the cotton cast is removed and quadriceps rehabilitation begins in earnest and continues until the circumference of both thighs is equal. The actual level of activity varies much with the individual patient. The agile, wiry person of relatively light weight may be allowed more freedom than the heavy lumbering giant whose ligaments are normally relaxed.

Running is permitted if synovitis is not marked. No contact is allowed until four months and not then if the quadriceps is not completely rehabilitated.

Naturally, each case must be strictly individualized both as to type of repair and postoperative management. A patient with a good, tight repair with intact ligament fibers can be permitted considerable liberty. Some patients need to be pushed in their rehabilitation (for example compensation cases and females) and the period of immobilization may be shortened. Other patients must be curbed (for example, 16 to 18 year old athletes) and their knees will require a full eight weeks of protection. The elastic bandage should be discarded early in the timorous and retained as a reminder in the overbold. If effusion persists the usual treatment for effusion is followed—namely, aspiration repeated as needed with injection of a corticoid and use of an elastic bandage—as long as moderate effusion persists. Some synovitis will ordinarily be present until essentially normal motion is recovered. In an occasional case there will be some difficulty in obtaining normal motion. This is made more probable by the fact that we suture each ligament as snugly as possible with the knee placed in the most relaxed position for that ligament. I would rather have some restriction of motion than any instability. Unfortunately the converse is more often true, more patients having persistent instability than limitation of motion.

If limitation of motion is intractable one may, under Pentothal anesthesia, carefully and slowly manipulate the knee to increase the range of flexion. Such a manipulation may require 40 to 60 minutes and good judgment is necessary to prevent injury. Manipulation must be followed by active physical therapy in order to maintain the motion obtained.

Such a regimen carefully followed with early examination, prompt decision, complete repair of all torn ligaments, followed by conscientious rehabilitation, will give increasingly gratifying results in the treatment of major injuries to the ligaments of the knee.

In a series of these cases, 80 per cent of the patients were under 25 years of age (Fig. 331), 60 per cent under 20 years of age. Since so many of these injuries occur in young people, we must try particularly to obtain the best possible recovery of function in the shortest time.

Following an injury to the ligaments of the knee, the question will arise as to whether or not the player should be allowed to compete. The answer must depend entirely upon the individual circumstances. There is no reason why patients with *mild* and the *moderate* sprains should not recover completely and be as strong as ever provided they had proper management at the time of injury. Obviously, for one reason or another, complete recovery in other cases will not always be attained. In these, decision must be made as to whether or not the remaining ligament function is adequate to withstand the rigors of athletic competition. The same decision must be made following an injury that has been treated surgically. If the operation was early and adequate ligament repair was carried out, the player may usually expect a normally functioning knee. But if complete rehabilitation is not obtainable, the vital decision must be made as to what level of athletic attainment should be permitted. If athletics have been an incidental factor in his life and competition is not truly important to him, he may want to abandon contact sports for fear the injury will be repeated. This might happen even though good recovery had been obtained. We have seen many players return to competitive athletics with no ap-

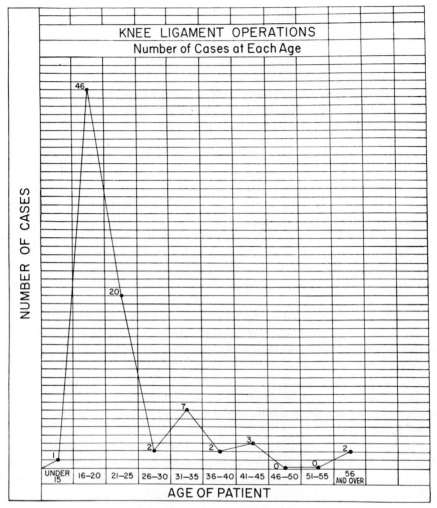

Figure 331.   Note that 60 per cent of the patients are under 20 years of age; 80 per cent are under 25. (O'Donoghue, D. H.: J. Bone & Joint Surg. 37-A:4.)

parent impairment following major injuries. The point I would like to make in this discussion is that one must not be casual one way or the other. The case must be carefully studied and a considered opinion given since this matter is of considerable importance to the persons most closely concerned. If chronic irritation persists with recurring synovitis, if there is slight instability, if there is pain on stress, these factors must be considered in advising the player on his athletic future.

CALCIFICATION

Periarticular calcification is not a common occurrence about the knee, but it does occur and may leave distressing sequelae. As with calcification elsewhere, I believe that one of its major causes is repeated irritation around the joint following infiltration of blood from an injury. In my experience, I have never seen gross calcification following early surgical repair of a knee ligament. I have seen it on many occasions after nonoperated sprains but it would be unfair to assume that surgical evacuation of the hematoma would have prevented calcification. It is my impression that calcification is more frequent following late operation that disrupts the organization of blood after it is well advanced (Fig. 332). This certainly has not been the rule, however, since in most cases calcification does not occur.

A moderate degree of calcification in the medial collateral ligament may not be troublesome. Major symptoms develop from calcification in the part of the ligament that glides back and forth over the condyle of the femur or the upper end of the tibia. Calcification here actually seems to give more trouble than calcification

A   B

Figure 332.   This 19 year old athlete with major injury to the knee was seen 24 hours after injury. He had tremendous swelling of the knee in the popliteal area extending down into the calf with obvious severance of the medial collateral ligament. Any attempt to straighten the knee beyond 60 degrees caused immediate pallor of the foot and cessation of arterial pulsation for a period of minutes. Because of the extreme swelling he was treated expectantly by aspiration of the hematoma, aspiration of the knee, elevation, ice pack, etc. He was operated upon ten days subsequent to the injury. The medial collateral ligament was avulsed from the tibia including the sartorious and semitendinosus; the posterior ligament was detached clear around to the midline; the posterior cruciate was torn off the medial femoral condyle; the anterior cruciate off the femur. There was excessive hemorrhage into the popliteal space with gross blood clot which was evacuated. He had good stability following ligament repair but developed tremendous calcification. This was later excised. Now a surgeon, the patient still has restriction of motion of the knee. Before the calcium was removed he could not flex the knee 90 degrees. Three years postoperative he had 15 degree restriction of flexion with a completely stable knee. This injury occurred over ten years ago. In a similar case I would now recommend immediate exploration of the popliteal space with evacuation of the hematoma and ligation or repair of whatever circulatory damage had been done.

A, Three years after the injury.

B, Three years after operation for calcium removal. No attempt was made to remove the calcium at the lower end of the ligaments since this was not symptomatic.

in the ligament attachment itself which we see occasionally following a moderate sprain.

Treatment. A nodule of calcium that causes persistent symptoms may be removed, but one should be particularly wary at removing the calcium when it is not symptomatic. A good test is the injection of a local anesthetic around the area to determine whether it relieves the pain. In removing the calcific plaque, great care should be taken to split the ligament fibers longitudinally, even if more than one split is necessary to get the calcium out. Transverse section offers extreme difficulty in repair and will necessitate another long period of immobilization, whereas if the ligament is divided along the line of its fibers a couple of weeks will be ample. There is a tendency to examine a patient, to take an x-ray which shows some calcification and to recommend removal of the calcium without any real analysis of the symptoms. Disappointment will usually result since there are, indeed, many areas of calcification in the body that cause no symptoms whatever. Many cases diagnosed by x-ray as calcium in the back of the knee have been referred to us for removal when actually the finding was a normal fabella that was perfectly innocent of any symptoms. Calcification of the lateral collateral ligament is not frequent. Calcification of the posterior ligament occurs but is usually not symptomatic since this ligament does not slide directly over the condylar surface.

PELLEGRINI-STIEDA DISEASE

A condition commonly called Pellegrini-Stieda disease consists of the formation of a plaque of calcium along the medial femoral condyle in the vicinity of the adductor tubercle, separated from the tibia by a band of radiolucency (Fig. 333). It is in some instances a reaction to a sprain in which there has been a forcible detachment of the medial collateral ligament at its attachment to the femoral condyle, and in other instances to partial avulsion of the adductor longus tendon.

Figure 333. Typical Pellegrini-Stieda disease caused by partial avulsion of the adductor muscle from the adductor tubercle of the femur and calcification within the hematoma. This particular case was persistently painful and the calcification was removed. This calcification is not within the medial collateral ligament. Early treatment here should have been protection against abduction or any adduction stress, together with local measures.

The symptoms are of sprain of the knee with tenderness high on the condyle in the one case and of adductor strain in the other. The presence of calcium is not necessarily of any consequence, the significant factor being the degree of pain. Frequently the area remains painful even after the injury has healed.

Treatment.   In some instances removal of the plaque of calcium is necessary. A word of warning is in order, however. If the surgeon is too eager and removes the calcium before it is entirely mature it will simply form again. If it is necessary to remove the calcium, great care should be taken that there is no interference with the attachment of the ligament to the femur. In a preponderance of cases removal of the calcium will not be necessary since the condition may mature and become quite inert with the passage of time.

DISLOCATION

Dislocations in the vicinity of the knee are of course the end result of a severe sprain since in order for any portion of a normal knee joint to dislocate certain groups of ligaments must be disrupted. Two basic dislocations of the knee occurring in athletic competition are the *patellofemoral dislocations* and *tibiofemoral dislocations*. In each instance we speak of the femur as being the stable bone with the other bone being displaced in relationship to it.

PATELLAR DISLOCATIONS

Patellar dislocations may be classified as acute and recurrent. In the athlete, chronic recurrent dislocation of the patella is not frequent since this condition ordinarily presumes a congenital or developmental anomaly which predisposes to the condition and would ordinarily discourage athletic competition.

Recurrent Dislocation of the Patella

Recurrent dislocation of the patella requires little discussion here beyond describing the type of lower extremity that predisposes to patellar dislocation and the mechanism of the disorder, with some words on treatment. The predisposing anatomical condition is an abnormally acute angle between the axis of the patellar ligament and the axis of the quadriceps mechanism. If the patellar ligament tends to angulate sharply laterally to reach its tibial attachment, this combined with the fact that the quadriceps mechanism tends to angulate medially at the knee results in a more acute angle between the patellar tendon and the long axis of the quadriceps so that, as the quadriceps muscle is contracted, there is a tendency for this angle to straighten by slipping of the patella laterally. This action may be inhibited by the prominence of the lateral femoral condyle anteriorly but the general tendency is for the patella to slide laterally with each forceful extension of the knee. The female with her wide pelvis and internally angulated femora is thus much more prone to patellar subluxation or dislocation than the male. A similar situation arises in a person with knock knee. A dislocated patella in a bowlegged individual is quite uncommon since in such a person the axis of the patellar tendon and quadriceps is essentially parallel.

One may, therefore, expect recurrent dislocation of the patella in a person with a wide pelvis, knock knee and a relatively flat lateral femoral condyle. Such a person as a rule is not an athlete. This recurring dislocation may arise gradually with the patella subluxating laterally, stretching the medial portion of the patellar retinaculum until the patella finally slips off either as a result of a relatively minor blow on its medial side or from a violent contraction of the quadriceps. Ordinarily in the initial instance the patella simply snaps off, slips right back on and there are few, if any, residual symptoms. The patient may describe his knee as having "given way." He may actually have fallen since his proprioceptive mechanism has warned him of the impending dislocation and relaxed the knee to prevent it.

On examination, findings will be entirely negative. One must not ascribe this locking knee to meniscus disorders. In fact, a well developed patellar subluxation and ultimate dislocation may occur with no actual tearing of the retinaculum. This patient soon learns that his activities must be curtailed and presents himself for treatment only when the recurrence becomes so frequent that it interferes with his ordinary activity. Surgical measures designed for correction of this condition must be carried out if the disability justifies them.

Treatment.   One must carefully analyze the characteristics of the injured extremity. Frequently what appears to be a recurrent dislocation of the patella may actually be one of repeated episodes of acute dislocation with no anatomical predisposition. This is particularly likely since the most commonly accepted treatment for the acutely dislocated patella at the present time is nonsurgical. After replacement of the dislocated bone the torn edges of the patellar retinaculum remain more or less widely separated. After healing, this inevitably results in a relaxed medial retinaculum so that as the knee flexes the patella does not receive as much pull medially as it does laterally and any additional force applied to the patella on the medial side will snap it over the lateral condylar ridge. This may occur as repeated episodes of subluxation with only an occasional complete dislocation. One must be on the alert, therefore, when examining a patient with such a history to determine whether or not there is actually a congenital or developmental defect since the remedial measures may be quite different in the two conditions.

If the anatomical characteristics are normal, all that may be necessary will be medial plication of the patellar retinaculum usually accompanied by division of the lateral patellar retinaculum, particularly if the condition has persisted over a long period of time. If on the other hand the angle of the patellar ligament is faulty, any of the capsuloplasty operations will give disappointing results since the predisposing cause is still present. Many procedures have been designed to correct the basic anatomic condition causing recurrent displacement. One may expect excellent results from any of them if the proper indication for it is present. Once successful correction is carried out, activity need not ordinarily be restricted. I recall a figure skater with bilateral recurrent dislocation of the patella symptomatic to the point that she had to give up her skating. Following transference of the tibial attachment of the patellar tendon medially and capsuloplasty of the knee she returned to her skating without further handicap. This particular patient was in her early 20's and one knee required almost a year for complete rehabilitation. I mention this to deprecate the all-too-prevalent tendency to warn a person that he must permanently decrease his activity when actually carefully designed treatment may permit normal use. The details of the various procedures are available in orthopedic textbooks and need not be described here.

Acute Dislocation of the Patella

The acute dislocation is of more pertinence than the recurrent type in any discussion of athletic injuries. The predisposing factors are the same as for chronic recurring dislocation, namely, knock knee with a shallow patellar groove and with the attachment of the patellar tendon well laterally on the tibia. The patient gives a history of severe pain in the knee following forceful extension or as a result of such exertion combined with a direct blow against the medial side of the patella. If the knee remains flexed the dislocation will persist.

On initial examination the patient will be in severe pain with the knee flexed, the tibia apparently abducted. He resists any attempt to manipulate the knee.

Careful examination makes the *diagnosis* obvious since the patella will be found to be riding lateral to the lateral condyle of the femur. Much more frequently the dislocation is spontaneously reduced as the knee extends so that the patient will give a story of an injury accompanied by severe pain and often describes the knee as having been "dislocated" and then having slipped back into place. It should be noted that this history is quite similar to that obtained from injury to the medial collateral ligament and not too different from that of an acute meniscus tear with locking spontaneously reduced.

If examination is done quite early there may be a palpable defect along the medial border of the patella with exquisite tenderness along the medial edge of this bone. The patient is extremely apprehensive of any attempt to push the patella laterally and will cry out and try to restrain the examiner's hand, particularly if manipulation is accompanied by a gesture toward flexing the knee. If examination is delayed the knee joint will be filled with fluid and there will be diffuse swelling, more severe anteriorly whereas in the case of a medial collateral tear it will be toward the medial side. On palpation of the knee one finds tenderness around the medial border of the patella with pain on flexion of the knee, which is pathognomonic. The negative findings are of considerable importance since there will be neither tenderness along the collateral ligaments nor pain on lateral motion of the tibia on the femur either with the knee extended or flexed. The patient with an acute patellar dislocation will permit a careful and considerate examiner to flex the knee a few degrees and externally rotate and abduct the tibia on the femur with no complaint, whereas in the acute case of medial collateral or indeed meniscus injuries this will not be possible. If hours elapse before the examination is carried out, the findings become less specific since muscle spasm tends to immobilize the knee, swelling becomes diffuse and tension within the capsule causes diffuse pain about the knee.

The lesion in acute dislocation is a rupture of the medial portion of the patellar retinaculum, which may be complete and may include a portion or all of the attachment of the vastus internus. In fact, the vastus aponeurosis and patellar retinaculum may be peeled away from the medial border of the patella, leaving it bare or actually tearing off a portion of the bone. Or the patellar retinaculum will split, much as a piece of cloth is torn, with the jagged tear extending anywhere along the medial aspect of the knee from the anterior edge of the deep layer of the medial collateral ligament to the patella.

X-ray is likely to be of little value except in a negative way (Fig. 334). Careful study of films may provide a clue particularly in regard to the general contour of

Figure 334.   Dislocation of the patella. Anteroposterior view shows the patella displaced to the lateral side. In the lateral view, note the overlapping of the patella and femoral
condyles. This picture could not be made of a normal knee.

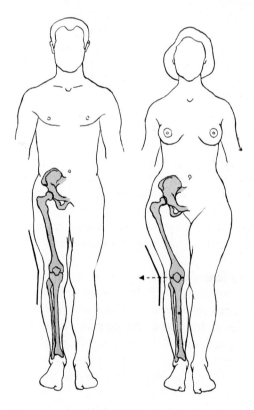

Figure 335.   Note that with the
broader pelvis in the female, it is necessary
for the femur to come inward at an increased angle in order to make the distal
end of the condyles parallel with the
ground. The quadriceps, patella and
patellar tendon make an angle centered at
the patella. As the quadriceps contracts,
this angle tends to straighten, which forces
the patella laterally.

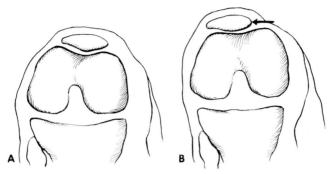

Figure 336.   A, Normal silhouette view of the patella. Note that the patella seats well in the groove with configuration between the undersurface of the patella and the femoral condyles. The lateral edge of the groove serves to help hold the patella in its normal position. B, Shallow groove with flat patella. The lateral buttress is lost, predisposing to dislocation.

bone, the anteroposterior view (Fig. 335) showing the increased tibiofemoral angle which predisposes to dislocation and the silhouette view (Fig. 336) the shallow patellar groove. More specifically, the latter may show the fragmentation along the medial border of the patella where there has been an avulsion of the ligament retinaculum (Fig. 337).

Treatment.   The treatment of acute dislocation of the patella is surgical. One has only to see the damage to tissues to realize that there can be no real substitute for accurate repositioning of the torn fibers and adequate repair. Research work is confirming more and more the conclusions that we have reached clinically, namely, that ligament or tendon heals by ligament or tendon if good apposition is secured whereas a gap that must be bridged in the healing process is likely to remain inadequate inelastic scar. I have seen separations of ¾ to 1 inch along the patellar retinaculum following acute dislocation with no tendency for the split fibers to fall spontaneously into apposition. Indeed, even slight flexion of the knee tends to force them further apart, the only acceptable position being complete extension or indeed hyperextension of the knee. This cannot or at least should not be tolerated for the length of time required for tissue repair. The operation is relatively simple, the

Figure 337.   A, Acute dislocation of patella with avulsion of a portion of the medial border of the patella. Note the shallow patellar groove with the flat undersurface of the patella so that there is little bony buttress to prevent dislocation. B, This was treated by removal of the medial one-fifth of the patella since the cartilage was entirely gone from this portion. This does not impair function of the knee.

lesion being essentially subcutaneous. With proper precautions in a well conditioned athlete, it should pose no undue hazard. The reward will be a prompt and complete recovery.

Since the acceptable treatment is surgical, the general management is consistent with this concept. After a careful examination and diagnosis, a compression bandage is applied and ice is used together with fixation of the knee until the operation can be carried out. The ideal time for surgical repair is immediately or at least as soon as proper preparation can be made. While a day or two delay does not completely preclude a good result, increasing experience indicates that there is no time like the present for surgical treatment of the ordinary acute injury. Ideally it is best treated the day it happens, but in no instance later than the following morning.

The operative technique will vary with the pathologic findings. As a general rule, a curved incision is made in the medial parapatellar area, beginning at the upper pole of the patella about ½ inch medial to it, extending along the border of the patella and paralleling the patellar tendon. On retraction of the skin edges the patellar retinaculum can be visualized and the nature of the damage ascertained. The incision may need to be extended higher if the vastus medialis has been avulsed, or swung lower and somewhat posteriorly if the medial flap must be reflected to expose the retinaculum further toward the inner side. Usually the capsule of the knee will be torn open. The joint should be carefully inspected, particularly the undersurface of the patella and the lateral edge of the lateral femoral condyle. An osteochondral fracture may be present in either location (Fig. 338). If there is a

Figure 338.   Acute dislocation of the patella in the oblique view with chondral fracture of the undersurface of the patella. Note the fragment lying just behind the femoral condyle slightly distal to the lower pole of the patella. Note also the defect on the underside of the patella. At operation an acute fracture with a fresh bleeding bed under the patella was found. The hooklike processes on the medial epicondylar ridge are a normal variant. This is the type of trauma that can cause apparent "patellar malacia" if unrecognized early.

chondral fracture or chondromalacia it should be carefully treated by chondrectomy or other measures, the exact technique depending upon the severity of the condition. One may suspect chondromalacia in a knee with a dislocated patella since the tendency for the patella to slide laterally on extension of the knee may be quite traumatic to the cartilage over a period of time. Malacia along the medial and superior facets of the patella is quite common and should be corrected at the time of operation. Treatment of the dislocation itself is relatively simple. By appropriate suture the defect is closed. If one is unable to suture to the edge of the patella, drill holes may be made along the edge of bone, carefully avoiding penetrating the patellar cartilage. Fixation is readily obtained in this manner.

Postoperatively the leg is placed in long leg posterior and lateral stirrup splints with the knee slightly flexed (10 to 15 degrees) for seven to ten days, at which time the sutures are removed and the knee is further protected against flexion by an appropriate splint with or without weight bearing depending upon the individual case. Healing will be prompt. The long leg cast can be removed after three weeks to be followed by a fourth week in a cotton cast while activity is gradually increased and the customary rehabilitative measures are initiated. A word of caution should be said. If the patient has the anatomical characteristics that predispose to recurrent dislocation, these should be carefully analyzed and a definite plan of management instituted. Either his activity should be sharply curtailed or reconstructive measures should be carried out to reduce the tendency toward lateral slipping. This is particularly important if there has been damage to the patella. One should have no hesitation in recommending transference of the patellar tendon attachment from the lateral to the medial aspect of the tibia in such a case, since without it recurrent trouble in later life is almost inevitable, even though athletic activities are curtailed. If the anatomical alignment is normal and no predisposing characteristics are manifest, further protection after the completion of healing is not indicated. In this instance there should be no more predilection for trouble than there would be following a broken tibia, for example.

TIBIOFEMORAL DISLOCATION

Tibiofemoral dislocation is a rare injury in athletes. There is some separation of the tibia from the femur in any complete tear of the collateral ligaments. Usually this dislocation is spontaneously reduced and by the time the patient is examined it appears to be what it indeed is, a ligament injury. In some instances the displacement is so complete that it does not reduce spontaneously. At other times a frank dislocation has been noted before it is reduced by a fellow player or some other individual on the field. With a history of complete dislocation one should investigate very carefully to determine whether it actually was tibiofemoral in character. A dislocation of the patella or indeed a dislocation of a meniscus with temporary locking may quite often be interpreted by the player himself as a dislocation of the knee.

The tibiofemoral displacement may be in any direction, and determination of this direction has important bearing on the surgical approach. If the tibia is displaced completely in front of the femur (Fig. 339), complete loss of both collateral ligaments, both cruciate ligaments and the posterior capsule is indicated. If the tibia

Figure 339.   Acute dislocation of the knee showing the femoral condyles completely posterior
to the tibia. Both cruciates and both collaterals must be torn. This is a severe sprain.

is dislocated behind the femur there is similar damage to the collaterals and cruciates
but the posterior capsule may be largely intact. Displacement of the tibia toward
the lateral side of the femur would indicate a complete tear of the medial collateral
and at least the medial portion of the posterior capsule and both cruciates while the
lateral collateral ligament may be intact. Conversely, if the displacement of the
tibia is toward the medial side of the femur, the major injury is on the lateral side
which would include both cruciates, the lateral collateral, the biceps, the popliteus
and peroneal nerve. It should be noted that in each of these injuries the cruciate
ligaments are torn. Attendant damage to other structures of the knee is usually
present. One or both of the menisci may be damaged. There may be chondral fracture of the patella or tibia. There may be damage to the blood vessels and nerves
about the knee which may take precedence over all else.

Diagnosis.   If the case is seen immediately a careful examination will be
highly informative. The first step should be to evaluate the circulation to the foot
and the second to determine the state of the nerve supply. It is extremely important
to know whether or not there has been immediate loss of innervation to any part
of the foot. Late paralysis will suggest pressure intrinsic or extrinsic on the nerve
and may well require different management than would early paralysis. The peroneal nerve is particularly vulnerable in dislocations.

After this preliminary survey of the condition of the leg and foot, attention is
directed to the knee. Careful inspection will reveal any persistent deformity and
its direction, thus providing a valuable guide to the pathology of the injury (see
above). If the deformity has been reduced either spontaneously or manually before
the examination it may be possible at this early date to determine the degree of
instability of the knee. This examination should be extremely careful, taking particular pains not to reproduce the dislocation. I remember one instance in which

the patient had a complete dislocation of the knee that was spontaneously reduced and re-dislocated three times before x-rays were made that showed the complete dislocation (see Fig. 339). Obviously, re-dislocation is a serious hazard and should be assiduously guarded against. After examination and some definition of the degree of pathology, measures for treatment should be promptly initiated.

Treatment. In the athlete the treatment of dislocation of the knee is surgical, and adequate repair requires all the skill one can muster. True enough, there have been cases treated nonsurgically with recovery of a useful degree of function of the knee, but I have never known of one so treated to end with anything approaching *normal* function. Immediate measures are as for any ligament injury of the knee. Following examination, aspiration of blood and injection of hyaluronidase and the application of a pressure bandage with ice are imperative. Then, without fail, the whole extremity must be protected by adequate splinting since irreparable damage may be done to the leg by careless handling. The patient should not walk from the field with assistance or be carried, leg dangling, with his arms over other players' shoulders. He should be tightly splinted manually, placed on a stretcher and not moved from the stretcher until proper support is applied to the knee.

Plans are now made for definitive treatment but the first consideration is the circulation of the leg, which is of vital importance. This should not be interpreted as meaning that repair should "wait until the swelling goes down." It means simply that one should assure himself of the adequacy of the circulation of the foot since if this is not adequate and does not respond to paravertebral sympathetic block and similar measures, the first step may well be exploration of the popliteal space. Rupture of the popliteal artery or vein is a distinct possibility. If it is necessary to explore posteriorly and if the circulation is not too disturbed, some degree of posterior repair may be carried out at this time. Repair of the posterior cruciate and posterior capsule may be feasible as part of this procedure. If the circulation of the extremity is intact, then a choice must be made between an approach to the knee from the medial and from the lateral side. This choice will depend upon where the major damage is suspected. One may obtain surprisingly good access to almost all parts of a badly torn knee with an incision on one side only. I have been able to repair the posterior cruciate to the tibia, the posterior capsule to the tibia, the anterior cruciate to the femur, and the medial collateral ligament to the femur and tibia, together with medial and lateral meniscectomy, all through a medial approach since the knee can be very carefully opened up in these circumstances to permit placement of sutures which can be tied after the joint is reduced and positioned. Tourniquet time must be carefully guarded. Indeed much of the closure may be carried out after the tourniquet is removed. Removal of the tourniquet before closure has the added advantage of permitting control of bleeding. It is good for one's peace of mind to know that no major vessel is the cause of the postoperative swelling which is almost inevitable.

Following a suitable period of recovery from the initial injury and the reparative surgery, a second operation may be carried out. If the peroneal nerve has been primarily damaged it should be explored and repaired within a relatively early period, say within two weeks. There is a degree of urgency of treatment of each of these structures and the priority is definitely in the following order: (1) circulatory embarrassment, (2) damage to the cruciate ligaments, (3) collateral ligament damage and (4) neurological deficit. Justification for this timing is quite evident with a little consideration. After the circulation I give second priority to the cruciates because the success of cruciate ligament repair varies inversely with the elapsed time after injury. It must be done within the first two weeks and the sooner the better.

A dislocation of the knee is an extremely serious injury. This is not sufficient justification for a negative approach to the problem since the dislocation need not necessarily terminate in a major disability. Time is of the very essence. The patient should be placed promptly in the hands of the specialist who will carry out definitive treatment.

A partial dislocation or subluxation has been amply covered in our discussion of sprain. A chronically subluxating knee is also a ligament problem.

MENISCUS INJURY

Another common condition is injury to the menisci. This injury goes hand in glove with ligament sprain. The general structural anatomy of the menisci is well known but it is well to recall certain significant differences between the two menisci in order to understand the damage one may expect from a given type of injury.

Medial Meniscus

The medial meniscus is "C" shaped (Fig. 340, A). Its anterior attachment is on the top of the tibia near the midline and in front of the tibial spine. The posterior attachment is on the top of the tibia behind the posterior spine. In each case the attachment is relatively near the periphery of the tibia so that the two ends are quite widely separated from each other. The meniscus is attached by means of the coronary ligament (which has its origin around the top of the tibia) to the medial collateral ligament and hence to the tibia. This attachment is firm and while it dose allow a little play there is no very extensive motion permitted in the normal medial meniscus.

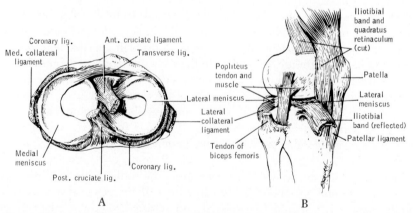

A   B

Figure 340.   A, Drawing of the top of the tibia showing the menisci and the coronary ligament. B, Drawing showing attachment of lateral meniscus to tensor fascia femoris which is frequently noted.

In sprain of the medial collateral ligament, the tibia and femur tend to separate on the medial side and stress is applied in the area of the attachment of the cartilage to the medial ligament. The cartilage may be forced to accompany either the femur or the tibia, depending upon the location of the ligament injury. Since the structure of the meniscus does not allow much bending stress, it will tear transversely or more commonly split around its periphery. If the tear is actually in the attachment to the ligament it will frequently heal. If it is within the substance of the meniscus it will not. In my experience meniscus injury accompanies repeated sprains to the knee more frequently than it does the initial single sprain. I know of no way to determine in an acute injury whether or not the meniscus is torn unless the knee is actually locked. If the knee is locked and the ligaments appear to be stable and the episode is the first, one may be justified in attempting to reduce the displacement by careful manipulation or by traction. If the meniscus has been detached at its periphery, this attachment may then heal. This possibility is much more likely if the meniscus has slipped into the knee and locked and the knee has been almost immediately unlocked. Such an incident occurs where the player hurts the knee and it is forcibly extended manually immediately following the injury and the meniscus snaps back in place. My own opinion is that if the knee actually locks even once the knee should be operated upon, the meniscus examined and, if torn, removed. However, I have no particular argument with the surgeon who prefers to wait for the second episode. There is nothing to be gained by waiting for repeated episodes of locking, and bragging of them by the patient cannot be condoned. We have been able to show that locking of the knee has a definitely deleterious effect upon the articular cartilage, not only on the condyles of the femur and tibia but more particularly on the patella. Careful explanation to the patient of the undesirable effects of the locking episodes will ordinarily convince him that he had better have his knee operated upon early with the prospect of an excellent result than postpone operation until malacia has become advanced.

Lateral Meniscus

Whereas the medial meniscus is "C" shaped with widely separated anterior and posterior attachments, the lateral meniscus is almost "O" shaped (Fig. 340, A), its anterior and posterior attachments being deep in the tibial notch and very close to each other. In many instances they are continuous with each other. The coronary ligament is much less firm and is more redundant. This meniscus is not attached to the fibular collateral ligament and as a consequence more motion is normally possible than in the case of the medial meniscus. Injury to the lateral side of the knee is less common than to the medial side. Furthermore, the lateral meniscus is much less likely to be damaged by acute lateral stress so that it is not frequent to see a lateral meniscus tear in conjunction with an acute sprain of the knee. On the other hand, by virtue of the looseness of the meniscus, particularly in its posterior portion, it is quite vulnerable to chronic damage so that it is more likely to be hurt by chronic overflexion of the knee. Frequently the damage comes on insidiously as a result of squatting with the heel against the buttock for long intervals on frequent occasions. I have been so impressed with the vulnerability of the lateral meniscus because of redundancy of its posterior one-third that I do not recommend deep knee bends or so-called "duck waddle" as conditioning exercises. As the knee moves into complete flexion the back of the meniscus may be caught between the impinging femoral condyle and tibial plateau and thrust forward, much as one would pinch an apple seed between his finger tips. This strains the posterior peripheral attachment until the meniscus may actually snap in front of the femoral condyle and finally progress to the typical bucket handle position and lie within the notch in front of and medial to the lateral articular condyle of the femur.

Although as a general rule the attachments of the lateral meniscus to the other lateral components of the knee are much less firm than is the case with the medial meniscus, this is not always true. In many instances there is a very firm attachment of the anterolateral section of the lateral meniscus to the iliotibial band. I have noted this to be almost always the case in partial or complete discoid menisci. Indeed, one often cannot distinguish a line of separation between the inner surface of the iliotibial band as it crosses the knee and the lateral margin of the lateral meniscus. This is almost always bilateral and predisposes markedly to injury. In this instance the front of the cartilage is firmly attached whereas the posterior part is relatively loose. As a consequence of this firm fixation as the stress occurs to adduct the leg on the thigh, the cartilage is actually dragged forward and its whole posterior portion may catch in front of the femoral condyle. This anatomical variant has real significance in the fact that the lateral compartment is extremely difficult to expose until the cartilage is separated from the iliotibial band (Fig. 340, B).

DIAGNOSIS

If one never makes the diagnosis of meniscus injury until the knee has undergone repeated locking he is overlooking many torn menisci! The diagnosis of meniscus injury may be made by history alone and it is extremely important that the history be carefully and objectively taken. It is not wise to put words in the patient's mouth. If he gives a definite, detailed and reliable history of locking of the knee, one may assume meniscus damage until he can prove it to be otherwise. More difficult is the case of chronic knee trouble with recurrent effusion and recurring periods of disability but with no locking or "giving way." One suspects meniscus damage. In this instance a very careful examination will be of extreme value. There is usually tenderness along the joint line in the damaged area. This may be posterior as a result of posterior tearing, or it may be midlateral or in front. The examiner should familiarize himself with the various manipulations that put stress on each meniscus. With the knee semiflexed, lateral stress will usually cause pain in acute injuries but not as consistently in chronic meniscus damage. There is usually pain on rotatory stress. With the knee flexed, the calf is grasped firmly and the leg rotated laterally and medially. Pain will frequently be noted at the exact site of the injury to the meniscus. One should at least be able to determine which side of the knee is involved. The various types of cartilage click, such as the Ledbetter tests, are of importance if elicitable. Another test which I think is quite valuable is carried out with the patient prone. The knee is placed in complete flexion and then hyperflexed to determine whether this causes pain and where the pain is located. Many cases of posterior tear will give a definite cartilage click on this maneuver. In fact, this maneuver may actually cause the cartilage to slip forward and the knee to be locked. In this same completely flexed position the foot is turned into external rotation and the knee flexed and extended a few degrees. The leg is then placed in internal rotation and the knee flexed and extended. Consistent clicking in these tests must be considered significant. In the final analysis, the knee that stubbornly resists conservative treatment and in which meniscus damage is suspected justifies arthrotomy. This is not to say that every painful knee should be operated upon for meniscus damage. The weight of the evidence must point toward meniscus damage to justify surgery under this preoperative diagnosis.

TREATMENT

I have previously stated that if the knee locks this in itself is justification for surgical treatment. The locking may be due to meniscus damage, or to a foreign body in the joint, displaced osteochondritis dissecans, etc. At arthrotomy one must be prepared to treat whatever lesion is found. If the knee locks, some presumptive cause must be found if the operation is to be successful. Removing a normal meniscus will not stop the knee from locking! (See Fig. 341.)

Some general principles referrable to surgery are important. There is no justification for removing a normal meniscus just because one has diagnosed meniscus damage preoperatively. It is true that the front of the meniscus upon examination may appear to be normal but there may be posterior damage that cannot be determined from in front, none the less it is pretty drastic to detach the anterior end of the meniscus in order to determine whether its posterior portion is torn. A better procedure is to enter the knee behind the medial collateral ligament to permit inspection of the posterior part of the meniscus. As stated, the removal of a normal meniscus is unjustifiable, and particularly so because it does not eliminate the cause of the trouble in the knee. If upon inspection no abnormality is found in either meniscus, the knee must be carefully explored for other lesions to account for the symptoms. These may or may not be remediable but are not helped by removing a normal meniscus.

A question that must be answered is, "What constitutes a 'normal' meniscus?" This is an area in which surgical experience counts heavily. I have no hesitation in

Figure 341. This case is of interest from a diagnostic standpoint. The boy had an abduction injury to the leg with symptoms of medial meniscus pathology. He actually did have a bucket-handle fracture of the medial meniscus. Survey x-rays revealed a tumor in the femoral condyle. It proved to be a benign chondroblastoma. In this instance the solid tumor was an incidental finding. Treatment of the tumor designed to improve the condition of the knee would have failed. The tumor was removed at a second operation.

removing a meniscus that is yellow and sclerotic or in which there is redundancy of one or the other attachments although there may be no obvious tear. However, I would feel extremely uneasy about removing a sclerotic meniscus in a knee in which there is a history of locking or giving way since certainly a sclerotic meniscus could not be expected to cause these symptoms. Frequently at arthrotomy there will be found a rather marked redundancy of the fat pad, the posterior margin of which may appear grossly sclerotic. This can be symptomatic, usually causing pain on forced or rapid extension of the knee as in place kicking. However, once again I would feel quite uneasy about simply trimming away the fat pad unless I could assure myself that there is no other pathologic condition in the knee. Fat pad symptoms should be around the pad and are elicited by pressure on this area.

I realize that this is vast oversimplification of the meniscus problem but would like to state a few of my own convictions.

1. A locking knee should be operated upon regardless of freedom from symptoms in the intervals between episodes.

2. Authentic "giving way" of the knee may be almost as significant of meniscus damage as is locking.

3. A careful history suggestive of meniscus damage supported by pertinent findings justifies arthrotomy provided there is real disability of the knee. If the symptoms are so mild as to cause no effusion, instability or actual disability from pain, arthrotomy may be postponed since the knee is not undergoing deterioration because of delay.

Technique for Medial Meniscectomy

The patient is placed in the supine position (Fig. 326) and given the usual meticulous preparation of the skin. The leg is draped. The footpiece (Fig. 342, A) of the table is then dropped to permit the leg to dangle off the table at a 90 degree angle. The surgeon drapes the front of his gown to entirely cover his feet and is seated at the foot of the table with the patient's foot between his knees. I prefer a straight incision (Fig. 342, B) which begins about ½ inch proximal to the lower pole of the patella and ¼ inch medial to the patellar tendon and proceeds parallel to the patellar tendon to terminate just opposite the patellar tubercle. This is actually the central portion of the anteromedial incision which we use for knee ligament repair (Fig. 327). Stockinette is fastened to the wound edges. The patellar retinaculum is split along the line of the incision and the synovium is opened. At this point the knee is carefully lavaged (Fig. 342, C) with warm sterile saline, particularly if blood is encountered. Through this short incision, a surprisingly good exploration of the knee can be carried out. The anterior attachment of the medial meniscus is examined. The anterior cruciate is checked. The posterior cruciate is noted. The knee is extended and the undersurface of the patella inspected by lifting it up with a toothed retractor and also by palpation with the finger.

Should there be attendant damage, particularly involvement of the lower end of the patella, the incision is extended proximally at this time to permit better exposure. It is not necessary to enlarge this incision in order to carry out adequate repair of the anterior cruciate ligament. If there is damage to the collateral ligament which should be repaired, the incision is extended distally.

The meniscus is now carefully examined. If it is possible to spring the knee

Figure 342.   The author's general set-up for medial meniscus surgery.

A, The leg is prepared and draped as shown in Figure 326. Note the knee flexed to 90 degrees with the foot lying between the operator's knees. The surgeon is draped with an extra double fan wrapped around as a skirt. Note the white double fan lying under the knee and not fannd out.

B, The short incision which is actually the central part of the general utility incision on the medial side of the knee (Fig. 327). This incision can be extended upward if it is desirable to expose the undersurface of the patella, downward if it is necessary to repair the medial ligament.

C, At the beginning and termination of the operation the knee is thoroughly lavaged with warm saline. The basin which catches the return flow will reveal many bits of foreign material which would be best out of the knee.

D, As the anesthetist extends the end of the table, the double fan which has been lying under the knee is extended out over the end of the table, thus, covering the whole end of the table which has been proximate to the floor.

E, Position for exploration of the patella or any other procedure needed with the knee extended. The skin and capsular incisions are more readily closed with the knee in extension.

Figure 343.   Anteroposterior and lateral views of the "cartilage feeler." Note the curve similar to a meniscotome and the short, blunt hook at the end. This can be deceptive if it is allowed to turn as it goes into the posterior compartment and then catches in the synovial sac, but it is a useful adjunct in the exploration.

open on the medial side, the entire cartilage may be visible. This is the exception rather than the rule. The periphery of the cartilage is palpated with a blunt Kelly forceps to determine whether there is a defect in the coronary ligament attachment or a split in the cartilage. I have devised a "feeler" for this purpose which is a small rod curved in the arc of the femoral condyle with a ⅜ inch right-angled blunt hook at its end (Fig. 343). This is to avoid any possibility that the point of the forceps will be forced through the coronary ligament rather than hooked into the defect. Anterior examination will ordinarily determine whether there has been damage to the meniscus. If the feeler hooks in the split in the cartilage or in its attachment, we assume the presence of a posterior tear. If the anterior part of the cartilage is friable, ecchymotic and redundant, we assume that the meniscus has been damaged somewhere. If this examination leads to the conclusion that the cartilage is pathological, it is removed as follows:

The anterior bony attachment is separated from the upper end of the tibia and the periphery of the cartilage is carefully divided from the coronary ligament as far back as convenient with the ordinary scalpel. At this point traction forward on the cartilage will confirm posterior damage. A curved cartilage knife or meniscotome is utilized to divide the meniscus from the coronary ligament as far back as the posterior bony attachment. This instrument must be exceedingly sharp and care must be taken that it follows the contour of the tibial rim, not the femoral condyle. If this instrument does not pass readily it should not be forced since damage can be done to the femoral condyle, the upper end of the tibia, the medial collateral ligament or the posterior cruciate ligament by unwise instrumentation. If the cartilage detaches readily it is pulled over into the notch. Using a very thin straight meniscotome, the bony attachment is divided, care being taken to get all of the meniscus. The operation to this point has all been done through the anterior incision which means that the pathologic characteristics were determined from in front, that the cartilage was readily divided by a curved meniscotome, that we removed all of the meniscus when we detached the posterior bony attachment. Failing any of these things, exposure of the posterior compartment of the knee must be made. This may be done in one or two ways. The anterior skin incision can be extended as for the ligament approach and the medial skin flap reflected subcutaneously. The posterior margin of the medial collateral ligament can be palpated as the curve of the tibial plateau swings posteriorly and a vertical split made along the line of its fibers. Dividing through the synovium will give access to the posterior compartment. This same area may be reached by making a short vertical incision through the skin paralleling the ligament fibers just at the posterior edge of the medial collateral ligament. The posterior ligament is relaxed in this flexed position and the posterior compartment can be readily visualized through this exposure. If no pathologic signs were present in front, the cartilage is particularly examined for them posteriorly. If we find no signs of damage to the cartilage it is not removed. If the removal from in front left a posterior tag or if the cartilage did not readily separate, we complete the meniscectomy posteriorly. Careful examination of this space is carried out to make sure there is no other damaged tissue. The posterior cruciate ligament can be palpated readily. The posterior femoral condyle can be inspected as can the upper end of the tibia. The wound is now thoroughly flushed with warm saline and closed in layers, 4-0 cotton in the synovium, 2-0 cotton in the ligament, 4-0 chromic in the subcutaneous tissue, No. 32 subcuticular wire for the skin.

Attention is next redirected to the anterior portion of the incision. The operative wound is thoroughly lavaged and the fat pad inspected. Any other morbid changes are noted and treated. If the patella is normal, the incision is then closed similarly to the posterior one. If it is necessary to treat the undersurface of the patella, the knee is then extended, the end of the table raised and draped as indicated (Fig. 342, D) and appropriate treatment to the patella is carried out: chondrectomy, partial patellectomy or patellectomy as the case may be. At the conclusion of the operation a cotton cast (Fig. 304) is applied and the tourniquet removed.

Technique for Lateral Meniscectomy

The lateral compartment is more difficult to expose than the medial. The leg is prepared and positioned as indicated above. The incision I prefer at present has a horizontal and a vertical component. The horizontal limb begins about 1½ inch lateral to the lower end of the patella and level with it, extends straight forward along the line of the iliotibial tract to the edge of the patellar tendon and then parallels the edge of the patellar tendon to the tubercle of the tibia (Fig. 329). The iliotibial band is split in the horizontal arm of the incision along the line of its fibers until the patellar tendon is reached, then the division parallels the patellar tendon. This permits the iliotibial band to be reflected backward without impairing its strength. The fat pad is troublesome but is incised to expose the knee. Electrocoagulation is used to seal obvious vessels. The lateral meniscus is now visualized. It is usually considerably more redundant than the medial. The same general rules are applied laterally as medially. There is one notable difference, however. This is in respect to the popliteal hiatus. There is normally a defect in the coronary ligament at the midlateral line of the meniscus through which traverses the popliteus tendon. One must not be misled into interpreting this as a tear. There is frequently a tear, sometimes difficult to detect, of the meniscus attachment from the popliteal hiatus back to the posterior meniscal attachment.

If the cartilage is found by anterior inspection to be pathological, it should be detached in front and pulled forward, whereupon the posterior characteristics can be readily determined. If the anterior part appears to be completely normal, a second incision must be made similar to that on the medial side, the approach being just in front of the fibular collateral ligament. This is somewhat more difficult than on the medial side since one encounters the popliteus tendon as it crosses the back of the knee laterally and care should be taken not to damage it.

Postoperative Care

Our postoperative care for meniscus injury is as follows: A cotton cast is applied and the tourniquet removed. An elastic bandage is placed from the toes to the bottom of the cotton cast. Rehabilitation is started immediately. The patient is expected to raise his leg that night; to exercise all of his muscles the next morning; be up in a chair the first postoperative day; be up on crutches with direct weight bearing the second postoperative day. Weight bearing without crutches is discouraged, however, because of the tendency to lurch and so strain the knee laterally. Since the cotton cast loosens up in a few days, the elastic bandage is removed from the foot and wrapped around the dressing.

The patient is allowed to go home in a few days and instructed to re-wrap the elastic bandage over the cotton cast every few days to keep it snug. When he reports back two weeks after the operation, the cotton cast and stitches are removed. If there is effusion the knee is aspirated, a corticoid injected and an elastic bandage provided. If there is no effusion, the patient is advised to wear an elastic bandage for another week. Rehabilitation is continued. No effort is made to force motion of the knee other than by the patient's voluntary effort. In the uncomplicated case recovery is rapid. Aspiration is repeated as often as indicated by effusion. It usually is not necessary at all. Athletic participation will be permitted as soon as the range of motion is normal and the strength of the operated leg is equal to that of the good leg. This may be at four weeks or may be later depending upon the many factors that influence recovery, such as the duration of symptoms prior to the operation, the degree of synovitis of the knee, and postoperative bleeding or effusion.

CHONDRAL AND OSTEOCHONDRAL FRACTURE

A chondral fracture is a fracture involving the articular cartilage and is particularly prevalent at the knee owing to the direct stresses and strains applied to the knee joint. A chondral fracture may be extremely difficult to diagnose and in many instances may be determined only after arthrotomy of the knee. If there is no fragment of underlying bone involved, the x-ray will be entirely negative.

The *diagnosis* must rest on history and clinical symptoms. If the fracture is complete and if a piece of cartilage is loose in the knee the symptoms will be those of a foreign body within the joint. While this fracture may be quite difficult to distinguish from a tear of one of the menisci or from osteochondritis dissecans, early differentation is somewhat academic since in any case arthrotomy is indicated. Many chondral fractures go completely unrecognized, particularly when they are incomplete so that the fragment is not actually dislodged. I feel quite sure that many cases of osteochondritis dissecans are in fact initiated by fractures of the cartilage. The most vulnerable areas in the joint are, first, the patella, and second, the two femoral condyles. The patella is particularly vulnerable because it is so common for the athlete to fall upon the flexed knee. The result may be a contusion to the articular cartilage, an actual fissuring of the cartilage, or in rare circumstances a complete chondral fracture with a piece of cartilage separated from the bone (Figs. 344 and 345).

The symptoms are those of damage to the undersurface of the patella, i.e., pain on flexion and extension, particularly against resistance, and pain on manual pressure of the patella against the femoral condyle, particularly on "rubbing" the patella against the condylar groove with the knee in complete extension. Such a fracture may cause actual catching or locking of the knee by an interuption of the normal glide pattern of the patella in the patellar groove.

I have recently operated in a case diagnosed as intrinsic injury to the knee with chondromalacia of the patella and was surprised to find two-thirds of the cartilage of the patella had been completely broken away and could be lifted

Figure 344. Acute chondral fracture of the patella with negative x-ray. The patient had a history of falling on the flexed knee with more than the usual amount of symptoms including hemarthrosis. Surgery revealed (A) acute chondral fracture of the patella with multiple fragments of cartilage. Definitely not degenerative. (B) The fragments may be lifted up revealing the hemorrhagic bleeding bone beneath an acute injury. (C) Further removal of the fragments and (D) fragments all removed and the vascular bed of the bone exposed. Note the apparently normal cartilage surrounding the defect with no evidence of fibrillation or malacia. This would later have been described as a typical osteochondritis dissecans or chondromalacia, either of which would have been wrong. This patient went on to a good recovery with no patellar symptoms at present.

Figure 345.   This is a case similar to that of Figure 344 seen much later. Note the typical
               osteochondritic fragment. Note also the defect under the patella.

up from its bed as a flap, exposing raw bone beneath. Another frequent chondral
injury is an avulsion type fracture of the cartilage and bone along the lateral margin
of the medial femoral condyle at the femoral attachment of the posterior cruciate
ligament (Fig. 367). I have seen many cases at operation which had been diagnosed
as osteochondritis dissecans of the medial femoral condyle, in which the loose body
was actually attached to the anterior end of the posterior cruciate ligament. Some
have been encountered in which the chondral body was completely free except for
the fact that it was still attached to the posterior cruciate ligament. These are, in
my opinion, chondral fractures rather than osteochondritis dissecans.

The primary diagnostic problem of chondral fracture will be to differentiate
it from other intrinsic conditions of the knee. It should be suspected if there is
persistent pain and persistent dysfunction around an otherwise normal appearing
patella. This is particularly true if acute symptoms have followed immediately upon
an injury. The orthopedist will see these patients relatively late since they are
usually treated for a contusion or a sprain and the question of chondral fracture
may arise only after the knee has failed to respond to ordinary therapeutic measures.

Proper *treatment* depends largely upon a proper diagnosis. If there is definitely
a subchondral fracture it is possible that protective immobilization will permit it to
heal. However, if the cartilage itself is broken without subchondral bone, the healing potential is so poor that it probably will not heal in any event. As a rule the exact
condition is not previously diagnosed and one must be prepared to carry out whatever definitive measure is indicated at the time of the arthrotomy of the knee.

Where a fragment of cartilage with some subchondral bone has been torn
away, including a portion of the posterior cruciate attachment, the treatment is
removal of this fragment and suture of the posterior cruciate to the cartilage bed
through drill holes. This will successfully restore posterior cruciate integrity. In
other cases in which the amount of cruciate ligament involved has been relatively
small, I have simply sutured the torn ligament to its uninvolved portion. The loose

fragment of bone and cartilage should be removed in any event and appropriate measures carried out to minimize the potential damage to the mechanism of the knee. Most of the young patients tolerate partial chondrectomy very well. One may smooth off the margins of the bed either on the patella or on the femoral condyle and expect a considerable degree of filling in as healing proceeds. Indeed, in many cases the fossa has pretty well smoothed itself out before arthrotomy has been accepted by the patient. I am extremely loath to sacrifice the patella in a young athlete. I would oppose even more the use of a metallic prosthesis since in either case the femoral condyle is exposed to considerable direct trauma. The small metallic prosthesis serves to concentrate the force in a small area and is potentially more dangerous than any direct trauma to the condyle protected by the quadriceps aponeurosis only, after removal of the patella.

FRACTURE

Fracture about the knee is not a frequent injury in the young athlete. The ordinary fracture is treated in the same manner as a similar fracture in any other patient, bearing in mind the general principles for treatment of the athlete particularly in reference to prompt diagnosis with the aid of x-ray. The aphorism in fracture treatment that "the nearer the joint the more perfect the reduction" is doubly true in the knee since the normally functioning knee joint will not tolerate any gross irregularity of its articular surfaces. This discussion will be confined to the treatment of those fractures about the knee which are more common to the athlete.

Fracture of the Patella

Fracture of the patella occurs in athletes but is not as common as chondral fracture of the patella. Fractures of either the upper (Fig. 346, A) or lower pole (Fig. 346, B) or along the medial or lateral margin (Fig. 346, C) usually are actually either strain fractures or sprain fractures and should be treated as such by removal of the fragment of bone and suture of the ligament or tendon to the patella. This should be done promptly and a perfectly functioning knee may be expected. It should be emphasized here that there is little place for bone repair in the treatment of fracture of the patella and I can think of few circumstances justifying the securing of bone-to-bone apposition and waiting for patellar union. The exception is in the incomplete fracture or possibly in the linear fracture extending from upper to lower pole. One should particularly suspect chondral fracture to accompany stellate fracture of the patella without displacement. It is not wise to carry out patellectomy in the athlete if it can be avoided since complete patellectomy is not compatible with such strenuous sport as soccer, football, etc., not because of failure of the quadriceps mechanism but because of the extreme vulnerability of the femoral condyles after removal of the patella. I would be even more fearful of permitting athletic participation following replacement of the patella by metallic prosthesis since this concentrates the force and in my opinion is more dangerous than complete patellectomy.

Fracture of the patella by direct contusion is not infrequent. The fracture usually involves the lateral portion of the patella since the bone is thinner in this area (Fig. 347). This fracture differs from the avulsion type in which the fragment is

Figure 346.   *A,* Avulsed quadriceps tendon and fragment from superior pole of patella. The shell of bone makes the diagnosis simple but the lesion is really a tendon avulsion rather than a fractured patella. Treated by repair of the quadriceps to the patella.

B, Avulsion fracture of lower pole of patella. In effect, a rupture of the tendon. Note that after removal of the fragments and repair of the tendon to the patella, there is essentially normal appearing patella remaining.

C, Fracture of lateral margin of the patella by a direct blow.

Figure 347.   This professional baseball player received a sharp blow on the knee with a baseball, had immediate swelling, pain and discomfort. He was treated for contusion. On examination some weeks later, the oblique view shows the fracture which had been overlooked in the anteroposterior and lateral views. The silhouette view (as in Figure 346, *C*) would demonstrate this even better.

torn away by the tendon or ligament. It is usually on the medial side and occurs as the patella is forced laterally. It also differs from the explosive type fracture caused by a forceful blow against the patella with the quadriceps in violent contraction, such as occurs when the knee hits the dashboard in a motor accident. This fracture is due to a sharp blow in a relatively localized area, as sometimes received by a baseball fielder. As he is squatted down with his knees flexed, the ball caroms to one side and hits directly on the patella. This same force may cause chondral damage. A typical example of this fracture is illustrated in Figure 346, C. The silhouette view made its diagnosis much easier since the small fragment is difficult to visualize in the anteroposterior view unless the x-ray is particularly good. This condition is treated by removal of the fragment and suture of the retinaculum to the patella. Uneventful recovery should be expected. At the time of repair the undersurface of the patella and the cartilage of the patellar groove should be carefully inspected for possible chondral damage.

Care should be taken not to confuse the *bipartite* or *tripartite patella* with acute injury (Fig. 348). The partite patella is usually bilateral and symmetrical, and is asymptomatic. Careful examination will demonstrate that the symptoms are not in the area of the anomaly. It should be borne in mind, however, that it is possible for the quadriceps lateralis to avulse or partially avulse the separate piece in which event the condition will become symptomatic. This ordinarily will respond well to rest and protection. If the symptoms persist, one is justified in removing the piece and suturing the tendon to the patella. This condition is quite analogous to avulsion of the accessory navicular in the foot. In both instances there is an underlying congenital anomaly on which is superimposed an acute injury.

Figure 348.   Bilateral bipartite patella. Note the completely separate portion of the patella on the superolateral margin. This should not be confused with acute fracture.

Figure 349.   Acute avulsion of anterior portion of upper surface of tibia including tibial spine. Anterior cruciate ligament did not actually attach to the tibial spine but the fragment usually includes it as it is peeled off backward. This was treated by double drill holes to the tibia into the bed and then through the fragment.

Avulsion Fracture

The *avulsion fracture of the tibial spine* (Fig. 349) is basically an avulsion of the anterior cruciate ligament and should be treated as such, the main emphasis being placed on the restoration of the anterior cruciate ligament to its normal length and function. Only in the exceptional case can this be done nonsurgically. I much prefer to expose the knee anteromedially, examine it carefully for other lesions and then carry out whatever measures will best restore the function of the anterior cruciate. The occasional "locking" caused by a displaced spine obviously demands reduction of the fragment. If there is a large fragment involving a portion of the articular cartilage on either side, it should be replaced and held in its bed by a transfixion screw or by suture passed through parallel drill holes running from in front of the tibia to the bed of the fragment and thence mattressed through the fragment. The sutures must be carefully placed so that the drill holes coincide in the fragment and in its bed or else the fragment will not be perfectly reduced.

If the fragment is relatively small or comminuted it should be removed and the cruciate ligament pulled down into the defect and firmly sutured, in which instance it will heal more rapidly than it will if the bone is replaced (Fig. 350). There is little purpose in leaving a small, thin fragment subject to necrosis. On the other hand, when the fragment is large and makes up a substantial portion of the upper tibia, as is frequently the case in younger persons, it should be preserved in the manner described. Normal function of the knee will not tolerate gross unreduced displacement of the tibial spine.

Avulsion fracture of the patellar tubercle of the tibia may occur. Diagnosis can readily be made by location of pain and tenderness and disturbance of the

Figure 350.   This nine year old girl fell from a bicycle, injuring her right knee. The doctor made x-rays, told her she had a "bone sliver" and told her to keep it at rest for two weeks. No support. No other treatment.

A, The acute injury showing a large fragment of the upper tibia avulsed by the anterior cruciate.

B, Four months later, the fragment in the same position. Film made with the knee at its maximum extension. Range of motion, 30 degrees.

C, Two months after removal of the fragment, some recurrence of the calcification. This knee has had very extensive physical therapy, active and passive motion. Range now (nine months post injury—five months postoperative) is 20-90 degrees. This disability could have been prevented by early adequate treatment.

quadriceps mechanism. It should be confirmed by x-ray. The most important consideration is the function of the tendon rather than the fragment of displaced bone. The tendon should be replaced surgically. If the bone fragment is small or comminuted it should be removed and the tendon repaired to its bed. If large it may be handled by repositioning of the fragment and internal fixation preferably by a transfixion screw.

There may also be *avulsion at the superior pole of the patella,* in which instance the quadriceps attachment is pulled away from the patella with or without a shell of the patellar bone. In incomplete avulsion the mechanism of injury is a powerful contraction of the quadriceps while the leg is being forcibly flexed. This is, in fact, a strain type injury and as the forces are arrested there may be greater or lesser damage to the attachment of the tendon to the upper pole of the patella. This will cause pain on active function of the quadriceps but will not interfere with extension of the knee otherwise. The incomplete injury is treated by protection, local injection and local heat. The degree of protection depends upon the extent of the damage.

If the force is severe enough, the whole quadriceps aponeurosis may be detached from the patella. This is a painful injury. Examination will reveal swelling about the upper end of the patella with tenderness along its superior margin. The patient will be unable to actively extend the knee. When he contracts the quadriceps a palpable defect may be felt above the patella. The patella will not be dis-

Figure 351.   Flexion injury of the knee with avulsion of the quadriceps tendon attachment from upper pole of the patella. Surgery revealed the whole quadriceps tendon pulled off the patella.

placed downward since there is no muscular mechanism attaching to the patella from below and its distance from the tibia will remain constant whether the knee is flexed or extended. X-ray may be of diagnostic value since often a shell of bone may be avulsed (Figs. 351 and 352). Treatment should be surgical repair with snug suture of the aponeurosis to the patella through drill holes. I recall one case in an older man in which he caught his heel on a step as he descended a stairway. Both of his knees flexed sharply and in a violent effort to regain his equilibrium he de-

Figure 352.   A, Interesting case of partial avulsion of the patellar tendon from the patella with marked calcification and painful nonunion. The calcium was removed and the patellar tendon repaired to the patella. B, Opposite patella for comparison. This is not a fractured patella.

Figure 353. Acute wrestling injury with avulsion of the popliteus tendon attachment from the femur with a relatively large fragment of bone. This was his only injury. Uneventful recovery following repair. The osteochondritis dissecans was an incidental finding, was asymptomatic and was not demonstrable surgically.

tached the quadriceps from the patella on both knees. Uneventful recovery followed surgical repair.

Major fractures about the knee are not particularly frequent as athletic injuries and are readily recognized by the accompanying major disability and by confirmatory x-ray. One should be particularly alert to the *associated ligament injuries.* Avulsion of the collateral ligament with a fragment of bone from the tibial plateau or femoral condyle is in reality a ligament injury and should be treated as such (Figs. 353 and 354). One must be aware that when a small fragment of bone has

Figure 354. Medial side injury. This is an avulsion of the femoral attachment of the medial collateral ligament. Notice this is definitely below the adductor tubercle. The medial joint space is somewhat wider than the lateral. This is likely to heal with a painful prominence and some redundancy of the ligament. Advise removal of the fragment and repair of the ligament to the fracture bed.

Figure 355.   Hyperextension injury with avulsion of posterior rim of tibia by posterior capsule.

been pulled off the condyle the probabilities are that the ligament is attached to it (Fig. 355). One must not assume that it is a chip fracture. For example, if the tip of the fibula is broken one should suspect avulsion of the biceps (Fig. 319, B) and/ or the fibular collateral ligament.

If the lateral table of the tibia is compressed, one should examine very carefully to determine the function of the medial collateral ligament which also was placed under strain by the force which caused the fracture (Fig. 356). The mechanism of this injury is force applied to the lateral side of the knee, very likely with the knee in extension. The medial collateral ligament and the posterior capsule hold the knee stable in this position and the relatively sharp edge of the lateral femoral condyle rotates slightly medially and drives into the central portion of the lateral tibial plateau. This force may split the edge of the plateau out laterally, may depress the central portion or cause any type of fracture of the upper tibia or, indeed, may snub off a portion of the femoral condyle. The same force, however, is being applied on the medial side of the knee. These fractures ordinarily occur in older people in whom the ligament is ordinarily stronger than the bone. In a young person there may be ligament damage as well. In the case which occurs with the knee slightly flexed the force is accepted mostly on the rounded portion of the condyle and no lateral bony damage occurs and the ligament tears on the medial side. If the leg is in extension with the support by the posterior capsule, the medial ligament holds for a period long enough that the bone breaks. If the force is continued on the femoral condyle, further compressing the tibia, the ligament may give way. We have, therefore, injuries on both sides of the knee, either one of which may be easily overlooked.

In checking a case with obvious medial collateral ligament damage, one should inspect the x-ray carefully to see whether there is some compression of the lateral plateau. Similarly, if the lateral plateau is compressed it is necessary to eliminate medial collateral ligament avulsion. The test of gross instability may be quite mis-

Figure 356. A, Torn medial collateral ligament. Note compression fractures of the lateral tibial plateau. The same force that tears the medial ligament drives the lateral condyle into the tibia. A disappointing result will be obtained if this fragment is not elevated. This is not common in the young athlete.

B, Postoperative film shows fragment completely elevated and held in place by a strut of bone bank bone. Medial collateral ligament was repaired. Good stability.

Figure 357. This patient received a forcible blow on the lateral side of the knee. A, Anteroposterior view showing depression of the central portion of the lateral tibial plateau. B, The stress picture reveals that his marked instability was due not only to depression of the plateau but to severance of the medial collateral ligament. Note that the femur has moved slightly medially and the edge of the condyle rests on the depression of the tibial plateau. This should be treated by elevation of the plateau but of equal importance is repair of the medial collateral ligament.

leading because either of these conditions alone will give instability of the knee with the leg going into more abduction than normal. Stress x-ray will in this instance be of great value since it will show whether or not the medial margin of the joint opens up (Fig. 357). It is extremely disappointing to fix the tibial plateau and find an unstable knee resulting from medial ligament damage. It will be equally disappointing to make a skillful repair of the medial collateral ligament, only to find that bony damage on the opposite side has impaired the result. The true importance of the treatment of fractures about the knee must be to obtain complete restoration of normal function by whatever method is most effective in a particular case.

Fracture of the Head of the Fibula

While, strictly speaking, fracture of the head of the fibula is not an injury to the knee, it does sometimes become a diagnostic problem. The head of the fibula may be broken by a direct blow in which there is an ordinary comminuted type fracture without gross displacement. Any fracture below the head, actually involving the neck, should cast immediate suspicion on the ankle joint rather than the knee. If the fracture is of the head of the bone one should determine particularly whether or not there is any displacement and check for involvement of the peroneal nerve as well as the biceps tendon and external collateral ligament. If the fracture involves the ligament and tendon attachments, treatment must be much more extensive than if it were simply a direct trauma type fracture of the bone.

There may occasionally be a *dislocation of the fibula from the tibia* (Fig. 358). Here, again, one should immediately suspect a twisting force with resultant damage to the ankle joint. The condition, however, may be localized at the knee and have been caused by direct trauma against the fibular head, knocking it away by tearing the relatively weak superior tibiofibular ligaments. In such an instance replacement should be accurate and, if there is any tendency whatever toward instability of the fibula, it may be fixed by internal fixation with a transfixion screw through

Figure 358. Fracture-dislocation of upper end of the fibula accompanying spiral fracture of the tibia. Because of peroneal nerve involvement, the area was explored and the end of the fibula fastened to the upper tibia after releasing the nerve.

Figure 359.   Epiphyseal fracture of upper tibia. Note slight separation of medial half of epiphysis with it split down the shaft. As a result of the injury the fractured part of the epiphysis closed, necessitating surgical closure of lateral tibia and fibula.

the fibula into the upper end of the tibia. This screw should be removed as soon as ligament healing is complete. Use of internal fixation will expedite rehabilitation. Careful attention should be paid to possible involvement of the peroneal nerve since it is in a very vulnerable location as it crosses around the fibular neck.

Epiphyseal Fractures

A word should be said about epiphyseal fractures about the knee since they do happen, particularly in children of secondary school age. These fractures are usually readily recognized by careful study of the x-ray. The incomplete fracture of the epiphysis may be overlooked and diagnosed a sprain (Figs. 359 to 362). A careful,

Figure 360.   Illustrating a case of slight epiphyseal subluxation of lower femur. Note the callus formation where the periosteum was stripped up laterally. This is the same mechanism as sprain of the medial collateral ligament and in fact was diagnosed as such until careful examination localized the tenderness on both sides of the lower femoral epiphysis and x-ray showed the fracture across the lateral corner of the metaphysis.

Figure 361.   This and the next case (Figure 362) represent a diagnostic problem. Both had what appeared to be medial instability of the knee joint. *A,* The original picture with suggestion of separation of the medial upper tibial epiphysis. *B,* Confirmed by stress x-ray under anesthesia. The apparent widening of the medial joint space is normal for this individual when compared with the opposite knee. This was treated by closed manipulation.

detailed examination will ordinarily solve this problem since the tenderness and pain will be completely around the epiphyseal plate and strain in any direction will tend to cause pain whereas ligament injury is quite unusual on both sides of the knee at once.

If no displacement is present, *treatment* generally given to injury about the knee will suffice, that is, local measures, compression bandage, ice followed by protection. It should be emphasized that the apparatus applied to protect the knee should result in elimination of pain on stress, otherwise it is not truly protective.

Figure 362.   Another medial side injury (see Figure 361) showing apparently normal upper tibial epiphysis but suspicious buckling of the lateral cortex. *A,* The normal side. *B,* The involved side. *C,* Oblique view confirms the true pathology, separation of the medial upper tibial epiphysis with compression of the lateral plateau. Closed manipulation corrected the deformity.

Growth disturbance may become a factor here as well as in the case presented in Figure 361.

Figure 363.   This 17 year old boy was sent in with diagnosis of acute rupture of the medial collateral ligament and instability of the knee. *A,* The picture sent in was interpreted as normal, but note the suspicious vertical line extending upward from the intercondylar notch. *B,* X-ray made with lateral stress under anesthesia revealed the true pathologic condition, an epiphyseal fracture across the medial condyle split down into the intercondylar notch. This was treated by transfixion screw in order to permit more rapid mobilization.

When effective it will be adequate for the ordinary incomplete epiphyseal fracture. Any displacement, even of a mild degree, should be corrected (Fig 363). Correction becomes increasingly difficult with the passage of time so that in any doubtful situation, x-rays should be made promptly and treatment carried out as soon as possible and under general anesthesia. Epiphyseal fractures do not necessarily affect the growth of the bone and they are much less likely to do so if reduction is ana-tomical and with a minimum amount of trauma. One should be able to reduce these fractures by closed manipulation. If open reduction is decided upon one must be particularly careful in handling the epiphyseal cartilage. Prying against the cartilage or levering the fragments into place with instruments may well do more damage than the injury itself. The epiphyseal cartilage as a rule remains with the epiphysis, the diaphyseal portion of bone being denuded, hence one must be particularly careful in handling the smaller fragment.

Fabella

The fabella (Fig. 305) is a sesamoid bone frequently found in the tendon of the lateral head of the gastrocnemius muscle as it passes under the femoral condyle. Fracture of the fabella is extremely uncommon but is of quite serious con-sequence when it occurs. One should be aware of the fabella and not mistake it for a foreign body or a loose fragment in the joint. If it is in two or more pieces the opposite knee should be carefully checked since as a rule the bipartite fabella will be bilateral. The location of the tenderness and pain on function of the gastroc-nemius are diagnostic points. The x-ray may be quite deceptive. If the fabella is actually involved, either by a fracture or by osteochondritis or chondromalacia, it should be removed. The approach is a lateral one in front of the fibular collateral ligament and behind the iliotibial band—the same approach utilized to expose the posterior horn of the lateral meniscus.

CHRONIC SYNOVITIS WITH EFFUSION ("Water on the Knee")

To be complete, any discussion of injuries to the knee in athletes requires comment on joint effusion. It must be recognized that this is not a specific diagnosis but a finding. In normal circumstances the fluid balance within the knee is finely adjusted with the fluid formed and absorbed in an equal ratio in order to keep the joint lubricated. There are many and varied causes for irritation of the synovia and recurrent effusion. I want to emphasize that there is no such thing as "water on the knee" as a disease or an injury. This excess fluid formation results from a pathologic condition within the knee. To examine the knee and say "He has an effusion" is like examining an abdomen and saying "He has rigidity." The effusion must be and ordinarily can be accounted for. If one is unable to explain the cause of the effusion, his management of the case must perforce be extremely inadequate. If the effusion followed an injury one may ordinarily dismiss the systemic and indeed most of the inflammatory causes of effusion. However, a word of caution is necessary since the active young athlete will almost always be able to explain the effusion in the knee on the basis of having injured the knee, since he is bumping his knees constantly. Unless the diagnosis is immediately obvious, measures must be made to rule out in succession the various causes of effusion. Here the routine examination of the knee becomes extremely valuable.

First, the *history*. Is there an immediately determinable cause for the fluid or did it develop insidiously? Has there been a change in the activity habits of the patient? For example, if a boy has run ten miles when he was not accustomed to this degree of activity, this might well account for the irritation and effusion. This cause could easily be overlooked since to him it might not suggest an injury. Inquire as to his general health. Are there signs of a rheumatic disturbance or an infectious process?

On *examination* observe the knee carefully. Is the knee swollen, tense and obviously inflamed, or is the suprapatellar pouch merely filled with fluid? On palpation much can be learned as to the nature of the effusion. The ordinary traumatic effusion, even with hemarthrosis, causes little local heat whereas an inflammatory knee will ordinarily be hot. Careful examination for tenderness around the menisci or over the condyles or around the patella may give a lead. Is there a local area of tenderness?

Careful manipulative examination of the knee will help to determine whether there has been ligament damage or whether there is persistent meniscus reaction. Is motion in the knee painful? After careful evaluation and x-ray study the knee joint should be aspirated and close attention given to the fluid. Cloudy, turgid, viscous fluid is very suggestive of acute inflammatory reaction, and conversely, clear, straw colored, thin fluid will pretty well eliminate this possibility. If there is gross blood one may immediately presume an injury. Careful study of the fluid is necessary to determine whether it is actually blood or bloody fluid or merely blood-tinged fluid. If the fluid is at first clear, then toward the end of the aspiration becomes bloody, one may assume the presence of an inflamed synovium in which the irritation from genupuncture has caused local bleeding at the site of the puncture. Culture of the fluid for the presence of infection is of undeniable importance. Routine microscopic or laboratory examination of knee joint fluid is of relatively little value in diagnosis but is a useful aid in eliminating systemic causes of effusion. The blood count is important and urinalysis may give a lead. The best single laboratory procedure is the sedimentation rate, which should be negative in cases of trauma.

The *treatment* of an effusion in the knee is the treatment of the underlying cause. This predicates accurate diagnosis. If the diagnosis must be deferred or is not possible, certain local measures are of value in the interim. The extent of treatment will vary considerably according to the symptoms. Certainly the joint should not be permitted to remain grossly distended over a long period of time since this very distention of the capsule will ofttimes perpetuate an effusion long after the causative lesion has been arrested. In general, then, the treatment should be aspiration, pressure and protection. Aspiration is repeated as often as the fluid recurs even though this may be every few days or, in certain very acute circumstances, daily. Injection of various medicaments into the joint may be indicated. I would not recommend injection of an antibiotic into the knee unless definite infection is demonstrable. In the case of gross blood, hyaluronidase may be of value in increasing absorption. In chronic inflammation the corticoid preparations are of value. In my opinion they should not be repeated more than once a week even though aspiration may be needed more frequently.

One of the most difficult decisions in the presence of chronic or so-called idiopathic effusion concerns the amount of protection necessary. If the condition seems to be relatively minor and there is no pain or other local symptoms, one may be under considerable pressure to permit unrestricted activity, particularly in the athlete. I believe that under certain circumstances athletic activity may be continued with an effusion in the knee, but I would feel extremely uneasy about permitting it unless I were sure of the underlying pathology. To be more specific, in a patient recovering from a meniscectomy where the rest of the knee appears to be in good condition, one might permit considerable activity in the presence of definite effusion since he can readily account for the symptoms. On the other hand, if the effusion is spontaneous one must be very sure of the nature of the pathology before permitting activity. This can ofttimes mean complete immobilization of the joint until either the diagnosis is determined or the effusion has been eliminated. While ordinary wrap-on elastic bandage is of little value in the knee for protection of the ligaments, it is of great importance in the presence of an effusion into the joint. Following aspiration of the fluid, if it is not necessary to immobilize the knee for other reasons a snug pressure bandage should be applied routinely, since it exerts the same restraining influence on intercapsular bleeding or effusion as does the pressure of a capsule full of fluid. I much prefer the wrap-on to the pull-on bandage since the pull-on bandage inevitably fits very few people. It is either too tight or too loose in its ordinary application.

Physical therapeutic measures are of considerable value in synovitis, whatever its cause. For this reason we recommend modalities such as diathermy, electric pad, whirlpool, hot packs and analgesic packs. It will be noted that with all of these measures the whole knee is encompassed by the heat. Such modalities as microtherm and infra-red or other rays are so restricted in their application that they tend to get the knee much too hot in one location and not hot enough in another. If only the bulb or infra-red ray is available, it should be used in the form of a baker so that the knee is exposed to the hot air rather than primarily to the ray.

Rehabilitative exercises would seem to be the antithesis of what is beneficial in effusion since effusion is encouraged by irritation of the synovium by motion. Obviously a compromise must be reached in a given case to decide what degree of rehabilitation will be compatible with recovery of the irritation. There are some rehabilitative measures, however, that are perfectly consistent with treatment of synovial irritation in the knee. These are the exercises for the foot, the hip and the rest of the body and also the isotonic contractions of the quadriceps and hamstrings that have been shown to be very effective in rehabilitation and yet do not entail any degree of motion of the knee and may be carried out with the knee straight.

OSGOOD-SCHLATTER DISEASE

Epiphysitis of the tibial tubercle is a particular type of involvement that is commonly called Osgood-Schlatter disease. The word "disease" is a misnomer since the condition is not a disease. Actually, three manifestations parade as Osgood-Schlatter disease. One is *bursitis of the infrapatellar tendon bursa* (Fig. 302). This bursa lies between the infrapatellar fat pad and the patellar tendon just proximal to the patellar tubercle of the tibia. The tenderness in this condition is elicited at a point slightly higher than the tubercle. The condition should be treated as a bursitis (see page 439).

The second type of Osgood-Schlatter disease is an *aseptic necrosis of the tip of the epiphysis* for the patellar tubercle of the tibia (Fig. 364). The necrosis occurs

Figure 364.   A, Normal tibial tubercle epiphysis. B, The excavated necrotic area with fragmentation which requires curettement.

Figure 365. Osgood-Schlatter disease, showing epiphysitis of the entire epiphysis with irregularity of the epiphyseal line. Since this epiphyseal cartilage is continuous with that of the upper tibia, it should not be disturbed. If surgery is utilized, exposure should be superficial to the cartilage.

in the patellar tendon attachment and is probably traumatic in origin since it is initiated by a fracture or by an avulsion of the tip of the patellar tubercle. Because of poor circulation the fragment fails to heal and the constant irritation or traction of the patellar tendon makes it symptomatic. The mass tends to enlarge with reactive inflammation so that a rather large tumor may result. The tumor is tender to touch and there is pain on active extension of the quadriceps against resistance.

The third type of Osgood-Schlatter disease is a *true epiphysitis involving the whole epiphysis* (Fig. 365). This type is not particularly frequent but generally is more severe than the others when it occurs.

The *symptoms* of the latter two conditions are pain on direct pressure and pain on active use of the quadriceps. Rather sharp limitation of the activity of the patient may result. As is true of epiphysitis in other areas, the reaction itself is self-limited but there may be considerable residual, usually in the form of a large patellar tubercle with separate fragments lying within the patellar tendon attachment (Fig. 366). This may or may not remain symptomatic after the active condition subsides.

Treatment varies with the type of pathology and until recently has usually been nonsurgical, an attempt being made to relieve the tension in the mass by measures reducing the activity of the knee. They may range from cutting down the patient's activity to putting his leg in a cast. However, following arrest of symptoms there is a strong tendency for them to recur, so that until the epiphysis closes it remains a constant source of irritation. Even after the growth period, local symptoms may persist. Surgical treatment will result in much more prompt and complete recovery in Types 2 and 3, once frank involvement has occurred.

At operation the patellar tendon is split over the area of the involvement and in the second type the sequestrated fragment is carefully removed and the area thoroughly curetted down to normal bone. The epiphyseal plate between the tubercle and tibia is not disturbed. The split tendon is resutured over the area and

Figure 366.   Old Osgood-Schlatter disease with fragmentation and painful, unsightly tumor. Treated by excision of the fragments, flattening of the tubercle and reattachment of the patellar tendon.

the knee protected for about four weeks by a cotton cast. If a large mass of bone and cartilage has developed it should be trimmed down with an osteotome to leave a fairly flat area. Following four weeks of immobilization and a few weeks of rehabilitation, recovery should be complete. On the other hand, if the condition is a true epiphysitis it may be necessary to drill through the epiphyseal cartilage into the tibia, great care being taken in the actively growing person that the epiphysis is not surgically closed. If the epiphysis is continuous with the proximal tibial epiphysis, back knee may develop owing to arrest of growth in front while growth persists in the posterior one-half of the plate. It should be emphasized to the parents that the condition is self-limited and will not develop into a malignant tumor, and if adequately treated it will not limit physical activity. Most parents and patients will accept surgical treatment if the alternatives are carefully explained. The recurrence rate is extremely small after surgical treatment and rather great after non-surgical treatment.

OSTEOCHONDRITIS DISSECANS (Osteochondral Fracture)

Over three-fourths of recognized cases of osteochondritis dissecans occur at the knee, and usually on the lateral margin of the medial condyle. They extend from the articular margin at the notch toward the medial side of the knee, a position coinciding almost exactly with the femoral attachment of the posterior cruciate ligament. The pathology of osteochondritis dissecans was discussed on page 68.

Etiology.   It cannot be doubted that some of these cases are caused by excessive traction on the attachment of the posterior cruciate ligament, resulting in fact in an avulsion or at least a partial avulsion of a fragment of bone by the ligament. I have seen many cases in which the osteochondritic fragment contained a major portion of the attachment of the posterior cruciate ligament (Fig. 367). It is not my contention that all of these cases are caused by trauma but simply that many of them are. Trauma would seem to account more plausibly for the frequent occurrence of the lesion in this location than any of the other stated explanations. The theory of spontaneous ischemia is not wholly tenable. This theory implies that ischemia is more marked in this particular location on the femoral condyle than elsewhere, but actually circulation should be somewhat better here because the posterior cruciate ligament attaches at this point. However, osteochondritis dissecans occurs occasionally in other areas in the knee and also in this same general area without actually including the attachment of the posterior cruciate, so that avulsion by the posterior cruciate cannot be the universal cause.

The lesion is most common at the extreme distal arch of the condyle, an area that is obviously quite subject to trauma, particularly in a fall on the flexed knee. With the knee flexed the patella rides directly over this area of the femoral condyle and the transmitted force strikes directly here. The principal argument against direct trauma as the occasional cause is that one would expect the lateral condyle to have received at least equal trauma whereas actually osteochondritis dissecans is quite unusual in the lateral condyle of the femur. The explanation may lie in the fact that the patella is so much thicker in its medial portion and so transmits the trauma more directly.

In summary, the cause of osteochondritis dissecans at the knee may be said to be (1) ischemia with loss of circulation to the bone of the epiphysis, (2) avulsion of the posterior cruciate ligament attachment, or (3) direct trauma transmitted through the patella directly against the condyle.

Diagnosis. Some cases give no positive clinical findings and are discovered incidentally in an x-ray examination for other conditions (Fig. 353). It should be

Figure 367.   A, Osteochondritis dissecans. Actually an osteochondral fracture of the femoral condyle with almost the entire femoral attachment of the posterior cruciate ligament remaining attached to the fragment. *B,* Three months following repair of posterior cruciate to femur. Excellent function. One probably cannot expect complete filling in of this defect at this age.

524   INJURIES OF THE KNEE

Figure 368.   Large osteochondritic fragment lodged in the posterior pouch.

recognized that the x-ray has been made for *some* reason and most frequently this is a chronic complaint of the knee, nonspecific in character and not suggesting meniscus damage, ligament injury or chronic synovitis. In such a case x-ray may show a well defined lesion of the medial femoral condyle on its articular surface and one may presume that the lesion may well be the cause of the slight complaint. As symptoms develop the condition becomes more acute with chronic synovitis and often mild effusion. Pain occurs after forced exertion. Examination at this time will reveal no specific findings. Tests for ligament injury are negative. Meniscus tests are negative. Occasionally percussion on the patella with the knee flexed to beyond 90 degrees will elicit discomfort. X-ray examination reveals the lesion. As the condition progresses, the bony sequestrum separates from its bed, the cartilage fissures and the fragment may become detached (Fig. 368). The symptoms then become that of a foreign body in the joint, occasionally a palpable foreign body with locking, increased synovitis, pain and loss of rhythmic motion of the knee (Fig. 369).

      Treatment.   If osteochondritis dissecans is seen incidentally without pre-existing symptoms the degree of needed protection will depend upon the size of the fragment and the extent of the necrosis. If the fragment is large, involves a considerable portion of the weight-bearing surface, and necrosis seems quite extensive, the treatment will vary according to the age of the patient. In a patient under 12, prevention of weight bearing and immobilization of the knee may well permit spontaneous healing. This will require a period of 8 to 18 months, which becomes quite disheartening to an active youth. In most cases a cast will be necessary with the knee flexed since the youngster can hardly be expected constantly to remember not to bear weight. In an older patient it is quite unlikely that complete resolution will occur. If it does, it will be so slow as to justify operative treatment to expedite recovery, if for no other reason. Surgery under these circumstances begins with arthrotomy of the knee and careful exploration of the area. If the fragment is completely detached it should be removed. If the cartilage appears to be intact

Figure 369.   Old neglected case of osteo-chondritis dissecans with multiple fragments and diffuse arthritis. Note calcareous layers surrounding the original piece.

without separation or depression one may be justified in drilling multiple 1/64 inch drill holes through the fragment into its bed in order to increase its circulation and encourage revascularization. It is difficult to assess this method because one can never be certain that healing would not have taken place without operative interference. If there appears to be a defect in the cartilage with any undermining at all, the case should be treated as if the fragment had been completely detached and the fragment should be removed. I have had little experience with replacement of the fragment and fixation by pins or screws. It does not appeal to me unless the fragment is large and vital to joint function.

If the condition is symptomatic, operative treatment is always the treatment of choice. The knee is exposed by a medial parapatellar incision with the knee flexed over the end of the table. The medial compartment is carefully explored, special attention being paid to the medial meniscus, to the fat pad and to the cruciate ligaments. Careful scrutiny is given to the femoral attachment of the posterior cruciate ligament. The condyle is then inspected and the defect examined. If the fragment is completely loose the knee should be searched until it is found and removed. At this stage it is important to examine the undersurface of the patella since frequently patellar malacia will be present, particularly if the osteochondritis dissecans has been present for a very long time. Following careful exploration in this position the end of the table is raised again with proper aseptic precautions to a position that directly presents the lesion itself in the wound (30 to 0 degrees). If the fragment is still in place, it is carefully removed by sharp dissection. If it includes the attachment of the posterior cruciate ligament this should be detached from the fragment, care being taken to preserve as much ligament as possible. The posterior cruciate ligament is carefully inspected and this detached portion sutured down to the remaining portion of the ligament. However, if as much as one-half of the attachment is torn it is advisable to make two parallel drill holes from the medial femoral epicondyle into the bed of the defect which is in the intercondylar notch at the articular margin (Fig. 367, B). The suture is passed through one of the drill holes, plicated through the loose end of the torn section of the posterior cruciate and passed out through the other drill hole to emerge on the medial epicondyle. Proper tension will permit close apposition of the cruciate ligament to the bone. Before this fixation the crater remaining following removal of the fragment is inspected and curetted down to fresh bleeding bone. The surrounding margins of the articular cartilage are trimmed down so that there is a beveled edge rather than a 90 degree margin. Great care is taken to remove any cartilage that is undermined. If the bone in the bed of the crater appears to be eburnated, multiple 1/64 inch drill holes are made through to fresh cancellous bone. The knee is now carefully lavaged by warm saline to wash out any fragments or debris. If the patella has been found to be irregular and malacic the knee is then extended completely, the patella elevated by grasping its margins with tenaculi and a chondroplasty carried out designed to leave firm, smooth cartilage. This is similar to the procedure done in primary patellar malacia (see below). The knee is then closed in layers in the usual manner and a cotton cast applied, followed by the usual postoperative care for arthrotomy of the knee.

The degree of activity permissible as healing occurs depends upon several factors. If the defect is relatively small and if there is good intact articular cartilage over at least one-half the breadth of the medial femoral condyle, early weight bearing should be permitted and in fact encouraged with the same plan for rehabilitation one would use following uncomplicated removal of the medial meniscus. The cotton cast and skin stitches are removed in 12 to 14 days and rehabilitation progresses as rapidly as the patient can tolerate progressively increasing exercises. Any postoperative effusion should be aspirated as frequently as is necessary. It ordinarily will not be necessary at all. Unlimited athletic participation is permissible as soon as the quadriceps is rehabilitated.

If, on the other hand, there is an extensive fragment involving more than one-half the width of the femoral condyle, it is my opinion that weight bearing should be prevented for a considerable period. This may seem rather difficult to justify since many months will probably be required for the condyle to heal and one could hardly deny weight bearing this long. However, it has seemed to me that a period of eight to ten weeks without weight bearing followed by careful crutch walking has given better results than attempts at earlier rehabilitation.

PATELLAR MALACIA

The term, "patellar malacia," has been used as a catch-all to include the many processes that involve the undersurface of the patella. Many of these conditions are not particularly pertinent to sports. True malacia is a softening or breaking down of a part or tissue. When chronic synovitis of the knee causes the patellar cartilage to break down and the bed to eburnate so that denuded bone is exposed the condition is called malacia. So also is fragmentation of the patellar cartilage in the young individual with no signs of arthritis. The previous discussion (page 67) of chondral fractures and their treatment applied particularly to the patella.

Etiologically, patellar malacia falls naturally into three groups.

GROUP I.   In the athlete, a relatively young individual, *trauma* may be the cause. This may be a chondral fracture or infraction either by acute trauma or by repeated lesser traumata to the patella. Infraction of the patellar cartilage subsequently causes irritation of the patellar groove on the femur and gradual changes supervene with fissuring, absorption and fragmentation of the cartilage. The findings at operation will depend upon the duration of symptoms. I have recently operated upon a young lady who was riding horseback. The horse got a little eager to turn into the barnyard and made a sharp turn that drove her patella forcibly into the gate post. She had an immediate severe reaction in the knee joint. The x-ray was consistently negative. At operation some four weeks later under diagnosis of chondral fracture of the patella, there was, indeed, a fracture of the cartilage of the patella which was already undergoing degenerative change. It was early enough, however, that there was still injection of cartilage with hemorrhage into the crater of the fragments so that there could be no question as to the etiology. Similar changes were present in the contiguous portion of the patellar groove. Had operation in this case been postponed for several months as in the ordinary case, typical chondromalacia of the patella would have been present. In my opinion trauma accounts for many of the cases of isolated patellar involvement in the young athlete (Fig. 338).

GROUP II.   Another etiological factor in involvement of the undersurface of the patella is *disturbance of rhythm of the patellar function*. This is the type of malacia that accompanies intrinsic injury to the knee (Fig. 370). Any condition that causes a disturbance in the rhythm of the knee action frequently results in involvement of the undersurface of the patella. The knee is checked abruptly and motion is reversed. The patella is driven against the femur. In fact, in an analysis of 350 cases* of intrinsic injury to the knee we were able to demonstrate some degree of patellar involvement in 65 per cent of the cases treated by operation, and in 15 per cent of these it was Grade 4. We were able to show a direct relationship

Figure 370.   Severe chondromalacia of the patella following neglected ligament injury.

* Bulletin of Hospital for Joint Diseases, Vol. 17, No. 1, April, 1956.

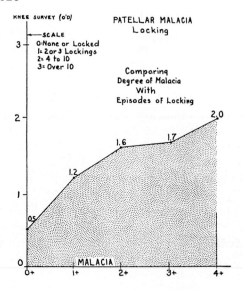

Figure 371. It should be noted in the above graph there is direct correlation in the number of times the knee locked prior to operative treatment and the degree of malacia. The knee which locked as many as ten times (category 2) showed 4+ malacia. (Hosp. for Joint Dis. Bull. 17:5.)

between the number of lockings of the knee and the degree of malacia (Fig. 371), and further, that the duration of symptoms and the degree of malacia (Fig. 372) also correlate. These two factors were much more important in indicating the amount of malacia present than was the age of the patient. This seemed so definite that we make a positive recommendation that surgical intervention should be prompt in intrinsic injury of the knee if for no other reason than to prevent damage to the undersurface of the patella. The exact mechanism of this breakdown of the patella has never been wholly explained. This condition also probably occurs as a result of various other causes including direct trauma, synovitis of the joint and general chondrolytic changes. The particular pathologic changes described usually accompany other intrinsic conditions of the knee.

Figure 372. The above chart shows that the great majority with symptoms of less than one week in duration showed no symptoms of patellar malacia; whereas only 2 per cent of those patients with symptoms of less than one week had 4+ malacia, 52 per cent of those with symptoms over three years showed 4+ patellar malacia. (Hosp. for Joint Dis. Bull. 17:10.)

GROUP III.   A third classification is *primary malacia of the patella*, usually bilateral without any demonstrable etiological factor. These cases are truly puzzling. One cannot rule out the effect of repeated traumata since the young patients are usually very active physically. They could be expected to traumatize their knee caps repeatedly. However, the simultaneous involvement of both knees with relative lack of involvement of other chondral surfaces equally susceptible to trauma prompts us to seek a cause other than simple contusion.

Diagnosis.   Group I caused by a single severe trauma is usually found in the knee that has been seriously contused to the point that a fractured patella is suspected. The findings remain localized about the patella: pain on pressure of the patella into the groove, pain on active extension of the knee particularly against resistance, pain on patellar ballottement. The severity of the symptoms will be increased by continued activity of the individual.

In Group II occurring coincidentally with other intrinsic conditions of the knee, the patellar symptoms may well be completely masked by the other condition so that the patient may present himself with his knee locked and swollen with effusion but with no demonstrable patellar symptoms. At arthrotomy one may be surprised to find extensive involvement of the undersurface of the patella. More frequently, however, careful examination prior to operation will reveal subpatellar crepitation and pain on pressure over the patella provided the condition is fairly severe.

In Group III with spontaneous degenerative changes, the joint is asymptomatic except for the patella. There will have been gradually increasing discomfort and disability in the knee centering around the patella without a history of previous trauma. The signs of involvement of the patella are quite obvious. If the undersurface of the patella is rough and irregular, the patella will not glide smoothly in the patellar groove and gross subpatellar crepitation is usually the first symptom. This is more severe on extension against resistance or on extension of the knee while the patella is held firmly against the patellar groove. There is also pain on going up or down stairs, squatting or anything that forces the patella against the patellar groove. This may become so severe as to become grossly disabling.

Treatment of the knee having these conditions of the patella is surgical. True enough, the symptoms may be ameliorated somewhat by nonsurgical treatment such as aspiration, injection of a corticoid, splinting and prevention of weight bearing but the future is bleak indeed since the defect in the patella remains and the symptoms will promptly recur with resumption of activity. Surgery may be directed primarily toward the patella or may be incidental to other operations. After arthrotomy by median parapatellar incision, the patella is carefully inspected with the examining finger and the extent of the pathologic involvement determined by palpation and observation. If the diagnosis is confirmed, the incision is enlarged sufficiently to permit the patella to be turned up on edge for thorough inspection of the undersurface. At this time a decision must be made on definitive treatment. This decision will be conditioned a great deal by the circumstances in each particular case and will vary from chondral shaving to patellectomy.

CHONDRAL SHAVING.   In the young athlete it is quite important to retain the patella if this is possible. With an extremely sharp knife blade the patellar cartilage is shaved down in attempt to reach firm, uninvolved cartilage. This is frequently possible in the young athlete since the patellar cartilage is relatively thick at this age. The degenerative changes may be found to be quite superficial. Care must be taken to remove all pathological cartilage even if this leaves denuded bone. After this step has been completed the patellar groove is carefully inspected and if necessary chondroplasty is done here also to eliminate all abnormal cartilage. At the conclusion of the chondroplasty the patella should slide smoothly in the patellar groove with minimal irregularity either of the patella or of the groove.

At this stage considerable surgical judgment is required to determine whether or not the patella should be retained. If the patient is young and otherwise has an excellent knee, one may be justified in leaving in a somewhat defective patella. On the other hand, if there are degenerative changes throughout the joint with marginal osteophytes and rather poor femoral cartilage, the patella probably should be sacrificed.

The cartilage of a young person has a great deal more regenerative power than the cartilage of an older individual and a crater such as is left following removal of an osteochondritis dissecans fragment may readily fill in in the former if it is curetted down to raw bone and no degenerated cartilage is left behind. In the older individual with very thin cartilage this regeneration does not occur. If there is severe malacia of the one or other margin of the patella only, it may be possible to remove completely the medial or lateral portion of the patella, leaving the bone narrower (Fig. 373). This is particularly important since frequently the malacia may be confined entirely to the medial facet of the patella.

PATELLECTOMY.   If one decides to remove the patella because of defective articular cartilage the technique of removal is extremely important. The patella should be removed by sharp dissection, care being taken to include all fragments of bone. The knee is then thoroughly lavaged and the quadriceps tendon and patellar tendon are inspected. At this stage it is important to remove with an osteotome the superolateral margin of the anterior articular surface of the femur since this stands up as a bony prominence upon which, later, the edge of the quadriceps lateralis tendon may catch with a painful snap. After this has been carefully taken off and the raw bone covered with bone wax, the adjacent tendons are inspected for roughness

Figure 373.   A, Injury 20 years old, apparently a chondral fracture of the patella, giving the appearance of osteochondritis dissecans of the patella. B, Treated by resection of medial border of patella because of irremediable cartilage damage.

or any undue thickening. If either is present the area is smoothed down. Imbrication sutures are then passed through the end of the quadriceps tendon, looped through the portion of the tendon over the patella down through the patellar tendon from behind-forward. About six of these sutures (cotton No. 1) are placed across the gap of the patellar bed. The superior and inferior portion of the parapatellar incision along the tendon is then closed leaving a 2 inch gap along the medial margin of the old patellar bed. The previously placed sutures are then tied with the knee in complete extension, closely approximating the quadriceps tendon to the patellar tendon and obliterating entirely the patellar fossa in the tendon. After these sutures are tied, a finger is passed underneath the suture line to make sure that the imbrication is smooth. After all these sutures are tied it should be possible to flex the knee to 90 degrees and determine whether or not the repaired tendon has a smooth gliding surface. By careful attention to this shortening of the quadriceps tendon mechanism, one will avoid the extremely disabling effect of loss of complete active extension of the knee which so frequently follows patellectomy. One can cheerfully sacrifice some degree of flexion in order to obtain complete active extension of the knee. Usually full motion is regained. Following operation the knee is immobilized in a cotton cast for two weeks, at which time the stitches are removed and weight bearing is begun in a cotton cast which is worn for about two more weeks. Rehabilitation begins on the first postoperative day.

The *prognosis* in patellar malacia depends largely on the etiology. If the cause was a chondral fracture the prognosis should be very good with no fear of recurrence provided a good patella was left. If the condition resulted from intrinsic pathology in the knee and this is corrected, the prognosis is also good. If the patellar malacia is a component of a generalized degenerative change in the knee or if it is a spontaneous type of degenerative change, the prognosis is much less favorable since the etiological factor probably has not been eliminated.

The question of athletic participation following involvement of the patella will inevitably arise. If one can be reasonably sure that he has left a relatively normal patella there should be no reason to forbid participation. Such would be the case in chondral fracture or malacia following rupture of the medial meniscus, for example. In the more chronic type one would hesitate to permit active competitive sports which cause overuse of the patella. If it is already questionable that the patella will withstand the rigors of ordinary use one is not justified in encouraging athletic participation, which would only precipitate the trouble. The decision here rests on the same considerations as following any other pathologic condition, and must remain a matter of personal judgment. Particularly to be considered is the importance to the individual of athletic competition. If his livelihood or his education depends upon it, if this is his career, greater effort should be made to permit him to participate. If on the other hand it is a casual thing and his interest can be diverted into less strenuous pursuits, this should be encouraged. Once again, it should be emphasized that treatment should be definitive and prompt in order that the proportion of cases responding by good recovery may be increased.

CHAPTER

19

Injuries of the Leg

For the purposes of this discussion the leg will be considered to be the area between the knee and the ankle and not immediately concerned with the two joints themselves.

ANATOMICAL CONSIDERATIONS

The upper portion of the leg receives the muscles from the thigh and involvement of these attachments has been discussed elsewhere (page 434). Likewise, the lower portion of the leg is intimately involved with the function of the ankle joint which also will be discussed in detail (page 552). The shafts of the tibia and fibula serve for origin of the muscles that move the ankle and foot. The tibia is the only weight-bearing bone since the fibula does not have a weight-bearing component. The fibula situated posterolaterally is not directly involved in the knee joint but forms a vital part of the ankle.

Throughout its length the fibula is bound to the tibia by the interosseous membrane. The interosseous membrane forms a "Y" above to surround the upper tibiofibular joint, the anterior division being called the anterosuperior tibiofibular ligament and the posterior division the posterosuperior tibiofibular ligament. A similar arrangement is formed below, the interosseous membrane thickening and dividing to surround the inferior tibiofibular syndesmosis, the two components being called the anterior and posterior inferior tibiofibular ligaments. Whereas the upper portion of the fibula is largely for muscle attachments and may serve to some extent as a brace, it has no vital function and in fact may be sacrificed without material loss of function provided proper security is made for the structures attaching at the top of the fibula. The lower one-third, as mentioned, is extremely important since it is vital in the formation of the ankle mortice.

The interosseous membrane serves as the floor of the anterior compartment of the leg (Fig. 375). This is a closed space, the boundaries being the anterior fascia of the leg in front, the interosseous membrane behind, the fibula laterally and the tibia medially. This space permits little, if any, expansion of the structures contained within. The posterior compartment on the contrary is a loosely contained space with a relaxed and redundant fascia. This space is not subject to constriction.

The tibia, the main weight-bearing bone, is roughly triangular in cross section and has muscle attachments at the posterolateral and posterior surfaces. The anterior border, the anteromedial surface and the posteromedial border are all subcutaneous.

CONTUSION

Contusion is extremely common in the lower leg since this part, particularly in athletics, is very much exposed to direct blows. The nature of the contusion will vary according to the location of the blow. If the blow is over the subcutaneous portion of the tibia the contusion is much more likely to be severe since the integument and periosteum are caught between the external force and extremely hard bone. This may result in a simple bruise with extravasation of blood in a localized area or the periosteal damage may result in severe traumatic periostitis, also usually localized. It is also possible to have contusion over the muscles of the anterior compartment; the resulting swelling within the compartment may be extremely uncomfortable owing to the closed nature of the space. Contusion of the muscles of the calf is also common but circulatory embarrassment is not usual here. An unusual type of contusion is of the peroneal nerve as it winds around the upper portion of the fibula. This may result in a painful neuritis or even transient paralysis of the peroneals with drop foot which may be very distressing to the athlete.

Contusion and Hematoma

Implicit in the pathology of a contusion is some degree of hematoma. In the lower leg this may be extremely disabling. A severe hematoma in the anterior enclosed space may become a surgical emergency since it may go on to actual ischemia and necrosis of the muscle (see Anterior Tibial Syndrome, page 537). A subperiosteal hematoma complicating contusion of the skin may also be painful and actually disabling if it is severe. Hematoma within the muscle is not as common in the calf as in other areas in the body.

Diagnosis.   Following injury of the lower leg, careful analysis should be made of the actual history to determine if possible the type of blow and the type of the instrument since a large blunt object such as a player's helmet will usually cause a different type of injury than a relatively sharp one such as a cleat or hard toe of a shoe. The part should be carefully examined to determine the degree of swelling and whether a hematoma is present. Function should be carefully checked since this may well give some indication as to whether the muscle is involved or whether there is involvement of a nerve. The leg should be carefully examined for a possible fracture from a direct blow on the tibia or fibula. The tibia is readily

palpable but it may be more difficult to examine the fibula since it is well surrounded
by muscle. If there is any question as to the degree of localized injury in either
bone, x-ray study should be done.

   Treatment.   If a diagnosis of contusion or hematoma is made, treatment will
depend upon the degree of involvement. If hematoma is present it should be
aspirated under aseptic technique and injected with hyaluronidase. These measures
should be immediately followed by pressure bandage and cold pack for six to eight
hours. Further analysis can then be made as to the severity of the injury. If fluid or
blood has recurred it should be re-aspirated. At the end of 12 to 24 hours, depending upon the degree of injury, heat should be substituted for cold. The degree of
protection of necessity will depend upon the location of injury. If the injury involves the bone and periosteum and is not severe, treatment should be by protective
pad and function need not be interfered with unless it is major injury. If, on the
other hand, the blow involves the muscle, the muscle should be kept at rest by
proper strapping or splinting until it is determined there is no major bleeding or
laceration within the muscle. Protective strapping should be used until such a time
as the part is symptom-free.

Contusion of the Peroneal Nerve

   As the peroneal nerve continues downward after leaving the popliteal space
and passes laterally, it crosses directly behind the neck of the fibula (Fig. 374),
winds around the lateral surface of the fibular neck to pass into the extensor
muscles anteriorly. It is extremely vulnerable to injury either posteriorly or laterally
since it lies directly between the skin and the bone. An ideal situation is present for
contusion of the nerve since the nerve will be caught between the hard contusing
object and the underlying bone. A relatively minor blow may cause serious nerve
injury.

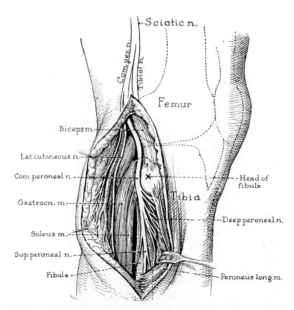

Figure 374.   Drawing showing relationship of peroneal nerve to the head of the fibula.

The *pathology* will vary greatly according to the severity of injury since the nerve may be only slightly shocked or may be crushed in two. The usual effects of contusion are congestion and edema with local swelling. Since the nerve is contained within a sheath, this swelling will cause pressure on the nerve fibers with resulting symptoms of pain, numbness and paresthesia. If there is actual hemorrhage into the sheath, the increased tension may proceed to actual paralysis due to intrinsic pressure. Indeed, this may result in necrosis of the nerve fibers with permanent functional loss. As a rule, the congestion diminishes, the swelling subsides and the nerve slowly returns to normal. If there has been actual damage to the nerve fibers themselves, they may be replaced by fibrous scar and greater or lesser loss of function results depending upon how many nerve filaments remain undamaged.

Contusion may cause hemorrhage in the surrounding tissues and this may cause secondary pressure on the nerve. This is not likely in this particular area.

The *symptoms* will be those of the local blow plus the effect on the nerve itself. The immediate symptom is almost always a "shocking feeling" with pain shooting throughout the distribution of the nerve to the lateral side of the leg and foot. Acute tingling and numbness remain after pain subsides. These may be transient and may disappear within seconds or minutes if actual damage to the nerve has not resulted. In such a case the patient may completely recover before he is ever examined by the doctor.

If the injury is more severe, a different pattern of symptomatology will emerge. The initial symptoms may be as indicated above but are followed by a completely asymptomatic period to be followed in turn by symptoms of pressure within the nerve. The pain and paresthesia will return and will increase in severity. As the pressure continues, signs of loss of function will develop. This will be evidenced by hypesthesia throughout the distribution and by weakness in dorsal flexion of the foot. This may progress to complete paralysis of the nerve with sensory loss and muscular afunction. There will follow a longer or shorter period during which the only symptoms will be loss of nerve function; namely, sensory and motor loss with no pain. This may develop within days or it may be several weeks before the painful stimuli have ceased. After a variable lapse of time, function will begin to return, usually in the sensory distribution first. One may be able to elicit a Tinel sign by tapping along the nerve distal to the injury and so get some idea as to the progression of recovery. This is rather difficult since the peroneal nerve becomes rather deep-seated a short distance below the knee. Recovery may be complete or may be only partial.

This whole train of symptoms may be interrupted at any time by the recovery process. The earlier the recovery begins, the more rapid and complete it will be. Very careful examination of the leg and foot in a case involving the peroneal nerve will be extremely rewarding since it is quite important to be able to follow accurately the succession of events. If the paralysis is immediate and complete, one may assume a major injury and govern treatment accordingly. Rapidly progressing development of signs of nerve pressure indicate increasing swelling within the sheath. The rate of its development is of considerable importance in determining the proper treatment. One should carefully outline the area of sensory involvement and determine not only touch but sharp and dull and hot and cold sensitivities although this is not as important here as it is in central nervous system lesions. A good practice is to outline in ink on the skin the area of involvement or to record it faithfully in notes. It is very gratifying to find on re-examination of such a patient that the area of his involvement has lessened and to be able to give him a favorable prognosis. On the contrary, if the area increases one can be prepared to modify his treatment accordingly.

When one is faced with involvement along the peroneal distribution without definite history of an injury, he may be able by careful palpation around the fibular head to locate areas of local tenderness that give some clue as to the possibility of a direct blow on the nerve. In the heat of an athletic contest, such a blow may be readily overlooked and the patient have no knowledge of an injury.

Treatment. The vast majority of these cases will require no specific treatment. If the blow is severe enough that the soft tissue contusion requires care, the customary treatment is in order—ice pack early, local heat later. However, as the nerve symptoms develop and there is motor paralysis or specific weakness, the muscles will require protection. Support of the ankle and foot must be provided by cast, splint or brace. A carefully applied drop-foot brace holding the foot to a right angle by a mechanical spring will permit ambulation without disconcerting drop foot. This will make walking easier and will prevent overstretching of the paralyzed muscles. Some such apparatus is also important in rehabilitation as the muscle strength returns. During the early phase of such a condition, we would recommend wearing the brace and shoe during sleeping hours to prevent contracture of the calf. Once the acute symptoms have subsided there is no particular interdiction of activities except that one can ill participate in sports with a drop foot. Overfatigue of any weakened muscle should be avoided and strength should be painstakingly restored by graduated exercises.

Should a blow be followed by a quiescent period and then by a rapidly developing paralysis, one is justified in exploring the peroneal nerve and performing neurolysis to be sure that the tight sheath is not constricting the nerve beyond the point of its tolerance. This is not often indicated. Even if the paralysis is immediate and complete, one is justified in a period of watchful waiting to give the nerve a chance to recover spontaneously. If there are no definite signs of recovery within three months I would recommend surgical exploration of the nerve with neurolysis or nerve suture as indicated.

In other instances, the quiescent period may be much longer only to be followed by the same pattern of progressively increasing nerve symptoms. This is due to scar formation with gradual constriction of some of the fibers of the nerve by the maturing scar. In such an instance, if the condition is steadily progressive there is no advantage in undue delay and early neurolysis should be done.

Another indication for surgery is the case in which there is intractable pain along the nerve that persists for several weeks. These cases should be treated by exploration of the nerve. The nerve should be carefully dissected free of all adhesions and appropriate neurolysis carried out, either surgically or by saline injection in order to expand the sheath.

STRAIN

Strain of the muscles and tendons about the ankle and foot will be discussed later (page 590). Here, in addition to the well delineated entities of strain involv-

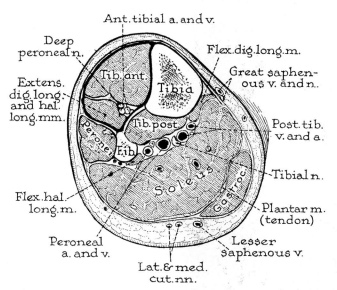

Figure 375. Cross section of leg showing its anterior compartment outlined by heavy line indicating muscles and vascular bundle within the compartment.

ing the leg proper, some rather unusual conditions will be covered although there may be some argument as to whether strain is actually the cause.

Anterior Tibial Syndrome

It will be recalled that in the anterior compartment of the leg the anterior tibial, the extensor hallucis and extensor digitorum longus muscles arise from the sides of the tibia, fibula and interosseous membrane, completely filling the anterior compartment. This compartment is tightly roofed by the anterior fascia of the leg (Fig. 375). In the anterior tibial syndrome for various reasons there is a rapid swelling of the muscle within this compartment. This may come on following active exercise alone and in theory is due to the fact that muscles which have not been previously conditioned are overused and respond by swelling and edema. It may also come on following direct injury in which there is excessive swelling and hemorrhage into the space. The condition can also be caused by localized infection within the space. In fact, anything that causes intractable swelling may cause this syndrome.

At onset there is severe pain over the involved area and loss of function so that contraction of the muscles contained in the space rapidly becomes impossible and a drop foot ensues (Fig. 376). Very soon even passive stretching of the muscles becomes quite painful. This is not ordinarily preceded by the symptoms of tenosynovitis, however. The skin over the area becomes red, glossy, warm and markedly tender with a feeling of woody tension even to the point of real hardness of the fascia over the space. There may occasionally be involvement of the peroneal nerve with sensory loss but the loss of muscle function is usually not due to nerve involvement but to pathologic change within the muscle itself. The muscles go on to ischemic necrosis, often called "Volkmann's ischemia of the leg,"

Figure 376.   Anterior tibial syndrome, late. This is an intractable deformity of the foot due to pressure of the vessels in the anterior compartment of the leg. Triple arthrodesis was necessary.

with swelling, edema, extravasation of red blood cells, destruction of blood cells and replacement of muscle tissue by fibrous scar. The result is a firm, inelastic, noncontractile muscle group. This can be extremely disabling and defies reconstructive treatment.

Treatment depends upon the extent of involvement. Any delay is disastrous. Early treatment should be prompt application of ice without pressure dressing. If the symptoms do not respond within a few hours, treatment must be surgical. If the anterior fascia of the leg is promptly sectioned, complete relief is obtained from pain and the other symptoms. If the operation is postponed until necrosis of the muscles has already occurred, fibrous replacement will still leave irreparable scarring.

This condition is not common but when it occurs it is an extreme emergency. The danger lies in the similarity of the early symptoms to so-called cramping, muscle spasm, "shin splints" or contusion. Any of these conditions that do not respond promptly to treatment should be carefully investigated. Of particular importance is the patient's complaint of constant, boring, aching pain made more severe by function but not disappearing under rest. The anterior tibial syndrome may spell the end of athletic competition for the affected individual.

Shin Splints

Another condition unique to the leg is so-called "shin splints." As with many names in common use, there is considerable and often raucous argument as to what is actually meant by the term. As is usual in these circumstances the title "shin splints" is a waste basket including many different conditions. The authors of various articles on the subject are inclined to state very definitely that it is caused by one particular thing to the exclusion of all others. This causes great confusion.

Shin splints ordinarily occurs early in the training period, frequently in training on hard floors such as indoor track. It also may occur on the hard ground in the early fall or on the basketball court. One of the conditions sometimes called "shin splints" is irritation of the attachment of the posterior tibial tendon along the posterior face of the tibia with resulting periostitis. Here the tenderness will be along the posterior medial angle of the tibia and pain will be on function of the posterior tibial muscle. Another cause is an actual tearing of the attachment of the posterior tibial muscle along the tibia. "Shin splints" may also be caused by irritation at the interosseous membrane in which case the symptoms are somewhat more posterior and seem to be deeper in the muscles of the calf. An ordinary periostitis along the posteromedial angle of the tibia may also be called "shin splints." Indeed, the involvement of the anterior tibial muscle at the anterior border of the tibia and onto its anterolateral face is by some called "shin splints." The last named condition may go on to serious involvement of the anterior compartment. A stress fracture of the tibia may also be misdiagnosed "shin splints" by the unwary.

Treatment. A condition having so many etiological factors must of necessity require varying types of treatment. However, certain basic measures are of importance regardless of the etiology, the primary ones being rest and local heat. A word of caution is nevertheless needed about use of heat in involvement of the anterior compartment since heat may only aggravate the tension within the space. In the ordinary case of "shin splints" local heat, rest of the part, and strapping to prevent stress of the posterior tibial muscle will give marked improvement. The outcome may be disappointing, however, since the condition has a great tendency to recur and may indeed keep a track man off the boards a whole season. A longer initial period of rest and protection will pay dividends in a more complete recovery. Various measures have been recommended such as binding of the leg with elastic or adhesive over foam rubber or various other types of padding. This has but little effect upon a condition that is basically due to overuse of the muscles. Physical therapeutic measures should be continued until the leg is symptom-free. Resumption of activity should be on a very carefully supervised basis and function should always be kept below the level that causes pain.

Rupture of the Plantaris Muscle

Another condition unique to the leg is rupture of the plantaris muscle. This is a pencil-sized muscle arising from the lateral condyle of the femur, passing beneath the gastrocnemius and soleus muscles to attach to the tendo achillis or the tubercle of the calcaneus on the medial side. The tendon is no larger than a piece of twine and is easily broken. To the freshman anatomy student it is the "fool's nerve." This muscle itself is frequently completely ruptured, in which case pain will be deep in the calf and may be quite disabling. Actually function of the muscle is of little importance in the human and there is no necessity for repair. A relatively short period of protection will result in complete recovery.

One must carefully distinguish between the above condition and *rupture of a portion of the calf,* in which case the symptoms will be much more severe and much longer lasting. Because of the extremely explosive action of the calf muscle, a vessel in the muscle or in the subcutaneous or fascial area will not infrequently be ruptured. This also gives a sharp stinging pain without serious disability but with development of ecchymosis which may be disquieting. This requires no treatment but should be distinguished from rupture of the plantaris.

Muscular Strain

The muscles of the lower leg are particularly subject to strain and this will be discussed at greater length later (see Ankle Strain, page 552). One of the most common locations for strain is at the musculotendinous junction of the calf. Much of the accustomed activity of the athlete involves forcible contraction of the calf so that the whole body weight is abruptly thrown on the calf mechanism. Strain here may be caused either by chronic overuse in the poorly conditioned calf or by a single violent stress. Strain in the calf mechanism may be extremely disabling.

Treatment.   Ordinarily strapping or taping is of little benefit except to prevent overstretching of the strained area. The athlete must be withdrawn from competition and instructed to do nothing that causes pain. The condition will frequently progress to chronic strain. Early treatment consists of rest, local heat, immobilization, followed by protective strapping and very gradual return to activity. In the early period the most efficient immobilization is a walking boot cast that will permit the patient to have fairly good activity and still prevent any possible strain on the calf. If the strain is less severe, primary plaster adhesive strapping will be adequate. Strapping is also used subsequent to removal of the cast (Fig. 377). This strapping is of the type designed to prevent dorsal flexion of the foot.

Figure 377.   A 3 inch strip of cross stretch elastic adhesive is run down the back of the calf and over the sole of the foot to the metatarsals. It is anchored in place by a Gibney type basket weave as shown on the right.

The foot should be placed in equinus and the major anchor strap should begin above the bulge of the calf and pass directly down the back of the leg, over the heel and along the sole of the foot to the toes. The recently developed cross stretch adhesive that stretches laterally rather than longitudinally serves well for this purpose. It has the advantage of rigidity in its long axis while the lateral stretch permits it to be molded well around the ankle and heel without wrinkling (Fig. 377). This can be so placed as to limit dorsal flexion to any desired degree and the foot may actually be held in plantar flexion. If the foot is held in plantar flexion by the strapping, the shoe heel must be built up a proportionate amount. Even after recovery it is advisable to elevate the heel of the street shoe and put a ½ inch pad in the heel of the athletic shoes to give some degree of relaxation to the calf. Once a strain has occurred it is advisable to strap the foot at each practice session or game so that it cannot be dorsiflexed beyond the point where it becomes painful or sensitive. By this means one may at least prevent the strain from excessive dorsal flexion although he cannot limit the strain caused by violent muscle contraction.

In a similar manner there may be strain to the anteromedial muscles of the foot, most often the anterior tibial, less frequently the posterior tibial except in relation to the muscle origins (see Shin Splints, page 538). In these instances the strapping should be so applied as to relieve the tension on the muscle involved. The peroneal group is infrequently involved since athletic activity does not ordinarily subject these muscles to the same tensions received by the posterior and medial groups.

Rupture of the Calf

The calf muscle may be ruptured partially or completely any place from its origin on the posterior part of the femoral condyles and back of the tibia to its attachment to the calcaneus. Usually the tear will be in the muscle belly itself: frequently in the musculotendinous junction between the gastrocnemius and the conjoined tendon with the soleus. The unit may occasionally rupture through the tendon itself or at the attachment to the heel, sometimes avulsing a fragment of bone. As in a muscle rupture anywhere, a determination of the location and extent of the injury is extremely important. The location is usually readily determined when the injury is examined early since the tenderness will be found to be quite localized. After several hours, swelling, edema and inflammation become diffuse and the exact location may be in doubt. Both active contraction of the muscle and passive stretching will cause pain. If there is complete severance of the whole muscle-tendon unit such as (1) the head of the gastrocnemius or (2) the entire gastrocnemius from the conjoined tendon, or (3) rupture of the tendon, loss of function will be noted so that the muscle on contraction will bunch up rather than flatten down as it normally does. If the rupture is in the tendon or musculotendinous junction a palpable defect can often be felt. The condition is quite disabling even with a relatively minor degree of tearing. It interdicts running or any activity that causes the athlete to be on his toes. This loss of function may be due to actual loss of continuity of the tendon but it is more frequently due to muscle spasm and pain. If the rupture is complete and seen early, repair is quite feasible even in the muscle belly.

Treatment. Surgical repair of the tendon is mandatory even if the case is seen late. In the early case incision is made directly over the involved area, the underlying muscles are inspected, the clot is evacuated and the muscle ends are apposed by mattress sutures placed with the knee flexed and the foot in plantar flexion. The extremity must be kept in this position for about three weeks if the repair is in the muscle itself. If the repair is in the tendon or tendon to bone, a much firmer internal fixation may be obtained and the extreme flexion position may not be necessary. In any instance, it is advisable to hold the foot in equinus for a period of time. When a fragment of bone is avulsed this fragment should be excised unless it is so large as to be vital to calcaneal function. The suture of tendon to bone bed directly through drill holes is preferable since tendon to bone union is much more prompt than bone to bone union.

A good bit of surgical judgment is required to determine just how long the foot needs to be kept in equinus after the repair. If it is held too long it may be difficult to get the calf muscle stretched out to its normal length. If the injury is fresh, the tissues strong and the suture material well placed, it may be possible to put the foot at right angles immediately after suture. If the strength of the fixation is questionable because of shreading of the tendon, the equinus position must be maintained longer. It should be borne in mind that at least three weeks are needed for the tendon to start to heal and even then union is quite insecure. In order to minimize morbidity a walking cast may be utilized after a week or ten days so that disability is not unduly prolonged. One should not anticipate return to competition in the same season in which the injury occurs. A little more time spent to get a complete recovery is well rewarded by the completeness of the recovery.

SPRAIN

Sprain occurs in the leg proper only at the upper end of the fibula. The upper end of the fibula does not participate primarily in the knee joint but may be involved in a knee injury. This is especially likely in relation to the fibular collateral ligament attachment (see page 447). There may be damage to the upper tibiofibular ligaments to the extent of an actual dislocation of the upper end of the fibula. The exact mechanism of isolated strain of this area is difficult to determine. It may be that some of the lesser sprains are caused by forcible traction of the biceps tendon with the knee in flexion (Fig. 378). The type of injury that damages the fibular collateral ligament of the knee would not ordinarily damage the tibiofibular ligament since its force tends to pull the fibula toward the tibia. If, however, the distracting force occurs with the knee flexed, the lateral collateral ligament may possibly pull the fibula backward in relation to the tibia. Certain it is that sprain to the extent of complete dislocation may occur from a direct blow to the upper end of the tibia, driving it away from its tibial attachment.

It may actually be possible manually to subluxate the head of the fibula back and forth or to dislocate it from the tibia if the ligament tear is severe, since the bone is subcutaneous and can be readily manipulated. Distinguishing symptoms are pain and tenderness around the anterior and posterior tibiofibular sulcis at the superior end.

Treatment.   If the fibula has dislocated and spontaneously replaced it may be difficult to determine that there has actually been a rupture of the ligaments.

Figure 378.   Drawing showing flexed knee, the biceps tendon pulling the fibula back.

Occasionally the dislocation remains unreduced (see Fig. 358, page 514). If it is seen early it may be readily reduced by manipulation. It may be held in place by simple splint fixation protecting the knee. The splint should extend from above the ankle to the groin. One must be extremely wary of trying to hold the fibula to the tibia by a constricting circumferential bandage because of the extreme vulnerability of the peroneal nerve. There may be a chronic dislocation of the upper end of the fibula and in many instances this will not be troublesome. However, the fact that the biceps and fibular collateral ligament attach to the fibula may cause this condition to become symptomatic. If it is symptomatic to the degree that it causes disability, surgical repair should be carried out by screw fixation across the upper end of the fibula into the tibia. This is rarely necessary.

FASCIAL HERNIA

Fascial hernia occurs in various areas of the body. One of the most common hernias of this type and one of the most likely to be symptomatic occurs in the anterior fascia of the leg. This rent usually takes place at the attachment of the anterior fascia to the anterior border of the tibia. The early symptoms will be those ordinarily connected with "shin splints," periostitis, or in fact simple contusion. As acute symptoms subside the patient will complain of a sharply localized mass that appears just lateral to the tibial crest but is not constant. It may or may not be tender. He may notice aching pain in the leg after continued use but at other times the condition may be almost wholly asymptomatic. Careful examination reveals a palpable defect in the fascia through which bulges a tumor mass particularly noticeable when the muscle is relaxed. When the anterior tibial muscle is contracted the mass will disappear since on contraction the tension in the muscle prevents it from bulging through the defect. The rim of the defect may readily be palpated.

Figure 379.   Exostosis of tibia. Note that the lateral view (A) is negative. The anteroposterior view (B) is inconclusive as to the nature of the mass, whereas the oblique (C) reveals the tumor very distinctly.

Treatment.   Ordinarily a careful, detailed explanation to the patient of the nature of his defect will suffice to reassure him and permit him to go on without further management. Occasionally, however, the condition is symptomatic enough that it causes disability by pain chronic in character involving the anterior tibial muscle. In these cases the defect is usually relatively small and there may be impingement of a portion of the muscle or soft tissue between the sharp edge of the fascia and edge of the bone. Here surgical interference is justified and consists in suture of the fascia to the tibia. This is successful if the sutured edge of fascial tissue is firm. Frequently, however, the edge of the fascia will be torn and effort to draw it to the tibia simply results in splitting it further. In this instance, extending the rent to a distance of 2 to 3 inches will give symptomatic relief so far as pain is concerned. The bulging will persist but its discrete character has been lost so that it no longer resembles a tumor mass.

EXOSTOSIS

There is no particular propensity toward traumatic exostoses in the leg. Although they frequently occur at the upper and lower ends of the tibia (Fig. 379) they are not frequent in its shaft. If they do occur they are managed as exostosis anywhere except that a much smaller exostosis will be symptomatic in a subcutaneous bone than in one surrounded completely by muscle. If the condition is symptomatic and cannot be handled by a simple protective pad, surgical excision should be entirely successful.

FRACTURE

It is not our intention to relate in detail the treatment of fracture of the bones of the leg. The tibia and fibula are both very subject to fracture from unusual forces.

Tibial Fracture

Fracture of the tibia is not common as an athletic injury but does occur. A complete fracture of the tibia will be symptomatic enough that x-ray studies will be made and the condition readily determined. Needless to say, treatment should be prompt and definitive. Competition within a season would not be expected following a fracture of the tibia even though it were an incomplete one.

Fibular Fracture

Whereas fracture of the tibia is relatively infrequent in athletic injury, fracture of the fibula is relatively common. In any fracture of the fibula, one is obligated to rule out associated injury to the ankle joint and I shall categorically state that any time there is a complete fracture of the fibula (see Ankle, page 555) above the level of the lower tibiofibular syndesmosis one is obligated to rule out accompanying complete rupture of the inferior tibiofibular ligaments. This is without doubt the most serious, most important consideration in the fracture of the fibula. The actual fracture of the fibula is usually quite inconsequential except that it does require a certain period for healing, but if the fracture is accompanied by a laceration of the tibiofibular ligament with resulting instability in or separation of the ankle mortice (see Fig. 392), the outcome is a serious permanent disability. The condition is readily handled if it is recognized early and treated promptly. It is very difficult to handle as a reconstructive measure. So the first step in considering the fracture of the fibula is to determine the integrity of the ankle joint.

The fibula is subject to fracture by direct blow. This is usually in the lower one-third and may be caused by contact with a shoe or other hard object. There is immediate severe pain but not necessarily severe disability. Upon examination local tenderness will be present at the site of the injury. There may or may not be local crepitation. There is prompt swelling with localized hematoma formation. The individual can usually walk quite well, in fact, may complete the football game since in a fracture of the fibula by direct blow the integrity of the ankle is not involved and disability is due to contraction of the muscle attachments on the fibular shaft. Diagnosis is confirmed by x-ray study which should always be made in a case of localized tenderness over any bone.

Treatment consists of management of the localized area and protection of the part. If there is definite hematoma with localized swelling, aspiration under surgically aseptic technique and infiltration of hyaluronidase is of some value. These measures are ordinarily not necessary. After a short period of packing in ice or compression bandage the extremity should be placed in a walking boot which should be worn for about three weeks. Union will not then be complete but by this time it is usually possible to so strap the extremity that some degree of function may be resumed. At least activity may be permitted to the point of starting rehabilitation but nonparticipation in contact sports probably is advisable for as long as six to eight weeks. One has a quite effective indicator in the degree of the patient's discomfort.

Stress Fracture (March Fatigue)

The fibula is particularly prone to stress fracture (Figs. 23 and 380), being second only to the metatarsals in this respect. This condition arises early in the training

Figure 380.   This boy was examined by a physician because of persistent pain in the lower fibula. X-ray was made (*A, B*) and he was advised that he had a malignant tumor and operation was scheduled. On seeing him in consultation a careful history elicited the fact that three weeks before he had sprinted off the curve of the track and up an incline and pulled up lame in this left leg. Two days later he ran in a race and had increased pain, particularly after the race. The pain and tenderness persisted but actually had seemed somewhat less in the past several days. He was advised that he probably had a stress fracture. The subsequent pictures (*C, D*) three weeks later show some increase in the extraperiosteal shadow but also some increased mottling. Meantime, the clinical symptoms had materially improved. Eight months later (*E, F*) the films show almost complete resolution. The patient had long been asymptomatic.

period and appears as aching pain, soreness and some distress on function, usually localized near the neck of the fibula. There is no history of injury. Examination will reveal localized tenderness over the bone. Early x-ray will usually be negative. The patient will be treated for contusion or sprain. The complaint persists and remains quite localized. X-rays after 10 to 14 days will often reveal a transverse crack across the bone. Possibly callus formation will appear with no fracture line visible. The significance of stress fracture of the fibula is not as important as that in the foot since the fibula is a nonweight-bearing bone but the patient should be carefully rehabilitated lest he develop chronic muscular disability in the leg. Frequently by the time the fracture is found the time for immobilization will be past and treatment will be by careful muscular rehabilitation and other physical therapeutic measures such as local heat and muscular massage.

Figure 381. Blown-up view of "fatigue" fracture of the tibia. Differential diagnosis here was of tumor because of no injury and the presence of severe aching pain. Time gave complete relief.

Stress fracture of the tibia has been known to occur but is very rare (Fig. 381). It is of necessity more disabling than in the fibula since the tibia is a weight-bearing bone. When the fracture is recognized a protective cast should be applied until union has progressed to the point of good stability with no pain.

Injuries of
the Ankle

ANATOMICAL CONSIDERATIONS

INJURIES to the ankle joint constitute one of the most common conditions encountered in the treatment of injuries to the athlete. There is no doubt that many ankle injuries are treated overcasually, which may account for the expression, "Once a sprain, always a sprain." It is my opinion that insufficient consideration has been given to the exact nature of the damage in the individual case. In order to be able to treat intelligently any injury of the ankle joint, a definitive diagnosis must be made. This predicates a working knowledge of the anatomy of the region involved.

Let us consider the anatomic characteristics of the ankle joint that have a direct bearing on the type of injury that occurs in response to various forces applied (Figs. 382, 383 and 384). The ankle joint is functionally a hinge joint with motion in only one plane—flexion and extension. The bony structure is designed as a mortice and tenon with considerable inherent stability (Fig. 382). The mortice is formed by the lateral malleolus, the undersurface of the tibia and the medial malleolus. The tenon is the body of the talus which is shaped to fit snugly into the mortice. It should be noted that the lateral malleolus is longer than the medial malleolus. Its distal tip extends to the bottom of the talus at the level of the talocalcaneal joint. It is roughly rectangular in outline but actually somewhat narrower at the level of the lower end of the tiba. The medial malleolus on the other hand is short and thick, being roughly pyramidal in shape with its base upward. Its distal tip extends only halfway down on the body of the talus.

548

Figure 382. Anatomical drawing of ankle, posterior view, showing the tibiofibular ligament which is heavy distally, thinning out to become the interosseous membrane proximally. The posterior and lateral fasciculi of the lateral collateral ligament and the posterior and medial fasciculi of the medial collateral ligament are shown. Note the different lengths of the two malleoli. The guide line indicates top of dome of talus.

The tibia and fibula are bound together by the anterior and posterior tibiofibular ligaments which are really thickened expansions of the same interosseous membrane that fastens the two bones together throughout their length. Although some motion is present in the articulation between the tibia and fibula at the lower end, there is to all practical purposes complete stability between the two bones. Definite motion has been demonstrated in the distal tibiofibular syndesmosis so that a certain amount of disability occurs from ankylosis between the tibia and fibula at the ankle joint. Thus, the ankle joint has stability from two sources: first, the mortice and tenon bony structure, and second, the extensive investiture of ligaments that surround the joint.

The ligaments become thin fore and aft (capsule) to permit flexion and extension of the joint, and thicken at sides to become the tibial and fibular collateral ligaments. The medial collateral, or deltoid, ligament is particularly strong, has a very broad attachment to the internal malleolus and extends downward in many bands to become intimately connected to the ligaments supporting the arch of the

Figure 383. Anatomical drawing of ankle, anterior view. Note massive deltoid ligament and very weak anterior talotibial ligament. Note no ligament from front of tibia to top of talus.

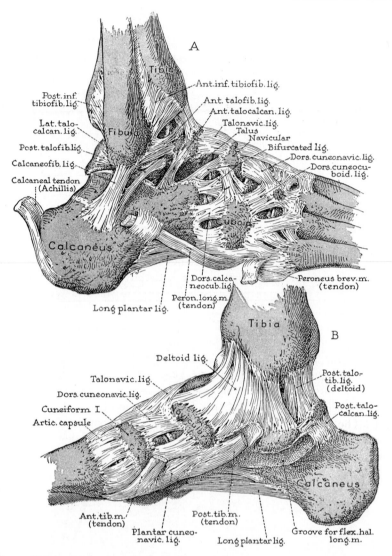

Figure 384.   Ligaments of the ankle and foot. *A*, Lateral side. Note very weak lateral ligaments. Distal end of fibula is at level of talocalcaneal joint. *B*, Medial side. Note massive deltoid ligament and short medial malleolus. Deltoid ligament extends down over medial side to support arch. The calcaneal tendon has been removed in *B*. (From Jones and Shepard, "A Manual of Surgical Anatomy," p. 116.)

foot. In addition to stabilizing the ankle joint on the medial side, it serves to support the arch and hence is a doubly vital structure.

It is possible to dissect the lateral collateral ligament into many separate ligaments but there are three primary fasciculi, one running forward to attach to the talus anteriorly (anterior talofibular), another backward to attach to the posterior portion of the talus (posterior talofibular), and one directly downward to attach to the calcaneus (calcaneofibular). These ligaments also blend into the lateral ligaments of the foot, extending forward onto the cuboid and to the base of the fifth metatarsal. Together the medial and lateral ligaments, acting in conjunction with the two malleoli, serve to prevent lateral rocking motion at the ankle joint.

The long lateral malleolus, with the medial ligament, prevents excess motion to the outer side. The length of the lateral malleolus firmly holds the body of the talus so that lateral motion in the tarsus is more restricted than is medial motion. A normal range of flexion-extension is permitted with its axis at the tip of the medial malleolus.

The talus is not rectangular in its general shape. The anterior portion of the body is distinctly wider than the posterior portion so that, as the foot goes into dorsal flexion, the wider part of the talus is forced between the two malleoli and the ankle is very stable in this position. As the foot goes into plantar flexion the narrower part of the body of the talus moves into the mortice and some lateral instability results in this position. On dorsiflexion of the foot the fibula is forced away from the tibia. On forcible dorsiflexion of the foot the anterior edge of the tibia nestles into the sulcus between the head and body of the talus. The anterior inferior angle of the tibia inclines slightly backward in order to prevent direct impingement between the talus and the tibia. As the foot dorsiflexes and everts, the talus is driven forcibly against the lateral malleolus. These factors are of considerable importance in the study of injuries to the ankle.

The two malleoli are subcutaneous and as such are subject to direct injury. The posterior tibial tendon and peroneal tendons lie in very intimate association with the back of the medial and the lateral malleolus respectively whereas the dorsiflexors and plantar flexors of the foot have a much less intimate relationship to the osseous structures in front of the ankle.

CONTUSION

There is nothing particularly significant in contusion about the ankle. The contusion will usually be on one or the other malleolus. The most immediate necessity is diagnosis of the injury. Once it has been confirmed that a contusion and not a fracture or a sprain is present, the treatment is simplified. A word of caution: In many sprains the maximum tenderness will be in the malleolus itself. A negative x-ray does not necessarily mean that the injury is a contusion only. An incomplete or fissure type fracture may simulate a contusion and one should be suspicious of the condition that is particularly slow to heal or causes pain on function. In an ordinary contusion of the ankle, ankle function is disturbed very little unless there has been a severe crushing injury of the soft tissues. A blow over the tendo achillis may lead to tenosynovitis complicating a contusion. A blow over the peroneal tendons may actually dislocate them from the groove—an injury very much more serious than simple contusion. These facts suggest that a careful examination should be made to eliminate other possible injuries before treatment for contusion is initiated.

Treatment is the same as for contusion elsewhere: aspiration of the hematoma, local injection (hyaluronidase), compression, cold packs to be followed in a few hours by heat. Support per se is not necessary. Protective appliances such as sponge rubber or felt doughnuts are important. Rehabilitation should be rapid and athletic participation is not unduly interfered with.

STRAIN

The ankle joint is subject to strain perhaps more than any other joint in the body. This is due to several factors. In the first place it is a weight-bearing joint and in the athlete is subject to very dynamic forces as a result of the explosive character of its motion under certain circumstances. The broad jumper, for example, not only takes off with a terrific drive but on landing forces both feet into extreme dorsal flexion with resultant strain on the tendo achillis. This strain may occur either at the attachment of the tendon to the calcaneus or frequently at the musculotendinous junction, occasionally along the course of the tendon. It is frequently complicated by tenosynovitis. Another tendon particularly subject to strain is the anterior tibial. A most annoying disability can arise from strain of this tendon at its attachment to the medial side of the foot. The peroneal tendons are much less frequently strained since the nature of the activity of the ankle does not require such forcible use of the everters as of the other muscles of the ankle.

Treatment of the acute condition is rest of the muscle involved, local heat, local injection with corticoid preparations, and protection against further injury. The proper degree of protection may be very difficult to decide. Since the condition involves the integrity of the muscle it is obvious that the strain cannot be well protected while activity of the muscle is permitted. An attempt to shorten the treatment period often results in prompt recurrence of the disability and the situation may become quite frustrating to the doctor—doubly so to the athlete. Certain protective measures can be used, however, the general rule being that no function should be allowed that causes pain. In sprain of the tendo achillis, for example, the pain may be caused mainly by overstretching of the tendon and this can be prevented by adequate strapping to prevent hyperdorsal flexion of the foot. With such protection the athlete may be able to jog or even run at a relatively steady pace but should not be allowed to charge out of the blocks or jump or hurdle. In short, he should do nothing that requires explosive activity of the muscle. Ordinarily the condition will require at least ten days of relative inactivity and sometimes much more than this. Unrestricted activity should be permitted only when it is entirely pain-free. Since pain is a relative thing it may be very difficult in a given case to decide just when unrestricted activity will be safe.

TENOSYNOVITIS

Tenosynovitis is quite frequent about the ankle and, as indicated in the above section, frequently follows strain. Tenosynovitis can result from contusion or infection but at the ankle the most common cause is overuse of the tendon. This causes irritation between the tendon and surrounding tissues with resulting loss of the smooth gliding pattern. The significant findings are pain on motion of the tendon particularly under tension, "snowball crepitation" on motion, tenderness along the involved area, local heat and redness and other signs of inflammatory reaction. Differentiation between tenosynovitis and strain may be extremely difficult but since their treatment is quite similar this is not a vital problem. In fact, the two often co-exist. When they do the condition becomes more resistant to treatment.

Treatment should be prompt. Complete rest of the involved tendon together with the use of local injection with corticoid is indicated. Local injection of anesthetic agents should not lull one into the conclusion that the inflammation has subsided since return to function under these circumstances will result in prompt exacerbation of the condition. Local injection is of value as a measure of treatment, not as a means of rehabilitation. Athletic participation is extremely difficult in case of tenosynovitis of the ankle since the only real way to prevent motion of the tendons of the ankle is to immobilize the ankle and this is not consistent with ordinary athletic endeavor. As rehabilitation progresses, protective measures should be designed to prevent extremes of motion in the involved tendon. If the heel cord is involved, strapping to prevent dorsal flexion will help (Fig. 377). If the anterior tibial or posterior tibial tendon is involved, strapping in inversion in the early stage (Fig. 385) and later a properly fitted arch support or wedging the shoe on the medial border of the sole and heel will serve to eliminate some of the static stress of this condition.

Tenosynovitis is more likely to be disastrous to a season's play than strain but for the same reason, namely, a marked tendency toward recurrence. The track man who develops a tenosynovitis running on the boards in the winter will frequently have a very ineffectual season since, when he puts out his maximum effort, he is likely to be pulled up short by recurrence of his tenosynovitis. As in so many other instances, early adequate treatment is the very best insurance of success. A period of complete nonparticipation may well be followed by a highly successful season whereas an attempt to continue athletics in spite of pain and discomfort can result only in continued ineffectual activity.

My best recommendation for treatment in severe acute tenosynovitis in the tendo achillis or anterior tibial is a period of elevation and hot packs until the acute redness has disappeared, followed by application of a walking boot cast to be worn for a period of 10 to 14 days. By this time the symptoms will have largely subsided

Figure 385.   Strapping in inversion. (Strips start on lateral border of dorsum of foot, pass under the sole of the foot and swing under the arch and up on medial aspect of leg.)

and adequate strapping can be applied to permit gradual return to function. Protective strapping should be continued for several weeks until one is sure there is no real likelihood of recurrence. The strapping must be specifically designed to protect the tendon involved. Great care must be taken that the adhesive straps do not actually constrict the tendon and so make the condition worse. For anterior tibial strain the strips should start on the lateral border of the dorsum of the foot, pass under the sole of the foot and swing under the arch and up the medial aspect of the leg (Fig. 385). They are applied with the foot in dorsal flexion and slightly inverted.

To support the tendo achillis the foot should be strapped in plantar flexion (Fig. 377).

DISLOCATION OR SUBLUXATION OF THE PERONEAL TENDONS

A condition unique to the ankle area is dislocation or subluxation of the peroneal tendons. This condition may be acute or chronic.

Acute

In the acute condition the history usually is of a blow back of the malleolus while the peroneal tendons are taut in dorsiflexion or eversion of the foot. The peroneal retinaculum gives way. One or both of the tendons pop out of the groove onto the lateral side of the malleolus. They usually spontaneously reduce. One may confuse this condition with an ankle sprain. Careful history and physical examination will eliminate the confusion, however. Tenderness is directly over the peroneal tendons and it may be confused with tenosynovitis. Indeed, tenosynovitis may be a sequel. In the acute case, it is usually not possible to displace the tendons at examination.

If the diagnosis can be made of an acute dislocation, the *treatment* is surgical. Incision posteriorly along the peroneal groove, replacement of the tendons with resuture of the retinaculum may be effective. In many cases there will be a shallow peroneal groove which predisposes to this condition. In this instance, repair should be accompanied by deepening of the groove in order to make the tendons more secure. Following surgery, fixation in a stirrup splint for two weeks, then a walking cast for two weeks, will give adequate protection. Active athletics should not be permitted under six weeks, however.

Chronic

Chronic subluxation of the peroneal tendons may be congenital or it may follow an acute episode that was untreated. In the latter instance there will be a history of acute injury with considerable soreness for many weeks, followed by recurrent episodes of something slipping out of place at the back of the ankle, with sharp pain. These occur as the athlete everts the foot with the tendons tight. They are quite distressing. The tendons slip back into position and all is well until the next episode. Careful history will usually reveal the original episode and the patient can describe the recurrent ones quite graphically. Physical examination will usually demonstrate the shallow groove with thickening of the retinaculum. The tendons can be slipped completely or partially out of the groove on manual examination.

This condition should be treated by surgical reconstruction of the groove with repair of the retinaculum, suitably reinforced by adjacent tissue. This is a very successful type of repair and should give prompt relief although six to eight weeks of immobilization will be needed for good stability.

SYNOVIAL HERNIA

Synovial hernia about the ankle will be discussed in the section dealing with the condition in the foot (page 597).

SPRAIN–DISLOCATION–FRACTURE

In this discussion these three conditions will be grouped together since there is no well defined way to differentiate between them at the ankle joint. This is particularly pertinent in the consideration of athletic injuries. While many fractures about the lower leg and ankle are primary, the result of terrific forces, in the athlete the injury is usually caused by stress forces which may result in either a sprain, or dislocation or a fracture—or all three.

MECHANICS OF INJURY

Since the ankle is functionally a hinge joint normally permitting only dorsal and plantar flexion, it follows that injuries to the ankle are primarily due to lateral stresses that force the ankle through a range of motion it does not normally possess. Less frequently they are due to hyperflexion or hyperextension. The injuries due to lateral stresses may readily be divided into two categories, namely, inversion injuries and eversion injuries.

Inversion Injury

Inversion injuries to the ankle (Fig. 386) are as a rule not due to pure inversion. They usually consist of inversion, internal rotation and plantar flexion of the foot in relation to the leg so that the foot is inverted and the ankle and leg are thrown to the outer side. It will be noted that the push is against the medial malleolus and that the pull is away from the lateral malleolus. As the foot inverts in relation to the leg, strain is put upon the external collateral ligament, which is the ligament primarily designed to restrict this motion. As a result of this overinversion the ligament will tear slightly, partially or completely according to the severity of the force. If the inverting force continues after the lateral ligament gives way the ankle "opens up" on the lateral side and the talus is forcibly thrust against the medial malleolus. The medial malleolus, being short and stubby and extending no more than half way down the vertical height of the body of the talus, will act as a fulcrum with its tip impinging against the central portion of the medial face of the talus. The talus thus rotates over the malleolus rather than pushing it off. In such a case the injury will probably be confined to the lateral side and there will be more or less complete laceration of the lateral collateral ligaments. It is unusual for this type of force to break off the lateral malleolus in the athlete.

Figure 386.   A, Mechanics of inversion injury of the ankle. Drawing showing talus rolling over medial malleolus. B, Inversion injury showing complete severance of the lateral collateral ligament permitting the talus to roll over the medial malleolus. There is no fracture. The ossicle on the medial side is the os trigonum. C, The same stress on the normal side.

In an elderly person in whom the bone is brittle and fragile, the malleolus may break rather than the ligament tear. If this same inversion force is continued as the talus is driven against the medial malleolus, the latter may break off (Fig. 387). In this instance the fracture line will ordinarily extend more or less vertically up the shaft of the tibia beginning at the lateral margin of the medial malleolus. There is injury on both sides of the ankle. This may be a bimalleolar fracture or perhaps a fracture of the medial malleolus plus an avulsion of the lateral collateral ligament.

Approximately 85 per cent of all injuries to the ankle consist of inversion injuries and are confined to ligament injury, so-called sprain or "sprain-fracture" of the ankle (Fig. 388). The vast majority of these may be classified as mild sprains without any particular loss of function of the ligament. If the force is violent, other fractures may occur such as fracture of the superomedial portion of the talus and fracture of the back of the articular surface of the tibia, but as a rule

Figure 387.   Inversion injury of the ankle. *A,* Drawing showing vertical fracture of the medial malleolus, with a split up the shaft and complete tear of the lateral ligament. *B,* Another inversion injury. In this instance the talus pushed the medial malleolus off instead of rolling over it. This should be treated by reduction and internal fixation.

Figure 388.   *A,* Drawing showing sprain-fracture of lateral malleolus. *B,* X-ray showing sprain-fracture of lateral margin of cuboid. This is really a sprain, not primarily a fracture.

Figure 389.   A, Drawing of eversion injury of the ankle. The talus pushes the fibula laterally, rupturing the tibiofibular ligament. The fibula may break at any level above the tibiofibular ligament. The medial collateral ligament is torn. B, X-ray showing normal ankle. C, Eversion injury. Lateral stress would displace the talus further.

injury is confined to the ligament injury on the lateral side with occasional instances of avulsion fracture of the tip of the fibula or "push-off" fracture of the medial malleolus.

Eversion Injury

If the opposite force is applied and the foot is carried outward in relationship to the leg, the talus is forced laterally and into dorsal flexion (Fig. 389). The anatomic difference between the two malleoli becomes doubly significant here. Whereas on the medial side the malleolus is short and the talus may rotate over it, on the lateral side the malleolus is at least as long as the height of the talus so that it is extremely difficult for the talus to rotate over the lateral malleolus with the

Figure 390.   Eversion injury. Showing fractured fibula without separation of ankle mortice. Note rupture of the deltoid ligament. Tibiofibular ligament is intact.

Figure 391.   X-ray views of injury shown in Figure 390. *A*, Carefully positioned anteroposterior view shows little or no pathology. *B*, Original deformity reproduced, clearly indicating nature of injury. *C*, Repair of deltoid ligament and fixation by transfixion screw. Correction not complete. *D*, Opposite ankle for comparison.

malleolar tip as the fulcrum. In eversion force, the push being toward the lateral side, the talus is driven forcibly against the lateral malleolus and severe pressure is applied to the malleolus before overstress of the short medial collateral ligament occurs which can permit some degree of lateral tilting of the talus. This stress applied to the lateral malleolus may cause one of several types of injuries but all are due to the same forces. Perhaps the most common injury is fracture of the fibula somewhere below the level of the lower end of the tibia, resulting in a single malleolar fracture (Figs. 390 and 391). This may occur without significant dam-

Figure 392.   A, Eversion injury. Fracture of fibula in which fibula is actually pushed off with separation of ankle mortice.

B, X-ray of same injury. Rupture of the medial ligament, separation of the tibiofibular ligament, lateral displacement of the talus, fracture of the fibula above the level of the joint. This fracture cannot occur without rupture of the medial ligament.

C, After repair of the medial ligament and fixation of the fibula to the tibia.

age to the deltoid ligament but it is more often accompanied by a rupture of this ligament. This same force may actually drive the fibula away from the tibia after rupturing the tibiofibular ligament and so permit separation of the ankle mortice (Fig. 392). In this instance as the force continues, the medial collateral ligament having given way, the tibiofibular ligaments having torn, the fibula is driven further away from the tibia and the fibula may break anywhere along its length. The common location of the break is somewhere in its lower third. If a fibular fracture appears above the level of the ankle joint, one may assume that the tibiofibular ligament has been torn and that the integrity of the ankle mortice has been lost. This is an extremely important point from the standpoint of treatment. Before this stress laterally is sufficient to push the fibula away from the tibia, something must give way on the medial side of the foot. This may consist in laceration of the medial collateral (deltoid) ligament or an avulsion of the medial malleolus.

Another common injury is the *bimalleolar fracture* (Fig. 393), namely, fracture of both malleoli at or below the level of the lower end of the tibia. This is also an eversion injury. If a fracture of the lower end of the fibula is observed at the level of the lower end of the tibia, one should check very carefully the integrity of the deltoid ligament. While the great majority of injuries of the ankle joint are sprains and the result of inversion injury, a great majority of fractures of the ankle are of the lateral malleolus and are caused by lateral motion or eversion.

From the description of the mechanics of injury it becomes quite apparent that it is of great importance in any individual case to determine if possible the type of forces involved and so be able to forecast to some extent the area upon which the strain is to be expected.

Figure 393. Bimalleolar fracture. All ligaments intact. This should be treated by replacement of the medial malleolus and internal fixation. In this case no treatment was necessary on the lateral side of the ankle since the fibula is relatively stable by virtue of its intact periosteum. In many cases fibular fixation is advisable (see Fig. 401).

Dorsiflexion Injury

Characteristically, the eversion injury is some combination of eversion, external rotation and dorsiflexion. Thus, strictly speaking, the dorsiflexion injury is a type of eversion injury, but it is so frequent that it merits individual description. As was indicated in the description of the anatomy of the ankle, the talus is broad in front and narrow behind. As the foot is pushed into dorsiflexion, the broad part of the talus seats firmly between the two malleoli and this stress is readily supported by the distal tibiofibular ligament. If the force continues or if some eversion component thrusts the talus more forcibly against the fibula, the result is unusual strain against this ligament, which binds the two bones together. This same force puts tension against the musculotendinous unit of the calf and may result in strain or actual rupture of this mechanism. Far more frequently the dorsiflexion simply springs the tibia and fibula apart, the force is resolved, the two bones fall back together and the disability does not seem to be severe. Simple dorsiflexion probably will not avulse the ligament completely.

Symptoms. The patient presents himself with a rather indefinite history. He may be able to say that his foot was pushed too far in dorsiflexion. Usually, he cannot be sure. He noticed that he experienced pain at the ankle and this subsided as the foot came down into the normal position. Contrary to the ordinary sprain of the ankle, local swelling is not manifested because the hemorrhage occurs deep in the leg and is not readily detectable under the skin. This is the patient who continues to play, tries to run, who has increasing pain and discomfort as he increases his activities. He may be able to run well at a normal pace but if he puts the pressure on, he will notice pain in the ankle. He will often be able to associate this pain with dorsiflexion of the foot.

Figure 394.   College athlete who had a dorsiflexion injury apparently resulting in a mild sprain. Inadequate treatment which did not prevent dorsiflexion resulted in persistent pain and repeated, unsatisfactory efforts to return to football. The player could not run all out. At the season's end, more thorough study revealed the true nature of the condition with calcification of the tibiofibular ligament over a considerable space. There was mild diastasis. Removal of the calcium and screw fixation for eight weeks resulted in improvement but some symptoms persisted.

A, Anteroposterior view showing slight tibiofibular diastasis with calcification.

B, Oblique view revealing the extent of the calcium deposit.

C, Postoperative view showing reduction of the diastasis and fixation.

Examination reveals a moderate degree of swelling with some fullness in the area back of the lateral malleolus, between it and the tendo achillis. Palpation directly along the sulcus between the tibia and fibula will demonstrate tenderness posteriorly and anteriorly. The findings at this stage are ordinarily not marked, however, unless the injury has been a severe one. On manipulation of the foot ordinary motion is free and pain-free. Inversion and eversion do not cause pain. Pain will be elicited on complete dorsiflexion of the foot, particularly with the knee flexed to relax the calf. These symptoms are very similar to those of talo-tibial exostosis, the distinction being that, in the sprain, pain is usually tibiofibular while in the exostosis it is ordinarily in front of the ankle. The two conditions may co-exist.

Treatment.   Early attention to this injury will result in prompt recovery since it is relatively easy to protect the injured part and even permit a relatively high degree of activity. Strapping of the foot to prevent dorsiflexion (Fig. 377), the use of an elevated heel on the shoe, in fact, those measures designed to prevent dorsiflexion will be effective. The foot should be strapped so that dorsiflexion cannot take place even under very severe stress. In too many instances the condition is minimized by both player and physician and only after weeks of frustration is the true nature of the injury recognized.

These cases account for the relatively high incidence of calcification noted between the tibia and fibula in x-rays of the ankle, since calcification is prone to occur where chronic irritation takes place (Fig. 394). The late manifestation of the chronic condition may be quite discouraging. I do not believe there is real justification for removing the calcification unless there is separation between the tibia and fibula making it advisable to restore the ankle mortice. Probably conservative treatment is better in the ordinary case. The foot should be carefully strapped to prevent the motion causing the pain.

DIAGNOSIS

History. Since the forces that cause ankle injuries are of such significance in the resulting damage, one must determine, if possible, the exact mechanics of the injury. Was the foot inverted or everted? How did the accident occur? Was disability immediate? Is disability the result of swelling and edema? Was there a primary deformity which was corrected by the patient, a friend or the x-ray technician before making the picture? How long ago did the injury occur? What was the treatment? Has heat or cold been applied? All these factors give important leads, not only as to the type and location of injury but as to its severity. They may be invaluable guides to the treatment indicated.

Examination. Examination of the injured ankle should be preceded by careful examination of the opposite leg in order that a normal may be obtained for comparison. One then proceeds with a meticulous but extremely gentle examination of the involved extremity. If one begins by simple observation, he can obtain the confidence of the apprehensive patient and with it more detailed information. Observation will reveal deformity, the location and amount of swelling, the degree of tension in the skin, and the extent of circulatory impairment. Following observation, by careful palpation one can determine the tension and the degree of swelling. There may be obvious bony crepitation on careful palpation through the skin. Then, by gentle manipulation the pain-free range of motion is determined and increased lateral motion is tested for. If abnormal lateral motion is elicited, note is made as to whether there is pain on attempting to force lateral motion. Any abnormal motion indicates serious ligament or bone injury.

X-ray Examination. X-ray examination should be carried out only after careful clinical examination by the surgeon. If possible, he should examine the foot before the x-ray is made. X-ray technicians are trained to position extremities in certain standard ways and often manipulation of the part to get proper x-ray position will reduce deformities or screen injuries that might otherwise be obvious. The x-ray technician should be instructed to make the original picture without correction of the position of the foot since this may provide an invaluable guide to the degree of injury (Fig. 395). Following this original picture, proper positioning can be made to obtain the standard views. At least three views should be made: an anteroposterior of the tarsus, an anteroposterior of the ankle, and a lateral of the ankle and foot. Oblique views are invaluable and may reveal fractures not seen in conventional views (Fig. 396). If abnormal motion can be elicited, an x-ray made in the abnormal position is of considerable value (Fig. 391). If the x-ray examination does not appear to be consistent with the clinical findings, a careful review of all findings must be made. Further x-ray views may be needed to clarify the situation.

Careful attention to all these details of history, physical examination and x-ray visualization will usually permit early diagnosis of a serious injury. Definitive treatment may then be carried out promptly rather than after a period of time pending

Figure 395. Original film of severe sprain, which illustrates dramatically the nature of this injury, namely, ruptured medial collateral ligament and ruptured tibiofibular ligament. Repair of medial ligament and fixation of fibula to tibia by long screw resulted in normal ankle.

Figure 396. Routine anteroposterior (*A*) and lateral (*B*) x-rays are apparently negative. Oblique view (*C*) reveals true condition, namely, fracture of medial malleolus and rupture of tibiofibular ligament. In this instance the clinical examination of the foot did not agree with the x-ray findings so further x-ray study was made.

determination that the injury is more serious than it was first considered to be. Although the majority of injuries to the ankle will be sprains without bone involvement, it is extremely embarrassing to discover after several weeks that treatment was woefully inadequate because of more extensive damage than was recognized at the time the treatment was begun.

TREATMENT

Before treatment can be properly initiated in any individual case, it is important to classify the injury not only as to type and to structures damaged but also as to severity. It is axiomatic that the closer an injury approaches the joint the more necessary it is to get completely accurate repositioning of the injured structures. One must not be satisfied with incomplete reduction or partial replacement of fractures or dislocations about the ankle any more than about any other joint. Indeed, it is more important to get accurate repositioning in a weight-bearing joint than in the nonweight-bearing joints in the upper extremity.

Complete reduction must be accomplished by the method that will insure the best result, not by the method that at the time seems the most convenient. A little extra care at the time of injury will save a great deal of time and trouble at a later date. It is well known that surgery will be required in a certain percentage of injuries about the ankle joint. Recognizing this fact, it is extremely important that surgery be considered as a method of treatment per primum. If it is going to be necessary for best results, it should be carried out promptly at the time of injury, rather than backed into after nonsurgical treatment has failed.

Sprains

Sprains, which comprise the majority of injuries about the ankle, can conveniently be classified into three groups—mild, moderate and severe. This arbitrary division is subject to a good deal of variation according to the views of the individual physician. The groups will, of necessity, overlap.

Mild Sprain.   A mild sprain (Fig. 397, A) is one in which there has been a partial tear of elements of one of the ligaments at the ankle joint without any actual functional weakening of the ligament as a whole. In such a case, one would expect to find minimal symptoms: local tenderness, local swelling and mild disability. Indeed, the disability may be so mild that the patient does not even seek advice from a physician.

A   **B**   **C**

Figure 397.   Drawings showing (A) partial tear of ligament, *mild* sprain; (B) *moderate* sprain, with more complete tear but still integrity of ligament; (C) *severe* sprain with tear and loss of integrity.

Examination will reveal no pain on normal motion, no abnormal motion and only a moderate degree of pain on reapplying the stress that caused the original injury. X-ray examination will be negative. This case requires no extensive treatment. This is the type of case that responds dramatically to the local treatment that was so popular a few years ago. Unfortunately, these local methods have been applied in many cases in which they were woefully inadequate.

Local application of ethyl chloride spray tends to break down the cycle of vessel spasm and reduce the local swelling and edema. It can have no effect on the strength of the ligament itself or on its healing. This should be kept in mind since, although it does tend to relieve the symptoms, it does not protect the joint against further damage. However, in the mild case, local injection of procaine and hyaluronidase will tend to permit rapid absorption of the hematoma and reduce pain. In this sense it is valuable in treatment.

In this group ideal treatment would be rest with application of ice followed by heat. However, in a mild sprain this is usually not mandatory. It is not justified if it interferes unnecessarily with the patient's occupation. Local injection followed by adequate strapping (Fig. 398) and a well fitted shoe is all the treatment that is necessary since there is no actual weakness of the ankle joint. It should be pointed out again, however, that if one is to permit activity, one must be extremely sure of the diagnosis. It is unwise in any case to use local treatment that relieves the symptoms and then permit the injured person to participate in active sports immediately. The lapse of several hours will determine more accurately the extent of injury.

Moderate Sprain.   A moderate sprain consists of one in which there has been an actual tear of a portion of the ligament but in which the integrity of the ligament has not been entirely lost. There is some weakness of the ligament but no abnormal motion is elicited. Ordinarily, the history is of sharp inversion of the foot followed by a fall with immediate severe pain. The patient is not necessarily wholly incapacitated for walking since direct weight bearing does not put strain on the injured ligament.

Figure 398.   Strapping for injury to lateral or medial ankle ligaments. Gibney type strapping.

Symptoms are usually so severe that medical aid is sought. On examination there is severe pain in the ankle, diffuse swelling through the ankle and foot and tenderness over the lateral side of the foot and ankle, usually sharply increased at the area of the damaged ligament. This may be at the attachment of the ligament to the foot, or at the malleolus, or it may be in the substance of the ligament. The patient may tend to hold the foot in an inverted position but any attempt to invert the foot beyond this point will cause severe pain. Even normal motion may be painful. An attempt to reproduce the forces that caused the injury will produce severe pain. However, there will be no abnormal motion since some portion of the ligament is still intact. X-ray is negative except as it may show a sprain-fracture at one or the other attachments of the ligament (Fig. 388).

In choosing treatment it should be borne in mind that whereas in the mild sprain there is no weakness and protection is not vital, in the moderate sprain there is definite weakness of the ligament. The first aim of treatment is to protect the ankle against further injury until healing occurs, the second to promote repair of the damage already present. Rather mild stresses superimposed over the already weakened ligament may cause complete avulsion.

Treatment consists in local injection of the area with hyaluronidase and procaine, followed by compression bandage and ice pack for several hours. Relief of symptoms by local injection should not permit early ambulation or early function of the part since this will have a detrimental effect upon healing. The patient should be put to bed with pressure bandage and ice pack for eight to ten hours. At the end of this time, further analysis should be made as to extent of the injury.

Following the period of ice packing, a posterior and a lateral stirrup splint (see Fig. 315) is applied from below the knee to the toes in order to maintain the part in the normal weight-bearing position. The patient is then allowed to get up on crutches but should be advised not to bear weight on the extremity. Several days later, after the swelling subsides, this splint should be replaced by a walking boot cast (see Fig. 317) which may be worn for ten days to three weeks depending upon the extent of the damage. Active weight bearing is encouraged as soon as this cast has dried.

It may be argued that a cast handicaps the patient needlessly. Usually, it will be found that, in a ligament injury of this degree, the patient will be substantially disabled in any event. He will actually get around more efficiently and with less pain in the walking cast than he will with ordinary wrapping or strapping. Some liberties with this regimen may be permitted in a well organized training program. For instance, during the early period of protective splinting, the splints may be removed daily for utilization of physical therapy. Whirlpool is at some disadvantage under these circumstances because it allows the foot to be pendant and so may increase the local swelling. It is not very feasible to remove the walking cast daily since it is difficult to replace it with sufficient security to permit pain-free weight bearing. Sometimes in the exceptional case under ideally controlled circumstances a very thorough strapping is utilized in place of a walking cast and this is removed each day for physical therapy and conscientiously replaced when treatment is finished.

Following removal of the cast after 10 to 20 days, it is advisable to apply well fitted adhesive strapping of the Gibney type (Fig. 398) to protect the ligament against further injury. This strapping should be worn until symptoms are minimal, ordinarily at least six weeks from the time of injury. If the original injury is treated adequately in this manner, there is little reason to expect recurrent injuries since the ligament will heal at its normal length and strength.

Severe Sprain.   A severe ankle sprain consists of one in which the integrity of the ligament has been lost completely. The ligament is either torn completely in two or one or the other of its attachments has pulled loose from the bone. History will be essentially the same as for moderate sprain but all complaints will be more severe. The patient will frequently volunteer the information that the foot had been out of place but had been reduced by manipulation and that pain was relieved by the reduction.

Examination will reveal more serious and extensive findings than in the other groups. The swelling will be more extreme. The pain will be more severe. Any attempt at motion of the foot will be resisted. The patient is extremely apprehensive. If the foot is examined very early, abnormal motion may be elicited without undue pain. It is justifiable, in certain cases, to inject procaine into the painful area or even to induce short general anesthesia in order to determine whether or not there is complete disruption of one of the ligaments of the ankle joint. An x-ray should be made in the abnormal position if possible (Fig. 386, A). These cases are relatively infrequent but when they occur the consequences may be extremely disastrous if the true condition is not recognized and appropriate treatment instituted. Many of the most disabling injuries reveal no demonstrable fracture but are caused by dislocation. Ligament injury may be extremely severe (Fig. 395).

An example of these serious injuries to the ankle is disruption of the medial collateral and tibiofibular ligaments, in which case the x-ray findings may be completely negative. Also the external collateral ligament may be completely torn and a normal x-ray picture seen. One must recognize the exact condition present in order to plan the best treatment, which obviously must be far more comprehensive than that for an ordinary sprain of the ankle. For this reason the diagnosis must be made at the earliest possible moment. If surgical repair of the ligament is to be carried out, it must be done promptly in order to secure the best results. If there is a complete severance of the medial collateral or tibiofibular ligament, or both, surgical treatment is certainly the treatment of choice.

A complete avulsion of the external collateral ligament may well heal in a satisfactory position without surgical intervention since snug support is not as necessary for the lateral ligament as for the medial or tibiofibular. However, it is the patient with this injury in whom recurrent sprain is prone to occur owing to overlength of the ligament. If it can be determined that a complete tear of this ligament is present, surgical repair will not only speed recovery but will improve the probability of obtaining a perfect functional result.

The warning is explicit that in these serious injuries one must not temporize but must make up his mind whether or not surgery is indicated. The time to carry out an operation is at the earliest possible moment after the need for one is determined. While late surgery is not nearly as favorable as is early operation, it should not be refused simply because the diagnosis was not made at time of the injury (Fig. 399). "Better late than never."

If nonsurgical treatment is the treatment of choice, then the same treatment is

Figure 399.   Fracture of tip of lateral malleolus with nonunion, resulting pain and disability from involvement of peroneal tendons as well as lateral collateral ligament. This patient was treated without immobilization. This is in reality a sprain-fracture, the tip having been avulsed by the lateral collateral ligament. Surgical removal of the fragment resulted in marked improvement. Early surgery should have given complete recovery. (*A*) Illustrating value of oblique view. (*B*) Stress film demonstrating no instability.

indicated as for a moderate sprain, namely local injection, compression, ice packs, splints, walking cast and adhesive strapping. All of these treatment phases must be somewhat more extensive and protection must be carried out for eight to ten weeks since there is marked functional loss in the ligament. If such a long period of immobilization is required, formal rehabilitation becomes necessary. Usually rehabilitation is required in direct proportion to the length of time it was necessary to immobilize the joint.

Following operative repair, posterior and lateral below-knee stirrup splints (see Fig. 315) are applied for about 10 to 12 days. Then stitches are removed and a walking boot cast (see Fig. 317) is applied which the patient will wear for three weeks. Then strapping and rehabilitation commence. Actually, rehabilitation will be much less necessary if a walking cast has been used since the muscles in the extremity that are not immobilized by the cast will be in good condition. I do not believe the oft-repeated statement that "Ligament injuries are worse than fractures." This aphorism has arisen from the fact that serious ligament injuries have been undertreated and so the consequences have been more severe than those from an adequately treated fracture. Careful investigation of the patient having painful recurrent sprains of the ankle will probably uncover an initial injury that was treated inadequately.

Figure 400.   This 19 year old boy received an injury to his right ankle two years ago which was seen here four months post-injury with complete instability of the lateral collateral ligament. A Watson-Jones reconstruction was done four months after the injury, resulting in good stability. The opposite (left) foot then had an identical situation. He hurt this left ankle one year ago and received the same casual treatment which he received on the first injury and again had complete loss of the lateral collateral ligament.

A, Anteroposterior view of both ankles. Note hole for the reconstruction in right fibula.

B, Stress film on both sides. Right shows good stability with tilt within the acceptable range. Left shows complete dislocation of the talus out of the mortice. The stress film on the right originally looked exactly like the present film on the left. More thorough treatment of the original injury might have prevented this chronic instability.

Fractures

I have noted above that while the most common injury to the ankle is sprain and is an inversion injury, the most common eversion injury to the ankle is actually fracture. The two most important factors in the treatment of fractures about the ankle are: (1) maintenance of the integrity of the ankle mortice, and (2) complete re-establishment of the weight-bearing surfaces of the talus and tibia.

Good function of the ankle will not follow uncorrected separation between the tibia and fibula with corresponding widening of the ankle mortice. While irregularity of the weight-bearing surface is usually quite obvious on x-ray examination, separation of the ankle mortice may not be so readily apparent. It is extremely important that one carefully analyze the relationship between the tibia and fibula in order to determine whether there is separation between the two with widening of the mortice. Actually, the vast majority of fractures around the ankle are malleolar fractures. If they are complete, they have been accompanied by some dislocation of the ankle.

If there is a fracture of the lateral malleolus with displacement and with no fracture of the medial malleolus there is usually avulsion of the medial collateral ligament. If there is a fracture of the medial malleolus by an inversion force, an avulsion of the lateral ligament must be present. If there has been a fracture of the medial malleolus because of an eversion force, either the lateral malleolus must be broken, or the tibiofibular ligament ruptured. The same force that causes a bimalleolar fracture may cause fracture of the medial malleolus with ruptured tibiofibular ligament or it may cause rupture of the medial ligament and rupture of the tibiofibular ligament with no fracture at all. Thus, it can be seen that the treatment of ligament injuries and fractures of the ankle are inseparable. If the two basic goals are borne in mind, namely, the integrity of the ankle mortice and the restoration of normal weight-bearing surfaces, the type of treatment indicated is clear.

Figure 401. Bimalleolar fracture with adequate internal fixation. In this instance the lateral screw transfixes the fibular fracture site and enters the tibia, coming through medially far enough that it can be removed from the opposite side if it breaks. In other instances an intramedullary pin may be placed in the fibula.

Actually, it is not common for the weight-bearing surfaces to be involved. Ordinarily the lower end of the tibia and the upper end of the talus are not fractured in ankle injuries so that the fracture that is actually being discussed here is the malleolar fracture. This is caused by the same forces that cause sprains.

In bimalleolar fractures, it is virtually impossible to obtain and maintain accurate reposition of both malleoli without internal fixation at least in one of them. In these cases, internal fixation has long been the rule. The excellent results obtained by this method have encouraged me to apply it to injuries apparently less severe. With fracture of the medial malleolus accompanied by a tibiofibular separation, I feel that open reduction should be carried out, and the internal malleolus accurately replaced and held by screw or some other method of fixation (Fig. 401). At the same time, the tibia and fibula should be held together by a long metal screw transfixing the lower fibula and crossing both cortices of the tibia. Since it has been demonstrated that under normal usage there is definite motion in the distal tibiofibular joint, I consider it advisable to remove the screw that holds the tibia and fibula together after a suitable interval for healing of the tibiofibular ligament. This period is usually between 8 and 12 weeks. It is not unusual for the screw to break in the interval between the two bones when normal activity is resumed earlier. If this happens it is extremely difficult to remove the tibial section of the screw (Fig. 402). This is of little consequence, however, since once the screw breaks normal motion is permitted and it is usually not necessary to remove either part of the broken screw. If the injury is a fracture of both malleoli, it is better to use internal fixation on both sides unless the lateral malleolus is quite stable after reduction with internal fixation of the medial malleolus.

Figure 402.   A, Fracture-dislocation of the ankle, treated by two transfixion screws.
Note that the upper screw is broken whereas the one which is slightly bent is intact. B, The
screws were later removed but the broken fragment was inaccessible. Note that it has freed
itself from the fibula by forming a cul-de-sac in the bone around the screw. This is visualized
even better in the lateral view (C). Note the *talotibial* spurs in this young athlete.

The techniques of these various surgical procedures are readily available elsewhere and need not be described here. Surgical treatment should be carried out only
by one well versed in the anatomy of the ankle. The proper surgical environment is
a *sine qua non* to success.

Since in many instances open surgery may be simpler to carry out and easier
to manage postoperatively than manipulative treatment, it follows that adequate
training is essential before any physician should attempt to manage a serious frac-
ure or dislocation about a joint.

Only by extreme care in examination, conscientious selection of the best
method of treatment and thorough preparation in technique can one expect to obtain optimum results in treatment of injuries about the ankle.

EXOSTOSES

This condition in its various manifestations appears quite frequently about the
ankle and foot, in fact, so frequently on the top of the talus and the front of the
tibia that it has been described as a separate entity namely, *talotibial exostoses.* An
exostosis should be distinguished from a marginal osteophyte. An exostosis is an
actual piling up of bone at the site of the irritative lesion whereas the marginal
osteophyte is an osteochondral ridge developing at the joint margin as a result of a
chronic synovitis or chronic arthritic change. An exostosis will characteristically
develop as a response to direct trauma so that it may be seen on the back or front
of the lower margin of the tibia, less frequently in front of the medial malleolus or
of the lateral malleolus due to impingement of the talus. On the talus the exostosis
forms just back of the head superiorly (Fig. 405). Here the trauma results from
repeated overflexion or overextension, overinversion or overeversion of the ankle
joint beyond its ordinary range. For example, with the foot driven into dorsiflexion,

Figure 403. Roentgenograms showing the area of opposition between the tibia and talus. A, The foot in a neutral position. B, The foot in dorsiflexion. C, The foot in hyperdorsiflexion.

the leading edge of the tibia impinges against the concavity of the neck of the talus. The resulting irritation causes a piling up of bone that simply serves to aggravate the condition.

It will be recalled that, in extreme dorsiflexion of the foot, the anterior lip of the tibia nestles into the sulcus which is located on top of the talus between its body and head. It should be noted that the leading edge of the lower end of the tibia normally inclines backward in order to prevent impingement against the talus during dorsiflexion (Fig. 403). There actually is no true ligamentous attachment at either of these locations. The anterior capsule of the joint attaches slightly higher on the tibia and runs forward to the navicular with little attachment to the superior surface of the neck of the talus. Spur formation in this region is the result of direct trauma during forcible dorsiflexion of the foot on the leg. It is not the late result of a ligament injury caused by extreme plantar flexion at the ankle, so-called "traction sprain." The injury occurs, not during ordinary running, but during the "drive" of the athlete when his cleats are fixed to the ground with the foot forcibly dorsiflexed and the neck of the talus in direct apposition to the tibia (Fig. 404).

In many instances, much more often than is usually noted, the reaction to direct trauma during such "driving" running is the formation of bone at the area of impingement. This reaction apparently is similar to the formation of calluses on the skin. This mass has an adverse rather than a protective effect, however, for the more bone that is piled up, the more easily the impingement occurs, and so a vicious cycle is formed resulting in gradually increasing disability.

Characteristically, the player loses his "drive." As a rule, he has rather vague complaints which do not seem sufficient to account for his disability. Ordinary examination reveals little; there is no swelling, no pain on inversion or eversion, and no tenderness around the malleoli. The impression grows among teammates and coaches that the player is "dogging it." This is especially likely since he can often run, cut and jump without pain so long as he does not go at full speed. The result may well be disappointment of the coaches, disheartenment of the player, and the ultimate blighting of an otherwise promising athletic career.

Figure 404.   Avulsion of the capsular attachment on top of the talus, together with fragment of bone 18 months after injury. This probably was a relatively big fragment to start with and since then has calcified. The patient's complaint now is on forceful running which impinges the fragment against the lower end of the tibia, similar to a talotibial spur.

Such a patient presents himself with a history of aching pain in the ankle sharply increased by "driving," often to the point that he feels he cannot "go all out." He is unable to explain his failure to get that extra push that differentiates the star from the ordinary athlete. He simply realizes that his previous speed and force have been unaccountably diminished.

Examination will almost uniformly elicit particular findings. One is pain on forcible dorsiflexion of the foot—an impingement type of pain located at the anterior talotibial sulcus. Another is pinpoint tenderness directly over the spur on the talus or tibia. Roentgenographic examination will reveal that the anterior margin of the lower end of the tibia has lost its slanted character and that the edge is sharp, often with an identifiable exostosis extending forward over the articular surface of the talus (Fig. 405, *A*). The condition may vary from a simple change in contour to a spur a centimeter or more long. This spur extends along the whole width of the bone and is in reality a ledge rather than a spur. In addition, an exostosis of a greater or lesser size may appear on the top of the neck of the talus. Upon dorsiflexion of the foot, the two will be seen to impinge (Fig. 405, *B*). Either one or both of these exostoses may be present.

These prominences are relatively small in the early stages but may be tremendous in the later stages, at which time the diagnosis becomes obvious. The condition may extend onto the front of the medial malleolus and, rarely, to the anterior edge of the fibula; in severe cases it may also occur in other areas of the foot in which there are impinging bones, such as the posterior part of the ankle. These exostoses appear to be similar to but are not etiologically the same as the spurring that is found on adjacent articular surfaces, such as the metatarsal-

Figure 405.   *A*, X-rays showing talotibial spurs, 3 plus. *B*, Showing impingement occurring when the foot is dorsiflexed.

cuneiform joints. The latter condition is almost always accompanied by degenerative change in the articular cartilage and an actual narrowing of the joint space and falls into the category of chronic arthritic change or so-called "marginal osteophytes." This is not the condition to which we are referring when we speak of impingement exostoses of the talus and tibia. The typical impingement exostosis is most common at the anterior edge of the tibia and neck of the talus and is not accompanied by marginal osteophytes, degenerative changes (Fig. 406), or other signs of chronic joint involvement. This is reflected in the prognosis since the result, from an athletic viewpoint, can hardly be classed as excellent if degenerative changes in the foot and ankle or, in fact, any other changes persist. The conditions may co-exist, but one is not necessarily the forerunner of the other. When severe, the impingement exostosis may be extremely disabling, precluding athletics or any real activity. In some instances the spur is broken off and is found as a loose body lying on top of the talar neck. As such, it may cause acute disability in an ankle already chronically impaired.

It seems doubtful that the condition is initiated by repeated mild sprain of the

Figure 406.   Advanced tibiotalar exostoses. Note degenerative change between talus and
fibula. Remaining tarsal joints are not degenerative. This is not degenerative arthritis.

very weak anterior capsule. Rather, it would appear that the reaction is initiated by
repeated mild traumata caused by direct impingement and is often made severe by
acute injury. There seems no question but that repeated insult is the definitive
factor in this progressive syndrome.

In order to determine its frequency we checked a long series of students of the
same age group and of the same general characteristics. One-half of them were athletes and one-half were nonathletes. We found that the presence of talotibial spurring was much more frequent in the athletes (Table 1), 45 per cent of them having

TABLE 1.   ROENTGENOGRAPHIC FINDINGS IN A SURVEY OF THE
ANKLES OF 120 ATHLETES AND NON-ATHLETES

ATHLETES		NON-ATHLETES	
No exostosis	66 (55%)	No exostosis	101 (84.2%)
Exostoses in only one bone		Exostoses in only one bone	
Talar		Talar	
Grade 1 14		Grade 1 8	
Grade 2 3		Grade 2 1	
17 (14.2%)		9 (7.5%)	
Tibial		Tibial	
Grade 1 4 (3.3%)		Grade 1 6 (5%)	
	21 (17.5%)		15 (12.5%)
Exostoses in both bones		Exostoses in both bones	
Grade 1 22		Grade 1 2	
Grade 2 7		Grade 2 2	
Grade 3 4			
	33 (27.5%)		4 (3.3%)
Total	120 (100%)	Total	120 (100%)

(From the Journal of Bone and Joint Surgery, Vol. 39A, p. 851.)

some degree of spurring while only 15 per cent of the nonathletes did. It should be understood these were nonsymptomatic cases.

The mere presence of a spur is not justification for *treatment* since the great majority of them are completely nonsymptomatic. Surgical treatment is highly successful in young, healthy adult males provided the proper indications for it are present. The athlete is, of course, the one to whom surgical correction has the most appeal since if he has to restrict his activity he is no longer an athlete. On the other hand, the casual player may well prefer to give up his athletic activities rather than to submit to surgical correction.

It should be re-emphasized that the condition we are calling talotibial exostosis is not accompanied by degenerative change in the joint. Frequently, as mentioned previously, the ankle joint will be surrounded by marginal osteophytes resulting from chronic degenerative changes in the articular cartilage. These are characterized by roughened joint space, eburnated articular cartilage, chronic pain in the joint and an altogether different picture than that of exostosis. Prognostically there is vast difference since cleaning up of the marginal osteophytes has little effect upon the chronic arthritis that is present, and will as a rule prove disappointing. It may be necessary in case the osteophyte is large or fragmented, but one should not be misled into believing that the ankle will be wholly cured by removing the loose fragment from a degenerative joint. This condition (marginal osteophytes) is also quite frequent in the joints of the foot and will be discussed in this section.

OSTEOCHONDRITIS DISSECANS (CHONDRAL FRACTURE)

Osteochondritis dissecans has not been recognized as frequently in the ankle as it has in the knee. It is probably true that it does not occur as frequently. I am sure, however, that a great many more cases are overlooked than are recognized since the lesion is readily confused with an ankle sprain followed by traumatic arthritis in the ankle. The most common cause of the condition is trauma. By far the most frequent location for chondral fracture of the ankle is the dome of the talus where it occurs either on the superolateral margin of the talus, usually in a central location, or on the superomedial margin of the talus, usually posteriorly.

The mechanism of the injury has been described by many authors. It is an inversion type of injury (Fig. 407). Dorsiflexion of the foot forces the broader anterior part of the body of the talus deeper into the tibiofibular mortice so that there is snug contact between the long lateral malleolus and the lateral surface of the talus. If sharp inversion occurs in this position, the superior margin of the talus impinges forcibly against the side of the fibula. The resulting lesion is a snubbing type of fracture in which the cartilage of the superior surface of the talus is "peeled off" the subchondral bone, usually taking a greater or lesser fragment of bone with it. The resulting lesion is a flap of cartilage similar to a piece of linoleum being peeled off the floor. The force may be enough to actually dislodge the whole fragment or may simply hinge it upward, leaving the medial portion of the cartilage flap intact (Fig. 408).

This same inversion force as it drives the talus against the side of the fibula may cause chondral damage to the medial side of the lateral malleolus. The fibular

Figure 407.   Osteochondritis dissecans showing mechanism of injury. (Journal of Bone &
Joint Surgery, Vol. 41-A, 1959; A. L. Berndt and Michael Hardy.)

cartilage may be damaged (Fig. 409) but is much less likely to be since there is no
margin or edge to be peeled away. I recall one case of an extremely resistant ankle
injury with symptoms along the anterior fibulotalar fissure in which surgical exposure revealed a completely loose fragment of articular cartilage with a corresponding defect in the fibular articular surface.

     When the lesion of the dome of the talus (Fig. 410) is on the medial side the
cause, strangely enough, also appears to be an inversion injury. Since it occurs at
the back end of the superior surface of the talus, one must assume that it occurs
in plantar flexion when the weight of the body is on the narrow posterior portion
of the talus. In this position of the ankle joint, the talus may rock to a considerable
degree before any tension is placed on the collateral ligaments since the narrow
posterior width of the talus does not provide good bony stability in the too wide
mortice. Landing from a jump may cause direct trauma to a relatively small area,
the typical instance being the basketball player who leaps in the air and lands on
his toes with his foot slightly inverted. The mechanism in this instance is a compres-

Figure 408.   Chondral fracture of superolateral border of the talus. This is an inversion injury catching the corner of the talus against the fibula.

Figure 409.   Osteochondral fracture of the articular cartilage of the fibula, old. *A,* The fragment is rounded off and displaced downward. *B,* Following removal.

Figure 410.   An 18 year old baseball pitcher with persistent "sprain" of both ankles. He had had extensive treatment for sprain with prompt recurrence of symptoms on resumption of activity. Examination revealed none of the classic symptoms of sprain. In fact, interim examination was essentially negative, except for some discomfort on forced inversion. X-ray revealed chondral fractures of the superomedial angle of the talus of each ankle. Surgery

Figure 411.   Osteochondral fragment between medial malleolus and talus. This is not in the deltoid ligament.

sion type which dislodges the talar cartilage, together with some subchondral bone, quite similar to that which we visualize as happening at the knee in a direct blow on the patella with the knee flexed. These osteochondral fractures may occur at other places in the ankle or foot (Fig. 411). I do not recall having seen a case involving the head of the talus unless there was an actual fracture of the talar head in which a relatively larger fragment of cartilage and bone was broken off.

Osteochondral fracture occasionally occurs at the superior margin of the posterior articular surface of the navicular with characteristic x-ray appearance of the small fragment with a translucent area between it and the parent bone, giving a scooped-out appearance at the cartilage surface (Fig. 412). One must presume that these same fractures occur on the inferior surface of the talus and on the superior surface of the calcaneus but if so they are difficult to recognize and must be rare.

The most important single factor in diagnosis of these injuries is an acute awareness that they occur. It is recommended that in any injury to the ankle, x-ray study should be made even though the injury does not appear to be severe. I know of no way to diagnose these conditions in the acute stage except by x-ray examination. We have for long years insisted that x-rays be made. Perhaps too little time has

---

through an anteromedial incision parallel to the anterior tibial tendon exposed a normal talar cartilage (A). Dorsiflexion of the foot revealed a chondral fracture with nonunion (B). This was a large fragment with only a very small segment of bone attached (C). It was removed leaving a wide gap. (D). The sclerotic bed after curettement, being drilled with multiple drill holes with a K wire. This patient resumed baseball pitching after a few months without symptoms. Earlier diagnosis might have saved many disheartening months.

Figure 412. A, Chondral fracture of navicular. B, Patient treated for sprain of the foot for many months primarily by manipulation and physical therapy. Note fracture through the tubercle of the navicular, unrecognized. Also note extreme atrophy in spite of misguided efforts at making him exercise. Removal of the fragment resulted in gradual improvement.

been spent in emphasizing that the films should be adequately studied after they are made. When these injuries occur they are often seen as emergencies. The pictures are frequently taken by a substitute technician. The films are usually examined briefly in the darkroom before they are completely fixed or dried. Such casual study will not reveal these lesions. Injuries to the ankle and foot should be x-rayed in at least three directions, namely, an anteroposterior view of the ankle, anteroposterior view of the foot and a lateral view showing foot and ankle. If there is the slightest doubt about complete visualization, oblique views should be made. In studying the film one should carefully outline each involved bone as a separate entity. In his mind's eye or actually with a pencil he should follow along the line of the superior dome of the talus, being particularly careful where it superimposes over the tibia. The appearance of a cloudy shadow, any type of irregularity or any extra fissure line demands further study from different angles.

Many of these cases are not suspected until the so-called "sprain" has not responded well to treatment. Indeed, the majority of them will not be examined by a doctor in the early stages since the sprain itself may be relatively minor. These fractures, particularly those of the medial surface of the talus, may occur without any actual tearing of the ligaments of the ankle. The usual history is for the patient to present himself with a painful ankle which has resisted all the usual modalities of treatment. Sometimes the treatment for the original injury was quite inadequate (Fig. 413). At other times completely adequate treatment for a sprain has been carried out. In spite of the measures used, the symptoms persist much longer than they should in a sprain. Careful examination at this time will soon determine that one is not dealing with a "chronic sprain" of the ankle. There is no tenderness along the lateral collateral ligaments. There are no symptoms involving the tip of the lateral malleolus or along the cuboid or superolateral surface of the foot. The local symptoms, if any, will be actually in the ankle joint, either at the anterolateral confluence of the talus, tibia and fibula or along a similar area on the posteromedial side of the joint. Such a case presenting with chronic symptoms that are aggravated by activity and that subside almost completely with rest is very frequently an osteochondral fracture. By that time the condition which we identify

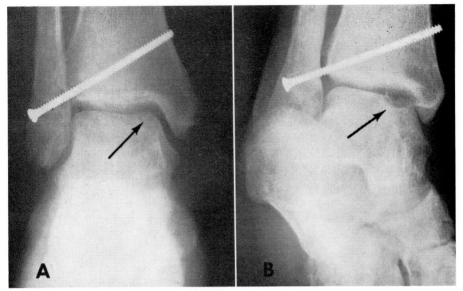

Figure 413. Case treated elsewhere for rupture of deltoid and tibiofibular ligament. Patient remained symptomatic. Examination of x-rays revealed chondral fracture of the superomedial surface of the talus. The patient improved after removal of this fragment and removal of the screw. Note incomplete reduction of tibiofibular diastasis.

as osteochondritis dissecans (although it is neither dissecting nor is it an osteo-chondritis) may be present. Careful x-ray study will reveal the typical appearance with a crater in the articular surface usually occupied by a line of opacity sur-rounded by an area of radiolucency (Fig. 414). In many instances only the crater appears since the fragment may be dislodged from the bone or may not throw

Figure 414. Osteochondritis dissecans of superolateral portion of the talus.

enough shadow to show in the film. This is particularly true in older cases. One should not withhold treatment simply because the opacity is not present.

Treatment.   It is my opinion that, in the vast majority of cases, treatment is surgical. True enough, we have learned (particularly at the knee and also at some nonweight-bearing joints) that a prolonged period of protection against weight bearing may permit these conditions to heal, particularly in the young individual. It has been suggested by some that this period should be at least six months and by others as long as a year. In my experience, the success of conservative treatment has not been great enough to justify denying weight bearing to an active young athlete for a period of a year. On the other hand, surgical treatment has been almost uniformly successful in those cases in which a pure lesion was involved. This qualification is made because a longstanding osteochondritis dissecans may cause irreversible chronic arthritic changes in the joint cartilage and in the capsular structures. In such an instance simple elimination of the primary lesion will not cure the condition even though it may result in marked improvement. It is my belief, therefore, that early operation is desirable.

In the unusual instance in which the injury is recognized at once, there may be some justification for conservative treatment. One should bear in mind, however, that no weight bearing can be permitted. Elimination of weight bearing is not accomplished in the walking cast. In fact, the only way I know for one to be relatively certain of no weight bearing is to use a long leg cast with the knee flexed to 90 degrees. Since all admit that many months of casting is necessary, this treatment is not without its hazards and is, to say the least, very onerous to the young and active athlete. It would not be tolerable in an adult. It might conceivably be tolerated by a youngster under 12. The only justification for such nonsurgical treatment would be the risk of surgery and the belief that surgery is not highly successful. Neither of these is a tenable presumption. Treatment, therefore, of these fractures is surgical at whatever stage they are seen.

In the lateral lesion the area may be approached by an extremely atraumatic incision over the anterolateral ankle parallel to and just lateral to the peroneus tertius tendon (Fig. 415). The dorsal retinaculum is divided, the anterior fasciculus

Figure 415.   Anterolateral approach: *A*, The skin incision. *B*, The skin has been separated, exposing the lateral edge of the extensor tendons. *C*, The tendon and muscles have been retracted and the capsule has been opened, exposing the spurs.

of the lateral collateral ligament is sectioned transversely and the capsule is exposed. Similarly, the medial side may be exposed by an incision medial to and paralleling the anterior tibial tendon. It is necessary to tie off the anterior division of the saphenous vein below the ankle. Both incisions may be made and the whole mass of tendons, vessels and nerves may be elevated forward out of harm's way. These approaches seem much better than the single incision directly anterior which involves the vascular bundle and the tendons.

In the early case, the capsule will be distended with blood. If the case is of longer duration, a diffuse synovitis will thicken the capsule. (The author recently operated in a case in which there was tremendously thickened synovium, at least ⅜ inch thick, which presented all the gross characteristics of a xanthomatous synovitis. A classical superolateral talar lesion was found and the other joint changes appeared to be confined to synovitis.) On dividing the capsule, the anterior margin of the lateral malleolus, the leading edge of the lower end of the tibia and the dome of the talus are exposed. On initial examination all of the cartilage appears to be intact and without any apparent defect, but as the foot is plantar flexed to expose the central portion of the talus, the defect comes into view. In the majority of instances the defect can readily be seen as a separate piece of cartilage, a depressed area with a cartilaginous wrinkle, or a fissure in the cartilage of the superior surface of the talus. In these cases the fragment can be readily lifted up and removed, using a small, curved hemostat or similar instrument. Since the fragment may be as long as 1 inch or more, it is frequently necessary to go back under the tibia to complete the removal. This can be more easily accomplished if its anterior portion is removed first since this allows ample room to explore the area completely. The chondral margin of the defect should be palpated carefully and any loose or undermined cartilage removed. The crater will present itself as an area lined with chronic granulation tissue which can be scraped away with a curette. The underlying bone is extremely sclerotic. The older the lesion, the more sclerotic the bed will be.

At the conclusion of this procedure there is a dished-out oval of bone including the superior lateral margin of the talus for a major portion of its middle one-third. This crater may be as large as ½ inch wide, ⅜ inch deep and 1 inch long, but as a rule it is smaller and is quite avascular even after brisk curetting. If this bed is sclerotic and avascular, it should be drilled (Fig. 28). Using a small size Kirschner wire and a hand drill, my own practice is to drill 8 to 12 holes in the bed deep enough to permit exudation of blood as the wire is removed. Several fresh drill points may be needed if the bone is extremely sclerotic. The area is not plugged with bone wax as in removal of marginal spurs since in this instance we want to encourage exudation of blood and formation of vascular buds at each of these drill holes. The wound is then closed in layers after thorough inspection and copious lavage of the whole operative area. One will be surprised to discover a considerable amount of debris in the basin after lavaging a joint which to the eye appeared quite clean. The lateral collateral ligament and the extensor retinaculum are carefully repaired. Posterior and lateral stirrup splints are applied to below the knee. At the end of 12 to 14 days the stirrup splints are removed, the stitches are removed and walking cast applied. This is worn for an additional two weeks depending to some extent upon the attendant joint changes since the ankle joint should be protected longer if there has been longstanding chronic synovitis.

Insofar as the bone lesion is concerned, I am convinced that early weight bearing and active use are better than prolonged protection. If the fragment is still in place, prolonged protection is needed to permit it to unite to the talus, but after its removal and curettage of the bed, active use will stimulate formation of granulation tissue followed by scar and in many cases by metamorphosis of the scar into fibrocartilage. So, as soon as the operative reaction and attendant arthritic changes have subsided, activity is encouraged. Nor do I see any reason to limit the patient's physical activity provided the ankle remains relatively symptom-free. However, in contact sports I think the ankle should be carefully strapped to prevent recurrence of the type of injury that caused the condition in the first place. The prognosis is extremely favorable in those cases which have not progressed to chronic joint changes. Similar lesions occurring elsewhere in the ankle and foot should be treated in a similar fashion.

Some surgeons have recommended that the osteochondral fragment be removed, the bed freshened up and the fragment replaced and pinned to its bed. This seems to me quite unsuitable in the talus. In the first place the lesion is not usually recognized early when the fracture is fresh and union could be expected to occur. In the second place, a major portion of the lesion is pretty well covered by the lower end of the tibia and, while it is available for removal and the bed may be reached for curetting and for drilling, it would be extremely difficult to replace the fragment and pin it adequately without more exposure than seems justified. Exposure can be obtained laterally by transection of the lateral malleolus and medially by transection of the medial malleolus. However, these measures are not without danger of complications and at the very best needlessly prolong convalescence. The success of re-pinning the fragment would seem to depend upon early recognition and treatment. These are the very cases in which removal of the fragment also gives very good results. Following pinning of the fragment, a prolonged period of nonweight bearing is desirable. As pointed out above, this presents difficulties and is not acceptable to many young patients, so that their cooperation is likely to be poor. For these reasons I do not recommend replacement and internal fixation of the fragment.

SYNOVITIS

Synovitis is much less of a problem at the ankle than it is at the knee. Actually, some degree of synovitis will occur with any injury involving the capsule of the ankle joint but as an isolated condition it is seldom encountered. One therefore has to deal very infrequently with "water on the ankle" per se. The very nature of the ankle joint is not consistent with extensive effusion. There is relatively little synovium in the ankle, the joint space is snug and tight and there is actually no area of the ankle joint where the synovial surfaces are in contact with each other as they are, for example, in the suprapatellar pouch. Effusion will occur with injury or with disease and if it does the treatment is the treatment of synovitis anywhere, namely, rest, heat, aspiration of fluid, injection of a corticoid. As the condition improves one permits resumption of activities with active rehabilitation but with protection against overuse.

Injuries of
the Foot

ANATOMICAL CONSIDERATIONS

THE FOOT is an extremely ingenious mechanism designed to transfer the body weight from the leg to the ground. The arch of the foot provides an elastic, springy connection so that the jar of weight bearing is dissipated to a large extent before it reaches the long bones of the leg and thigh. It also has the function of improving locomotion by adding speed and agility to the gait. Additionally the foot is capable of rolling from side to side when contacting surface imperfections, so permitting the leg to remain vertical while the foot rolls into inversion or eversion.

The leg contacts the foot, not in the center of the foot but in its posterior one-third, so that the longer lever arm from the heads of the metatarsals to the ankle has a marked advantage over the shorter lever arm from the ankle to the back of the calcaneus. Space does not permit a full description of all the many joints of the foot or of its multiplicity of ligaments and tendons, each designed to improve function. A careful study of the anatomy of the foot is extremely interesting and quite rewarding to the surgeon who has to treat injuries to this area.

Basically, the foot is divided into three divisions: the posterior part, consisting of the talus and calcaneus; the central part consisting of the navicular, cuboid and the three cuneiforms; and the anterior part consisting of the metatarsals and the phalanges (Figs. 416, 417 and 418). Each of these areas has characteristics that serve to account for distinctive types of injuries. Thus, injuries to the posterior

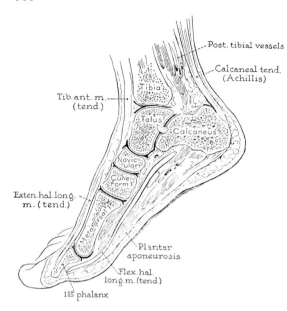

Figure 416. Sagittal section of right foot and ankle, showing bony structure and superficial muscles. (From Jones and Shepard, "Manual of Surgical Anatomy.")

division are usually of the compression type as the forceful drive of the leg into the foot collapses the bone. In the central portion of the foot, the injury is usually an avulsion type as the foot is forced through a range of motion beyond its capacity and either the ligament tears, the bone fractures, or both. In the anterior part, the injury is like that occurring in long bones anywhere.

The ankle is basically a hinge joint permitting flexion and extension of the foot on the leg. Lateral motion and circumduction occur largely on the pivot of

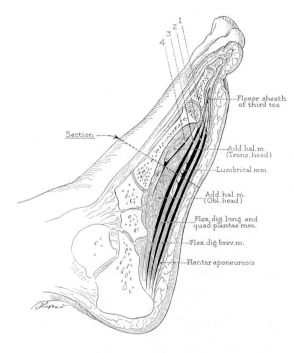

Figure 417. Sagittal section through plantar spaces (1, 2, 3, 4) of right foot. (From Jones and Shepard, "Manual of Surgical Anatomy.")

Figure 418. The bones of the right foot, viewed from below. (From Jones and Shepard, "Manual of Surgical Anatomy.")

the talonavicular joint, which is essentially a universal joint. This rotatory motion is permitted by the talocalcaneal and talonavicular joints, which in many motions act as a single unit. There is but slight motion in the remaining joints of the mid-foot, particularly the calcaneocuboid, the naviculocuneiform, the intercuneiform and the tarsometatarsal joints. This entire area of the foot is firmly bound together by ligaments from the front of the talus to the metatarsal heads. In dissection of the foot it is difficult to delineate the actual joint lines in the cuneiform-metatarsal areas, so close is the fit. Since there is such intricate apposition of the many bones of the foot, it is very important that the joint surfaces be maintained in the proper position and without undue irregularity. Failures in these respects account for the severity of the disability following what appears to be a relatively minor injury.

The general contour of the foot is that of a longitudinal arch resting posteriorly on the bottom of the calcaneus and anteriorly on the metatarsal heads. This arch is supported by the plantar ligament arising from the calcaneus and extending forward to attach near the metatarsal heads. In the normal foot the lateral portion of this arch rests on the ground, giving additional support to the foot. The plantar ligament is reinforced by the short flexors and other intrinsic muscles and ligaments of the foot. Thus, the integrity of the longitudinal arch is preserved by bony architecture, by strong ligaments and by active muscle.

The undersurface of the foot is covered with unusually heavy skin. The underlying fat pad is compartmented by dense, fibrous bands so that it makes a very adherent contact with the deep fascia. The skin of the sole does not slide back and forth as does the skin on top of the foot.

Muscle attachments are arranged to move the foot through its various ranges of active motion and still give static support. The synchronous action of the muscles of the foot is not dissimilar to that of the hand and wrist. The muscle assumes a different function depending upon the starting position of the foot and the motion involved. So also there are different functions of the muscles and varying tensions on the joint depending upon the position of the foot—in equinus, calcaneus, inversion or eversion. The rapidly reversing motions by the athlete cause excessive strain on the various components of the foot.

CONTUSION

Contusion of the foot is a frequent occurrence and may be caused by any sort of direct trauma as by a dropped weight or trampling or striking by another player. Contusion of the dorsum of the foot may be quite distressing because of the extremely sensitive nature of this area. Thin integument overlies the tendons, blood vessels and nerves so that they are caught between the underlying bone and the blow over thin skin.

The complications of contusion may be more important than the contusion itself. The blow may cause damage to a nerve causing intractable pain over the dorsum of the foot, damage to the blood vessels with phlebitis or hemorrhage, damage to the tendons with resulting tenosynovitis, damage to the periosteum or to the joints. Each of these conditions should be treated appropriately, the important element being recognition of the complication so that one will not continue to reassure the patient that he has a minor condition that will promptly recover when the patient is convinced that he has a rather severe condition that definitely is not recovering. This is particularly true of tenosynovitis which has the same tendency to recur here as elsewhere.

Contusions of the undersurface of the foot have the added complication of weight bearing. These frequently are caused by a faultily placed spike, a loose cleat, or even a wrinkle in the sock so that the subcutaneous tissue lying between the thick plantar skin and underlying bone and muscle becomes ecchymotic and reacts by inflammation, forming the characteristic "stone bruise." Under the heel or under the metatarsal heads this may be very persistent. The remedy is to relieve weight bearing until the condition has become arrested. This is frequently incompatible with athletic participation. It is particularly distressing to the track man or basketball player since it seems to him to be a minor condition yet it interferes with his effective competition. Early local injection with a long-acting anesthetic agent followed by one of the corticoid preparations is a valuable adjunct in the treatment. Certain ingenuity can be utilized to prevent weight bearing of the tender part and so permit running. This is a good deal more feasible in football shoes than it is in track or basketball shoes. The usual physical therapeutic measures are of some value in expediting recovery since they serve to improve the local circulation, relieve congestion and promote absorption.

STRAIN

Strain is particularly common in the foot. The complex of intrinsic muscles making up the foot is extremely extensive and is subjected to great forces by athletic activity. Some areas are much more frequently involved than others, one of the most common being the insertion of the TENDO ACHILLIS to the calcaneus. Strain here may be severely incapacitating since, each time the calf is contracted in walking or running, severe pain occurs at the attachment of the tendon to the heel. Another common location is at the attachment of the ANTERIOR TIBIAL on the medial side of the foot. Strain is particularly likely to occur here if there is a tendency for the athlete to pronate the heel so that the talus tends to rotate downward and inward in relation to the foot. The anterior tibial is the most active muscle in dorsiflexing the foot and is the opponent of the tendo achillis. Early in the season, running will frequently cause irritation at either site. Less frequently there will be strain at the attachment of the PERONEALS or of the POSTERIOR TIBIAL or of the FLEXORS OF THE TOES.

Treatment of strain has been detailed elsewhere (page 56). Elimination of stress is of prime importance. In the heel, strapping to prevent dorsiflexion of the foot and elevation of the heel by a pad in the shoe or an extra rubber heel will serve to relieve the condition provided violent activity is prevented. Physical therapy, especially local heat, is of value but protection is the true remedy for the condition. A longer period of complete disability will be rewarded by complete recovery whereas temporizing measures often will result in repeated recurrence. If the patient has had a strain of the attachment of the tendo achillis he probably should keep the foot strapped throughout the remainder of the season to prevent forcible dorsiflexion. True enough, this will not prevent active traction by the calf. It will reduce passive stretching which may be an important factor, particularly in contact sports. On the other hand, if the anterior tibial is injured the foot should be strapped to prevent extreme plantar flexion. The shoe should be wedged on the inner side of the heel to throw the weight toward the outer side of the foot (page 540).

While discussing strain of the tendo achillis attachment, one should mention APOPHYSITIS OF THE CALCANEUS (Fig. 419). This is another of the group of aseptic necroses which occur at various places in the epiphyses of the young athlete. At the calcaneus it is not ordinarily as disabling as at the hip or knee. The calcaneal epiphysis has a wide attachment to the calcaneus and therefore is not particularly subject to extensive irreversible necrosis. Faulty circulation is manifested by sclerosis of the epiphysis, frequently accompanied by fragmentation, but the condition is self-limited and usually does not demand drastic treatment. Symptomatically there is pain at the posterior point of the heel, usually somewhat below the actual attachment of the tendo achillis. Pain is elicited by forcible activity so that the adolescent can usually go about his regular activity without trouble only to have recurrence of pain if he starts to run or jump, or violently exercises his foot.

Unlike strain of the tendo achillis, this condition can usually be completely relieved by restricting dorsiflexion of the foot so that adequate strapping down the back of the leg and over the sole of the foot anchored properly around the ankle, combined with elevation of the shoe heel, is usually all the treatment that is necessary. In my experience a few weeks' reduction of activity will usually result in complete relief from symptoms although the x-ray evidence of apophysitis will persist for many months. The very acute or resistant case may require a walking cast for six to eight weeks. There is no residual except occasionally some prominence of the back of the heel which may cause symptoms by pressure against the heel of the shoe. During the acute stage, if the tenderness is quite acute it may be necessary to cut the counter out of the back of the shoe in order to relieve pressure

Figure 419. *A,* Typical calcaneal apophysitis indicated by sclerosis and fragmentation. *B,* Another manifestation of calcaneal apophysitis with irregular and delayed epiphyseal formation.

here, and to apply suitable felt padding. Obviously, if the condition is acute, athletics are contraindicated.

SPRAIN

We have defined sprain as a ligament injury and have discussed it particularly from the standpoint of the acute sprain. However, in the foot one must definitely distinguish between static sprain and the acute traumatic sprain.

Traumatic Sprain

Traumatic sprain of the foot is similar to sprain elsewhere and may be acute or chronic. It is caused by violent overstretching of a ligament or ligaments by forcing the involved joint through a wider range of motion than the ligaments will normally permit. The same force applied repeatedly may result in a chronic irritative lesion in the ligament itself. It is basically due to abnormal motion.

Treatment is similar to that of sprain anywhere. In the early stage local injection into the hematoma, compression, ice, followed by adequate support and local heat, is the treatment of choice. Usually support can be accomplished by adequate strapping and elimination of weight bearing, the exact type of support depending upon the ligament involved. Thus, if the sprain involves the calcaneocuboid ligament, it will be treated much like sprain of the ankle. In the plantar ligament it will be treated by support under the arch to prevent distraction between the heads of the metatarsals and the calcaneus. Acute sprain should be evaluated as to its severity since this will to a considerable extent determine the degree of immobilization and its duration. If the sprain has been due to inversion or eversion of the foot, suitable strapping of the ankle type (Fig. 398) is advisable since it is difficult to immobilize the foot properly without including the lower leg. This is particularly true of sprain of the arch where it is important to keep the foot inverted (Fig. 385). Additional support can be given by a wedge on the shoe heel so that, if an arch sprain is present, a medial heel wedge to invert the foot will relieve tension. If the sprain is in the lateral ligaments of the foot a lateral wedge on the heel or lateral Dutchman on the sole worn on a temporary basis for a matter of a few weeks will be of considerable value in relieving the strain until healing is complete.

If the injury appears to be quite severe at the time of the initial examination, careful x-ray study must be made to rule out any fracture or dislocation. The proper local treatment should then be instituted followed by elevation of the foot, compression bandage and ice pack overnight. Evaluation the next day will permit one to determine somewhat better the extent of injury. In some instances it may be necessary to continue elevation and cold followed by heat until swelling subsides sufficiently to permit application of plaster splint for a few days, followed by a plaster boot. This boot should be worn for ten days and followed by adequate strapping, arch support and wedge on the shoe heel until the foot is symptom-free.

The acute sprain may involve the intermetatarsal ligaments at the distal end of the metatarsal. It is particularly likely to occur in the track man who runs in a very light shoe or may run barefooted and receive an injury to his anterior ligaments. This should be treated in the usual manner but the strapping in this case should be circumferential around the forefoot. This must not be confused with chronic sprain of the intermetatarsal ligaments, which may be extremely resistant to treatment. Once the acute sprain occurs, the forefoot should be strapped for the remainder of the season.

Static Sprain

Static conditions of the foot constitute a comprehensive subject matter and will not be dwelt upon at length here. However, one will be called upon frequently to distinguish between a chronic sprain of the foot and a static sprain of the arch. Whereas the chronic sprain is due to repeated episodes of over-motion, the static sprain is due to the constant stress of superimposed weight on the arch of the foot. This is most frequently manifested by pain along the plantar ligament from the attachment of the calcaneus to its attachment near the metatarsal heads. It is promptly relieved by elimination of weight bearing. There is no history of any particular injury. The condition is more likely to occur early in the season when the patient abruptly changes from his regular shoes which have considerable support in the arch to the flat shoes of athletic equipment. This plus the superimposed weight of his equipment and more violent exercise plus long hours on his feet may combine to cause a sprain of the arch. The diagnosis is often suggested by the fact that the player has had foot trouble before and frequently is wearing arch support shoes or arch supports in his street shoes.

Treatment.   Static sprain of this type will not respond well to treatment indicated for acute sprains but should receive the treatment given for flatfoot, namely, support of the arch, improvement of the posture of the foot and reconstructive exercises (Fig. 420) to improve the muscle tone of the foot. When one recalls that the muscles of the foot are closely similar to those of the hand, he will recognize the importance of proper specific exercises for the so-called weak foot or chronic sprain. Participation in sports cannot be permitted without adequate support either by means of arch supports or adequate strapping since every recurrence of symptoms simply makes it more difficult to effect a complete recovery. This type of condition is not at all limited to "flatfoot." In fact, some of the most painful arches are the very high ones in which cases most of the body weight is carried on the metatarsal

Figure 420.   Reconstructive exercises for foot. Position: The patient sitting with the feet on a smooth, flat surface. These exercises should be done slowly and forcibly with maximum effort maintained for three seconds, 1-2-3.

A, Actively lift the toes, keeping the ball of the foot on the floor. This should be done 30 times.

B, Slide the foot forward so that the toes protrude beyond the edge. Flex toes downward 30 times.

C, Spread the toes widely 30 times. At first it may be necessary to assist this movement with the hands.

D, Raise the inner margin of the foot with the weight thrown on the outer margin. Curl the toes downward and backward in attempt to "make a fist."

E, Holding one foot firmly on the floor, place the other foot forward until it rests on the opposite heel. In this position, rotate the anterior part of the foot from the outside inward, so the tip of the right big toe makes a complete circle in a clockwise direction. Definite effort must be made to force this motion to the extreme. The left should turn counterclockwise.

These exercises must be done slowly to the count of 1-2-3 seconds, with a similar period between each movement. Distinct effort must be made to get the most possible motion and if this is done a definite strain will be felt upon the involved muscles. Exercises should be begun at about ten times apiece, gradually increasing it to 30 times apiece. They should be done twice daily.

You must not hurry through these exercises.

heads and on the heel. This subjects the plantar ligament and other inferior ligaments of the foot to considerable stress on weight bearing. A carefully outlined
program meticulously followed by the patient will give gratifying results. It should
be emphasized again that during the violent exercise of athletics the arch should
be protected by flexible cork and leather arch supports once it has been subject to
chronic sprain.

Chronic sprain of the intermetatarsal ligaments is evidenced by pain in the
area of the metatarsal heads. This may be a sequela of acute sprain or may be due
to static stretching of the ligaments. It must be treated by circumferential strapping,
metatarsal pad and anterior heel, but here again the treatment will likely be incompatible with athletic activity. Chronic sprain may be accompanied by or confused with plantar neuroma.

PLANTAR NEUROMA (Morton's Toe)

Plantar neuroma is a static condition of the foot that is relatively frequent in
athletes (Fig. 421). The player usually complains of a "sprain" of the anterior
arch. The symptom that distinguishes it from sprain is intermittent, excruciating
pain in the lateral part of the forefoot usually running into the adjacent sides of
the third and fourth toes and occasionally up the dorsum of the foot toward the
ankle. The condition is not ordinarily brought on by any specific motion or any
specific sprain. It comes on spontaneously when least expected. The patient is
usually much more comfortable barefooted whereas in sprain of the arch the foot
is not comfortable without the support of shoes. On examination tenderness will
be found between the third and fourth metatarsal heads, and it will be exquisite
on localized pressure in the plantar surface of the web between the third and
fourth toes when pressure is directed back toward the third and fourth heads. This
finding is best elicited by pressure of the rubber end of a pencil. Compression of
the metatarsal heads, particularly by rolling the heads across each other by lateral
pressure, will often elicit a definite click accompanied by pain, usually referred to
the third and fourth toes.

The cause of this condition is a neuroma of the plantar nerve at the point
where the medial and lateral branches join and then separate to pass to the adjacent sides of the third and fourth toes. The thickened area where the "x" is formed

Figure 421.   Plantar neuroma. Plantar aspect.

is subject to trauma when caught between the metatarsal heads. A predisposing factor is relaxation of the intermetatarsal ligaments which permits splaying of the forefoot. As a result of this irritative pressure an extremely large mass of nerve and fibrous tissue may gradually be formed. The larger the mass the more frequently it is caught between the metatarsal heads and the more severe the symptoms.

Once plantar neuroma has developed, the *treatment* is surgical by excision of the tumor mass. Relief is ordinarily dramatic. However, athletic competition will be interdicted for a matter of four to six weeks in order to permit recovery from the effects of the operation.

TENOSYNOVITIS

The foot is quite subject to tenosynovitis since its tendons are charged with the responsibility not only of motion but also of supporting considerable weight. The cause of tenosynovitis here is the same as in other locations, namely, a direct blow or chronic overuse. The latter is more important in the athlete. Frequently tenosynovitis is combined with other conditions such as strain of the tendon attachment. The resultant irritation causes friction between the tendon and its surrounding sheath with edema, inflammation and adhesions, all of which cause pain on active function. Characteristic findings are pain on passive stretching of the involved tendon, pain on active motion of the involved tendon, and tenderness over the tendon at the point of the irritation. Careful palpation over the tendon while active motion is carried out will often elicit "snowball" crepitation, which is diagnostic of tenosynovitis. The tendon sheath does not usually distend with excess fluid as does the joint in synovitis. Tenosynovitis is particularly prone to occur in the early phases of training, being especially frequent in track men particularly when they are training on the boards.

Treatment.   Tenosynovitis is another of those conditions which can be treated well only by elimination of the stress involved. This of necessity means elimination of competitive athletics. Other measures of importance in expediting the cure are local injection, local physical therapy and protection. In the foot it is difficult to prevent stress on the tendon without giving support to the arch. These cases frequently should be treated by a splint to prevent motion altogether, followed later by adequate strapping and wrapping to prevent excess motion. At the same time the splint and the strapping should support the arch of the foot. Caution should be used in application of the strapping so that it does not compress the tendon between it and the underlying bone since this may increase the irritation rather than diminish it.

Tenosynovitis involving the dorsiflexors, namely, the anterior tibial, peroneus tertius and toe extensors, should be treated by strapping the foot to prevent plantar flexion (see Fig. 13). Tenosynovitis of the posterior structures such as the calf, peroneals and posterior tibial should be strapped so that the foot will not dorsiflex beyond neutral and also to give lateral support (see Fig. 377). All too often, however, the irritating factor is function of the muscle rather than passive stretching of the tendon and continued forcible motion is incompatible with prompt recovery. Once recovery is complete, strapping is of great importance in preventing recurrence.

BURSITIS

Bursitis is not a common problem in injury to the foot although it is well to bear in mind that it may occur. A particularly distressing type of bursitis is involvement of the bursa lying between the calcaneus and skin on the plantar surface of the heel. This can be readily mistaken for strain of the attachment of the plantar ligament, particularly if spurs happen to be demonstrable at this attachment. It can usually be distinguished by the fact that tenderness is considerably further posterior on the heel than is usually the case in involvement of the plantar ligament. *Treatment* is by local injection, local application of heat, protective sponge rubber in the shoes and in severe cases by excision of the bursa. There may be a bursitis of the bunion joint but this is not frequent in athletes and requires no discussion here.

Another bursa frequently involved in the foot is that lying between the tendo achillis and the back of the calcaneus. The symptoms here may be readily confused with those of strain of the attachment of the tendo achillis. However, active contraction of the calf should not cause increase of symptoms in bursitis although local pressure does. Careful examination will usually distinguish the condition, the pain being just proximal to the attachment of the tendon to the calcaneus and anterior to the tendon. Tenderness may also be elicited by pressure in the space anterior to the tendo achillis. Rarely does the bursa enlarge enough to permit the fluid to be palpated or aspirated. *Treatment* consists of local injection and protection against pressure. In the acute phase, dorsiflexion of the foot should be prevented by strapping. This bursitis is not usually as resistant as apophysitis and not as recurrent as strain of the tendo achillis attachment.

SYNOVIAL HERNIA

Whereas synovial hernia is not particularly common in the ankle, it is frequent in the foot. This is explained by the multiplicity of joints and tendons in the foot, making legion the areas where chronic sprain followed by weakness of the capsule and herniation of the synovium may occur. It is not necessary to discuss these in detail in their various locations, but one or two deserve special mention here. One frequent area is near the peroneal tendon distal to the lateral malleolus. In this instance the herniation may be of extremely large size as in the case recently operated upon in which the mass was about the size and shape of one's long finger but came down to a single defect in the tendon sheath no larger than the point of a lead pencil (Fig. 421A). Another frequent area of involvement is the dorsum of the foot in the long extensor tendons where it may come off the tendon sheath or from the tarsal joints.

The *treatment* is the same as treatment of synovial hernia elsewhere (page 64). It cannot be overemphasized that if surgical treatment is undertaken it should be done as a major procedure under general anesthesia so that the sac can be meticulously dissected out and if at all possible repair made of the defect in the sheath or capsule if one is found. Chopping off the top of the mass through a ½ inch "medical" incision only results in scarring which makes a surgical procedure extremely diffi-

Figure 421A.   Lateral side injury of the peroneal tendons with resulting painful tumor alongside peroneal tendons. Section proved it to be a synovial hernia off the tendon sheath. *A,* The exposed mass. *B,* The dissection. *C,* Down to match-stem pedicle. *D,* The intact mass removed.

cult at a later time. Surgical excision should be followed by complete immobilization for at least the three weeks needed for ligament or capsule to heal. Resulting stiffness is not as common in the foot as it is in the wrist. No particular rehabilitation is necessary other than for the muscles which have been immobilized.

One can only condemn the treatment of these lesions by violent direct trauma, such as a sharp blow. Aspiration of the mass followed by pressure dressing can be readily done in the foot and is an acceptable measure. Some have reported unbelievably good results from injection of steroids but in my experience this has rarely had any more effect than simple aspiration of the lesion. Repeated aspiration particularly in the foot entails the hazard of ultimate infection and is probably not justified by the results. In several cases in which surgery has followed corticoid injections we have seen plaques of calcific-like material within the sac or in the adjacent tissues. These have been ascribed to irritation from the injection but the matter will require further investigation.

A synovial hernia of moderate size is not incompatible with athletic activity. There is really no objection to permitting athletic competition and postponing removal of the hernia to a later time, provided adequate strapping is utilized and symptoms are not severe enough to interdict active use.

DISLOCATION

Dislocation of the foot is not frequent in athletics. It is much more infrequent than ankle dislocation for obvious reasons. The foot is protected by the shoe and frequently by wrapping and is not subject to the violent disruption stresses that may dislocate the ankle or knee. When a severe injury to the foot occurs, careful study of the x-rays should be carried out, comparing them with films of the opposite foot. Particularly to be looked for is a possible separation of the tarsal joints. A common type of dislocation is one extending along the foot between the first and second metatarsal bases, along the internal and middle cuneiforms, and across the foot laterally at the level of the metatarsal cuboid joints (Fig. 422). This may be suspected from a tendency of the foot to be broader in this area with characteristic widening of the joint space, the wider space angulating across the foot. The base of the fifth metatarsal is more prominent than normal and pressure here is quite painful. The tip of the base of the metatarsal may be broken off so that the shaft is actually lateral to the proximal tip. This represents a serious disruption of the ligaments of the foot and should be treated by complete reduction and internal fixation. If it is not treated or is treated overcasually, the result is broadening of the forefoot,

Figure 422.   A, Dislocation through the first and second metatarsal, the inner and middle cuneiform, between the middle cuneiform and navicular, the navicular and cuboid. Note definite increase in space between the middle and medial cuneiform and the medial cuneiform and distal side of the navicular. This is an old dislocation and was relieved by reduction and surgical fusion between the inner and middle cuneiform.

B, Postoperative picture showing dislocation between the medial and middle cuneiform held with two fine staples. Fusion of this joint was carried out.

Figure 423.   Result of unreduced dislocation similar to that in Figure 422 with gross disability. Note the displacement between the first and second metatarsals extending along the metatarsal cuneiform and cuboid joints with lateral displacement. *Right,* The normal foot for comparison.

chronic strain of the tarsal joints and marked incapacity which is extremely difficult to treat at a later stage (Fig. 423). In such obviously severe injuries of the forefoot a particular effort must be made to be sure that the swelling, pain and disability are not actually due to a persistent displacement or to a spontaneously reduced dislocation.

Other examples of dislocation are illustrated in Figures 424, 425 and 426.

Figure 424.   Fracture-dislocation of the foot. Note fracture extending across the bases of metatarsals 2-3-4 with lateral dislocation of the base of M-5. The whole unit is displaced laterally. This is a disabling type injury if not reduced by approximating the shaft of M-2 to M-1. This is similar to the injury in Figure 422.

Figure 425.   Unusual case of compound dislocation of ankle and foot. Note that the talus is tipped out of the ankle mortice but the deltoid ligament is apparently intact. Talus is also dislocated on the tarsus.

Figure 426.   A, Fracture-dislocation in tarsal-metatarsal region. This is similar to that of Figure 422 except that the defect continued back through the navicular by breaking its middle third. B, The follow-up shows good healing of the navicular but widening of the space between the first and second rays. This probably could have been prevented by early open reduction and internal fixation.

Dislocations of the toes are not frequent but should be promptly recognized and completely reduced. Support is usually provided adequately by strapping the injured toe to the adjacent toes, which are used as a splint. With well fitted shoes and firm soles, continued activity is justifiable. The habit of playing competitive sports in sock feet is to be deplored since the shoe is an excellent protection for the foot.

FRACTURE

The anatomical division of the foot into posterior, middle and anterior portions has definite clinical value in consideration of fractures.

Fracture of the Posterior Portion of the Foot

This section of the foot, including as it does the talus and calcaneus, is rarely fractured in athletics if sprain-fractures are excluded. The ordinary fracture here is by direct compression as in a fall from a height or from driving the foot into the floor board of a car (Figs. 427 and 428). Fortunately, neither of these causes is common in athletics. Certain fractures do occur in special situations such as have been described in the section on the ankle. Abnormal forceful motion may cause avulsion (Figs. 429, 430 and 431) or snubbing fractures of the talus (Fig. 432). So also the sustentaculum tali may be broken by forceful eversion of the foot (Fig. 427). It is extremely important to restore the contour of the calcaneus and particularly the integrity of the talocalcaneal joint. Adduction or abduction of the foot may cause a snubbing (Fig. 433) or avulsion fracture of the superior portion of the calcaneus at the calcaneocuboid joint. If the fragment is large and displaced it should be replaced surgically if necessary. The smaller fragment may be treated as a sprain and recovery will be good (Fig. 434).

Figure 427.   Compression fracture in talocalcaneal area as the pole vaulter landed on the edge of the pit. Note the fracture of the sustentaculum tali in the lateral view. This could be easily overlooked.

Figure 428. Persistently painful heel after sharply striking the ground. *A,* The negative lateral film. *B,* Two weeks later showing condensation at the ball of the calcaneus indicating a compression fracture.

Figure 429. Avulsion of the posterior portion of the talus in blown-up view. Note the shape of the avulsed fragment which would fit right on the posterior end of the talus. This is not an os trigonum. This is the result of a dorsiflexion injury, the same forces that cause tibiofibular separation.

Figure 430. A forcible dorsiflexion injury. Note the separate fragment at the back of the talus. This is an actual fracture of the posterior process of the talus, not os trigonum. Note normal foot (*right*) showing unusually long posterior process. The mechanism here is probably snapping off of this posterior process as the back of the talus comes forcibly against the top of the calcaneus. This patient had been treated for a "minor strain" and was still very symptomatic three months later. Removal of the fragment relieved the symptoms.

Figure 431. Avulsion of the superior margin of the head of the talus. Detachment of the anterior capsule.

Figure 432. A, Fracture through anterior portion of the body of the talus, result of forcible plantar flexion injury. B, Result nine months after open reduction and internal fixation.

Figure 433.   Snubbing fracture of overhanging anterosuperior margin of calcaneus, caused by plantar flexion of the foot forcing the cuboid upward. The same force caused partial avulsion of the superior lip of the navicular.

Figure 434.   Sprain-fracture of lateral margin of calcaneus, an inversion injury.

Fracture of the Central Portion of the Foot

This portion of the foot includes the navicular, cuboid, and first, second and third cuneiforms. This section is extremely well bound together by the various ligaments and moves almost as a unit. Compression fractures may occur in these bones but they are usually not recognized as such unless there has been a major injury to the foot. A much more common fracture in athletics is avulsion of an adjacent fragment of bone by the ligament at the time of dislocation or subluxation of the joint. This may be between the cuneiforms or between the cuneiforms and the cuboid or navicular. In the dislocation between the first and second metatarsals, then between the first and second cuneiforms and then across between the navicular and cuboid, there may be one or more areas of fracture (Fig. 426). That is, the injury may split the middle cuneiform rather than cause dislocation between the first and second; the posterior portion of the cuboid may fracture rather than dislocate between the cuboid and navicular. These are modifications of the same injury and require the same treatment; namely, firm fixation in perfect position until union occurs. Surgery may be necessary to accomplish this end. Bony fusion of the joint is considerably more functional than hypermobility or painful motion and results in no particular handicap. Several weeks will be needed for union and during this period the foot should be carefully immobilized in a cast that molds the arch into perfect position. A walking cast is not advisable. When the cast is removed and tape applied, protection should be supplied by a molded arch support for many months since chronic disability of the foot is frequent following fractures in this area.

Fracture of the Anterior Portion of the Foot

By far the most common area for fracture is the anterior portion of the foot which consists of the long bones of the metatarsals and phalanges.

Fracture of the Metatarsals. The five metatarsals are long bones that are firmly bound together by overlapping layers of ligament at their bases, held together in the midshaft by the interosseous membrane and at the distal ends by the plantar and dorsal divisions of the distal intermetatarsal ligament.

Figure 435.   Typical avulsion fracture at base of the fifth metatarsal.

Figure 436.   Fracture of the bases of the second, third and fourth metatarsals caused by a sharp hyperflexion injury as the player was hit on the leg from behind. This is one of the hazards of "clipping."

FRACTURE OF THE BASE OF THE METATARSAL.   The most frequent fracture is at the base of the fifth metatarsal (Fig. 435). This conical base with its tip posterior is considerably weaker than the quadrilateral bases of the other metatarsals (Fig. 436). The strong attachment of the peroneus brevis plus the massive lateral ligament attachments tend to fix the base of this metatarsal as the forefoot is sharply inverted and adducted and a greater or lesser fragment of the base of

Figure 437.   *A,* Metatarsal fractures resulting from a fall from a horse when the foot caught between the horse and road. *B,* Skeletal traction was ineffectual. *C,* Open reduction with transfixion pin and threaded wire resulted in a normal foot. There is no epiphyseal disturbance of the metatarsals as yet. (The line across the base of the proximal phalanx of the first toe in *A* is an artifact.)

Figure 438.   *A,* Comminuted fracture of shaft of first metatarsal. *B,* Postoperative view
after traction.

this bone may be pulled away. This is essentially a sprain-fracture and may be treated as such. Nonunion of the fragment is not unusual and while not necessarily disabling it may be quite painful. Immobilization in plaster splints followed by a walking cast for a total of four weeks will usually give firm enough fixation that taping and a good stout shoe may then be used for support. If painful nonunion persists the fragment, if small, may be removed and the attachments replaced to the metatarsal. If the fragment is large, internal fixation may be necessary.

On the opposite side of the foot the base of the first metatarsal is not often the site of fracture, owing not only to its sturdy structure but to the fact that the stresses applied to this side are not as great as those on the lateral side.

The metatarsal bases may be involved in fracture-dislocation in which a portion of the base is snubbed off as the shaft is forced away from its normal position (Fig. 424). These fractures are usually caused by sharp dorsiflexion or forcible plantar flexion of the foot. The result may be extremely distressing particularly if the lesion is not recognized. Careful x-ray study will usually reveal the fracture, particularly when one's attention is called to it by sharply localized tenderness. It is important that the integrity of the joint surfaces be restored as fully as possible, particularly if there is tendency for a portion of the bone to subluxate. In these cases reduction should be followed by fixation with transfixion Kirschner wire, the wire being passed across the bases of the intact bones and through the involved bone after complete reduction.

FRACTURE OF THE SHAFT OF THE METATARSAL.   Metatarsal shaft fractures are similar to those of long bones elsewhere. The presence of five bones in the same plane allows each one to protect the other to some extent. The cause may be a crushing force applied over the dorsum of the foot as it is resting on the ground, or forcible torsion of the forefoot on the tarsus. Examination reveals tenderness over the involved area with swelling and hematoma formation. Diagnosis can be confirmed by x-ray study. If there is gross displacement, the fracture should be reduced and held in good position. This may require open reduction. Frequently if only one shaft is involved it may hold well without internal fixation (Figs. 438 and 439). In a comminuted, oblique or spiral fracture of several shafts, skeletal traction may be needed through the toes to secure proper alignment of the bones (Fig. 437). Particular attention should be paid to the space between the metatarsals, best judged by comparison with the opposite foot. If the bases of these bones tend to separate they can frequently be held in good position by threaded Kirschner wires transfixed through several metatarsals after the bones have been placed in normal position. Fracture of the metatarsals is an extremely disabling injury to an athlete and complete healing must be secured before competition is permitted. An arch support should be worn, particularly in athletic shoes.

Isolated fatigue fracture of the metatarsal shaft may occur from strain (pages 65 and 616). Indeed, excessive strain may cause complete fracture with displacement as the leverage is applied to the metatarsal heads with the foot in equinus.

Figure 439. Fracture of proximal end of the shaft of the fifth metatarsal. Note bipartite medial sesamoid to first toe.

Figure 440.   Typical fracture of the neck of the fourth metatarsal. This view shows a little plantar rotation of the head of the metatarsal and clinically the head was quite prominent in the sole of the foot. This deformity should be corrected to prevent painful metatarsal head. There is an incomplete fracture of M-3.

FRACTURE OF THE HEAD AND NECK OF THE METATARSAL.   Fracture through this area in the foot is not nearly so frequent as in the hand. Ordinarily there is little displacement and simple fixation and protection from weight bearing will suffice (Fig. 440). However, if the fracture is unrecognized and malunion or nonunion occurs, the metatarsal head may be removed. This is not to be recommended for an acute injury since union can usually be obtained without it if good fixation is secured. It may be necessary to pass a Kirschner wire through the head of the metatarsal and down into the shaft in order to hold the head in proper position.

Fracture of the articular cartilage of the metatarsal head is infrequent in athletics and does not constitute a serious hazard. If a portion of the head is broken off in any way and heals in an irregular manner, that head may be removed. It is not advisable to remove more than one head or to remove the first or fifth in an athlete.

Fracture of the Toes.   Fractures of the toes do not present as serious a problem as do fractures of the fingers in spite of the fact that similar anatomical structures are involved. While fracture of the toe seems to arouse a sardonic amusement in the minds of everyone but the victim, to the athlete the fractured toe may be extremely disturbing, even to the point of missing a season's play. While it is usually not necessary to carry out the methods for fixation in the toes that are used in the fingers, one should at least take pains enough in the treatment of these conditions to be sure that the end result will be compatible with normal and not unduly delayed function. Many of these accidents occur in the dressing room rather than on the playing field, as by slipping on the wet floor or stubbing the toes against articles of furniture. The tendency for a certain amount of horseplay to work off excess exuberance makes this more probable. Direct forces, as when a bench tips over on the bare toes, may also result in painful injuries. While the ordinary person may get by pretty well with a heavy shoe, the athlete with his extremely flexible shoes and with the ever present necessity for forcible flexion and extension of the toes presents a wholly different problem.

FRACTURE OF THE FIRST TOE.   The first toe should be considered separately since it is much more vital in the mechanics of the foot than the smaller toes. Even in normal stride, considerable stress is applied to the first toe so that after the strike phase when the first toe reaches the ground, it is forcibly flexed to assist in the walkover from heel to toe. As the opposite leg is moved forward, the big toe of the hind foot is kept on the ground in a marked degree of dorsiflexion; and as the toe leaves the ground to swing the leg forward again, sharp flexion of the toe aids in propulsion. A stiff or painful metatarsophalangeal or interphalangeal joint in the first toe that is disabling for ordinary walking is usually remedied by a stiff sole or an anterior heel, but this is not compatible with athletics.

The first toe may be injured by direct force as when the locker room bench falls on it. This results in a more severe contusion with or without comminuted fracture of the distal or proximal phalanx. This is a painful injury with blood extravasation into the tissues, swelling, throbbing and severe discomfort. Careful x-ray study is demanded to determine whether there is fracture involving the joint since this has much more serious implications than fracture of the tuft or shaft (Fig. 441). If the x-ray is negative, careful study of the toe itself will reveal the extent of the hematoma. Any blood under the nail should be drained, preferably by drilling through the nail rather than lifting the nail further away from the nail bed unless avulsion has already taken place. The foot should be elevated and

Figure 441.   Tuft-fracture of distal phalanx of first toe. Note also avulsion fracture of lateral margin of the articular surface of the distal phalanx.

packed in ice and walking forbidden. Concentrated treatment the first few hours or days may well save a long period of disability.

A FRACTURE OF THE DISTAL PHALANX probably will not require manipulation or even rigid immobilization. If it is at the base of the distal phalanx (Fig. 442) particularly if it extends into the joint, careful reduction should be carried out and a toe spica cast applied. If the fracture is of the articular surface, the fragment may require pinning in place with a small wire. The same rules for treatment of fracture about the joint applies to the first toe as to weight-bearing joints anywhere.

FRACTURE OF THE PROXIMAL PHALANX is much more serious than of the distal. The fracture may be of the head, the neck (Fig. 443), the shaft or the base. Any deformity should be corrected and held with intramedullary fixation by a Kirschner wire. This is a satisfactory method and obviates the necessity for long periods in plaster. Athletic competition cannot be permitted in these injuries as long as there is a danger of stress causing recurrence of the deformity.

An extremely painful fracture of the first toe comes as the result of a forceful kick that drives the base of either the distal (Fig. 444) or proximal phalanx into the opposing head. This results in osteochondral damage and occasionally comminu-

Figure 442.   Avulsion fracture of the lateral margin of the proximal end of the distal phalanx of the first toe caused by forcing the distal phalanx inward.

Figure 443. Fracture of neck of proximal phalanx of first toe, treated by plaster cast and later by shoe with a metal plate. The stability of the fracture permitted it to be held without internal fixation.

tion of the base of the bone. In some cases the displacement from a comminuted fracture of the proximal phalanx will be enough to require traction with a wire through the distal phalanx and on an outrigger.

Should a painful traumatic arthritis of the interphalangeal joint occur, it can be best treated by removal of the articular surface and fusion of the joint in the straight position. This results in little disability.

Involvement of the METATARSOPHALANGEAL JOINT is much more serious since

Figure 444. Osteochondral damage of base of distal phalanx of first toe from soccer kicking.

Figure 445.   Spur over the dorsum of the distal end of the first metatarsal, apparently the result of kicking. The opposite foot and the rest of the joints are normal. Complete relief followed excision.

fusion of this joint is not compatible with the best function of the foot. In this joint one is justified in attempting to remove the irregularity rather than to fuse the joint. Occasionally from sprain or sprain-fracture an irregularity forms around the bases of the bones. Spurs may arise which seriously interfere with dorsiflexion (Fig. 445). Good function may be expected following resection of these spurs provided they are not manifestations of chronic degenerative arthritis involving the articular cartilage.

FRACTURES OF THE SMALLER TOES.   While fractures of the smaller toes are much less disabling than those of the first toe, they can be extremely exasperating. The most common is fracture of the proximal phalanx of the fifth toe from a night-time attempt to move the furniture with the toe (Fig. 446). This causes sharp abduction of the toe resulting in a spiral, oblique fracture. In the second, third and

Figure 446.   Spiral fracture of shaft of little toe involving the interphalangeal joint. In this toe this fracture can be treated by simple coaptation dressing.

Figure 447. Spiral fracture of proximal phalanx of third toe. Treated by strapping of the second, third and fourth toes together. The forefoot should also be strapped and a hard-soled shoe worn.

fourth toes the fracture is usually from overflexion or overextension and is usually a transverse fracture, often near the joint (Fig. 447). Avulsion of a portion of the articular surface frequently occurs. These fractures have a tendency to heal with the toe in flexion so that a painful hammer toe may result which will require definitive treatment. X-ray study will reveal the fracture.

An effort should be made to realign the toe. In the fifth toe, abduction deformity usually persists. This can be corrected without anesthesia by inserting a pencil or pen shaft between the fourth and fifth toes at the base and exerting quick, firm pressure outward on the pencil and inward on the head of the first phalanx. Perfect position, while not necessary, is desirable. Following reduction, the toe should be strapped to its fellow if it is the fifth toe or to the toe on either side if it is one of the others. Because of swelling extending back into the forefoot and difficulty in gait, it is also advisable to extend the strapping backward and circumferentially to include the forefoot (Fig. 448). This will result in less disability in

Figure 448. Strapping for fractured third toe. Note that the adjacent toes are strapped to the broken one. The whole is strapped to the forefoot.

the toe and a great deal more comfort on weight bearing. The patient should be able to walk in a shoe that has been cut out to relieve the pressure at the tender area. The decision as to athletic competition may be a difficult one since the player may feel very good as he walks or even runs. To his dismay, he may find as he goes full speed or cuts sharply, throwing the foot into varus or valgus, that he will experience sharp pain which may cause him to fall or lose stride and so cost him a great deal of his effectiveness. A period of rest is probably well worthwhile. In such an injury, packing in ice overnight may mean the difference between rapid, uneventful healing and tedious convalescence since, once the toe becomes badly swollen and edematous, the restoration of pain-free function becomes increasingly difficult.

Avulsion fractures of the toes (Fig. 442) are, strictly speaking, tendon or ligament injuries, and here again there is a tendency for hammer toe deformity to occur. A common avulsion is that of the extensor aponeurosis by sharp plantar flexion. The toe is flexed and painful. At the time of the initial injury, the toe should be strapped straight if the condition is recognized. Usually this condition is not seen by the doctor until persistence of pain brings the patient in weeks later. At this time fusion of the involved joint is the best treatment.

Fatigue Fracture (March Fracture)

It was in the foot that the fatigue fracture was first described. The so-called "march" fracture was reported following mobilization for World War II when many young males who were unaccustomed to being on their feet were equipped with a pack and asked to walk long distances in heavy shoes. The resulting stresses on bones not used to this degree of activity caused a great deal of strain, particularly in the area of the metatarsal necks. The patient develops symptoms similar to those of an arch strain with pain along the forepart of the arch, increased on weight bearing or other activity and relieved by rest. Examination reveals local tenderness over the metatarsals with pain on stretching of the plantar arch but usually none on other motions of the foot. X-ray examination made in an early stage is usually negative. The patient is treated for arch sprain with pads and heat but the condition persists with local tenderness and increasing disability. Subsequent x-rays made after a few weeks will show callus formation around the metatarsal shaft (Fig. 449). This is sometimes accompanied by evidence of a crack across the shaft but there may be absolutely no indication of a break in the continuity of the bone. This condition has frequently been confused with bone tumor and instances have been reported in which amputation had been recommended under the diagnosis of osteogenic sarcoma with periosteal reaction. A little patience will usually answer the question since in march fracture callus rapidly consolidates, becomes harder and smaller and ultimately disappears.

This condition is incompatible with active competitive sports during the acute stage and competition should be permitted only after consolidation of the mass of callus is complete. If the lesion is recognized early the best treatment is with a plaster boot for two to three weeks followed by adequate strapping for a week or ten days, then the use of an arch support and a firm shoe. This type of condition illustrates graphically the value of re-examination by x-ray. If the initial x-rays have been negative but the symptoms persist, careful follow-up films will often reveal

Figure 449. Typical "march" fracture in a young athlete. Note complete absence of any fracture line as such. Uneventful healing.

the pathologic changes. It should be emphasized again that x-ray is simply an adjunct to the diagnosis and a negative x-ray by no means rules out a bone lesion.

OTHER CONDITIONS OF THE FOOT

Hammer Toe

There is no necessity to detail the treatment of hammer toe. This condition results from a combination of contracture of the flexor and extensor tendons so that one or more joints is in flexion and another in extension (Fig. 450). A frequent combination is for the interphalangeal joints to be in flexion and the metatarsophalangeal joint in extension. This causes pressure on the tip of the distal phalanx and on the dorsum of the proximal interphalangeal joint. Painful corns may result. Hammer toes may come from unrecognized poliomyelitis, from a high arched, cavus type foot, as a result of short shoes or socks, or from previous injury. Proper care of the primary condition should minimize the deformity. Hammer toes can be successfully treated and athletics can be resumed. In the meantime, a properly fitted shoe with the leather split at the pressure point, or the application of suitable pads may add materially to the patient's comfort.

Subungual Exostosis

This is a painful condition of the distal phalanx, usually of the first toe, which is not uncommon in athletes (Fig. 451). Pathologically an exostosis develops on top of the distal phalanx extending up under the nail bed. Trauma may be a definite etiological factor. The condition may develop in a basketball player as a result of having his toe repeatedly trampled. Once the exostosis develops it is extremely sensitive to pressure or trauma. The patient will present himself with a very painful,

Figure 450.   Hammer toes, corrected by fusion of the proximal interphalangeal joints. The severe hallux valgus has been corrected.

Figure 451.   Subungual exostosis. Note the sharp spurring upward of the distal end of the distal phalanx. This was treated by resection of the tuft of the distal phalanx.

swollen, edematous toe. In many instances the nail has been cut away to permit the tumor mass to push up without the pressure of the nail over it. While these lesions look vicious clinically, they are always benign and may be cured by removal of the exostosis. If it is extensive and the nail bed has been destroyed, removal of the distal one-half of the distal phalanx with plastic closure of the toe after removal of the entire nail and nail bed may be the best solution. This condition is often confused with ingrown toenail or simple contusion and hematoma. The frightening appearance may suggest a malignant type tumor.

Ingrown Toenail

Ingrown toenail may occur on any toe but is most severe on the first. Basically, the cause is a rolling of the toenail in a scroll-like fashion so that the two lateral margins tend to roll under the central portion to make a tube rather than a flat plane. This is a natural tendency of the nail as evidenced in some species of mammals in which a conical claw is formed by a complete circling of the toenail. The resulting convexity causes the edge of the nail to dig into the side of the toe. The paronychial fold bulges to the outside and extends out over the dorsum of the nail.

Treatment. In the early stages ingrown toenail can usually be managed conservatively. Prophylaxis is of prime importance; well fitted shoes and socks, careful hygiene to avoid inflammation and proper trimming of the nail will many times prevent serious deformity. The nail should be trimmed straight across without the rounding off and pointing of the nail that is so popular in the hand. If the nail tends to be heavy, the center portion may be thinned by the emory board or suitable nail file so that, in the middle of the nail extending from the root to the tip, the substance is quite thin. This permits the lateral margins to roll upward by breaking the arc of the nail. A similar thing has been done by misguided individuals who split the nail down its center but this often results in serious complications. The flattening may be aided by placing very small pellets of cotton under the nail corners, once the tendency for ingrowing is noted. This must be carefully done, otherwise the pellets may break off the corner of the nail and do more harm than good. They should not be made large enough to lift the nail away from the nail bed lest the problem be further complicated. If infection occurs, it should be adequately treated by drainage, application of hot packs and suitable antibiotics, both local and general. The patient should be barred from the general dressing room while his toe is acutely infected. The necessity for surgery of a toenail can usually be prevented by adequate attention in the early stages.

If the deformity persists and defies conservative treatment, surgery will usually give very satisfactory results. I cannot condemn too strongly the prevalent custom of simply removing the nail. In the first place this is not simple and in the second place, when the nail regenerates it is even more curled than before so that the problem is only magnified. A suitable procedure is illustrated in Figure 452, great care being taken to eliminate all of the nail root and nail bed lest a recurrence or spur formation occurs that will require further treatment.

Active competition in the presence of a serious ingrown toenail is scarcely permissible since excruciating pain may result from the foot being trod upon. Active forcible flexion and extension may cause pain and increased inflammation.

Figure 452.   Surgical treatment of ingrown toenail. Care is taken to eliminate all the nail
                   root and nail bed to prevent recurrence or spur formation.

Ingrown toenail involving the smaller toes is much less serious but should receive essentially the same treatment. This, however, is more difficult to carry out in the small toes. Surgical removal of all or part of the nail bed is not a mutilating operation and is far more acceptable in the small toes than a similar procedure on the first toe.

Corns

The best way to prevent disability in an athlete from a corn is to prevent the corn. The shoe must be carefully fitted and no pressure points permitted to develop. The most common locus is the toes where definite pressure occurs between the toe and shoe. The little toe particularly is an offender since it will frequently tend to curl up in the hammer toe position. Many athletes have a very high arch with some degree of hammer toe in all the small toes. These tend to get corns along the dorsum of the proximal interphalangeal joints. It does little good to remove a corn and not eliminate the situation that caused it. The area should be padded to protect it from pressure. The corn should be softened up by lanolin. If necessary, judicious trimming may be done. Careless application of medicated corn plasters has often resulted in painful ulcers. Careful fitting of the shoe and sock and avoidance of wrinkles are important.

Calluses

Calluses of the foot are the result of friction and pressure. They tend to be extremely disabling since the piling up of keratin, presumably as a protective measure, results in interposition of a very hard mass between the bone and the shoe. Painful bruising of the underlying tissues or periosteum may result. The obvious measure is to prevent the imbalance of the foot and get more even distribution of weight by building up or padding the shoe in such a manner as to relieve the weight on the involved area. The most frequent pressure on the foot is under the metatarsal heads. Painful callus under the first head may be relieved by shifting the weight to the lateral side of the foot. An anterior heel or metatarsal bar may protect against direct weight bearing. In running on the toes, however, the metatarsal bar which ordinarily protects a person by taking the weight off the metatarsal head is, of course, not functioning. Careful attention to the callus by softening it with lanolin, buffing it down with an emory board, etc., will pay dividends. In an intractable case the metatarsal head may be removed.

Athlete's Foot

Fungus infections of the foot are endemic in almost the entire population. They are particularly prevalent in the locker room where too often little attention is paid to ordinary precautionary measures. For details of prevention and treatment, see page 56. Enteric medication seems to offer definite promise in resistant cases.

Verrucae

The verruca or wart must be distinguished from callus. The callus arises as a direct result of too much pressure on a certain area. The verruca, on the other hand, is a skin disease probably caused by a virus which may spread over the entire sole of the foot and be extremely disabling. Confusion may arise when the verruca is at a weight-bearing point and is surrounded by callus. Treatment should be carried out by one especially proficient in the treatment of conditions of the foot. Radiation should be used only under the careful guidance of an expert and probably not more than one series given to any one area.

Freiberg's Disease

Freiberg's disease is an osteochondritis of the metatarsal head, usually before the epiphysis closes, similar to Perthes' disease at the hip (Fig. 453). Early

Figure 453. Freiberg's disease. *A,* The unaffected foot. Note extra long second metatarsal shaft with large head which bears undue proportion of the weight. This contributes to the osteochondritis. *B,* The healed osteochondritis of the metatarsal head (Freiberg's disease) with joint irregularity and pain. *C,* Removal of the second metatarsal head relieved the condition.

Freiberg's disease should be treated by prevention of weight bearing but this condition is frequently not recognized until it is well advanced. If the bone is seriously deformed, the painful metatarsal head should be removed. If it heals without deformity, it is of no consequence.

Figure 454.   Congenital hallux valgus, right. Note bifid epiphysis on the proximal phalanx of first toe, left. This is not pathologic.

Figure 455.   Congenital short first metatarsal with separation of the first and second heads. This throws unusual weight on the second head and is likely to cause a painful foot.

Figure 456.   Note accessory navicular at the medial border of right foot. This should not
be interpreted as an injury. Note the much smaller one on the left side.

Congenital Deformities of the Foot

There are many other deformities of the foot that are simply developmental
and of little significance. They may at times be the precursors of later disability due
to static imbalance but should not bar participation in athletics. The congenital
hallux valgus (Fig. 454) or bunion is amenable to surgical treatment if necessary.
In the male it usually can be handled without surgery. Congenital short first metatarsal (Fig. 455) may be helped by suitable padding of the shoe. Pronation or
supination similarly can be improved by improving the weight-bearing stance. The
accessory navicular (Fig. 456) or prehallux may become symptomatic by pronation
of the foot and may be completely relieved by application of a suitable arch support.
The athletic shoes with little or no arch, often with no heel, may often give inadequate support to the pronated or flat foot and need to be supplemented by a molded
arch support.

Fracture of a Sesamoid

Various sesamoid bones in the foot are subject to injury.

Accessory Navicular.   The most common sesamoid injury occurs in the
prehallux or accessory navicular. In an eversion injury with a tight posterior tibial
tendon, an avulsion force is applied to the accessory bone and it is pulled away
from its attachment to the navicular or, in the occasional case, pulled in two. This
is similar to avulsion of the tendon attachment to the navicular. It may be misleading since the accessory navicular will be recognized as being an extra bone and the

injury may be overlooked. A history of forceful eversion of the foot or of active contraction of the posterior tibial is characteristic. On examination, tenderness will be sharply localized to the accessory bone and to the navicular. Forced passive eversion or strong active inversion against resistance is painful. X-rays may be confirmatory.

TREATMENT for this condition may be nonsurgical. The patient is placed in a cast with the foot inverted for about three weeks, followed by inversion type strapping for another three weeks. However, if there is separation of the fragment or if the navicular is large, it will be advisable to remove the accessory navicular and complete the sling operation by positioning the posterior tibial tendon under the navicular. This type of operation is particularly gratifying since the arch is usually good and correction of the pronation will give markedly improved function of the foot.

Figure 457.   Unrecognized fracture of sesamoid. Note the difference from bipartite sesamoid with irregular fracture line and calcification around the area. This sesamoid was removed.

While this condition may be overlooked, the contrary situation also must be guarded against. One must not interpret an accessory navicular as being a fracture of the tubercle of the navicular. Careful comparison with the opposite foot and careful analysis of the clinical findings will usually distinguish between the two conditions. As indicated above, the two may coincide and require sharp diagnostic acumen. In case the accessory bone remains persistently painful, it should in any event be removed.

Sesamoid in the Flexor Tendon to the Big Toe. The medial sesamoid under the first metatarsophalangeal joint is subject to trauma when the toe is in forced dorsal flexion and a blow is applied to the ball of the foot. The mechanics of this injury resembles that of patellar fracture in which the combination of tension on the patella plus a localized blow fractures the bone. This injury can be extremely distressing, since it prevents the athlete from running on his toes. He may have very persistent pain and the true pathology is readily overlooked. This history of sudden, severe pain under the ball of the foot with tenderness and inability to "drive" are significant. Examination will reveal sharply localized tenderness with localized swelling, pain on dorsiflexion of the toe and pain on active plantar flexion of the toe. X-ray is confirmatory.

TREATMENT consists of immobilization of the foot for several weeks. Usually the acute condition is not recognized and it is seen as a chronic condition at which time the best treatment will be excision of the sesamoid (Fig. 457).

Bipartite Sesamoid

This is a congenital condition in which the medial and occasionally the lateral sesamoid will show transverse separation of the two segments at the midline (Fig. 439). This must not be confused with fracture, which is much less frequent. Since many fractures are not recognized until late, they may, indeed, under x-ray resemble the rounded-off margins of the partite bone. The history will be quite different as a rule, however, in that discomfort in the case of the bipartite sesamoid will be gradual in onset and mild in character. The symptoms are ordinarily those of accompanying metatarsal arch strain and the bipartite sesamoid is found coincidentally and usually is of no significance whatever. Careful analysis of the case and comparison with the opposite foot will give a lead as to the true nature of the condition. Chronic symptoms definitely localized in the sesamoid merit its surgical removal. Disappointment will follow removal without these clear indications.

Index

The *italicized folios* refer to the page numbers of illustrations.

627